MEDICAL RECORDS.

INTERNATIONAL CLASSIFICATION OF DISEASES

MANUAL
OF THE INTERNATIONAL
STATISTICAL CLASSIFICATION
OF DISEASES, INJURIES, AND
CAUSES OF DEATH

Based on the Recommendations
of the Ninth Revision Conference, 1975,
and Adopted by the Twenty-ninth World Health Assembly

Volume 1

WORLD HEALTH ORGANIZATION

GENEVA

1977

Reprinted 1974, 1980, 1986

Volume 1 Introduction

    List of Three-digit Categories

    Tabular List of Inclusions and Four-digit Sub-categories

    Medical Certification and Rules for Classification

    Special Lists for Tabulation

    Definitions and Recommendations

    Regulations

Volume 2 Alphabetical Index

ISBN 92 4 154004 4

© World Health Organization 1977

PRINTED IN SWITZERLAND

86/6847 — Presses Centrales — 7000 (R)

TABLE OF CONTENTS

INTRODUCTION

INTRODUCTION

General principles

A classification of diseases may be defined as a system of categories to which morbid entities are assigned according to some established criteria. There are many possible choices for these criteria. The anatomist, for example, may desire a classification based on the part of the body affected whereas the pathologist is primarily interested in the nature of the disease process, the public health practitioner in aetiology and the clinician in the particular manifestation requiring his care. In other words there are many axes of classification and the particular axis selected will be determined by the interest of the investigator. A statistical classification of disease and injury will depend, therefore, upon the use to be made of the statistics to be compiled.

Because of this conflict of interests, efforts to base a statistical classification on a strictly logical adherence to any one axis have failed in the past. The various titles will represent a series of necessary compromises between classifications based on aetiology, anatomical site, circumstances of onset, etc., as well as the quality of information available on medical reports. Adjustments must also be made to meet the varied requirements of vital statistics offices, hospitals of different types, medical services of the armed forces, social insurance organizations, sickness surveys, and numerous other agencies. While no single classification will fit all the specialized needs, it should provide a common basis of classification for general statistical use; that is storage, retrieval and tabulation of data.

A statistical classification of disease must be confined to a limited number of categories which will encompass the entire range of morbid conditions. The categories should be chosen so that they will facilitate the statistical study of disease phenomena. A specific disease entity should have a separate title in the classification only when its separation is warranted because the frequency of its occurrence, or its importance as a morbid condition, justifies its isolation as a separate category. On the other hand, many titles in the classification will refer to groups of separate but usually related morbid conditions. Every disease or morbid condition, however, must have a definite and appropriate place as an inclusion in one of the categories of the statistical classification. A few items of the statistical list will be residual titles for other and miscellaneous conditions which cannot be classified under the more specific titles. These miscellaneous categories should be kept to a minimum.

It is this element of grouping in a statistical classification that distinguishes it from a nomenclature, a list or catalogue of approved names for morbid conditions, which must be extensive in order to accommodate all pathological conditions. The concepts of classification and nomenclature are, nevertheless, closely related in the sense that some classifications (e.g. in zoology) are so detailed that they become nomenclatures. Such classifications, however, are generally unsuitable for statistical analysis.

The aims of a statistical classification of disease cannot be better summarized than in the following paragraphs written by William Farr[1] a century ago:

" The causes of death were tabulated in the early Bills of Mortality (Tables mortuaires) alphabetically; and this course has the advantage of not raising any of those nice questions in which it is vain to expect physicians and statisticians to agree unanimously. But statistics is eminently a science of classification; and it is evident, on glancing at the subject cursorily, that any classification that brings together in groups diseases that have considerable affinity, or that are liable to be confounded with each other, is likely to facilitate the deduction of general principles.

" Classification is a method of generalization. Several classifications may, therefore, be used with advantage; and the physician, the pathologist, or the jurist, each from his own point of view, may legitimately classify the diseases and the causes of death in the way that he thinks best adapted to facilitate his inquiries, and to yield general results.

" The medical practitioner may found his main divisions of diseases on their treatment as medical or surgical; the pathologist, on the nature of the morbid action or product; the anatomist or the physiologist on the tissues and organs involved; the medical jurist on the suddenness or the slowness of the death; and all these points well deserve attention in a statistical classification.

" In the eyes of national statists the most important elements are, however, brought into account in the ancient subdivision of diseases into plagues, or epidemics and endemics, into diseases of common occurrence (sporadic diseases), which may be conveniently divided into three classes, and into injuries, the immediate results of violence or of external causes. "

Historical Review

Early history

François Bossier de Lacroix (1706-1777), better known as Sauvages, first attempted to classify diseases systematically. Sauvages' comprehensive treatise was published under the title Nosologia Methodica. A contemporary of Sauvages was the great methodologist Linnaeus (1707-1778), one of whose treatises was entitled Genera Morborum. At the beginning of the 19th century, the classification of disease in most general use was one by William Cullen (1710-1790), of Edinburgh, which was published in 1785 under the title Synopsis Nosologiae Methodicae.

The statistical study of disease, however, began for all practical purposes with the work of John Graunt on the London Bills of Mortality a century earlier. In an attempt to estimate the proportion of liveborn children who died before reaching the age of six years, no records of age at death being available, he took all deaths classed as thrush, convulsions, rickets, teeth and worms, abortives, chrysomes, infants, livergrown, and overlaid and added to them half the deaths classed as smallpox, swine pox, measles, and worms without convulsions. Despite the crudity of this classification his estimate of a 36 per cent mortality before the age of six years appears from later evidence to have been a good one. While three centuries have contributed something to the scientific accuracy of disease classification, there are many who doubt the usefulness of attempts to compile statistics of disease, or even causes of death, because of the difficulties of classification. To these, one can quote Major Greenwood[2]: " The scientific purist, who will wait for medical statistics until they are nosologically exact, is no wiser than Horace's rustic waiting for the river to flow away ".

Fortunately for the progress of preventive medicine, the General Register Office of England and Wales, at its inception in 1837, found in William Farr (1807-1883)—its first medical statistician—a man who not only made the best possible use of the imperfect classifications of disease available at the time, but laboured to secure better classification and international uniformity in their use.

Farr found the classification of Cullen in use in the public services of his day. It had not been revised so as to embody the advances of medical science, nor was it deemed by him to be satisfactory for statistical purposes. In the first Annual Report of the Registrar General, therefore, he discussed the principles that should govern a statistical classification of disease and urged the adoption of a uniform classification.

Both nomenclature and statistical classification received constant study and consideration by Farr in his annual " Letters " to the Registrar General published in the Annual Reports of the Registrar General. The utility of a uniform classification of causes of death was so strongly recognized at the first International Statistical Congress, held at Brussels, in 1853, that it requested William Farr and Marc d'Espine, of Geneva, to prepare " une nomenclature uniforme des causes de décès applicable à tous les pays ". [3] At the next Congress, at Paris in 1855, Farr and d'Espine submitted two separate lists which were based on very different principles. Farr's classification was arranged under five groups: Epidemic diseases, Constitutional (general) diseases, Local diseases arranged according to anatomical site, Developmental diseases, and diseases that are the direct result of violence. D'Espine classified diseases according to their nature (gouty, herpetic,

haematic, etc.). The Congress adopted a compromise list of 138 rubrics.
In 1864, this classification was revised at Paris " sur le modèle de celle de
W. Farr ", and was subsequently revised in 1874, 1880, and 1886. Although there was never any universal acceptance of this classification,
the general arrangement, including the principle of classifying diseases by
anatomical site, proposed by Farr has survived as the basis of the International List of Causes of Death.

Adoption of International List of Causes of Death

The International Statistical Institute, the successor to the International Statistical Congress, at its meeting in Vienna in 1891, charged a
committee, of which Jacques Bertillon (1851-1922), Chef des Travaux
statistiques de la ville de Paris, was chairman, with the preparation of a
classification of causes of death. It is of interest to note that Bertillon was
the grandson of Achille Guillard, a noted botanist and statistician,
who had introduced the resolution requesting Farr and d'Espine to
prepare a uniform classification at the First Statistical Congress in 1853.
The report of this committee was presented by Bertillon at the meeting of
the International Statistical Institute at Chicago in 1893 and adopted by it.
The classification prepared by Bertillon was based on the classification of
causes of death used by the City of Paris, which, since its revision in 1885,
represented a synthesis of English, German, and Swiss classifications. The
classification was based on the principle, adopted by Farr, of distinguish-
ing between general diseases and those localized to a particular organ or
anatomical site. In accordance with the instructions of the Vienna
Congress made at the suggestion of L. Guillaume, the Director of the
Federal Bureau of Statistics of Switzerland, Bertillon included three
classifications: the first, an abridged classification of 44 titles; the second,
a classification of 99 titles; and the third, a classification of 161 titles.

The Bertillon Classification of Causes of Death, as it was at first
called, received general approval and was adopted by several countries,
as well as by many cities. The classification was first used in North
America by Jesús E. Monjarás for the statistics of San Luis de Potosí,
Mexico. [4] In 1898, the American Public Health Association, at its meeting in Ottawa, Canada, recommended the adoption of the Bertillon Classification by registrars of Canada, Mexico, and the United States. The
Association further suggested that the classification be revised every ten
years.

At the meeting of the International Statistical Institute at Christiania
in 1899, Bertillon presented a report on the progress of the classification,
including the recommendations of the American Public Health Associa-

tion for decennial revisions. The International Statistical Institute then adopted the following resolution:

" The International Statistical Institute, convinced of the necessity of using in the different countries comparable nomenclatures:

" Learns with pleasure of the adoption by all the statistical offices of North America, by some of those of South America, and by some in Europe, of the system of cause of death nomenclature presented in 1893:

" Insists vigorously that this system of nomenclature be adopted in principle and without revision, by all the statistical institutions of Europe;

" Approves, at least in its general lines, the system of decennial revision proposed by the American Public Health Association at its Ottawa session (1898);

" Urges the statistical offices who have not yet adhered, to do so without delay, and to contribute to the comparability of the cause of death nomenclature." [5]

The French Government therefore convoked at Paris, in August 1900, the first International Conference for the revision of the Bertillon or International Classification of Causes of Death. Delegates from 26 countries attended this Conference. A detailed classification of causes of death consisting of 179 groups and an abridged classification of 35 groups were adopted on 21 August 1900. The desirability of decennial revisions was recognized, and the French Government was requested to call the next meeting in 1910. Actually the next conference was held in 1909, and the Government of France called succeeding conferences in 1920, 1929, and 1938.

Bertillon continued as the guiding force in the promotion of the International List of Causes of Death, and the revisions of 1900, 1910, and 1920 were carried out under his leadership. As Secretary-General of the International Conference, he sent out the provisional revision for 1920 to more than 500 persons, asking for comments. His death in 1922 left the International Conference without a guiding hand.

At the 1923 session of the International Statistical Institute, Michel Huber, Bertillon's successor in France, recognized this lack of leadership and introduced a resolution for the International Statistical Institute to renew its stand of 1893 in regard to the International Classification of Causes of Death and to co-operate with other international organizations in preparation for subsequent revisions. The Health Organization of the League of Nations had also taken an active interest in vital statistics and appointed a Commission of Statistical Experts to study the classification of diseases and causes of death, as well as other problems in the field of medical statistics. E. Roesle, Chief of the Medical Statistical Service of the German Health Bureau and a member of the Commission of Expert Statisticians, prepared a monograph that listed the expansion in the rubrics of the 1920 International List of Causes of Death that would be required if the classification was to be used in the tabulation of statistics of morbidity. This careful study was published by the Health Organization of the League of Nations in 1928. [6] In order to co-ordinate the work of both agencies, an international commission, known as the " Mixed Commission ", was created with an equal number of representatives from the International Statistical Institute and the Health Organization of the League of Nations. This Commission drafted the proposals for the Fourth (1929) and the Fifth (1938) revisions of the International List of Causes of Death.

The Sixth, Seventh and Eighth Revisions

The International Health Conference held in New York City in 1946 entrusted the Interim Commission of the World Health Organization with the responsibility of undertaking preparatory work for the next decennial revision of the International Lists of Causes of Death and for the establishment of International Lists of Causes of Morbidity [7]. The International Conference for the Sixth Revision of the International Lists of Diseases and Causes of Death was convened in Paris in April 1948 by the Government of France and its secretariat was entrusted jointly to the competent French administrations and to the World Health Organization which had carried out the preparatory work under the Arrangement concluded by the governments represented at the International Health Conference in 1946 [7].

The Sixth Decennial Revision Conference marked the beginning of a new era in international vital and health statistics. Apart from approving a comprehensive list for both mortality and morbidity and agreeing on international rules for selecting the underlying cause of death it recommended the adoption of a comprehensive programme of international co-operation in the field of vital and health statistics, including the establishment of national committees on vital and health statistics for the purpose of co-ordinating statistical activities in the country and to serve as a link between the national statistical institutions and the World Health Organization [8].

The International Conference for the Seventh Revision of the International Classification of Diseases was held in Paris under WHO auspices in February 1955 [9]. In accordance with a recommendation of the WHO Expert Committee on Health Statistics [10] this revision was limited to essential changes and amendments òf errors and inconsistencies.

The Eighth Revision Conference convened by WHO met in the Palais des Nations, Geneva, from 6 to 12 July 1965 [11]. This revision was of a

more radical nature than the Seventh but left unchanged the basic structure of the Classification and the general philosophy of classifying diseases
according to their aetiology rather than a particular manifestation.

Report of the International Conference for the Ninth Revision

The International Conference for the Ninth Revision of the International Classification of Diseases convened by the World Health Organization met at WHO headquarters in Geneva from 30 September to
6 October 1975. The Conference was attended by delegations from 46
Member States:

Algeria	Nigeria
Australia	Norway
Austria	Poland
Belgium	Portugal
Brazil	Saudi Arabia
Canada	Singapore
Chad	Spain
Denmark	Sudan
Egypt	Sweden
Finland	Switzerland
France	Thailand
German Democratic Republic	Togo
Germany, Federal Republic of	Trinidad and Tobago
Guatemala	Tunisia
Hungary	Union of Soviet Socialist Republics
India	United Arab Emirates
Indonesia	United Kingdom of Great Britain
Ireland	and Northern Ireland
Israel	United Republic of Cameroon
Italy	United States of America
Japan	Venezuela
Libyan Arab Republic	Yugoslavia
Luxembourg	Zaire
Netherlands, Kingdom of the	

The United Nations, the Organization for Economic Cooperation and
Development, the International Labour Organisation and the International Agency for Research on Cancer sent representatives to participate
in the Conference, as did the Council for International Organizations of
Medical Sciences and ten other international non-governmental organizations concerned with dental health, dermatology, gynaecology and
obstetrics, mental health, neurosurgery, ophthalmology, paediatrics,
pathology, radiology, and rehabilitation of the disabled.

The Conference was opened by Dr A. S. Pavlov, Assistant Director-
General, on behalf of the Director-General. Dr Pavlov reviewed the
history of the ICD, reminding delegates that it had developed from an

International List of Causes of Death, first agreed in 1893. WHO took over responsibility with the Sixth Revision and its concern with the ICD is written into its Constitution. Since WHO took over, there had been a great extension of use of the ICD for the indexing and retrieval of records and for statistics concerning the planning, monitoring and evaluation of health services, besides its traditional use in epidemiology.

The Conference elected the following officers:

Chairman:	Dr R. H. C. Wells (Australia)
Vice-Chairmen:	Dr J. M. Avilan-Rovira (Venezuela)
	Dr G. Cerkovnij (USSR)
	Dr I. M. Moriyama (United States of America)
	Mr G. Paine (United Kingdom)
Rapporteurs:	Dr M. A. Heasman (United Kingdom)
	Dr (Mlle) M. Guidevaux (France)
Secretariat:	Dr A. S. Pavlov (Assistant Director-General, WHO)
	Mr K. Uemura (Director, Division of Health Statistics, WHO)
	Dr K. Kupka (Chief Medical Officer, International Classification of Diseases, WHO) (Secretary)
	Mr H. G. Corbett (Statistician, International Classification of Diseases, WHO)
	Professor G. G. Avtandilov (USSR) (Temporary Adviser)

The Conference adopted an agenda dealing with the Ninth Revision of the International Classification of Diseases, with several provisional supplementary classifications intended for use in conjunction with it, and with allied topics.

1. Ninth Revision of the International Classification of Diseases

1.1 Review of activities in the preparation of the proposals for the Ninth Revision

The procedures leading up to the Ninth Revision commenced in 1969 with the calling of a Study Group. The work had been planned and carried out so that the proposals before the Conference were in a much more advanced state of preparation than had been the case at earlier revisions. The intention was to have the completed manual, with its alphabetical index, in the hands of users in good time to allow for adequate training and familiarization in countries before its introduction. The progress of preparations for revision had been guided by further meetings of the Study Group and by meetings of Heads of Centres for Classification of Diseases. The first meeting of the Study Group considered that the revision ought to be a limited one. It soon became clear, however, that a much more radical revision was being demanded by specialists in many fields of medicine. Views were sought from individual consultants, international specialists bodies, the WHO Centres for Classification of Diseases and headquarters units. Regional offices arranged meetings so that representatives of Member States could give their views. The third meeting of the Study Group considered proposals incorporating views from all these sources, and on the basis of their recommendations draft proposals were circulated to Member States in mid-1973. Comments on the proposals were considered by the WHO Expert Committee on Health Statistics in June 1974 [12], and the final proposals before the Conference were the results of its recommendations. Delegates from several countries spoke in support of the revision as proposed. In particular it was reiterated that clinical pressures had demanded an extensive revision at this stage on the grounds that the structure of several of the ICD chapters was out of touch with modern clinical concepts. The delegation from Sweden, on behalf of the five Nordic countries (Denmark, Finland, Iceland, Norway and Sweden), put forward the view that the problems and cost associated with so extensive a change would be substantial since these countries had established a 5-digit version based on the ICD-8 which was widely used in computerized health information systems. They considered that this 5-digit version met to a large extent the clinical demands for greater specificity which the Ninth Revision was aiming at. The Conference noted the concern of the Nordic countries but, recognizing the need pointed out by several countries to satisfy clinical requirements by structural changes as well as by providing increased specificity, in general supported the scope of the proposed revision as presented to the Conference.

1.2 *History and development of uses of the ICD*

The Conference was reminded of the impressive history of the classification. Its origins lay in a list of causes of death, which was used for many years. At the Sixth Revision, the classification was extended to cover non-fatal conditions. Later the classification had been shown to be useful for the purposes of hospital indexing, particularly if adapted by means of some extra subdivision. More recently adaptations had been made for use in medical audit systems. The Ninth Revision proposals include a device designed to improve its suitability for use in statistics for the evaluation of medical care. For the future, it would have to be decided what kind of adaptation of the ICD would render it usable for Health Insurance Statistics, and whether it was possible to adapt it as a basis for central payment for medical services. All these uses tended to push the classification in the direction of more detail. At the other end of the scale it had to be remembered that there were demands from countries and areas where such sophistication was irrelevant but which nevertheless would like a classification based on the ICD so as to assess their progress in health care and in the control of sickness.

1.3 *General characteristics of the proposed Ninth Revision*

The general arrangement of the proposals for the Ninth Revision considered by the Conference was much the same as in the Eighth Revision, though with much additional detail. Care had been taken to ensure that the categories were meaningful at the 3-digit level. There were certain innovations:

(i) Optional fifth digits were provided in certain places: for example, for the mode of diagnosis in tuberculosis, for method of delivery in Chapter XI, for anatomical site in musculoskeletal disorders and for place of accident in the E code.

(ii) An independent 4-digit coding system was provided to classify histological varieties of neoplasm, prefixed by the letter M (for morphology) and followed by a fifth digit indicating behaviour. This code was for optional use in addition to the normal code indicating topography.

(iii) The role of the E code for external causes had changed. In the Sixth, Seventh and Eighth Revisions, Chapter XVII consisted of two alternative classifications, one according to the nature of the injury (the N code) and one according to external cause (the E code). In the Ninth Revision it was proposed to drop the N prefix and consider only the nature of injury as part of the main classification. The E code becomes a supplementary classification to be used, where relevant, in conjunction with codes from any part of the classification. For mortality statistics, however, the E code should still be used in preference to Chapter XVII in presenting underlying causes of death, when only one is used.

(iv) The Ninth Revision proposals included dual classification of certain diagnostic statements. The Conference heard that the system had been introduced into the 1973 proposals after it had become obvious that there was a demand to classify diseases according to important manifestations, e.g. to classify numps encephalitis to a category for encephalitis. It would have been unwise to change the whole axis of the ICD to this basis, so the first proposal was to make the positioning according to manifestation alternative to the traditional placing according to aetiology. As a result of criticism, it is now proposed that the " traditional " aetiology codes, those marked with a †, should be considered primary, and the new codes, positioned in the classification according to manifestation and marked with an *, should be secondary, for use in applications concerned with the planning and evaluation of medical care. This system applies only to diagnostic statements that contain information about both etiology and manifestation and when the latter is important in its own right.

(v) Categories in the Mental Disorders Chapter include descriptions of their content with a view to overcoming the particular difficulties in this field, where international terminology is not standard.

The V code (formerly the Y code) continues to appear in Volume 1.

These characteristics of the proposed revision were accepted by the Conference.

1.4 *Adoption of Ninth Revision of the International Classification of Diseases*

The Conference,

Having considered the proposals prepared by the Organization on the recommendations of the Expert Committee on Health Statistics [12],

Recognizing the need for a few further minor modifications to meet the comments on points of detail submitted by Member States during the Conference,

Recommends that the revised Detailed List of Categories and Sub-Categories in Annex I* to this report constitute the Ninth Revision of the International Classification of Diseases.

2. *Classification of Procedures in Medicine*

In response to requests from a number of Member States, the Organization had drafted a classification of therapeutic, diagnostic and prophylactic procedures in medicine, covering surgery, radiology, laboratory and other procedures. Various national classifications of this kind had been studied and advice sought from hospital associations in a number of countries. The intention was to provide a tool for use in the analysis of health services provided to patients in hospitals, clinics, outpatient departments, etc.

The Conference congratulates the Secretariat on this important development and

Recommends that the provisional procedures classifications should be published as supplements to, and not as integral parts of, the Ninth

---

* The Annexes to the Report are not reproduced here. They are represented by the contents of this Volume.

Revision of the International Classification of Diseases. They should be published in some inexpensive form and, after two or three years' experience, revised in the light of users' comments.

3. *Classification of Impairments and Handicaps*

The ICD provided the means of classifying current illness or injury; the classification of procedures provided a means of coding the treatment or other services consumed by the patient. There remained a need to classify impairments and the consequent handicaps or disadvantages.

This was an area in which much development was occurring and a draft classification had been prepared by the Organization although this was to a large extent experimental and exploratory. It had been drafted after much consultation with agencies responsible for social services and rehabilitation.

The Conference having considered the classification of Impairments and Handicaps believes that these have potential value and accordingly

Recommends that the Impairments and Handicaps classifications be published for trial purposes as a supplement to, and not as an integral part of, the Ninth Revision of the International Classification of Diseases.

4. *Adaptations of ICD for the Use of Specialists*

The Conference noted three adaptations of the ICD which had been designed for the use of specialists.

The first was an adaptation for oncology – ICD-O. Coding was on three axes indicating the topography, morphology and behaviour of tumours. The 4-digit topography code was based on the list of sites of the malignant neoplasm section of Chapter II of the Ninth Revision of the ICD, but was to be used for any type of neoplasm. To this would be added a 4-digit code indicating histological variety of neoplasm, and a single-digit code indicating behaviour. It was intended that the code should be used by centres requiring to record extra detail about tumours, as an alternative to the Ninth Revision of ICD, with which it was entirely compatible. (A conversion guide would be available, enabling translation of codes by computer if desired.)

Other adaptations had been produced for dentistry and stomatology and for ophthalmology. Each of these contains, in a small volume, all conditions of interest to the specialist, selected from all chapters of the ICD, and provides additional detail by means of a fifth digit.

5. Lay Reporting

The Conference discussed the problem of securing badly needed morbidity and mortality statistics in countries still suffering from a lack of sufficiently qualified personnel. There was a divergence of opinion concerning the system of classification to be used where information about sickness or causes of death is necessarily furnished by persons other than physicians. Some delegates considered that the International Classification of Diseases in some simplified form (e.g. one of the tabulation lists) would serve this purpose while others believed that a system independent of the ICD needed to be established.

A small working party, consisting of delegates from Member States with experience of the problem, was convened to consider the question in more detail and in the light of its report

The Conference,

Realizing the present problem involved in the full utilization of ICD by the developing countries in most of the regions;

Recognizing the need for introducing a system which could provide useful and objective morbidity and mortality data for efficient health planning;

Appreciating the field trials conducted in some countries for collection of morbidity and mortality information through non-medical health or other personnel and the experience thus obtained;

Noting the concern of the World Health Organization for development and promotion of health services, particularly in the developing countries, as contained in resolutions EB55.R16[13], WHA28.75[14], WHA28.77[15] and WHA28.88 [16],

Recommends that the World Health Organization should

(1)   become increasingly involved in the attempts made by the various developing countries for collection of morbidity and mortality statistics through lay or paramedical personnel;

(2)   organize meetings at regional level for facilitating exchange of experiences between the countries currently facing this problem so as to design suitable classification lists with due consideration to national differences in terminology;

(3)   assist countries in their endeavour to establish or expand the system of collection of morbidity and mortality data through lay or paramedical personnel.

6. Statistics of Death in the Perinatal Period and Related Matters

The Conference considered with interest the reports of the Scientific Group on Health Statistics Methodology relating to Perinatal Events [17] and the recommendations of the Expert Committee [12] on this subject. These were the culmination of a series of special WHO meetings attended by specialists from many disciplines. It had become clear that a review of the situation was needed in the light of certain developments in medical sciences, notably those leading to the improved survival of infants born at a very early gestational age.

After discussion, the Conference

Recommends that, where practicable, statistics in relation to perinatal deaths should be derived from a special certificate of perinatal death (instead of the normal death certificate) and presented in the manner set out in Annex II, which also includes relevant definitions. This annex also includes recommendations in respect of maternal mortality statistics.

7. Mortality Coding Rules

The Conference was made aware of the problems arising in selecting the underlying cause of death where this was the result of factors connected with surgical or other treatment. It was proposed that where an untoward effect of treatment is responsible for death then this should be coded rather than the condition for which the treatment was given. Although there were views expressed by some delegates that this interfered with the traditional underlying cause concept, the Conference preferred the former view and accordingly

Recommends that the modification rule in Annex III be added to the existing rules for selection of cause of death for primary mortality tabulation.

The Conference was also informed that additional guidelines for dealing with certificates of death from cancer had been drafted and were being tested in several countries. If the tests showed that the guidelines improved consistency in coding, they would be incorporated into the Ninth Revision.

8. Selection of a Single Cause for Statistics of Morbidity

No rules had hitherto been incorporated into the ICD concerning the tabulation of morbidity. Routine statistics are normally based upon a single cause and the Conference considered that the application of the ICD to routine morbidity statistics had reached a point where international recommendations for selection of a single cause for presentation of morbidity statistics was appropriate and accordingly

Recommends that the condition to be selected for single-cause analysis for health-care records should be the main condition treated or investigated during the relevant episode of hospital or other care. If no diagnosis was made, the main symptom or problem should be selected instead. Whenever possible, the choice should be exercised by the responsible medical practitioner or other health-care professional and the main condition or problem distinguished from other conditions or problems.

It is desirable that, in addition to the selection of a single cause for tabulation purposes, multiple condition coding and analysis should be attempted wherever possible, particularly for data relating to episodes of health care by hospitals (inpatient or outpatient), health clinics and family practitioners. For certain other types of data, such as from health examination surveys, multiple cause analysis may be the only satisfactory method.

9. *Short Lists for Tabulation of Mortality and Morbidity*

Difficulties had become apparent in the use of the present short lists A, B, C and D for the tabulation of mortality and morbidity. Their construction and numbering was such that confusion often arose and comparability of statistics based on different lists presented some difficulties. Proposed new lists were presented to the Conference in which totals were shown for groups of diseases and for certain selected individual conditions. Minimum lists of 55 items were recommended for the tabulation of mortality and morbidity and countries could add to these further items from a basic list of 275 categories.

The Conference

Recommends that the Special Tabulation Lists set out in Annex IV to this report should replace the lists for tabulation of morbidity and mortality and should be published as part of the International Classification of Diseases together with appropriate explanation and instruction as to their use.

10. *Multiple Condition Coding and Analysis*

The Conference noted with interest the extended use of multiple condition coding and analysis in a number of countries with a variety of ends in view. One example was the study of the interrelationship of various conditions recorded on a death certificate; another was to permit computer selection of the underlying cause of death. The Conference also

noted the value of a store of multiple-coded national data on mortality
and morbidity. The Conference expressed encouragement of such work
but did not recommend that the ICD should contain any particular rules
or methods of analysis to be followed.

11. *Different Disease-Coding Systems*

The Conference was reminded of the existence of other disease classifications and reviewed their attributes as a preliminary to discussion of
the possible form of the Tenth Revision. Some of these classifications
are developments from the International Classification of Diseases;
others are multi-axial, enabling retrieval from different viewpoints but
not primarily designed with the presentation of routine statistics in mind.
In others, a unique code is given to each disease or term, enabling
retrieval of specific conditions and assembly into alternative classifications
according to need. These developments seemed to indicate some desire
for greater flexibility and to raise doubts as to whether a single multi-
purpose classification was any longer practicable. It was felt that multi-
axial classification often destroyed the ability to retrieve disease terms.
Allocating a unique code to a disease or term might be one way of overcoming problems caused by changes in classification.

12. *The Tenth Revision of the International Classification of Diseases*

The Conference recognized the need to make an early start in planning the next revision of the classification and discussed a number of
questions that needed to be settled before detailed work could begin.
The most fundamental point was that the Organization's programme
was no longer confined to disease classification alone. Many other reasons,
social and economic, for contact with health services were now included
in the main classification and supplementary classifications of procedures
in medicine and of impairments and handicaps had been added. These
needed to be further developed and incorporated into a comprehensive
and coordinated system of classifications of health information. The
name of the Organization's programme should reflect the wider scope
of its activities.

Standardization of nomenclature on a multilingual basis was essential
for conformity in diagnosis, and glossaries similar to the one developed
for psychiatry might be provided for other specialities where diagnostic
concepts were unclear. A lack of balance in the Eight Revision, which
contained 140 categories for infectious diseases but only 20 for the whole
of perinatal morbidity, had been retained in the Ninth Revision because
ot its essentially conservative nature, but such a restriction should not
necessarily hold for the next revision.

It was acknowledged that conflicts existed between the need for a fairly broad classification for the purposes of international comparisons and the desire for a very high degree of specificity for diagnostic indexing and for epidemiological research, and between the requirements of a classification usable at the community level in developing countries and one suitable for a national morbidity programme with access to a computer. The structure of the Tenth Revision was another question for urgent decision; should the present uni-axial system be retained or should there be a move to a multi-dimensional approach; should the coding and classification elements be separated so that the former could remain constant while the latter could be revised at shorter intervals than at present?

The view of the Conference was that these questions should be decided within the next two or three years by the construction and trial of model classifications of various types. It was recognized that this would be an additional task to the normal work of the Organization in this area and would require the provision of extra resources.

The Conference recognized the great value of the work already done and still being done on ICD; it also recognized the rapidly increasing demands for more flexibility than is available in the present structure of this classification.

The Conference,

Noting that the ICD, despite the present constraints upon resources, which it completely absorbs, is one of the most influential activities of WHO,

Recommends that:

(1) WHO should continue its work in developing revisions of the ICD and related classifications and that the Organization's activity in connexion with the revision of the ICD should be expanded;

(2) the ICD programme should be given sufficient resources to enable it simultaneously to explore the needs for new departures in the realm of health classifications and how these can be met without detracting from the present revision process; the programme should also be enabled to carry out extensive field trials of the various alternative approaches that exist or which may emerge.

The Conference expressed the hope that efforts would be made to retain the continuity of expertise that had been developed in the Organization, in the centres for classification of diseases and among numerous organizations and individuals throughout the world.

13. *Publication of the Ninth Revision*

The Conference was informed that, although the Tabular List of the ICD (Volume 1) in English and French could be made available in published form by the end of 1976, it was unlikely that the Alphabetical Index (Volume 2) could be published before the middle of 1977. The Russian and Spanish versions should follow the English and French fairly closely.

Member States intending to publish national language versions would receive pre-publication copies of the various parts of the classification as and when they were completed by the Secretariat to enable them to adhere as nearly as possible to this timetable.

Several delegates pointed out that the late appearance of the alphabetical indexes at the Eight Revision had resulted in a high rate of coding errors during the first year of use.

Because of the large amount of work still to be done before the Ninth Revision can be published and because the training of coders requires that both volumes, including the alphabetical index, should be in the hands of users some 12 months before it is due to come into use,

The Conference

Recommends that the Ninth Revision of the International Classification of Diseases should come into effect on 1 January 1979.

14. *Familiarization and Training in the Use of the Ninth Revision*

There were many aspects of the proposed revision, besides the change in the categories themselves, which would require very careful explanation to coders and to users of statistics based on the ICD. It was planned that familiarization courses would be organized by the WHO regional offices, to help Member countries in planning their own courses. The Conference noted with interest that WHO hoped to prepare a set of training material covering an instructional course for coders of approximately two weeks, to make sure that the instruction was as consistent as possible. WHO would also make available explanatory material for users of statistics.

Adoption of the Ninth Revision

The Twenty-ninth World Health Assembly, meeting in Geneva in May 1976, adopted the following resolution with regard to the Manual of the International Classification of Diseases (Resolution WHA29.34) [18].

The Twenty-ninth World Health Assembly,

Having considered the report of the International Conference for the Ninth Revision of the International Classification of Diseases,

1. *Adopts* the detailed list of three-digit categories and optional four-digit sub-categories recommended by the Conference as the Ninth Revision of the International Classification of Diseases, to come into effect as from 1 January 1979;

2. *Adopts* the rules recommended by the Conference for the selection of a single cause in morbidity statistics;

3. *Adopts* the recommendations of the Conference regarding statistics of perinatal and maternal mortality, including a special certificate of cause of perinatal death for use where practicable;

4. *Requests* the Director-General to issue a new edition of the *Manual of the International Statistical Classification of Diseases, Injuries and Causes of Death.*

The Assembly adopted a further resolution concerning activities related to the International Classification of Diseases (Resolution WHA29.35) [19].

The Twenty-ninth World Health Assembly,

Noting the recommendations of the International Conference for the Ninth Revision of the International Classification of Diseases in respect of activities related to the Classification,

1. *Approves* the publication, for trial purposes, of supplementary classifications of Impairments and Handicaps and of Procedures in Medicine as supplements to, but not as integral parts of, the International Classification of Diseases;

2. *Endorses* the recommendation of the Conference concerning assistance to developing countries in their endeavour to establish or expand the system of collection of morbidity and mortality statistics through lay or paramedical personnel;

3. *Endorses* the request made by the Executive Board in resolution EB57.R34 [20] to the Director-General that he investigate the possibility of preparing an International Nomenclature of Diseases as an improvement to the Tenth Revision of the International Classification of Diseases.

Manual of the Ninth Revision

Conventions used in the Tabular List

The Tabular List makes special use of parentheses and colons which needs to be clearly understood. When parentheses are used for their

normal function of enclosing synonyms, alternative wordings or explanatory phrases, square brackets [...] are employed. Round brackets (...)
are used to enclose supplementary words which may be either present
or absent in the statement of a diagnosis without affecting the code number
to which it is assigned. Words followed by a colon [:] are not complete
terms, but must have one or other of the understated modifiers to make
them assignable to the given category. " NOS " is an abbreviation for
"not otherwise specified" and is virtually the equivalent of "unspecified"
and" unqualified ".

As an example of the use of the above conventions, category 464.0,
Acute laryngitis, includes the following terms:

Laryngitis (acute):
  NOS
  Haemophilus influenzae [H. influenzae]
  oedematous
  pneumococcal
  septic
  suppurative
  ulcerative

This signifies that to this category should be assigned laryngitis, with
or without the adjective " acute ", if standing alone or if accompanied by
one or other of the modifiers: Haemophilus influenzae [of which H.
influenzae is an alternative wording], oedematous, pneumococcal, septic,
suppurative, or ulcerative. Influenzal, streptococcal, diphtheritic, tuberculous, and chronic laryngitis will be found in other categories.

Dual classification of certain diagnostic statements

The Ninth Revision of the ICD contains an innovation in that there
are two codes for certain diagnostic descriptions which contain elements
of information both about a localised manifestation or complication and
about a more generalised underlying disease process. One of the codes
—marked with a dagger (†)—is positioned in the part of the classification
in which the diagnostic description is located according to normal ICD
principles, that relating to the underlying disease, and the other—marked
with an asterisk (*)—is positioned in the chapter of the classification
relating to the organ system to which the manifestation or complication
relates. Thus tuberculous meningitis has its dagger code in the chapter
for infectious and parasitic diseases, and its asterisk code in the nervous
system chapter.

The necessity for this arose from the desire of specialists and those
concerned with statistics of medical care to have certain manifestations

which are medical-care problems in their own right classified in the chapters relating to the relevant organ system. The ICD has traditionally classified generalised diseases and infectious disease entities which may affect several parts of the body to special chapters of the classification, and their manifestations are normally assigned to the same place, so that until now tuberculous meningitis has been classifiable only to the infectious and parasitic diseases chapter.

The dagger and asterisk categories are in fact alternative positionings in the classification for the relevant conditions, enabling retrieval or statistical analysis from either viewpoint. It is, however, a principle of ICD classification that the dagger category is the primary code and that the asterisk code is secondary, so it is important where it is desired to work with the asterisk code, and both are used, to use some special mark or a predetermined positioning in the coded record, to identify which is the dagger, and which the asterisk, code for the same entity.

The criteria adopted in the Ninth Revision are that asterisk categories are provided:

(i) if the manifestation or complication represents a medical-care problem in its own right and is normally treated by a specialty different from the one which would handle the underlying condition, and

(ii) if the information about both the manifestation and the underlying condition is customarily contained in one diagnostic phrase (such as " diabetic retinitis "), or

(iii) if the category relating to the manifestation is subdivided according to the cause—an example is arthropathy in which the subdivisions relate to broad groups of causes.

Other underlying condition/manifestation combinations exist which do not cause coding and retrieval problems and have therefore not been incorporated in the " dagger and asterisk " system. Examples are:

(i) situations where the two elements are customarily recorded as discrete diagnostic phrases and can be dealt with simply by coding the two terms separately, e.g. certain types of anaemia which may be the consequence of other diseases; the classification of the anaemia is usually according to its morphological type and does not depend on the cause;

(ii) where the manifestation is an intrinsic part of the basic disease and is not regarded as a separate medical-care problem; for example, cholera, dysentery, etc. in the infectious and parasitic diseases chapter do not have asterisk categories in the digestive system chapter; lower genito-urinary tract manifestations of venereal diseases, in the infectious and parasitic diseases chapter, do not have asterisk categories in the genitourinary diseases chapter, although gonococcal salpingitis and orchitis do;

(iii)   where the ICD has traditionally classified the condition according to the manifestation, e.g. anaemia due to enzyme defect.

The areas of the Classification where the dagger and asterisk system operates are limited; there are about 150 rubrics of each in which asterisk- or dagger-marked terms occur. They may take one of three different forms:—

(i)   if the symbol († or *) and the alternative code both appear in the title of the rubric, all terms classifiable to that rubric are subject to dual classification and all have the same alternative code, e.g.

049.0†   *Lymphocytic choriomeningitis* (321.6*)

Lymphocytic:
  meningitis (serous)
  meningoencephalitis (serous)

321.2*   *Meningitis due to ECHO virus* (047.1†)

Meningo-eruptive syndrome

(ii)   if the symbol appears in the title but the alternative code does not, all terms classifiable to that rubric are subject to dual classification but they have different alternative codes (which are listed for each term), e.g.

074.2†   *Coxsackie carditis*

Aseptic myocarditis of   Coxsackie:
     newborn (422.0*)   endocarditis (421.1*)
                                     myocarditis (422.0*)
                                     pericarditis (420.0*)

420.0*   *Pericarditis in diseases classified elsewhere*

Pericarditis (acute):   Pericarditis (acute):
  Coxsackie (074.2†)   tuberculous (017.8†)
  meningococcal (036.4†)   uraemic (585†)
  syphilitic (093.8†)

(iii)   if neither the symbol nor the alternative code appear in the title, the rubric as a whole is not subject to dual classification but individual inclusion terms may be; if so, these terms will be marked with the symbol and their alternative codes, e.g.

078.5   *Cytomegalic inclusion disease*

Cytomegalic inclusion virus hepatitis† (573.1*)
Salivary gland virus disease

424.3   *Pulmonary valve disorders*

Pulmonic regurgitation:
  NOS
  syphilitic* (093.2†)

The use of asterisk coding is entirely optional. It should never be employed in coding the underlying cause of death (only dagger coding should be used for this purpose) but may be used in morbidity coding and in multiple-condition coding whether in morbidity or mortality. Any published tabulations, whether according to the detailed list or one of the short lists, of frequencies based on asterisk coding should be clearly annotated " Based on ICD asterisk coding ".

Role of the E Code

As explained in the Report of the International Revision Conference (see paragraph 1.3 (iii), page XVI), the E Code is now a supplementary classification that may be used, if desired, to code external factors associated with morbid conditions classified to any part of the main classification. For single-cause tabulation of the underlying cause of death, however, the E Code should be used as the primary code if, and only if, the morbid condition is classifiable to Chapter XVII (Injury and Poisoning).

Gaps in the numbering system

It will be noticed that certain code numbers have not been used, leaving gaps in the numbering system. The reason for this practice was to avoid unnecessary changes in code numbers familiar to coders who have been using the Eighth Revision. For example, gangrene (category 445 in the Eighth Revision) has been moved to category 785.4; in order to avoid changing the code numbers of categories 446 (Polyarteritis nodosa and allied conditions), 447 (Other disorders of arteries and arterioles) and 448 (Diseases of capillaries), it was preferred to leave the code number 445 unused in the Ninth Revision.

Glossary of mental disorders

A glossary describing and defining the content of rubrics in Chapter V (Mental Disorders) was published separately from the Eighth Revision of the International Classification of Diseases. In the Ninth Revision, the glossary has been incorporated into the Classification itself (see pages 177-213).

The glossary descriptions are not intended as an aid for the lay coder, who should code whatever diagnostic statement appears on a medical record according to the provisions of the Tabular List and Alphabetical Index. Their purpose is to assist the person making the diagnosis, who should do so on the basis of the descriptions rather than the category titles, which may differ in meaning from place to place.

Adaptations of the ICD

Several adaptations or applications of the ICD to specific specialties have been published or are in preparation. They are briefly described below.

Dentistry and Stomatology

The "Application of the ICD to Dentistry and Stomatology" (ICD-DA), based on the Eighth Revision of the ICD, was prepared by the Oral Health Unit of WHO and first published in 1969. It brings together those ICD categories that include "diseases or conditions that occur in, have manifestations in, or have associations with the oral cavity and adjacent structures". It provides greater detail by means of a fifth digit, but the numbering system is so organized that the relationship between an ICD-DA code and the ICD code from which it is derived is immediately obvious and frequencies for ICD-DA categories can be readily aggregated into ICD categories.

ICD-DA has been revised to concord with the Ninth Revision of the ICD and this revision was published by the World Health Organization in 1977.

Oncology

The "International Classification of Diseases for Oncology" (ICD-O) was published by the World Health Organization in 1976. Developed in collaboration with the International Agency for Research on Cancer (WHO) and the United States National Cancer Institute, with input from many other countries and extensive field trials, the ICD-O is intended for use in cancer registries, pathology departments and other agencies specializing in cancer.

ICD-O is a dual-axis classification, providing coding systems for topography and morphology. The topography code uses for *all* neoplasms the same three- and four-digit categories that the Ninth Revision of ICD uses for *malignant* neoplasms (categories 140-199), thus providing increased specificity of site for other neoplasms, where the ICD provides a more restricted topographical classification or none at all.

The morphology code is identical to the neoplasms section of the morphology field of the Systematized Nomenclature of Medicine (SNOMed) [21] and is compatible with the 1968 Edition of the Manual of Tumor Nomenclature and Coding (MOTNAC) [22] and the Systematized Nomenclature of Pathology (SNOP) [23]. It is a five-digit code, the first four digits identifying the histological type and the fifth the behaviour of the neoplasm (malignant, in situ, benign, etc.). The ICD-O morphology code also appears in this Volume (see pages 667-690) and in the Alphabetical Index.

In addition to the topography and morphology codes, ICD-O also includes a list of tumour-like lesions and conditions. A table explaining the method of converting ICD-O codes into ICD codes will be published in due course.

Ophthalmology

The International Council of Ophthalmology, supported by ophthalmological groups in many countries, has prepared a Classification of Disorders of the Eye, based on the Ninth Revision of the ICD.

In addition to the ICD section "Disorders of the eye and adnexa" (categories 360-379), it includes all other ICD categories that classify eye disorders, from infectious diseases to injuries. It is a five-digit classification, being identical with ICD at the three- and four-digit level but introducing additional detail at the fifth digit for the use of specialists.

The classification was published in the "International Nomenclature of Ophthalmology" by the American Academy of Ophthalmology and Otolaryngology [24] in 1977, which also includes definitions or short descriptions of all terms, synonyms and equivalent terms in French, German and Spanish, and reference terms to facilitate literature retrieval.

WHO Centres for Classification of Diseases

Six WHO Centres have been established to assist countries with problems encountered in the classification of diseases and, in particular, in the use of the ICD. They are located in institutions in Paris (for French language users), São Paulo (for Portuguese), Moscow (for Russian) and Caracas (for Spanish); there are two Centres for English language users, in London and, for North America, in Washington, DC., USA. Communications should be addressed as follows:—

Head, WHO Centre for Classification of Diseases
Office of Population Censuses and Surveys
St. Catherine's House
10 Kingsway
London WC2B 6JP
United Kingdom

or

Head, WHO Center for Classification of Diseases for North America
National Center for Health Statistics
US Public Health Service
Department of Health, Education and Welfare
Washington, DC.,
United States of America

REFERENCES

1. Registrar General of England and Wales, *Sixteenth Annual Report, 1856*, Appendix, 75–76

2. GREENWOOD, M. (1948) *Medical statistics from Graunt to Farr.* Cambridge, p. 28

3. Registrar General of England and Wales, *Sixteenth Annual Report, 1856*, Appendix, p. 73

4. BERTILLON, J. (1912) Classification of the causes of death. (Abstract). *Trans. 15th Int. Cong. Hyg. Demog.,* Washington, pp. 52–55

5. *Bull. Inst. int. Statist. 1900,* **12,** 280

6. ROESLE, E. (1928) *Essai d'une statistique comparative de la morbidité devant servir à établir les listes spéciales des causes de morbidité.* Geneva (League of Nations Health Organization, document C. H. 730)

7. *Off. Rec. Wld Hlth Org.,* 1948, **2,** 110

8. *Off. Rec. Wld Hlth Org.,* 1948, **11,** 23

9. World Health Organization (1955) *Report of the International Conference for the Seventh Revision of the International Lists of Diseases and Causes of Death,* Geneva (unpublished document WHO/HS/7 Rev. Conf./17 Rev. 1)

10. *Wld Hlth Org. techn. Rep. Ser.,* 1952, **53**

11. World Health Organization (1965) *Report of the International Conference for the Eighth Revision of the International Classification of Diseases,* Geneva (unpublished document WHO/HS/8 Rev. Conf./11.65)

12. World Health Organization, Expert Committee on Health Statistics (1974) *Ninth Revision of the International Classification of Diseases,* Geneva (unpublished document WHO/ICD9/74.4)

13. *Off. Rec. Wld Hlth Org.,* 1975, **223,** 10

14. *Off. Rec. Wld Hlth Org.,* 1975, **226,** 42

15. *Off. Rec. Wld Hlth Org.,* 1975, **226**, 44

16. *Off. Rec. Wld Hlth Org.,* 1975, **226**, 53

17. World Health Organization, Scientific Group on Health Statistics Methodology related to Perinatal Events (1974), Geneva (unpublished document ICD/PE/74.4)

18. *Off. Rec. Wld Hlth Org.,* 1976, **233**, 18

19. *Off. Rec. Wld Hlth Org.,* 1976, **233**, 18

20. *Off. Rec. Wld Hlth Org.,* 1976, **231**, 25

21. College of American Pathologists (1976), *Systematized Nomenclature of Medicine,* Chicago, Illinois

22. American Cancer Society, Inc. (1968), *Manual of Tumor Nomenclature and Coding,* New York, NY

23. College of American Pathologists (1965), *Systematized Nomenclature of Pathology,* Chicago, Illinois

24. American Academy of Ophthalmology and Otolaryngology (1977), *International Nomenclature of Ophthalmology,* 15 Second Street, S.W., Rochester, Minnesota 55901.

LIST OF THREE-DIGIT CATEGORIES

I. INFECTIOUS AND PARASITIC DISEASES

Intestinal infectious diseases (001-009)

001 Cholera
002 Typhoid and paratyphoid fevers
003 Other salmonella infections
004 Shigellosis
005 Other food poisoning (bacterial)
006 Amoebiasis
007 Other protozoal intestinal diseases
008 Intestinal infections due to other organisms
009 Ill-defined intestinal infections

Tuberculosis (010-018)

010 Primary tuberculous infection
011 Pulmonary tuberculosis
012 Other respiratory tuberculosis
013 Tuberculosis of meninges and central nervous system
014 Tuberculosis of intestines, peritoneum and mesenteric glands
015 Tuberculosis of bones and joints
016 Tuberculosis of genitourinary system
017 Tuberculosis of other organs
018 Miliary tuberculosis

Zoonotic bacterial diseases (020-027)

020 Plague
021 Tularaemia
022 Anthrax
023 Brucellosis
024 Glanders
025 Melioidosis
026 Rat-bite fever
027 Other zoonotic bacterial diseases

Other bacterial diseases (030-041)

030 Leprosy
031 Diseases due to other mycobacteria
032 Diphtheria

033   Whooping cough
034   Streptococcal sore throat and scarlatina
035   Erysipelas
036   Meningococcal infection
037   Tetanus
038   Septicaemia
039   Actinomycotic infections
040   Other bacterial diseases
041   Bacterial infection in conditions classified elsewhere and of unspecified site

Poliomyelitis and other non-arthropod-borne viral diseases of central nervous system (045-049)

045   Acute poliomyelitis
046   Slow virus infection of central nervous system
047   Meningitis due to enterovirus
048   Other enterovirus diseases of central nervous system
049   Other non-arthropod-borne viral diseases of central nervous system

Viral diseases accompanied by exanthem (050-057)

050   Smallpox
051   Cowpox and paravaccinia
052   Chickenpox
053   Herpes zoster
054   Herpes simplex
055   Measles
056   Rubella
057   Other viral exanthemata

Arthropod-borne viral diseases (060-066)

060   Yellow fever
061   Dengue
062   Mosquito-borne viral encephalitis
063   Tick-borne viral encephalitis
064   Viral encephalitis transmitted by other and unspecified arthropods
065   Arthropod-borne haemorrhagic fever
066   Other arthropod-borne viral diseases

Other diseases due to viruses and Chlamydiae (070-079)

070 Viral hepatitis
071 Rabies
072 Mumps
073 Ornithosis
074 Specific diseases due to Coxsackie virus
075 Infectious mononucleosis
076 Trachoma
077 Other diseases of conjunctiva due to viruses and Chlamydiae
078 Other diseases due to viruses and Chlamydiae
079 Viral infection in conditions classified elsewhere and of un-
    specified site

Rickettsioses and other arthropod-borne diseases (080-088)

080 Louse-borne [epidemic] typhus
081 Other typhus
082 Tick-borne rickettsioses
083 Other rickettsioses
084 Malaria
085 Leishmaniasis
086 Trypanosomiasis
087 Relapsing fever
088 Other arthropod-borne diseases

Syphilis and other venereal diseases (090-099)

090 Congenital syphilis
091 Early syphilis, symptomatic
092 Early syphilis, latent
093 Cardiovascular syphilis
094 Neurosyphilis
095 Other forms of late syphilis, with symptoms
096 Late syphilis, latent
097 Other and unspecified syphilis
098 Gonococcal infections
099 Other venereal diseases

Other spirochaetal diseases (100-104)

100 Leptospirosis
101 Vincent's angina

102 Yaws
103 Pinta
104 Other spirochaetal infection

Mycoses (110-118)

110 Dermatophytosis
111 Dermatomycosis, other and unspecified
112 Candidiasis
114 Coccidioidomycosis
115 Histoplasmosis
116 Blastomycotic infection
117 Other mycoses
118 Opportunistic mycoses

Helminthiases (120-129)

120 Schistosomiasis [bilharziasis]
121 Other trematode infections
122 Echinococcosis
123 Other cestode infection
124 Trichinosis
125 Filarial infection and dracontiasis
126 Ancylostomiasis and necatoriasis
127 Other intestinal helminthiases
128 Other and unspecified helminthiases
129 Intestinal parasitism, unspecified

Other infectious and parasitic diseases (130-136)

130 Toxoplasmosis
131 Trichomoniasis
132 Pediculosis and phthirus infestation
133 Acariasis
134 Other infestation
135 Sarcoidosis
136 Other and unspecified infectious and parasitic diseases

Late effects of infectious and parasitic diseases (137-139)

137 Late effects of tuberculosis
138 Late effects of acute poliomyelitis
139 Late effects of other infectious and parasitic diseases

II. NEOPLASMS

Malignant neoplasm of lip, oral cavity and pharynx (140-149)

140 Malignant neoplasm of lip
141 Malignant neoplasm of tongue
142 Malignant neoplasm of major salivary glands
143 Malignant neoplasm of gum
144 Malignant neoplasm of floor of mouth
145 Malignant neoplasm of other and unspecified parts of mouth
146 Malignant neoplasm of oropharynx
147 Malignant neoplasm of nasopharynx
148 Malignant neoplasm of hypopharynx
149 Malignant neoplasm of other and ill-defined sites within the lip, oral cavity and pharynx

Malignant neoplasm of digestive organs and peritoneum (150-159)

150 Malignant neoplasm of oesophagus
151 Malignant neoplasm of stomach
152 Malignant neoplasm of small intestine, including duodenum
153 Malignant neoplasm of colon
154 Malignant neoplasm of rectum, rectosigmoid junction and anus
155 Malignant neoplasm of liver and intrahepatic bile ducts
156 Malignant neoplasm of gallbladder and extrahepatic bile ducts
157 Malignant neoplasm of pancreas
158 Malignant neoplasm of retroperitoneum and peritoneum
159 Malignant neoplasm of other and ill-defined sites within the digestive organs and peritoneum

Malignant neoplasm of respiratory and intrathoracic organs (160-165)

160 Malignant neoplasm of nasal cavities, middle ear and accessory sinuses
161 Malignant neoplasm of larynx
162 Malignant neoplasm of trachea, bronchus and lung
163 Malignant neoplasm of pleura
164 Malignant neoplasm of thymus, heart and mediastinum
165 Malignant neoplasm of other and ill-defined sites within the respiratory system and intrathoracic organs

Malignant neoplasm of bone, connective tissue, skin and breast (170-175)

170 Malignant neoplasm of bone and articular cartilage
171 Malignant neoplasm of connective and other soft tissue
172 Malignant melanoma of skin
173 Other malignant neoplasm of skin
174 Malignant neoplasm of female breast
175 Malignant neoplasm of male breast

Malignant neoplasm of genitourinary organs (179-189)

179 Malignant neoplasm of uterus, part unspecified
180 Malignant neoplasm of cervix uteri
181 Malignant neoplasm of placenta
182 Malignant neoplasm of body of uterus
183 Malignant neoplasm of ovary and other uterine adnexa
184 Malignant neoplasm of other and unspecified female genital organs
185 Malignant neoplasm of prostate
186 Malignant neoplasm of testis
187 Malignant neoplasm of penis and other male genital organs
188 Malignant neoplasm of bladder
189 Malignant neoplasm of kidney and other and unspecified urinary organs

Malignant neoplasm of other and unspecified sites (190-199)

190 Malignant neoplasm of eye
191 Malignant neoplasm of brain
192 Malignant neoplasm of other and unspecified parts of nervous system
193 Malignant neoplasm of thyroid gland
194 Malignant neoplasm of other endocrine glands and related structures
195 Malignant neoplasm of other and ill-defined sites
196 Secondary and unspecified malignant neoplasm of lymph nodes
197 Secondary malignant neoplasm of respiratory and digestive systems
198 Secondary malignant neoplasm of other specified sites
199 Malignant neoplasm without specification of site

Malignant neoplasm of lymphatic and haematopoietic tissue (200-208)

200 Lymphosarcoma and reticulosarcoma
201 Hodgkin's disease
202 Other malignant neoplasm of lympoid and histiocytic tissue
203 Multiple myeloma and immunoproliferative neoplasms
204 Lymphoid leukaemia
205 Myeloid leukaemia
206 Monocytic leukaemia
207 Other specified leukaemia
208 Leukaemia of unspecified cell type

Benign neoplasms (210-229)

210 Benign neoplasm of lip, oral cavity and pharynx
211 Benign neoplasm of other parts of digestive system
212 Benign neoplasm of respiratory and intrathoracic organs
213 Benign neoplasm of bone and articular cartilage
214 Lipoma
215 Other benign neoplasm of connective and other soft tissue
216 Benign neoplasm of skin
217 Benign neoplasm of breast
218 Uterine leiomyoma
219 Other benign neoplasm of uterus
220 Benign neoplasm of ovary
221 Benign neoplasm of other female genital organs
222 Benign neoplasm of male genital organs
223 Benign neoplasm of kidney and other urinary organs
224 Benign neoplasm of eye
225 Benign neoplasm of brain and other parts of nervous system
226 Benign neoplasm of thyroid gland
227 Benign neoplasm of other endocrine glands and related structures
228 Haemangioma and lymphangioma, any site
229 Benign neoplasm of other and unspecified sites

Carcinoma in situ (230-234)

230 Carcinoma in situ of digestive organs
231 Carcinoma in situ of respiratory system
232 Carcinoma in situ of skin

233 Carcinoma in situ of breast and genitourinary system
234 Carcinoma in situ of other and unspecified sites

Neoplasms of uncertain behaviour (235-238)

235 Neoplasm of uncertain behaviour of digestive and respiratory systems
236 Neoplasm of uncertain behaviour of genitourinary organs
237 Neoplasm of uncertain behaviour of endocrine glands and nervous system
238 Neoplasm of uncertain behaviour of other and unspecified sites and tissues

Neoplasms of unspecified nature (239)

239 Neoplasm of unspecified nature

III. ENDOCRINE, NUTRITIONAL AND METABOLIC DISEASES AND IMMUNITY DISORDERS

Disorders of thyroid gland (240-246)

240 Simple and unspecified goitre
241 Nontoxic nodular goitre
242 Thyrotoxicosis with or without goitre
243 Congenital hypothyroidism
244 Acquired hypothyroidism
245 Thyroiditis
246 Other disorders of thyroid

Diseases of other endocrine glands (250-259)

250 Diabetes mellitus
251 Other disorders of pancreatic internal secretion
252 Disorders of parathyroid gland
253 Disorders of the pituitary gland and its hypothalamic control
254 Diseases of thymus gland
255 Disorders of adrenal glands
256 Ovarian dysfunction
257 Testicular dysfunction
258 Polyglandular dysfunction and related disorders
259 Other endocrine disorders

Nutritional deficiencies (260-269)

260   Kwashiorkor
261   Nutritional marasmus
262   Other severe protein-calorie malnutrition
263   Other and unspecified protein-calorie malnutrition
264   Vitamin A deficiency
265   Thiamine and niacin deficiency states
266   Deficiency of B-complex components
267   Ascorbic acid deficiency
268   Vitamin D deficiency
269   Other nutritional deficiencies

Other metabolic disorders and immunity disorders (270-279)

270   Disorders of amino-acid transport and metabolism
271   Disorders of carbohydrate transport and metabolism
272   Disorders of lipoid metabolism
273   Disorders of plasma protein metabolism
274   Gout
275   Disorders of mineral metabolism
276   Disorders of fluid, electrolyte and acid-base balance
277   Other and unspecified disorders of metabolism
278   Obesity and other hyperalimentation
279   Disorders involving the immune mechanism

IV.   DISEASES OF BLOOD AND BLOOD-FORMING ORGANS

280   Iron deficiency anaemias
281   Other deficiency anaemias
282   Hereditary haemolytic anaemias
283   Acquired haemolytic anaemias
284   Aplastic anaemia
285   Other and unspecified anaemias
286   Coagulation defects
287   Purpura and other haemorrhagic conditions
288   Diseases of white blood cells
289   Other diseases of blood and blood-forming organs

V. MENTAL DISORDERS

Organic psychotic conditions (290-294)

290   Senile and presenile organic psychotic conditions
291   Alcoholic psychoses
292   Drug psychoses
293   Transient organic psychotic conditions
294   Other organic psychotic conditions (chronic)

Other psychoses (295-299)

295   Schizophrenic psychoses
296   Affective psychoses
297   Paranoid states
298   Other nonorganic psychoses
299   Psychoses with origin specific to childhood

Neurotic disorders, personality disorders and other nonpsychotic mental disorders (300-316)

300   Neurotic disorders
301   Personality disorders
302   Sexual deviations and disorders
303   Alcohol dependence syndrome
304   Drug dependence
305   Nondependent abuse of drugs
306   Physiological malfunction arising from mental factors
307   Special symptoms or syndromes not elsewhere classified
308   Acute reaction to stress
309   Adjustment reaction
310   Specific nonpsychotic mental disorders following organic brain damage
311   Depressive disorder, not elsewhere classified
312   Disturbance of conduct not elsewhere classified
313   Disturbance of emotions specific to childhood and adolescence
314   Hyperkinetic syndrome of childhood
315   Specific delays in development
316   Psychic factors associated with diseases classified elsewhere

Mental retardation (317-319)

317   Mild mental retardation
318   Other specified mental retardation
319   Unspecified mental retardation

VI. DISEASES OF THE NERVOUS SYSTEM AND SENSE ORGANS

Inflammatory diseases of the central nervous system (320-326)

320 Bacterial meningitis
321 Meningitis due to other organisms
322 Meningitis of unspecified cause
323 Encephalitis, myelitis and encephalomyelitis
324 Intracranial and intraspinal abscess
325 Phlebitis and thrombophlebitis of intracranial venous sinuses
326 Late effects of intracranial abscess or pyogenic infection

Hereditary and degenerative diseases of the central nervous system (330-337)

330 Cerebral degenerations usually manifest in childhood
331 Other cerebral degenerations
332 Parkinson's disease
333 Other extrapyramidal disease and abnormal movement disorders
334 Spinocerebellar disease
335 Anterior horn cell disease
336 Other diseases of spinal cord
337 Disorders of the autonomic nervous system

Other disorders of the central nervous system (340-349)

340 Multiple sclerosis
341 Other demyelinating diseases of central nervous system
342 Hemiplegia
343 Infantile cerebral palsy
344 Other paralytic syndromes
345 Epilepsy
346 Migraine
347 Cataplexy and narcolepsy
348 Other conditions of brain
349 Other and unspecified disorders of the nervous system

Disorders of the peripheral nervous system (350-359)

350 Trigeminal nerve disorders
351 Facial nerve disorders

352   Disorders of other cranial nerves
353   Nerve root and plexus disorders
354   Mononeuritis of upper limb and mononeuritis multiplex
355   Mononeuritis of lower limb
356   Hereditary and idiopathic peripheral neuropathy
357   Inflammatory and toxic neuropathy
358   Myoneural disorders
359   Muscular dystrophies and other myopathies

Disorders of the eye and adnexa (360-379)

360   Disorders of the globe
361   Retinal detachments and defects
362   Other retinal disorders
363   Chorioretinal inflammations and scars and other disorders of
        choroid
364   Disorders of iris and ciliary body
365   Glaucoma
366   Cataract
367   Disorders of refraction and accommodation
368   Visual disturbances
369   Blindness and low vision
370   Keratitis
371   Corneal opacity and other disorders of cornea
372   Disorders of conjunctiva
373   Inflammation of eyelids
374   Other disorders of eyelids
375   Disorders of lacrimal system
376   Disorders of the orbit
377   Disorders of optic nerve and visual pathways
378   Strabismus and other disorders of binocular eye movements
379   Other disorders of eye

Diseases of the ear and mastoid process (380-389)

380   Disorders of external ear
381   Nonsuppurative otitis media and Eustachian tube disorders
382   Suppurative and unspecified otitis media
383   Mastoiditis and related conditions
384   Other disorders of tympanic membrane
385   Other disorders of middle ear and mastoid

386   Vertiginous syndromes and other disorders of vestibular system
387   Otosclerosis
388   Other disorders of ear
389   Deafness

VII.   DISEASES OF THE CIRCULATORY SYSTEM

Acute rheumatic fever (390-392)

390   Rheumatic fever without mention of heart involvement
391   Rheumatic fever with heart involvement
392   Rheumatic chorea

Chronic rheumatic heart disease (393-398)

393   Chronic rheumatic pericarditis
394   Diseases of mitral valve
395   Diseases of aortic valve
396   Diseases of mitral and aortic valves
397   Diseases of other endocardial structures
398   Other rheumatic heart disease

Hypertensive disease (401-405)

401   Essential hypertension
402   Hypertensive heart disease
403   Hypertensive renal disease
404   Hypertensive heart and renal disease
405   Secondary hypertension

Ischaemic heart disease (410-414)

410   Acute myocardial infarction
411   Other acute and subacute form of ischaemic heart disease
412   Old myocardial infarction
413   Angina pectoris
414   Other forms of chronic ischaemic heart disease

Diseases of pulmonary circulation (415-417)

415   Acute pulmonary heart disease
416   Chronic pulmonary heart disease
417   Other diseases of pulmonary circulation

Other forms of heart disease (420-429)

420 Acute pericarditis
421 Acute and subacute endocarditis
422 Acute myocarditis
423 Other diseases of pericardium
424 Other diseases of endocardium
425 Cardiomyopathy
426 Conduction disorders
427 Cardiac dysrhythmias
428 Heart failure
429 Ill-defined descriptions and complications of heart disease

Cerebrovascular disease (430-438)

430 Subarachnoid haemorrhage
431 Intracerebral haemorrhage
432 Other and unspecified intracranial haemorrhage
433 Occlusion and stenosis of precerebral arteries
434 Occlusion of cerebral arteries
435 Transcient cerebral ischaemia
436 Acute but ill-defined cerebrovascular disease
437 Other and ill-defined cerebrovascular disease
438 Late effects of cerebrovascular disease

Diseases of arteries, arterioles and capillaries (440-448)

440 Atherosclerosis
441 Aortic aneurysm
442 Other aneurysm
443 Other peripheral vascular disease
444 Arterial embolism and thrombosis
446 Polyarteritis nodosa and allied conditions
447 Other disorders of arteries and arterioles
448 Diseases of capillaries

Diseases of veins and lymphatics, and other diseases of circulatory system (451-459)

451 Phlebitis and thrombophlebitis
452 Portal vein thrombosis
453 Other venous embolism and thrombosis
454 Varicose veins of lower extremities

455 Haemorrhoids
456 Varicose veins of other sites
457 Noninfective disorders of lymphatic channels
458 Hypotension
459 Other disorders of circulatory system

VIII. DISEASES OF THE RESPIRATORY SYSTEM

Acute respiratory infections (460-466)

460 Acute nasopharyngitis [common cold]
461 Acute sinusitis
462 Acute pharyngitis
463 Acute tonsillitis
464 Acute laryngitis and tracheitis
465 Acute upper respiratory infections of multiple or unspecified sites
466 Acute bronchitis and bronchiolitis

Other diseases of upper respiratory tract (470-478)

470 Deflected nasal septum
471 Nasal polyps
472 Chronic pharyngitis and nasopharyngitis
473 Chronic sinusitis
474 Chronic disease of tonsils and adenoids
475 Peritonsillar abscess
476 Chronic laryngitis and laryngotracheitis
477 Allergic rhinitis
478 Other diseases of upper respiratory tract

Pneumonia and influenza (480-487)

480 Viral pneumonia
481 Pneumococcal pneumonia
482 Other bacterial pneumonia
483 Pneumonia due to other specified organism
484 Pneumonia in infectious diseases classified elsewhere
485 Bronchopneumonia, organism unspecified
486 Pneumonia, organism unspecified
487 Influenza

Chronic obstructive pulmonary disease and allied conditions (490-496)

490   Bronchitis, not specified as acute or chronic
491   Chronic bronchitis
492   Emphysema
493   Asthma
494   Bronchiectasis
495   Extrinsic allergic alveolitis
496   Chronic airways obstruction, not elsewhere classified

Pneumoconioses and other lung diseases due to external agents (500-508)

500   Coalworkers' pneumoconiosis
501   Asbestosis
502   Pneumoconiosis due to other silica or silicates
503   Pneumoconiosis due to other inorganic dust
504   Pneumopathy due to inhalation of other dust
505   Pneumoconiosis, unspecified
506   Respiratory conditions due to chemical fumes and vapours
507   Pneumonitis due to solids and liquids
508   Respiratory conditions due to other and unspecified external
        agents

Other diseases of respiratory system (510-519)

510   Empyema
511   Pleurisy
512   Pneumothorax
513   Abscess of lung and mediastinum
514   Pulmonary congestion and hypostasis
515   Postinflammatory pulmonary fibrosis
516   Other alveolar and parietoalveolar pneumopathy
517   Lung involvement in conditions classified elsewhere
518   Other diseases of lung
519   Other diseases of respiratory system

IX.   DISEASES OF THE DIGESTIVE SYSTEM

Diseases of oral cavity, salivary glands and jaws (520-529)

520   Disorders of tooth development and eruption

521 Diseases of hard tissues of teeth
522 Diseases of pulp and periapical tissues
523 Gingival and periodontal diseases
524 Dentofacial anomalies, including malocclusion
525 Other diseases and conditions of the teeth and supporting structures
526 Diseases of the jaws
527 Diseases of the salivary glands
528 Diseases of the oral soft tissues, excluding lesions specific for gingiva and tongue
529 Diseases and other conditions of the tongue

Diseases of oesophagus, stomach and duodenum (530-537)

530 Diseases of oesophagus
531 Gastric ulcer
532 Duodenal ulcer
533 Peptic ulcer, site unspecified
534 Gastrojejunal ulcer
535 Gastritis and duodenitis
536 Disorders of function of stomach
537 Other disorders of stomach and duodenum

Appendicitis (540-543)

540 Acute appendicitis
541 Appendicitis, unqualified
542 Other appendicitis
543 Other diseases of appendix

Hernia of abdominal cavity (550-553)

550 Inguinal hernia
551 Other hernia of abdominal cavity, with gangrene
552 Other hernia of abdominal cavity with obstruction, without mention of gangrene
553 Other hernia of abdominal cavity without mention of obstruction or gangrene

Noninfective enteritis and colitis (555-558)

555 Regional enteritis
556 Idiopathic proctocolitis
557 Vascular insufficiency of intestine
558 Other noninfective gastroenteritis and colitis

Other diseases of intestines and peritoneum (560-569)

560   Intestinal obstruction without mention of hernia
562   Diverticula of intestine
564   Functional digestive disorders, not elsewhere classified
565   Anal fissure and fistula
566   Abcess of anal and rectal regions
567   Peritonitis
568   Other disorders of peritoneum
569   Other disorders of intestine

Other diseases of digestive system (570-579)

570   Acute and subacute necrosis of liver
571   Chronic liver disease and cirrhosis
572   Liver abscess and sequelae of chronic liver disease
573   Other disorders of liver
574   Cholelithiasis
575   Other disorders of gallbladder
576   Other disorders of biliary tract
577   Diseases of pancreas
578   Gastrointestinal haemorrhage
579   Intestinal malabsorption

X.   DISEASES OF THE GENITOURINARY SYSTEM

Nephritis, nephrotic syndrome and nephrosis (580-589)

580   Acute glomerulonephritis
581   Nephrotic syndrome
582   Chronic glomerulonephritis
583   Nephritis and nephropathy, not specified as acute or chronic
584   Acute renal failure
585   Chronic renal failure
586   Renal failure, unspecified
587   Renal sclerosis, unspecified
588   Disorders resulting from impaired renal function
589   Small kidney of unknown cause

Other diseases of urinary system (590-599)

590   Infections of kidney
591   Hydronephrosis

592   Calculus of kidney and ureter
593   Other disorders of kidney and ureter
594   Calculus of lower urinary tract
595   Cystitis
596   Other disorders of bladder
597   Urethritis, not sexually transmitted, and urethral syndrome
598   Urethral stricture
599   Other disorders of urethra and urinary tract

Diseases of male genital organs (600-608)

600   Hyperplasia of prostate
601   Inflammatory diseases of prostate
602   Other disorders of prostate
603   Hydrocele
604   Orchitis and epididymitis
605   Redundant prepuce and phimosis
606   Infertility, male
607   Disorders of penis
608   Other disorders of male genital organs

Disorders of breast (610-611)

610   Benign mammary dysplasias
611   Other disorders of breast

Inflammatory disease of female pelvic organs (614-616)

614   Inflammatory disease of ovary, fallopian tube, pelvic cellular
        tissue and peritoneum
615   Inflammatory diseases of uterus, except cervix
616   Inflammatory disease of cervix, vagina and vulva

Other disorders of female genital tract (617-629)

617   Endometriosis
618   Genital prolapse
619   Fistulae involving female genital tract
620   Noninflammatory disorders of ovary, fallopian tube and broad
        ligament
621   Disorders of uterus, not elsewhere classified

622 Noninflammatory disorders of cervix
623 Noninflammatory disorders of vagina
624 Noninflammatory disorders of vulva and perineum
625 Pain and other symptoms associated with female genital organs
626 Disorders of menstruation and other abnormal bleeding from female genital tract
627 Menopausal and postmenopausal disorders
628 Infertility, female
629 Other disorders of female genital organs

XI. COMPLICATIONS OF PREGNANCY, CHILDBIRTH AND THE PUERPERIUM

Pregnancy with abortive outcome (630-639)

630 Hydatidiform mole
631 Other abnormal product of conception
632 Missed abortion
633 Ectopic pregnancy
634 Spontaneous abortion
635 Legally induced abortion
636 Illegally induced abortion
637 Unspecified abortion
638 Failed attempted abortion
639 Complications following abortion and ectopic and molar pregnancies

Complications mainly related to pregnancy (640-648)

640 Haemorrhage in early pregnancy
641 Antepartum haemorrhage, abruptio placentae, and placenta praevia
642 Hypertension complicating pregnancy, childbirth and the puerperium
643 Excessive vomiting in pregnancy
644 Early or threatened labour
645 Prolonged pregnancy
646 Other complications of pregnancy, not elsewhere classified
647 Infective and parasitic conditions in the mother classifiable elsewhere but complicating pregnancy, childbirth and the puerperium
648 Other current conditions in the mother classifiable elsewhere but complicating pregnancy, childbirth and the puerperium

Normal delivery, and other indications for care in pregnancy, labour and delivery (650-659)

650   Delivery in a completely normal case
651   Multiple gestation
652   Malposition and malpresentation of fetus
653   Disproportion
654   Abnormality of organs and soft tissues of pelvis
655   Known or suspected fetal abnormality affecting management of mother
656   Other fetal and placental problems affecting management of mother
657   Polyhydramnios
658   Other problems associated with amniotic cavity and membranes
659   Other indications for care or intervention related to labour and delivery and not elsewhere classified

Complications occurring mainly in the course of labour and delivery (660-669)

660   Obstructed labour
661   Abnormality of forces of labour
662   Long labour
663   Umbilical cord complications
664   Trauma to perineum and vulva during delivery
665   Other obstetrical trauma
666   Postpartum haemorrhage
667   Retained placenta or membranes, without haemorrhage
668   Complications of the administration of anaesthetic or other sedation in labour and delivery
669   Other complications of labour and delivery, not elsewhere classified

Complications of the puerperium (670-676)

670   Major puerperal infection
671   Venous complications in pregnancy and the puerperium
672   Pyrexia of unknown origin during the puerperium
673   Obstetrical pulmonary embolism
674   Other and unspecified complications of the puerperium, not elsewhere classified
675   Infections of the breast and nipple associated with childbirth
676   Other disorders of the breast associated with childbirth, and disorders of lactation

XII. DISEASES OF THE SKIN AND SUBCUTANEOUS TISSUE

Infections of skin and subcutaneous tissue (680-686)

680 Carbuncle and furuncle
681 Cellulitis and abscess of finger and toe
682 Other cellulitis and abscess
683 Acute lymphadenitis
684 Impetigo
685 Pilonidal cyst
686 Other local infections of skin and subcutaneous tissue

Other inflammatory conditions of skin and subcutaneous tissue (690-698)

690 Erythematosquamous dermatosis
691 Atopic dermatitis and related conditions
692 Contact dermatitis and other eczema
693 Dermatitis due to taken internally substances
694 Bullous dermatoses
695 Erythematous conditions
696 Psoriasis and similar disorders
697 Lichen
698 Pruritus and related conditions

Other diseases of skin and subcutaneous tissue (700-709)

700 Corns and callosities
701 Other hypertrophic and atrophic conditions of skin
702 Other dermatoses
703 Diseases of nail
704 Diseases of hair and hair follicles
705 Disorders of sweat glands
706 Diseases of sebaceous glands
707 Chronic ulcer of skin
708 Urticaria
709 Other disorders of skin and subcutaneous tissue

XIII.   DISEASES OF THE MUSCULOSKELETAL SYSTEM AND CONNECTIVE TISSUE

Arthropathies and related disorders (710-719)

710   Diffuse diseases of connective tissue
711   Arthropathy associated with infections
712   Crystal arthropathies
713   Arthropathy associated with other disorders classified elsewhere
714   Rheumatoid arthritis and other inflammatory polyarthropathies
715   Osteoarthrosis and allied disorders
716   Other and unspecified arthropathies
717   Internal derangement of knee
718   Other derangement of joint
719   Other and unspecified disorder of joint

Dorsopathies (720-724)

720   Ankylosing spondylitis and other inflammatory spondylopathies
721   Spondylosis and allied disorders
722   Intervertebral disc disorders
723   Other disorders of cervical region
724   Other and unspecified disorders of back

Rheumatism, excluding the back (725-729)

725   Polymyalgia rheumatica
726   Peripheral enthesopathies and allied syndromes
727   Other disorders of synovium, tendon and bursa
728   Disorders of muscle, ligament and fascia
729   Other disorders of soft tissues

Osteopathies, chondropathies and acquired musculoskeletal deformities (730-739)

730   Osteomyelitis, periostitis and other infections involving bone
731   Osteitis deformans and osteopathies associated with other disorders classified elsewhere
732   Osteochondropathies
733   Other disorders of bone and cartilage
734   Flat foot
735   Acquired deformities of toe

736 Other acquired deformities of limbs
737 Curvature of spine
738 Other acquired deformity
739 Nonallopathic lesions, not elsewhere classified

XIV. CONGENITAL ANOMALIES

740 Anencephalus and similar anomalies
741 Spina bifida
742 Other congenital anomalies of nervous system
743 Congenital anomalies of eye
744 Congenital anomalies of ear, face and neck
745 Bulbus cordis anomalies and anomalies of cardiac septal closure
746 Other congenital anomalies of heart
747 Other congenital anomalies of circulatory system
748 Congenital anomalies of respiratory system
749 Cleft palate and cleft lip
750 Other congenital anomalies of upper alimentary tract
751 Other congenital anomalies of digestive system
752 Congenital anomalies of genital organs
753 Congenital anomalies of urinary system
754 Certain congenital musculoskeletal deformities
755 Other congenital anomalies of limbs
756 Other congenital musculoskeletal anomalies
757 Congenital anomalies of the integument
758 Chromosomal anomalies
759 Other and unspecified congenital anomalies

XV. CERTAIN CONDITIONS ORIGINATING IN THE PERINATAL PERIOD

760 Fetus or newborn affected by maternal conditions which may be unrelated to present pregnancy
761 Fetus or newborn affected by maternal complications of pregnancy
762 Fetus or newborn affected by complications of placenta, cord and membranes
763 Fetus or newborn affected by other complications of labour and delivery

764 Slow fetal growth and fetal malnutrition
765 Disorders relating to short gestation and unspecified low birth-weight
766 Disorders relating to long gestation and high birthweight
767 Birth trauma
768 Intrauterine hypoxia and birth asphyxia
769 Respiratory distress syndrome
770 Other respiratory conditions of fetus and newborn
771 Infections specific to the perinatal period
772 Fetal and neonatal haemorrhage
773 Haemolytic disease of fetus or newborn, due to isoimmunization
774 Other perinatal jaundice
775 Endocrine and metabolic disturbances specific to the fetus and newborn
776 Haematological disorders of fetus and newborn
777 Perinatal disorders of digestive system
778 Conditions involving the integument and temperature regulation of fetus and newborn
779 Other and ill-defined conditions originating in the perinatal period

XVI. SYMPTOMS, SIGNS AND ILL-DEFINED CONDITIONS

Symptoms (780-789)

780 General symptoms
781 Symptoms involving nervous and musculoskeletal systems
782 Symptoms involving skin and other integumentary tissue
783 Symptoms concerning nutrition, metabolism and development
784 Symptoms involving head and neck
785 Symptoms involving cardiovascular system
786 Symptoms involving respiratory system and other chest symptoms
787 Symptoms involving digestive system
788 Symptoms involving urinary system
789 Other symptoms involving abdomen and pelvis

Nonspecific abnormal findings (790-796)

790 Nonspecific findings on examination of blood
791 Nonspecific findings on examination or urine

792 Nonspecific abnormal findings in other body substances
793 Nonspecific abnormal findings on radiological and other exam-
        ination of body structure
794 Nonspecific abnormal results of function studies
795 Nonspecific abnormal histological and immunological findings
796 Other nonspecific abnormal findings

Ill-defined and unknown causes of morbidity and mortality (797-799)

797 Senility without mention of psychosis
798 Sudden death, cause unknown
799 Other ill-defined and unknown causes of morbidity and mortality

XVII. INJURY AND POISONING

Fracture of skull (800-804)

800 Fracture of vault of skull
801 Fracture of base of skull
802 Fracture of face bones
803 Other and unqualified skull fractures
804 Multiple fractures involving skull or face with other bones

Fracture of spine and trunk (805-809)

805 Fracture of vertebral column without mention of spinal cord
        lesion
806 Fracture of vertebral column with spinal cord lesion
807 Fracture of rib(s), sternum, larynx and trachea
808 Fracture of pelvis
809 Ill-defined fractures of trunk

Fracture of upper limb (810-819)

810 Fracture of clavicle
811 Fracture of scapula
812 Fracture of humerus
813 Fracture of radius and ulna
814 Fracture of carpal bone(s)
815 Fracture of metacarpal bone(s)
816 Fracture of one or more phalanges of hand
817 Multiple fractures of hand bones

818   Ill-defined fractures of upper limb
819   Multiple fractures involving both upper limbs, and upper limb
      with rib(s) and sternum

Fracture of lower limb (820-829)

820   Fracture of neck of femur
821   Fracture of other and unspecified parts of femur
822   Fracture of patella
823   Fracture of tibia and fibula
824   Fracture of ankle
825   Fracture of one or more tarsal and metatarsal bones
826   Fracture of one or more phalanges of foot
827   Other, multiple and ill-defined fractures of lower limb
828   Multiple fractures involving both lower limbs, lower with upper
      limb, and lower limb(s) with rib(s) and sternum
829   Fracture of unspecified bones

Dislocation (830-839)

830   Dislocation of jaw
831   Dislocation of shoulder
832   Dislocation of elbow
833   Dislocation of wrist
834   Dislocation of finger
835   Dislocation of hip
836   Dislocation of knee
837   Dislocation of ankle
838   Dislocation of foot
839   Other, multiple and ill-defined dislocations

Sprains and strains of joints and adjacent muscles (840-848)

840   Sprains and strains of shoulder and upper arm
841   Sprains and strains of elbow and forearm
842   Sprains and strains of wrist and hand
843   Sprains and strains of hip and thigh
844   Sprains and strains of knee and leg
845   Sprains and strains of ankle and foot
846   Sprains and strains of sacroiliac region
847   Sprains and strains of other and unspecified parts of back
848   Other and ill-defined sprains and strains

Intracranial injury, excluding those with skull fracture (850-854)

850 Concussion
851 Cerebral laceration and contusion
852 Subarachnoid, subdural and extradural haemorrhage, following injury
853 Other and unspecified intracranial haemorrhage following injury
854 Intracranial injury of other and unspecified nature

Internal injury of chest, abdomen and pelvis (860-869)

860 Traumatic pneumothorax and haemothorax
861 Injury to heart and lung
862 Injury to other and unspecified intrathoracic organs
863 Injury to gastrointestinal tract
864 Injury to liver
865 Injury to spleen
866 Injury to kidney
867 Injury to pelvic organs
868 Injury to other intraabdominal organs
869 Internal injury to unspecified or ill-defined organs

Open wound of head, neck and trunk (870-879)

870 Open wound of ocular adnexa
871 Open wound of eyeball
872 Open wound of ear
873 Other open wound of head
874 Open wound of neck
875 Open wound of chest (wall)
876 Open wound of back
877 Open wound of buttock
878 Open wound of genital organs (external), including traumatic amputation
879 Open wound of other and unspecified sites, except limbs

Open wound of upper limb (880-887)

880 Open wound of shoulder and upper arm
881 Open wound of elbow, forearm and wrist
882 Open wound of hand except finger(s) alone
883 Open wound of finger(s)
884 Multiple and unspecified open wound of upper limb
885 Traumatic amputation of thumb (complete) (partial)

886 Traumatic amputation of other finger(s) (complete) (partial)
887 Traumatic amputation of arm and hand (complete) (partial)

Open wound of lower limb (890-897)

890 Open wound of hip and thigh
891 Open wound of knee, leg [except thigh] and ankle
892 Open wound of foot except toe(s) alone
893 Open wound of toe(s)
894 Multiple and unspecified open wound of lower limb
895 Traumatic amputation of toe(s) (complete) (partial)
896 Traumatic amputation of foot (complete) (partial)
897 Traumatic amputation of leg(s) (complete) (partial)

Injury to blood vessels (900-904)

900 Injury to blood vessels of head and neck
901 Injury to blood vessels of thorax
902 Injury to blood vessels of abdomen and pelvis
903 Injury to blood vessels of upper extremity
904 Injury to blood vessels of lower extremity and unspecified sites

Late effects of injuries, poisonings, toxic effects and other external causes (905-909)

905 Late effects of musculoskeletal and connective tissue injuries
906 Late effetcs of injuries to skin and subcutaneous tissues
907 Late effects of injuries to the nervous system
908 Late effects of other and unspecified injuries
909 Late effects of other and unspecified external causes

Superficial injury (910-919)

910 Superficial injury of face, neck and scalp except eye
911 Superficial injury of trunk
912 Superficial injury of shoulder and upper arm
913 Superficial injury of elbow, forearm and wrist
914 Superficial injury of hand(s) except finger(s) alone
915 Superficial injury of finger(s)
916 Superficial injury of hip, thigh, leg and ankle
917 Superficial injury of foot and toe(s)
918 Superficial injury of eye and adnexa
919 Superficial injury of other, multiple and unspecified sites

Contusion with intact skin surface (920-924)

920 Contusion of face, scalp, and neck except eye(s)
921 Contusion of eye and adnexa
922 Contusion of trunk
923 Contusion of upper limb
924 Contusion of lower limb and of other and unspecified sites

Crushing injury (925-929)

925 Crushing injury of face, scalp and neck
926 Crushing injury of trunk
927 Crushing injury of upper limb
928 Crushing injury of lower limb
929 Crushing injury of multiple and unspecified sites

Effects of foreign body entering through orifice (930-939)

930 Foreign body on external eye
931 Foreign body in ear
932 Foreign body in nose
933 Foreign body in pharynx and larynx
934 Foreign body in trachea, bronchus and lung
935 Foreign body in mouth, oesophagus and stomach
936 Foreign body in intestine and colon
937 Foreign body in anus and rectum
938 Foreign body in digestive system, unspecified
939 Foreign body in genitourinary tract

Burns (940-949)

940 Burn confined to eye and adnexa
941 Burn of face, head and neck
942 Burn of trunk
943 Burn of upper limb, except wrist and hand
944 Burn of wrist(s) and hand(s)
945 Burn of lower limb(s)
946 Burns of multiple specified sites
947 Burn of internal organs
948 Burns classified according to extent of body surface involved
949 Burn, unspecified

Injury to nerves and spinal cord (950-957)

950 Injury to optic nerve and pathways
951 Injury to other cranial nerve(s)
952 Spinal cord lesion without evidence of spinal bone injury
953 Injury to nerve roots and spinal plexus
954 Injury to other nerve(s) of trunk excluding shoulder and pelvic girdles
955 Injury to peripheral nerve(s) of shoulder girdle and upper limb
956 Injury to peripheral nerve(s) of pelvic girdle and lower limb
957 Injury to other and unspecified nerves

Certain traumatic complications and unspecified injuries (958-959)

958 Certain early complications of trauma
959 Injury, other and unspecified

Poisoning by drugs, medicaments and biological substances (960-979)

960 Poisoning by antibiotics
961 Poisoning by other anti-infectives
962 Poisoning by hormones and synthetic substitutes
963 Poisoning by primarily systemic agents
964 Poisoning by agents primarily affecting blood constituents
965 Poisoning by analgesics, antipyretics and antirheumatics
966 Poisoning by anticonvulsants and anti-Parkinsonism drugs
967 Poisoning by sedatives and hypnotics
968 Poisoning by other central nervous system depressants
969 Poisoning by psychotropic agents
970 Poisoning by central nervous system stimulants
971 Poisoning by drugs primarily affecting the autonomic nervous system
972 Poisoning by agents primarily affecting the cardiovascular system
973 Poisoning by agents primarily affecting the gastrointestinal system
974 Poisoning by water, mineral and uric acid metabolism drugs
975 Poisoning by agents primarily acting on the smooth and skeletal muscles and respiratory system
976 Poisoning by agents primarily affecting skin and mucous membrane, ophthalmological, otorhinolaryngological and dental drugs
977 Poisoning by other and unspecified drugs and medicaments

978 Poisoning by bacterial vaccines
979 Poisoning by other vaccines and biological substances

Toxic effects of substances chiefly nonmedicinal as to source (980-989)

980 Toxic effect of alcohol
981 Toxic effect of petroleum products
982 Toxic effect of solvents other than petroleum-based
983 Toxic effect of corrosive aromatics, acids and caustic alkalis
984 Toxic effect of lead and its compounds (including fumes)
985 Toxic effect of other metals
986 Toxic effect of carbon monoxide
987 Toxic effect of other gases, fumes or vapours
988 Toxic effect of noxious substances eaten as food
989 Toxic effect of other substances, chiefly nonmedicinal as to source

Other and unspecified effects of external causes (990-995)

990 Effects of radiation, unspecified
991 Effects of reduced temperature
992 Effects of heat and light
993 Effects of air pressure
994 Effects of other external causes
995 Certain adverse effects not elsewhere classified

Complications of surgical and medical care not elsewhere classified (996-999)

996 Complications peculiar to certain specified procedures
997 Complications affecting specified body systems, not elsewhere classified
998 Other complications of procedures, not elsewhere classified
999 Complications of medical care, not elsewhere classified

SUPPLEMENTARY CLASSIFICATION OF EXTERNAL CAUSES OF INJURY AND POISONING

Railway accidents (E800-E807)

E800 Railway accident involving collision with rolling stock

E801 Railway accident involving collision with other object

E802 Railway accident involving derailment without antecedent collision

· E803 Railway accident involving explosion, fire or burning

E804 Fall in, on or from railway train

E805 Hit by rolling stock

E806 Other specified railway accident

E807 Railway accident of unspecified nature

Motor vehicle traffic accidents (E810-E819)

E810 Motor vehicle traffic accident involving collision with train

E811 Motor vehicle traffic accident involving re-entrant collision with another motor vehicle

E812 Other motor vehicle traffic accident involving collision with another motor vehicle

E813 Motor vehicle traffic accident involving collision with other vehicle

E814 Motor vehicle traffic accident involving collision with pedestrian

E815 Other motor vehicle traffic accident involving collision on the highway

E816 Motor vehicle traffic accident due to loss of control, without collision on the highway

E817 Noncollision motor vehicle traffic accident while boarding or alighting

E818 Other noncollision motor vehicle traffic accident

E819 Motor vehicle traffic accident of unspecified nature

Motor vehicle nontraffic accidents (E820-E825)

E820 Nontraffic accident involving motor-driven snow vehicle

E821 Nontraffic accident involving other off-road motor vehicle

E822 Other motor vehicle nontraffic accident involving collision with moving object

E823 Other motor vehicle nontraffic accident involving collision with stationary object

E824 Other motor vehicle nontraffic accident while boarding and alighting

E825 Other motor vehicle nontraffic accident of other and unspecified nature

Other road vehicle accidents (E826-E829)

E826 Pedal cycle accident

E827 Animal-drawn vehicle accident

E828 Accident involving animal being ridden

E829 Other road vehicle accidents

Water transport accidents (E830-E838)

E830 Accident to watercraft causing submersion

E831 Accident to watercraft causing other injury

E832 Other accidental submersion or drowning in water transport accident

E833 Fall on stairs or ladders in water transport

E834 Other fall from one level to another in water transport

E835 Other and unspecified fall in water transport

E836 Machinery accident in water transport

E837 Explosion, fire or burning in watercraft

E838 Other and unspecified water transport accident

Air and space transport accidents (E840-E845)

E840 Accident to powered aircraft at takeoff or landing

E841 Accident to powered aircraft, other and unspecified

E842 Accident to unpowered aircraft

E843 Fall in, on or from aircraft

E844 Other specified air transport accidents

E845 Accident involving spacecraft

Vehicle accidents not elsewhere classifiable (E846-E848)

E846 Accidents involving powered vehicles used solely within the buildings and premises of an industrial or commercial establishment

E847 Accidents involving cable cars not running on rails

E848 Accidents involving other vehicles not elsewhere classifiable

Accidental poisoning by drugs, medicaments and biologicals (E850-E858)

E850 Accidental poisoning by analgesics, antipyretics, antirheumatics
E851 Accidental poisoning by barbiturates
E852 Accidental poisoning by other sedatives and hypnotics
E853 Accidental poisoning by tranquillizers
E854 Accidental poisoning by other psychotropic agents
E855 Accidental poisoning by other drugs acting on central and autonomic nervous systems
E856 Accidental poisoning by antibiotics
E857 Accidental poisoning by anti-infectives
E858 Accidental poisoning by other drugs

Accidental poisoning by other solid and liquid substances, gases and vapours (E860-E869)

E860 Accidental poisoning by alcohol, not elsewhere classified
E861 Accidental poisoning by cleansing and polishing agents, disinfectants, paints and varnishes
E862 Accidental poisoning by petroleum products, other solvents and their vapours, not elsewhere classified
E863 Accidental poisoning by agricultural and horticultural chemical and pharmaceutical preparations other than plant foods and fertilizers
E864 Accidental poisoning by corrosives and caustics, not elsewhere classified
E865 Accidental poisoning from foodstuffs and poisonous plants
E866 Accidental poisoning by other and unspecified solid and liquid substances
E867 Accidental poisoning by gas distributed by pipeline
E868 Accidental poisoning by other utility gas and other carbon monoxide
E869 Accidental poisoning by other gases and vapours

Misadventures to patients during surgical and medical care (E870-E876)

E870 Accidental cut, puncture, perforation or haemorrhage during medical care
E871 Foreign object left in body during procedure
E872 Failure of sterile precautions during procedure
E873 Failure in dosage

E874 Mechanical failure of instrument or apparatus during procedure

E875 Contaminated or infected blood, other fluid, drug or biological substance

E876 Other and unspecified misadventures during medical care

Surgical and medical procedures as the cause of abnormal reaction of patient or later complication, without mention of misadventure at the time of procedure (E878-E879)

E878 Surgical operation and other surgical procedures as the cause of abnormal reaction of patient, or of later complication, without mention of misadventure at the time of operation

E879 Other procedures, without mention of misadventure at the time of procedure, as the cause of abnormal reaction of patient, or of later complication

Accidental falls (E880-E888)

E880 Fall on or from stairs or steps
E881 Fall on or from ladders or scaffolding
E882 Fall from or out of building or other structure
E883 Fall into hole or other opening in surface
E884 Other fall from one level to another
E885 Fall on same level from slipping, tripping or stumbling
E886 Fall on same level from collision, pushing or shoving, by or with other person
E887 Fracture, cause unspecified
E888 Other and unspecified fall

Accidents caused by fire and flames (E890-E899)

E890 Conflagration in private dwelling
E891 Conflagration in other and unspecified building or structure
E892 Conflagration not in building or structure
E893 Accident caused by ignition of clothing
E894 Ignition of highly inflammable material
E895 Accident caused by controlled fire in private dwelling
E896 Accident caused by controlled fire in other and unspecified building or structure
E897 Accident caused by controlled fire not in building or structure
E898 Accident caused by other specified fire and flames
E899 Accident caused by unspecified fire

Accidents due to natural and environmental factors (E900-E909)

E900 Excessive heat

E901 Excessive cold

E902 High and low air pressure and changes in air pressure

E903 Travel and motion

E904 Hunger, thirst, exposure, neglect

E905 Venomous animals and plants as the cause of poisoning and toxic reactions

E906 Other injury caused by animals

E907 Lightning

E908 Cataclysmic storms, and floods resulting from storms

E909 Cataclysmic earth surface movements and eruptions

Accidents caused by submersion, suffocation and foreign bodies (E910-E915)

E910 Accidental drowning and submersion

E911 Inhalation and ingestion of food causing obstruction of respiratory tract or suffocation

E912 Inhalation and ingestion of other object causing obstruction of respiratory tract or suffocation

E913 Accidental mechanical suffocation

E914 Foreign body accidentally entering eye and adnexa

E915 Foreign body accidentally entering other orifice

Other accidents (E916-E928)

E916 Struck accidentally by falling object

E917 Striking against or struck accidentally by objects or persons

E918 Caught . 'identally in or between objects

E919 Accident. ᵈd by machinery

E920 Accidents caused by cutting and piercing instruments or objects

E921 Accident caused by explosion of pressure vessel

E922 Accident caused by firearm missile

E923 Accident caused by explosive material

E924 Accident caused by hot substance or object, caustic or corrosive material and steam

E925 Accident caused by electric current

E926 Exposure to radiation

E927 Overexertion and strenuous movements

E928 Other and unspecified environmental and accidental causes

Late effects of accidental injury (E929)

E929   Late effects of accidental injury

Drugs, medicaments and biological substances causing adverse effects in therapeutic use (E930-E949)

E930   Antibiotics
E931   Other anti-infectives
E932   Hormones and synthetic substitutes
E933   Primarily systemic agents
E934   Agents primarily affecting blood constituents
E935   Analgesics, antipyretics and antirheumatics
E936   Anticonvulsants and anti-Parkinsonism drugs
E937   Sedatives and hypnotics
E938   Other central nervous system depressants
E939   Psychotropic agents
E940   Central nervous system stimulants
E941   Drugs primarily affecting the autonomic nervous system
E942   Agents primarily affecting the cardiovascular system
E943   Agents primarily affecting gastrointestinal system
E944   Water, mineral and uric acid metabolism drugs
E945   Agents primarily acting on the smooth and skeletal muscles and respiratory system
E946   Agents primarily affecting skin and mucous membrane, ophthalmological, otorhinolaryngological and dental drugs
E947   Other and unspecified drugs and medicaments
E948   Bacterial vaccines
E949   Other vaccines and biological substances

Suicide and selfinflicted injury (E950-E959)

E950   Suicide and selfinflicted poisoning by solid or liquid substances
E951   Suicide and selfinflicted poisoning by gases in domestic use
E952   Suicide and selfinflicted poisoning by other gases and vapours
E953   Suicide and selfinflicted injury by hanging, strangulation and suffocation
E954   Suicide and selfinflicted injury by submersion [drowning]
E955   Suicide and selfinflicted injury by firearms and explosives
E956   Suicide and selfinflicted injury by cutting and piercing instruments
E957   Suicide and selfinflicted injuries by jumping from high place

E958 Suicide and selfinflicted injury by other and unspecified means
E959 Late effects of selfinflicted injury

Homicide and injury purposely inflicted by other persons (E960-E969)

E960 Fight, brawl, rape
E961 Assault by corrosive or caustic substance, except poisoning
E962 Assault by poisoning
E963 Assault by hanging and strangulation
E964 Assault by submersion [drowning]
E965 Assault by firearms and explosives
E966 Assault by cutting and piercing instrument
E967 Child battering and other maltreatment
E968 Assault by other and unspecified means
E969 Late effects of injury purposely inflicted by other person

Legal intervention (E970-E978)

E970 Injury due to legal intervention by firearms
E971 Injury due to legal intervention by explosives
E972 Injury due to legal intervention by gas
E973 Injury due to legal intervention by blunt object
E974 Injury due to legal intervention by cutting and piercing instruments
E975 Injury due to legal intervention by other specified means
E976 Injury due to legal intervention by unspecified means
E977 Late effects of injuries due to legal intervention
E978 Legal execution

Injury undetermined whether accidentally or purposely inflicted (E980-E989)

E980 Poisoning by solid or liquid substances, undetermined whether accidentally or purposely inflicted
E981 Poisoning by gases in domestic use, undetermined whether accidentally or purposely inflicted
E982 Poisoning by other gases, undetermined whether accidentally or purposely inflicted
E983 Hanging, strangulation or suffocation, undetermined whether accidentally or purposely inflicted
E984 Submersion [drowning], undetermined whether accidentally or purposely inflicted
E985 Injury by firearms and explosives, undetermined whether accidentally or purposely inflicted

E986   Injury by cutting and piercing instruments, undetermined whether accidentally or purposely inflicted

E987   Falling from high place, undetermined whether accidentally or purposely inflicted

E988   Injury by other and unspecified means, undetermined whether accidentally or purposely inflicted

E989   Late effects of injury, undetermined whether accidentally or purposely inflicted

Injury resulting from operations of war (E990-E999)

E990   Injury due to war operations by fires and conflagrations

E991   Injury due to war operations by bullets and fragments

E992   Injury due to war operations by explosion of marine weapons

E993   Injury due to war operations by other explosion

E994   Injury due to war operations by destruction of aircraft

E995   Injury due to war operations by other and unspecified forms of conventional warfare

E996   Injury due to war operations by nuclear weapons

E997   Injury due to war operations by other forms of unconventional warfare

E998   Injury due to war operations but occuring after cessation of hostilities

E999   Late effects of injury due to war operations

SUPPLEMENTARY CLASSIFICATION OF FACTORS INFLUENCING HEALTH STATUS AND CONTACT WITH HEALTH SERVICES

Persons with potential health hazards related to communicable diseases (V01-V07)

V01   Contact with or exposure to communicable diseases

V02   Carrier or suspected carrier of infectious diseases

V03   Need for prophylactic vaccination and inoculation against bacterial diseases

V04   Need for prophylactic vaccination and inoculation against certain viral diseases

V05   Need for other prophylactic vaccination and inoculation against single diseases

V06 Need for prophylactic vaccination and inoculation against com-
       binations of diseases
V07 Need for isolation and other prophylactic measures

Persons with potential health hazards related to personal and family history (V10-V19)

V10 Personal history of malignant neoplasm
V11 Personal history of mental disorder
V12 Personal history of certain other diseases
V13 Personal history of other diseases
V14 Personal history of allergy to medicinal agents
V15 Other personal history presenting hazards to health
V16 Family history of malignant neoplasm
V17 Family history of certain chronic disabling diseases
V18 Family history of certain other specific conditions
V19 Family history of other conditions

Persons encountering health services in circumstances related to reproduction and development (V20-V28)

V20 Health supervision of infant or child
V21 Constitutional states in development
V22 Normal pregnancy
V23 Supervision of high-risk pregnancy
V24 Postpartum care and examination
V25 Contraceptive management
V26 Procreative management
V27 Outcome of delivery
V28 Antenatal screening

Healthy liveborn infants according to type of birth (V30-V39)

V30 Singleton
V31 Twin, mate live born
V32 Twin, mate stillborn
V33 Twin, unspecified
V34 Other multiple, mates all live born
V35 Other multiple, mates all stillborn
V36 Other multiple, mates live- and stillborn
V37 Other multiple, unspecified
V39 Unspecified

Persons with a condition influencing their health status (V40-V49)

V40 Mental and behavioural problems
V41 Problems with special senses and other special functions
V42 Organ or tissue replaced by transplant
V43 Organ or tissue replaced by other means
V44 Artificial opening status
V45 Other postsurgical states
V46 Other dependence on machines
V47 Other problems with internal organs
V48 Problems with head, neck and trunk
V49 Problems with limbs and other problems

Persons encountering health services for specific procedures and aftercare (V50-V59)

V50 Elective surgery for purposes other than remedying health states
V51 Aftercare involving the use of plastic surgery
V52 Fitting and adjustment of prosthetic device
V53 Fitting and adjustment of other device
V54 Other orthopaedic aftercare
V55 Attention to artificial openings
V56 Aftercare involving intermittent dialysis
V57 Care involving use of rehabilitation procedures
V58 Other and unspecified aftercare
V59 Donors

Persons encountering health services in other circumstances (V60-V68)

V60 Housing, household and economic circumstances
V61 Other family circumstances
V62 Other psychosocial circumstances
V63 Unavailability of other medical facilities for care
V64 Persons encountering health services for specific procedures, not carried out
V65 Other persons seeking consultation without complaint or sickness
V66 Convalescence
V67 Follow-up examination
V68 Encounters for administrative purposes

Persons without reported diagnosis encountered during examination and investigation of individuals and populations (V70-V82)

V70 General medical examination

V71 Observation and evaluation for suspected conditions

V72 Special investigations and examinations

V73 Special screening examination for viral diseases

V74 Special screening examination for bacterial and spirochaetal diseases

V75 Special screening examination for other infectious diseases

V76 Special screening for malignant neoplasms

V77 Special screening for endocrine, nutritional, metabolic and immunity disorders

V78 Special screening for disorders of blood and blood-forming organs

V79 Special screening for mental disorders and developmental handicaps

V80 Special screening for neurological, eye and ear diseases

V81 Special screening for cardiovascular, respiratory and genito-urinary diseases

V82 Special screening for other conditions

TABULAR LIST OF INCLUSIONS
AND
FOUR-DIGIT SUBCATEGORIES

I. INFECTIOUS AND PARASITIC DISEASES

Includes: diseases generally recognized as communicable or trans-
missible as well as a few diseases of unknown but
possibly infectious origin

Excludes: acute respiratory infections (460-466)
influenza (487.–)
carrier or suspected carrier of infectious organism (V02.–)
certain localized infections

Note: Categories for "late effects" of infectious and parasitic diseases
are to be found at 137.– to 139.–

INTESTINAL INFECTIOUS DISEASES (001-009)

Excludes: helminthiases (120-129)

001 Cholera

001.0 *Due to Vibrio cholerae*

001.1 *Due to Vibrio cholerae el tor*

001.9 *Unspecified*

002 Typhoid and paratyphoid fevers

002.0 *Typhoid fever*

Typhoid (fever) (infection) [any site]

002.1 *Paratyphoid fever A*

002.2 *Paratyphoid fever B*

002.3 *Paratyphoid fever C*

002.9 *Paratyphoid fever, unspecified*

003 Other salmonella infections

Includes: infection or food poisoning by Salmonella [any serotype]

003.0 *Salmonella gastroenteritis*

Salmonellosis

003.1 *Salmonella septicaemia*

003.2 *Localized salmonella infections*

Salmonella:
  arthritis † (711.3*)
  meningitis † (320.7*)

Salmonella:
  osteomyelitis † (730.2*)
  pneumonia † (484.8*)

— 49 —

003.8 *Other*

003.9 *Unspecified*
Salmonella infection NOS

004 Shigellosis

Includes: bacillary dysentery

004.0 *Shigella dysenteriae*
Infection by group A Shigella (Schmitz) (Shiga)

004.1 *Shigella flexneri*
Infection by group B Shigella

004.2 *Shigella boydii*
Infection by group C Shigella

004.3 *Shigella sonnei*
Infection by group D Shigella

004.8 *Other*

004.9 *Unspecified*

005 Other food poisoning (bacterial)

Excludes: salmonella infections (003.–)
toxic effect of noxious foodstuffs (988.–)

005.0 *Staphylococcal food poisoning*
Staphylococcal toxaemia specified as due to food

005.1 *Botulism*
Food poisoning due to Clostridium botulinum

005.2 *Food poisoning due to Clostridium perfringens [Cl. welchii]*
Enteritis necroticans

005.3 *Food poisoning due to other Clostridia*

005.4 *Food poisoning due to Vibrio parahaemolyticus*

005.8 *Other bacterial food poisoning*
Food poisoning due to Bacillus cereus
Excludes: salmonella food poisoning (003.–)

005.9 *Food poisoning, unspecified*

006 Amoebiasis

Includes: infection due to Entamoeba histolytica

Excludes: amoebiasis due to organisms other than Entamoeba histoly-
tyca (007.8)

006.0 *Acute amoebic dysentery without mention of abscess*

Acute amoebiasis

006.1 *Chronic intestinal amoebiasis without mention of abscess*

Chronic:
  amoebiasis
  amoebic dysentery

006.2 *Amoebic nondysenteric colitis*

006.3 *Amoebic liver abscess*

006.4 *Amoebic lung abscess*

Amoebic abscess of lung (and liver)

006.5 *Amoebic brain abscess*

Amoebic abscess of brain (and liver) (and lung)

006.6 *Amoebic skin ulceration*

006.8 *Amoebic infection of other sites*

Amoebic: Amoeboma
  appendicitis
  balanitis

Excludes: specific infections by free-living amoebae (136.2)

006.9 *Amoebiasis, unspecified*

Amoebiasis NOS

007   Other protozoal intestinal diseases

Includes: protozoal:
          colitis
          diarrhoea
          dysentery

007.0 *Balantidiasis*

Infection by Balantidium coli

007.1 *Giardiasis*

Infection by Giardia lamblia   Lambliasis

007.2 *Coccidiosis*

Infection by Isospora belli and Isospora hominis
Isosporosis

007.3 *Intestinal trichomoniasis*

007.8 *Other protozoal intestinal diseases*

007.9 *Unspecified*
Flagellate diarrhoea   Protozoal dysentery NOS

008   Intestinal infections due to other organisms

Includes: any terms listed in 009.– with mention of the responsible
            organisms
Excludes: food poisoning by these organisms (005.–)

008.0 *Escherichia coli*

008.1 *Arizona*

008.2 *Aerobacter aerogenes*

008.3 *Proteus (mirabilis) (morganii)*

008.4 *Other specified bacteria*
Staphylococcal enterocolitis

008.5 *Bacterial enteritis, unspecified*

008.6 *Enteritis due to specified virus*
Enteritis due to:
  adenovirus
  enterovirus

008.8 *Other organism, not elsewhere classified*
Viral:
  enteritis NOS
  gastroenteritis
Excludes: influenza with involvement of gastrointestinal tract (487.8)

009   Ill-defined intestinal infections

Excludes: diarrhoeal disease due to specified organism (001-008)
            diarrhoea following gastrointestinal surgery (564.4)
            intestinal malabsorption (579.–)
            ischaemic enteritis (557.–)
            other noninfective gastroenteritis and colitis (558)
            regional enteritis (555.–)
            ulcerative colitis (556)

009.0 *Infectious colitis, enteritis and gastroenteritis*

Colitis		Dysentery:
Enteritis	} septic	NOS
Gastroenteritis		catarrhal
		haemorrhagic

009.1 *Colitis, enteritis and gastroenteritis of presumed infectious origin*

Catarrh, enteric or intestinal

Colitis ⎤
Enteritis ⎬ NOS
Gastroenteritis ⎦ haemorrhagic

009.2 *Infectious diarrhoea*

Diarrhoea: Infectious diarrhoeal disease NOS
  dysenteric
  epidemic

009.3 *Diarrhoea, of presumed infectious origin*

Diarrhoea NOS   Diarrhoeal disease NOS

Note: In countries where any term listed in 009.1 and 009.3 without further specification can be assumed to be of noninfectious origin, the term should be classified to 558.–.

TUBERCULOSIS (010–018)

Includes: infection by Mycobacterium tuberculosis (human) (bovine)

Excludes: congenital tuberculosis (771.2)

The following fifth-digit subclassification may be used, if desired, with categories 010–018:

  .0 Bacteriological or histological examination not done
  .1 Bacteriological or histological examination unknown (at present)
  .2 Tubercle bacilli found (in sputum) by microscopy
  .3 Tubercle bacilli not found (in sputum) by microscopy, but found
     by culture
  .4 Tubercle bacilli not found by bacteriological examination, but
     tuberculosis confirmed histologically
  .5 Tubercle bacilli not found by bacteriological or histological
     examination but tuberculosis confirmed by other methods
     [inoculation in animals]
  .9 Unspecified

010   **Primary tuberculous infection**

010.0 *Primary tuberculous complex*

010.1 *Tuberculous pleurisy in primary progressive tuberculosis*

010.8 *Other primary progressive tuberculosis*

Excludes: tuberculous erythema nodosum (017.1)

010.9 *Unspecified*

011 Pulmonary tuberculosis

Use additional code, if desired, to identify any associated silicosis (502)

011.0 *Tuberculosis of lung, infiltrative*

011.1 *Tuberculosis of lung, nodular*

011.2 *Tuberculosis of lung with cavitation*

011.3 *Tuberculosis of bronchus*
Excludes: isolated bronchial tuberculosis (012.2)

011.4 *Tuberculous fibrosis of lung*

011.5 *Tuberculous bronchiectasis*

011.6 *Tuberculous pneumonia [any form]*

011.7 *Tuberculous pneumothorax*

011.8 *Other pulmonary tuberculosis*

011.9 *Unspecified*
Respiratory tuberculosis NOS
Tuberculosis of lung NOS

012 Other respiratory tuberculosis

Excludes: respiratory tuberculosis, unspecified (011.9)

012.0 *Tuberculous pleurisy*
Tuberculosis of pleura   Tuberculosis hydrothorax
Tuberculous empyema
Excludes: pleurisy with effusion without mention of cause (511.9)
              tuberculous pleurisy in primary progressive tuberculosis
              (010.1)

012.1 *Tuberculosis of intrathoracic lymph nodes*
Tuberculosis of lymph nodes:
  hilar
  mediastinal
  tracheobronchial
Excludes: when specified as primary (010.–)

012.2 *Isolated tracheal or bronchial tuberculosis*

012.3 *Tuberculous laryngitis*
Tuberculosis of glottis

012.8 *Other*
Tuberculosis of: Tuberculosis of:
  mediastinum   sinus [any nasal]
  nasopharynx
  nose (septum)

013   Tuberculosis of meninges and central nervous system

013.0† *Tuberculous meningitis* (320.4*)

Tuberculosis of meninges (cerebral)   Tuberculous:
   (spinal)   leptomeningitis
                                     meningoencephalitis

Excludes: tuberculoma of meninges (013.1)

013.1† *Tuberculoma of meninges* (349.2*)

013.8   *Other*

Tuberculoma† ⎫
Tuberculosis† ⎬ of brain (348.8*)
Tuberculous:
  abscess of brain† (324.0*)
  myelitis† (323.4*)

013.9   *Unspecified*

Tuberculosis of central nervous system NOS

014   Tuberculosis of intestines, peritoneum and mesenteric glands

Tuberculosis (of):   Tuberculous:
  anus   ascites
  intestine (large) (small)   enteritis
  rectum   peritonitis† (567.0*)
  retroperitoneal (lymph nodes)

015   Tuberculosis of bones and joints

Includes: tuberculous:
          arthritis† (711.4*)
          necrosis of bone† (730.-*)
          osteitis† (730.-*)
          osteomyelitis† (730.-*)
          synovitis† (727.0*)
          tenosynositis† (727.0*)

015.0† *Vertebral column*

Pott's: Tuberculous:
  curvature (737.4*)   kyphosis (737.4*)
  disease (730.4*)   spondylitis (720.8*)

015.1   *Hip*

015.2   *Knee*

015.7   *Other bone*

Tuberculous dactylitis   Tuberculous mastoiditis† (383.1*)

015.8   *Other joint*

015.9   *Unspecified*

016   Tuberculosis of genitourinary system

016.0   *Kidney*

Tuberculous pyelitis† (590.8*)   Tuberculous pyelonephritis†
(590.8*)

016.1   *Other urinary organs*

Tuberculosis of bladder† (595.4*)   Tuberculosis of ureter† (593.8*)

016.2†   *Epididymis* (604.9*)

016.3   *Other male genital organs*

Tuberculosis of: Tuberculosis of testis† (608.8*)
  prostate† (601.4*)
  seminal vesicle† (608.8*)

016.4   *Female genital organs*

Tuberculous:
  oophoritis† (614.2*)
  salpingitis† (614.2*)

016.9   *Unspecified*

017   Tuberculosis of other organs

017.0   *Skin and subcutaneous cellular tissue*

Lupus: Tuberculosis:
  NOS   colliquativa
  exedens   cutis
  vulgaris   lichenoides
Scrofuloderma   papulonecrotica
       verrucosa cutis

Excludes: lupus erythrematosus (695.4)
          disseminated (710.0)

017.1   *Erythema nodosum with hypersensitivity reaction in tuberculosis*

Bazin's disease   Tuberculosis indurativa
Erythema:
  induratum
  nodosum, tuberculous

Excludes: erythema nodosum NOS (695.2)

017.2   *Peripheral lymph nodes*

Scrofula   Tuberculous adenitis
Scrofulous abscess

Excludes: tuberculosis of lymph nodes:
              bronchial and mediastinal (012.1)
              mesenteric and retroperitoneal (014)
              tuberculous tracheobronchial adenopathy (012.1)

017.3 *Eye*

Tuberculous:
  chorioretinitis, disseminated† (363.1*)
  episcleritis† (379.0*)
  interstitial keratitis† (370.5*)
  iridocyclitis, chronic† (364.1*)
  keratoconjunctivitis (phlyctenular)† (370.3*)

017.4 *Ear*

Tuberculosis of ear† (382.3*)
Tuberculous otitis media† (382.3*)

Excludes: tuberculous mastoiditis (015.7)

017.5 *Thyroid gland*

017.6† *Adrenal glands* (255.4*)

Addison's disease, tuberculous

017.7 *Spleen*

017.8 *Other*

Tuberculosis of:
  endocardium [any valve]† (424.–*)
  oesophagus† (530.1*)

Tuberculosis of:
  myocardium† (422.0*)
  pericardium† (420.0*)

018   Miliary tuberculosis

Includes: tuberculosis:
           disseminated
           generalized
           miliary, whether of a single specified site, multiple sites or
                unspecified site
           polyserositis

018.0 *Acute*

018.8 *Other*

018.9 *Unspecified*

ZOONOTIC BACTERIAL DISEASES (020-027)

020   Plague

Includes: infection by Yersinia pestis

020.0 *Bubonic*

020.1 *Cellulocutaneous*

020.2 *Septicaemic*

020.3 *Primary pneumonic*

020.4 *Secondary pneumonic*

020.5 *Pneumonic, unspecified*

020.8 *Other*

Abortive plague   Pestis minor
Ambulatory plague

020.9 *Unspecified*

021 Tularaemia

Includes: infection by Francisella tularensis

Deer fly fever   Rabbit fever

022 Anthrax

022.0 *Cutaneous anthrax*

Malignant pustule

022.1 *Pulmonary anthrax*

Respiratory anthrax   Wool-sorters' disease

022.2 *Gastrointestinal anthrax*

022.3 *Anthrax septicaemia*

022.8 *Other manifestations*

022.9 *Unspecified*

023 Brucellosis

Includes: fever:
     Malta
     Mediterranean
     undulant

023.0 *Brucella melitensis*

023.1 *Brucella abortus*

023.2 *Brucella suis*

023.3 *Brucella canis*

023.8 *Other*

Infection by more than one organism

023.9 *Unspecified*

024　　Glanders

Infection by:
　Actinobacillus mallei
　Malleomyces mallei
　Pseudomonas mallei

Farcy
Malleus

025　　Melioidosis

Infection by:
　Malleomyces pseudomallei
　Pseudomonas pseudomallei
　Whitmore's bacillus

Pseudoglanders

026　　Rat-bite fever

026.0 *Spirillary fever*

Rat-bite fever due to Spirillum minor [S. minus]
Sodoku

026.1 *Streptobacillary fever*

Epidemic arthritic erythema
Haverhill fever

Rat-bite fever due to Streptobacil-
　lus moniliformis

026.9 *Unspecified*

027　　Other zoonotic bacterial diseases

027.0 *Listeriosis*

Excludes: congenital listeriosis (771.2)

Infection
Meningitis† (320.7*)
Meningoencephalitis† (320.7*)
Septicaemia
} by Listeria monocytogenes

027.1 *Erysipelothrix infection*

Erysipeloid (of Rosenbach)
Infection
Septicaemia
} by Erysipelothrix insidiosa [E. rhusiopathiae]

027.2 *Pasteurellosis*

Pasteurella pseudotuberculosis infection
Mesenteric adenitis   ⎤ by Pasteurella multocida
Septic infection (cat-bite) (dog-bite) ⎦   [P. septica]

Excludes: infection by:
               Francisella tularensis (021)
               Yersinia pestis (020.–)

027.8 *Other*

027.9 *Unspecified*

OTHER BACTERIAL DISEASES (030-041)

Excludes: bacterial venereal diseases (098.–, 099.–)
               bartonellosis (088.0)

030   Leprosy

Includes: Hansen's disease
               infection by Mycobacterium leprae

030.0 *Lepromatous [type L]*

Lepromatous leprosy (macular) (diffuse) (infiltrated) (nodular) (neuritic)

030.1 *Tuberculoid [type T]*

Tuberculoid leprosy (macular) (maculoanaesthetic) (major) (minor)
    (neuritic)

030.2 *Indeterminate [group I]*

Indeterminate leprosy (macular) (neuritic)

030.3 *Borderline [group B]*

Borderline or dimorphous leprosy (infiltrated) (neuritic)

030.8 *Other*

030.9 *Unspecified*

031   Diseases due to other mycobacteria

031.0 *Pulmonary*

Infection by Mycobacterium:
    avium
    intracellulare [Battey bacillus]
    kansasii
Battey disease

031.1   *Cutaneous*

Buruli ulcer
Infection by Mycobacterium:
 marinum [M. balnei]
 ulcerans

031.8   *Other*

031.9   *Unspecified*

Atypical mycobacterium infection NOS

032   Diphtheria

Includes: infection by Corynebacterium diphtheriae

032.0   *Faucial diphtheria*

Membranous angina, diphtheritic

032.1   *Nasopharyngeal diphtheria*

032.2   *Anterior nasal diphtheria*

032.3   *Laryngeal diphtheria*

Laryngotracheitis, diphtheritic

032.8   *Other*

Cutaneous diphtheria

032.9   *Diphtheria, unspecified*

033   Whooping cough

033.0   *Bordetella pertussis [B. pertussis]*

033.1   *Bordetella parapertussis [B. parapertussis]*

033.8   *Other specified organism*

033.9   *Whooping cough, unspecified organism*

034   Streptococcal sore throat and scarlatina

034.0   *Streptococcal sore throat*

Streptococcal:
 angina
 laryngitis
 pharyngitis
 tonsillitis

Septic:
 angina
 sore throat

034.1   *Scarlatina*

Scarlet fever

035 Erysipelas

Excludes: postpartum or puerperal erysipelas (670)

036 Meningococcal infection

036.0† *Meningococcal meningitis* (320.5*)

Cerebrospinal fever
  (meningococcal)

Meningitis:
  cerebrospinal
  epidemic

036.1† *Meningococcal encephalitis* (323.4*)

036.2 *Meningococcaemia*

Meningococcal septicaemia

036.3† *Waterhouse-Friderichsen syndrome, meningococcal* (255.5*)

Meningococcal haemorrhagic
  adrenalitis
Meningococcic adrenal syndrome

Waterhouse-Friderichsen
  syndrome NOS

036.4† *Meningococcal carditis*

Meningococcal:
  endocarditis (421.1*)
  pericarditis (420.0*)

036.8 *Other*

Meningococcal optic neuritis† (377.3*)

036.9 *Unspecified*

Meningococcal infection NOS

037 Tetanus

Excludes: tetanus:
      complicating abortion (634-638 with fourth digit .0, 639.0)
      complicating ectopic or molar pregnancy (639.0)
      neonatorum (771.3)
      puerperal (670)

038 Septicaemia

Excludes: during labour (659.3)
      following ectopic or molar pregnancy (639.0)
      following infusion, injection, transfusion or vaccination
        (999.3)
      postoperative (998.5)
      postpartum, puerperal (670)
      when complicating abortion (634-638 with fourth digit
        .0, 639.0)

038.0 *Streptococcal septicaemia*

038.1 *Staphylococcal septicaemia*

038.2 *Pneumococcal septicaemia*

038.3 *Septicaemia due to anaerobes*

Excludes: anaerobic streptococci (038.0)
gas gangrene (040.0)

038.4 *Septicaemia due to other gram-negative organisms*

Gram-negative septicaemia NOS

038.8 *Other specified septicaemias*

Excludes: septicaemia (due to):
anthrax (022.3)
gonococcal (098.8)
herpetic (054.5)
meningococcal (036.2)
septicaemic plague (020.2)

038.9 *Unspecified septicaemia*

Septicaemia NOS

Excludes: bacteraemia NOS (790.7)

039 Actinomycotic infections

Includes: actinomycotic mycetoma
infection by Actinomycetales such as species of Actinomyces,
Actinomadura, Nocardia, Streptomyces
maduromycosis (actinomycotic)

039.0 *Cutaneous*

Erythrasma   Trichomycosis axillaris

039.1 *Pulmonary*

039.2 *Abdominal*

039.3 *Cervicofacial*

039.4 *Madura foot*

Excludes: madura foot due to mycotic infection (117.4)

039.8 *Of other specified sites*

039.9 *Of unspecified site*

Actinomycosis NOS   Nocardiosis NOS
Maduromycosis NOS

040 Other bacterial diseases

Excludes: bacteraemia NOS (790.7)
bacterial infection NOS (041.9)

040.0 *Gas gangrene*

Infection by Clostridium:
  histolyticum
  oedematiens
  perfringens [welchii]
  septicum
  sordellii

Gas bacillus infection or gangrene
Malignant oedema
Myositis, clostridial

040.1 *Rhinoscleroma*

040.2 *Whipple's disease*
Intestinal lipodystrophy

040.3 *Necrobacillosis*

040.8 *Other bacterial diseases*
Tropical pyomyositis† (728.0*)

041 Bacterial infection in conditions classified elsewhere and of unspecified site

Excludes: bacteraemia NOS (790.7)
         septicaemia (038.–)

Note: This category will rarely be used for primary coding. It is provided as an additional code where it is desired to identify the bacterial agent in diseases classified elsewhere. This category will also be used in primary coding to classify bacterial infections of unspecified nature or site.

041.0 *Streptococcus*

041.1 *Staphylococcus*

041.2 *Pneumococcus*

041.3 *Friedländer's bacillus*

041.4 *Escherichia coli*

041.5 *Haemophilus influenzae [H. influenzae]*

041.6 *Proteus (mirabilis) (morganii)*

041.7 *Pseudomonas*

041.8 *Other*

Aerobacter aerogenes
Eaton's agent
Mima polymorpha
Mycoplasma

Pleuropneumonia-like organisms
  [PPLO]
Other cocci, not elsewhere classified

041.9 *Bacterial infection, unspecified*

POLIOMYELITIS AND OTHER NON-ARTHROPOD-BORNE VIRAL
DISEASES OF CENTRAL NERVOUS SYSTEM (045-049)

045†   Acute poliomyelitis (323.2*)

045.0† *Acute paralytic poliomyelitis specified as bulbar* (323.2*)

Infantile paralysis (acute)   ⎫ specified as bulbar
Poliomyelitis (acute) (anterior) ⎬
Polioencephalitis (acute) (bulbar)
Polioencephalomyelitis (acute) (anterior) (bulbar)

045.1† *Acute poliomyelitis with other paralysis* (323.2*)

Paralysis:
   acute atrophic, spinal
   infantile, paralytic
Poliomyelitis (acute) ⎫
   anterior   ⎬ with paralysis except bulbar
   epidemic   ⎭

045.2† *Acute nonparalytic poliomyelitis* (323.2*)

Poliomyelitis (acute) ⎫
   anterior   ⎬ specified as nonparalytic
   epidemic   ⎭

045.9† *Acute poliomyelitis, unspecified* (323.2*)

Infantile paralysis
Poliomyelitis (acute) ⎫
   anterior   ⎬ unspecified whether paralytic or nonparalytic
   epidemic   ⎭

046   Slow virus infection of central nervous system

046.0† *Kuru* (323.0*)

046.1† *Jakob-Creutzfeldt disease* (331.5*)

Subacute spongioform encephalopathy

046.2† *Subacute sclerosing panencephalitis* (323.1*)

Dawson's inclusion body encephalitis
Van Bogaert's sclerosing leucoencephalitis

046.3† *Progressive multifocal leucoencephalopathy* (331.6*)

Multifocal leucoencephalopathy NOS

046.8   *Other*

046.9   *Unspecified*

047   Meningitis due to enterovirus

Includes: meningitis:
            abacterial
            aseptic
            viral

Excludes: meningitis due to:
            adenovirus (049.1†, 321.7*)
            arthropod-borne virus (060-066†, 321.7*)
            leptospira (100.8†, 321.8*)
            virus of:
                herpes simplex (054.7†, 321.4*)
                herpes zoster (053.0†, 321.3*)
                lymphocytic choriomeningitis (049.0†, 321.6*)
                mumps (072.1†, 321.5*)
                poliomyelitis (045.–†, 321.7*)
            any other infection specifically classified elsewhere

047.0† *Coxsackie virus* (321.1*)

047.1† *ECHO virus* (321.2*)

047.8† *Other* (321.7*)

047.9† *Unspecified* (321.7*)
Viral meningitis NOS

048   Other enterovirus diseases of central nervous system

Boston exanthem

049   Other non-arthropod-borne viral diseases of central nervous system

049.0† *Lymphocytic choriomeningitis* (321.6*)
Lymphocytic:
    meningitis (serous)
    meningoencephalitis (serous)

049.1† *Meningitis due to adenovirus* (321.7*)

049.8 *Other*

Encephalitis: von Economŏ's disease† (323.4*)
    acute:
        inclusion body† (323.4*)
        necrotizing† (323.4*)
    epidemic† (323.4*)
    lethargica† (323.4*)
    Rio Bravo† (323.4*)

049.9 *Unspecified*
Viral encephalitis NOS† (323.4*)

VIRAL DISEASES ACCOMPANIED BY EXANTHEM (050-057)

Excludes: arthropod-borne viral diseases (060-066)

050 Smallpox

050.0 *Variola major*
Haemorrhagic (pustular) smallpox   Malignant smallpox
Purpura variolosa

050.1 *Alastrim*
Variola minor

050.2 *Modified smallpox*

050.9 *Smallpox, unspecified*

051 Cowpox and paravaccinia

051.0 *Cowpox*
Vaccinia not from vaccination
Excludes: vaccinia (generalized) (from vaccination) (999.0)

051.1 *Pseudocowpox*
Milkers' node

051.2 *Contagious pustular dermatitis*
Ecthyma contagiosum   Orf

051.9 *Paravaccinia, unspecified*

052 Chickenpox

Varicella

053 Herpes zoster

Includes: shingles
zona

053.0† *With meningitis (321.3*)*

053.1 *With other nervous system complications*
Geniculate herpes zoster   Post-herpetic:
Herpetic geniculate ganglionitis†   polyneuropathy† (357.4*)
(351.1*)   trigeminal neuralgia† (350.0*)

053.2† *With ophthalmic complications*

Herpes zoster:
  dermatitis of eyelids (373.5*)
  iridocyclitis (364.0*)

Herpes zoster:
  keratoconjunctivitis (370.4*)

053.7 *With other complications*

053.8 *With unspecified complication*

053.9 *Herpes zoster without mention of complication*

054 Herpes simplex

Excludes: congenital herpes simplex (771.2)

054.0 *Eczema herpeticum*

Kaposi's varicelliform eruption

054.1 *Genital herpes*

Herpetic vulvovaginitis† (616.1*)

Herpetic ulceration of vulva†
  (616.5*)

054.2 *Herpetic gingivostomatitis*

054.3† *Herpetic meningoencephalitis* (323.4*)

Herpes encephalitis

Simian B disease

054.4† *With ophthalmic complications*

Herpes simplex:
  dermatitis of eyelid (373.5*)
  keratitis (370.4*)
  keratoconjunctivitis (370.4*)
Iritis due to herpes simplex (364.0*)

Keratitis:
  dendritic (370.1*)
  disciform (370.5*)

054.5 *Herpetic septicaemia*

054.6 *Herpetic whitlow*

054.7 *With other complications*

Meningitis due to herpes simplex† (321.4*)
Visceral herpes simplex

054.8 *With unspecified complication*

054.9 *Herpes simplex without mention of complication*

055 Measles

Includes: morbilli
         rubeola

055.0† *Postmeasles encephalitis* (323.6*)

055.1† *Postmeasles pneumonia (484.0*)*

055.2† *Postmeasles otitis (382.0*)*

055.7   *With other complications*

055.8   *With unspecified complication*

055.9   *Measles without mention of complication*

056   Rubella

Includes: German measles
Excludes: congenital rubella (771.0)

056.0   *With neurological complications*
Encephalomyelitis† (323.4*)

056.7   *With other complications*
Rubella arthritis† (711.5*)

056.8   *With unspecified complications*

056.9   *Rubella without mention of complication*

057   Other viral exanthemata

057.0   *Erythema infectiosum [fifth disease]*

057.8   *Other*
Dukes(-Filatow) disease   Pseudoscarlatina
Exanthema subitum   Roseola infantum
Fourth disease   Sixth disease
Parascarlatina

057.9   *Unspecified*

ARTHROPOD-BORNE VIRAL DISEASES (060-066)

060   Yellow fever

060.0   *Sylvatic*
Jungle yellow fever

060.1   *Urban*

060.9   *Unspecified*

061·   Dengue

Breakbone fever
Excludes: haemorrhagic fever caused by dengue virus (065.4)

062 †   Mosquito-borne viral encephalitis (323.3*)

062.0† *Japanese encephalitis* (323.3*)

062.1† *Western equine encephalitis* (323.3*)

062.2† *Eastern equine encephalitis* (323.3*)

Excludes: Venezuelan equine encephalitis (066.2)

062.3† *St. Louis encephalitis* (323.3*)

062.4† *Australian encephalitis* (323.3*)

Australian arboencephalitis   Australian X disease

062.5† *California virus encephalitis* (323.3*)

Encephalitis: Tahyna fever
  California
  La Crosse

062.8† *Other* (323.3*)

Encephalitis by Ilheus virus

062.9† *Unspecified* (323.3*)

063†   Tick-borne viral encephalitis (323.3*)

Includes: diphasic meningoencephalitis

063.0† *Russian spring-summer [taiga] encephalitis* (323.3*)

063.1† *Louping ill* (323.3*)

063.2† *Central European encephalitis* (323.3*)

063.8† *Other* (323.3*)

Langat encephalitis   Powassan encephalitis

063.9† *Unspecified* (323.3*)

064†   Viral encephalitis transmitted by other and unspecified arthropods (323.3*)

Arthropod-borne viral encephalitis, vector unknown
Negishi virus encephalitis

Excludes: viral encephalitis NOS (049.9)

065   Arthropod-borne haemorrhagic fever

065.0 *Crimean haemorrhagic fever [CHF Congo virus]*
Central Asian haemorrhagic fever

065.1 *Omsk haemorrhagic fever*

065.2 *Kyasanur Forest disease*

065.3 *Other tick-borne haemorrhagic fever*

065.4 *Mosquito-borne haemorrhagic fever*

Chikungunya haemorrhagic fever   Dengue haemorrhagic fever

Excludes: Chikungunya fever (066.3)
           dengue (061)
           yellow fever (060.–)

065.8 *Other*

065.9 *Unspecified*

Arbovirus haemorrhagic fever NOS

066   Other arthropod-borne viral diseases

066.0 *Phlebotomus fever*

Sandfly fever   Changuinola fever

066.1 *Tick-borne fever*

Nairobi sheep disease   Tick fever:
Tick fever: Kemerovo
  American mountain   Quaranfil
  Colorado

066.2 *Venezuelan equine fever*

066.3 *Other mosquito-borne fever*

Fever (viral):   Fever (viral):
  Bunyamwera   Oropouche
  Bwamba   Pixuna
  Chikungunya   Rift valley
  Guama   Wesselsbron
  Mayaro   West Nile
  Mucambo   Zika
  O'nyong-nyong

Excludes: dengue (061)
           yellow fever (060.–)

066.8 *Other*

Chandipura fever   Piry fever

066.9 *Unspecified*

Arbovirus infection NOS

OTHER DISEASES DUE TO VIRUSES AND CHLAMYDIAE (070-079)

070†   Viral hepatitis (573.1*)

Excludes: cytomegalic inclusion virus hepatitis (078.5†, 573.1*)

070.0† *Viral hepatitis A with hepatic coma* (573.1*)

070.1† *Viral hepatitis A without mention of hepatic coma* (573.1*)
Infectious hepatitis

070.2† *Viral hepatitis B with hepatic coma* (573.1*)

070.3† *Viral hepatitis B without mention of hepatic coma* (573.1*)
Serum hepatitis

070.4† *Other specified viral hepatitis with hepatic coma* (573.1*)

070.5† *Other specified viral hepatitis without mention of hepatic coma* (573.1*)

070.6† *Unspecified viral hepatitis with hepatic coma* (573.1*)

070.9† *Unspecified viral hepatitis without mention of hepatic coma* (573.1*)
Viral hepatitis NOS

071   Rabies

Hydrophobia   Lyssa

072   Mumps

072.0† *Mumps orchitis* (604.9*)

072.1† *Mumps meningitis* (321.5*)

072.2† *Mumps encephalitis* (323.4*)
Mumps meningoencephalitis

072.3† *Mumps pancreatitis* (577.0*)

072.7   *Mumps with other complications*

072.8   *Mumps with unspecified complication*

072.9   *Mumps without mention of complication*
Epidemic parotitis   Infectious parotitis

073   Ornithosis

Parrot fever   Psittacosis

074   Specific diseases due to Coxsackie virus

Excludes: Coxsackie virus:
                    infection NOS (079.2)
                    meningitis (047.0†, 321.1*)

074.0   *Herpangina*

Vesicular pharyngitis

074.1   *Epidemic pleurodynia*

Bornholm disease   Epidemic:
Devil's grip   myalgia
                                                            myositis

074.2†   *Coxsackie carditis*

Aseptic myocarditis of newborn   Coxsackie:
      (422.0*)   endocarditis (421.1*)
                                                            myocarditis (422.0*)
                                                            pericarditis (420.0*)

074.3   *Hand, foot and mouth disease*

Vesicular stomatitis and exanthem

074.8   *Other*

Acute lymphonodular pharyngitis

075   Infectious mononucleosis

Glandular fever   Pfeiffer's disease
Monocytic angina

076   Trachoma

Excludes: late effect of trachoma; see category 139.1

076.0   *Initial stage*

Trachoma dubium

076.1   *Active stage*

Granular conjunctivitis   Trachomatous:
      (trachomatous)   follicular conjunctivitis
                                                            pannus

076.9   *Unspecified*

Trachoma NOS

077   Other diseases of conjunctiva due to viruses and Chlamydiae

Excludes: ophthalmic complications of viral diseases classified elsewhere

077.0† *Inclusion conjunctivitis* (372.0*)

Paratrachoma   Swimming pool conjunctivitis

Excludes: inclusion blennorrhoea (neonatal) (771.6)

077.1† *Epidemic keratoconjunctivitis* (370.4*)

Shipyard eye

077.2† *Pharyngoconjunctival fever* (372.0*)

Viral pharyngoconjunctivitis

077.3† *Other adenoviral conjunctivitis* (372.0*)

Acute adenoviral follicular conjunctivitis

077.4† *Epidemic haemorrhagic conjunctivitis* (372.0*)

Apollo: Conjunctivitis due to enterovirus
  conjunctivitis   type 70
  disease   Haemorrhagic conjunctivitis
                                            (acute) (epidemic)

077.8† *Other viral conjunctivitis*

Newcastle conjunctivitis (372.0*)

077.9† *Unspecified*

Viral conjunctivitis NOS (372.0*)

078   Other diseases due to viruses and Chlamydiae

Excludes: Viraemia NOS (790.8)
          viral infection NOS (079.–)

078.0   *Molluscum contagiosum*

078.1   *Viral warts*

Condyloma acuminatum   Warts (infectious)
Verruca (vulgaris) (plana) (plantaris)

078.2   *Sweating fever*

Miliary fever   Sweating disease

078.3   *Cat-scratch disease*

Benign lymphoreticulosis (of inoculation)
Cat-scratch fever

078.4   *Foot and mouth disease*

Epizootic:
  aphthae
  stomatitis

078.5 *Cytomegalic inclusion disease*

Cytomegalic inclusion virus hepatitis† (573.1*)
Salivary gland virus disease

Excludes: congenital cytomegalovirus infection (771.1)

078.6† *Haemorrhagic nephrosonephritis* (581.8*)

Haemorrhagic fever:	Haemorrhagic fever:
epidemic	Russian
Korean	with renal syndrome

078.7 *Arenaviral haemorrhagic fever*

Haemorrhagic fever:	Haemorrhagic fever:
Argentine	Junin virus
Bolivian	Machupo virus

078.8 *Other*

Epidemic:	Marburg disease
cervical myalgia	Tanapox
vertigo† (386.1*)	Winter vomiting disease
vomiting syndrome	

079   **Viral infection in conditions classified elsewhere and of unspecified site**

,Note: This category will rarely be used for primary coding. It is provided as an additional code where it is desired to identify the viral
agent in diseases classified elsewhere. This category will also be
used in primary coding to classify virus infection of unspecified
nature or site.

079.0 *Adenovirus*

079.1 *ECHO virus*

079.2 *Coxsackie virus*

079.3 *Rhinovirus*

079.8 *Other*

079.9 *Unspecified*

Viral infection NOS

Excludes: viraemia NOS (790.8)

RICKETTSIOSES AND OTHER ARTHROPOD-BORNE DISEASES
(080-088)

Excludes: arthropod-borne viral diseases (060-066)

080 Louse-borne [epidemic] typhus

Typhus (fever):
  classical
  epidemic

Typhus (fever):
  exanthematic NOS
  louse-borne

081 Other typhus

081.0 *Murine [endemic] typhus*

Typhus (fever):
  endemic
  flea-borne

081.1 *Brill's disease*

Brill-Zinsser disease

Recrudescent typhus (fever)

081.2 *Scrub typhus*

Japanese river fever
Kedani fever

Mite-borne typhus
Tsutsugamushi

081.9 *Unspecified*

Typhus (fever) NOS

082 Tick-borne rickettsioses

082.0 *Spotted fevers*

Rocky Mountain spotted fever

São Paulo fever

082.1 *Boutonneuse fever*

African tick typhus
India tick typhus
Kenya tick typhus

Marseilles fever
Mediterranean tick fever

082.2 *North Asian tick fever*

Siberian tick typhus

082.3 *Queensland tick typhus*

082.8 *Other*

Lone star fever

082.9 *Unspecified*

Tick-borne typhus NOS

083 Other rickettsioses

083.0 *Q-fever*

083.1   *Trench fever*
Quintan fever   Wolhynian fever

083.2   *Rickettsialpox*
Vesicular rickettsiosis

083.8   *Other*

083.9   *Unspecified*

084   Malaria

Excludes: congenital malaria (771.2)
Note: Subcategories 084.0-084.6 exclude the listed conditions with mention of pernicious complications (084.8, 084.9).

084.0   *Falciparum malaria [malignant tertian]*
Malaria (fever):
  by Plasmodium falciparum
  subtertian

084.1   *Vivax malaria [benign tertian]*
Malaria (fever) by Plasmodium vivax

084.2   *Quartan malaria*
Malaria (fever) by Plasmodium   Malariae malaria
  malariae

084.3   *Ovale malaria*
Malaria (fever) by Plasmodium ovale

084.4   *Other malaria*
Monkey malaria

084.5   *Mixed*
Malaria (fever) by more than one parasite

084.6   *Unspecified*
Malaria (fever) NOS

084.7   *Induced malaria*
Therapeutically induced malaria
Excludes: accidental infection from syringe, blood transfusion, etc.
                (084.0-084.6, above, according to parasite species)
              transmission from mother to child during delivery (771.2)

084.8   *Blackwater fever*
Haemoglobinuric: Malarial haemoglobinuria
  fever (bilious)
  malaria

084.9   *Other pernicious complications of malaria*

Algid malaria
Cerebral malaria

Malarial:
    hepatitis† (573.2*)
    nephrosis† (581.8*)

085   Leishmaniasis

085.0   *Visceral [kala-azar]*

Dumdum fever
Infection by Leishmania:
    donovani
    infantum

Leishmaniasis:
    dermal, post-kala-azar
    Mediterranean
    visceral (Indian)

085.1   *Cutaneous, urban*

Aleppo boil
Baghdad boil
Delhi boil
Infection by Leishmania tropica
Oriental sore

Leishmaniasis, cutaneous:
    dry form
    late
    recurrent
    ulcerating

085.2   *Cutaneous, Asian desert*

Infection by Leishmania tropica
    major

Leishmaniasis, cutaneous:
    acute necrotizing
    rural
    wet form
    zoonotic form

085.3   *Cutaneous, Ethiopian*

Infection by Leishmania ethiopica

Leishmaniasis, cutaneous:
    diffuse
    lepromatous

085.4   *Cutaneous, American*

Chiclero ulcer
Infection by Leishmania mexicana

Leishmaniasis tegumentaria diffusa

085.5   *Mucocutaneous (American)*

Espundia
Infection by Leishmania brasiliensis

Uta

085.9   *Unspecified*

086   Trypanosomiasis

Includes: with meningoencephalitis† (323.4*)

086.0† *Chagas's disease with heart involvement* (425.6*)

Any condition in 086.2 with heart involvement

086.1 *Chagas's disease with other organ involvement*
Any condition in 086.2 with involvement of organ other than heart

086.2 *Chagas's disease without mention of organ involvement*
American trypanosomiasis   Infection by Trypanosoma cruzi

086.3 *Gambian trypanosomiasis*
Infection by Trypanosoma   Gambian sleeping sickness
   gambiense

086.4 *Rhodesian trypanosomiasis*
Infection by Trypanosama   Rhodesian sleeping sickness
   rhodesiense

086.5 *African trypanosomiasis, unspecified*
Sleeping sickness NOS

086.9 *Unspecified*

087   Relapsing fever
Recurrent fever

087.0 *Louse-borne*

087.1 *Tick-borne*

087.9 *Unspecified*

088   Other arthropod-borne diseases

088.0 *Bartonellosis*
Carrion's disease   Verruga peruana
Oroya fever

088.8 *Other*

088.9 *Unspecified*
Arthropod-borne disease, not elsewhere classified

SYPHILIS AND OTHER VENEREAL DISEASES (090-099)

Excludes: nonvenereal endemic syphilis (104.0)
           urogenital trichomoniasis (131.0)

090   Congenital syphilis

090.0 *Early congenital syphilis, symptomatic*
Congenital syphilitic: Syphilitic (congenital):
   choroiditis   epiphysitis
   coryza (chronic)   osteochondritis
   hepatomegaly   pemphigus
   mucous patches   Any congenital syphilitic condition
   periostitis   specified as early or manifest
   splenomegaly   less than two years after birth

090.1 *Early congenital syphilis, latent*

Congenital syphilis without clinical manifestations, with positive serological reaction and negative spinal fluid test, less than two years after birth

090.2 *Early congenital syphilis, unspecified*

Congenital syphilis NOS, less than two years after birth

090.3† *Syphilitic interstitial keratitis* (370.5*)

Syphilitic keratitis:
  parenchymatous
  punctata profunda

Excludes: interstitial keratitis NOS (370.5)

090.4 *Juvenile neurosyphilis*

Congenital:
  neurosyphilis
  syphilitic:
    encephalitis† (323.4*)
    meningitis† (320.7*)

Dementia paralytica juvenilis
Juvenile:
  general paresis
  tabes
  taboparesis

Use additional code, if desired, to identify any associated mental disorder

090.5 *Other late congenital syphilis, symptomatic*

Gumma due to congenital syphilis
Hutchinson's teeth
Syphilitic saddle nose

Any congenital syphilitic condition specified as late or manifest two years or more after birth

090.6 *Late congenital syphilis, latent*

Congenital syphilis without clinical manifestations, with positive serological reaction and negative spinal fluid test, two years or more after birth

090.7 *Late congenital syphilis, unspecified*

Congenital syphilis NOS, two years or more after birth

090.9 *Congenital syphilis, unspecified*

091 **Early syphilis, symptomatic**

Excludes: early cardiovascular syphilis (093.–)
          early neurosyphilis (094.–)

091.0 *Genital syphilis (primary)*

Genital chancre

091.1 *Primary anal syphilis*

091.2   *Other primary syphilis*

Primary syphilis of: Primary syphilis of tonsils
  fingers
  lip

091.3   *Secondary syphilis of skin or mucous membranes*

Condyloma latum   Secondary syphilis of:
Secondary syphilis of: skin
  anus   tonsil
  mouth   vulva
  pharynx

091.4   *Adenopathy due to secondary syphilis*

Syphilitic adenopathy   Syphilitic lymphadenitis
  (secondary)   (secondary)

091.5†   *Uveitis due to secondary syphilis*

Syphilitic chorioretinitis (secondary) (363.1*)
Syphilitic iridocyclitis (secondary) (364.1*)

091.6   *Secondary syphilis of viscera and bone*

Secondary syphilis of liver† (573.2*) Secondary syphilitic:
                                          hepatitis† (573.2*)
                                          periostitis† (730.3*)

091.7   *Secondary syphilis, relapse*

Secondary syphilis, relapse (treated) (untreated)

091.8   *Other forms of secondary syphilis*

Acute syphilitic meningitis† (320.7*) Syphilitic alopecia

091.9   *Unspecified secondary syphilis*

092   **Early syphilis, latent**

Includes: syphilis (acquired) without clinical manifestations, with pos-
            itive serological reaction and negative spinal fluid test,
            less than two years after infection

092.0   *Early syphilis, latent, serological relapse after treatment*

092.9   *Early syphilis, latent, unspecified*

093   **Cardiovascular syphilis**

093.0†   *Aneurysm of aorta, specified as syphilitic* (441.7*)

Dilatation of aorta, specified as syphilitic

093.1†   *Syphilitic aortitis* (447.7*)

093.2† *Syphilitic endocarditis* (424.–*)

Syphilitic:
  aortic incompetence or stenosis
  ostial coronary disease

093.8   *Other*

Syphilitic:
  myocarditis† (422.0*)
  pericarditis† (420.0*)

093.9   *Unspecified*

094   Neurosyphilis

Use additional code, if desired, to identify any associated mental disorder

094.0   *Tabes dorsalis*

Arthropathy: Locomotor ataxia (progressive)
  neurogenic (Charcot)† (713.5*)   Posterior spinal sclerosis
  tabetic† (713.5*)   (syphilitic)
Charcot's joint disease† (713.5*)   Tabetic neurosyphilis

094.1   *General paresis*

Dementia paralytica   Paretic neurosyphilis
General paralysis (of insane)   Taboparesis
  (progressive)

094.2† *Syphilitic meningitis* (320.7*)

Meningovascular syphilis

094.3   *Asymptomatic neurosyphilis*

094.8   *Other*

Syphilitic: Syphilitic:
  acoustic neuritis† (388.5*)   Parkinsonism† (332.1*)
  disseminated retinochoroiditis†   retrobulbar neuritis† (377.3*)
    (363.1*)   ruptured cerebral aneurysm†
  encephalitis† (323.4*)   (430*)
  optic atrophy† (377.1*)

094.9   *Unspecified*

Gumma (syphilitic)   ⎫
Syphilis (early) (late) ⎬ of central nervous system NOS
Syphiloma   ⎭

095   Other forms of late syphilis, with symptoms

Gumma (syphilitic)   ⎫ any site except those classifiable in 093.–
Syphilis, late or tertiary ⎭   and 094.–

Gumma (syphilitic) NOS
Syphilis [stage unspecified]:
  bone† (730.8*)
  kidney† (583.8*)
  liver† (573.2*)
  lung† (517.8*)
  muscle† (728.0*)
Syphilitic:
  episcleritis† (379.0*)
  peritonitis† (567.0*)

096   Late syphilis, latent

Syphilis (acquired) without clinical manifestations, with positive sero-
    logical reaction and negative spinal fluid test, two years or more
    after infection

097   Other and unspecified syphilis

097.0 *Late syphilis, unspecified*

097.1 *Latent syphilis, unspecified*

Positive serological reaction for syphilis

097.9 *Syphilis, unspecified*

Syphilis (acquired) NOS

Excludes: syphilis NOS causing death under two years of age (090.9)

098   Gonococcal infections

098.0 *Acute, of lower genitourinary tract*

Gonococcal: Gonorrhoea (acute):
  Bartholinitis (acute)   NOS
  urethritis (acute)   genitourinary (tract) NOS
  vulvovaginitis (acute)

098.1 *Acute, of upper genitourinary tract*

Gonococcal: Gonorrhoea (acute):
  endometritis (acute)† (615.–*)   bladder† (595.4*)
  orchitis (acute)† (604.9*)   cervix† (616.0*)
  prostatitis (acute)† (601.4*)   seminal vesicle† (608.0*)
  salpingitis, acute† (614.0*)

098.2 *Chronic, of lower genitourinary tract*

Any condition in 098.0 specified as chronic or with duration of two months
    or over

098.3 *Chronic, of upper genitourinary tract*
Any condition in 098.1 specified as chronic or with duration of two months
   or over
Gonococcal salpingitis (chronic)† (614.1, 614.2*)

098.4† *Of eye*
Gonococcal:
   conjunctivitis (neonatorum) (372.0*)
   iridocyclitis (364.0*)
   ophthalmia (neonatorum) (372.0*)

098.5† *Of joint*
Gonococcal:
   arthritis (711.4*)
   bursitis (727.3*)

Gonococcal:
   synovitis (727.0*)
   tenosynovitis (727.0*)

098.6 *Of pharynx*

098.7 *Of anus and rectum*

098.8 *Of other sites*
Gonococcaemia
Gonococcal:
   endocarditis† (421.1*)
   keratosis (blenorrhagica)† (701.1*)

Gonococcal:
   meningitis† (320.7*)
   peritonitis† (567.0*)

099   Other venereal diseases

099.0 *Chancroid*
Bubo (inguinal):
   chancroidal
   due to Haemophilus ducreyi
Ulcus molle (cutis) (skin)

Chancre:
   Ducrey's
   simple
   soft

099.1 *Lymphogranuloma venereum*
Climatic or tropical bubo
(Durand-)Nicolas-Favre disease

Esthiomene
Lymphogranuloma inguinale

099.2 *Granuloma inguinale*
Donovanosis
Granuloma pudendi (ulcerating)

Granuloma venereum

099.3 *Reiter's disease*
Reiter's syndrome

099.4 *Other nongonococcal urethritis*
Nonspecific and nongonococcal urethritis so stated

099.8 *Other*

099.9 *Unspecified*

OTHER SPIROCHAETAL DISEASES (100-104)

100   Leptospirosis

100.0   *Leptospirosis icterohaemorrhagica*

Leptospiral or spirochaetal jaundice (haemorrhagic)
Weil's disease

100.8   *Other*

Fever:
  Fort Bragg
  pretibial
  swamp

Infection by Leptospira:
  australis
  bataviae
  pyrogenes
Leptospiral meningitis (aseptic)†
  (321.8*)

100.9   *Unspecified*

101   Vincent's angina

Acute necrotizing ulcerative:
  gingivitis
  stomatitis
Fusospirochaetal pharyngitis

Spirochaetal stomatitis
Trench mouth
Vincent's:
  gingivitis
  infection [any site]

102   Yaws

Includes: framboesia
             pian

102.0   *Initial lesions*

Chancre of yaws
Framboesia, initial or primary

Initial framboesial ulcer
Mother yaw

102.1   *Multiple papillomata and wet crab yaws*

Butter yaws
Framboesioma

Pianoma
Plantar or palmar papilloma of
  yaws

102.2   *Other early skin lesions*

Early yaws (cutaneous) (macular) (papular) (maculopapular) (micro-
  papular)
Framboeside of early yaws
Cutaneous yaws, less than five years after infection

102.3   *Hyperkeratosis*

Ghoul hand
Hyperkeratosis, palmar or plantar (early) (late) due to yaws
Worm-eaten soles

102.4 *Gummata and ulcers*

Nodular late yaws (ulcerated)   Gummatous framboeside

102.5 *Gangosa*

Rhinopharyngitis mutilans

102.6 *Bone and joint lesions*

Goundou
Gumma, bone
Gummatous osteitis or periostitis } of yaws (late)
Ganglion
Hydrarthrosis
Osteitis } of yaws (early) (late)
Periostitis (hypertrophic)

102.7 *Other manifestations*

Juxta-articular nodules of yaws   Mucosal yaws

102.8 *Latent yaws*

Yaws without clinical manifestations, with positive serology

102.9 *Yaws, unspecified*

103   Pinta

103.0 *Primary lesions*

Chancre (primary)
Papule (primary) } of pinta [carate]
Pintid

103.1 *Intermediate lesions*

Erythematous plaques
Hyperchromic lesions } of pinta [carate]
Hyperkeratosis

103.2 *Late lesions*

Cardiovascular lesions
Skin lesions:
  achromic
  cicatricial } of pinta [carate]
  dyschromic
Vitiligo

103.3 *Mixed lesions*

Achromic and hyperchromic skin lesions of pinta [carate]

103.9 *Unspecified*

104   Other spirochaetal infection

104.0   *Nonvenereal endemic syphilis*

Bejel   Njovera

104.8   *Other*

Excludes: relapsing fever (087.–)
            syphilis (090-097)

104.9   *Unspecified*

MYCOSES (110-118)

Excludes: infection by Actinomycetales such as species of Actinomyces,
            Actinomadura, Nocardia, Streptomyces (039.–)

110   Dermatophytosis

Includes: infection by species of Epidermophyton, Microsporum and
            Trichophyton
            tinea, any type except those in 111

110.0   *Of scalp and beard*

Kerion   Trichophytic tinea, scalp [black
Sycosis, mycotic   dot tinea]

110.1   *Of nail*

Dermatophytic onychia   Tinea unguium
Onychomycosis

110.2   *Of hand*

Tinea manuum

110.3   *Of groin and perianal area*

Dhobie itch   Eczema marginatum

110.4   *Of foot*

Athlete's foot   Tinea pedis

110.5   *Of the body*

Herpes circinatus   Tinea imbricata [Tokelau]

110.6   *Deep seated dermatophytosis*

Granuloma trichophyticum   Majocchi's granuloma

110.8   *Of other sites*

110.9   *Of unspecified site*

Favus NOS   Ringworm NOS
Microsporic tinea NOS

111   Dermatomycosis, other and unspecified

111.0   *Pityriasis versicolor*

Infection by Malassezia [Pityrosporum] furfur
Tinea flava
Tinea versicolor

111.1   *Tinea nigra*

Infection by Cladosporium species   Pityriasis nigra
Keratomycosis nigricans   Tinea palmaris nigra
Microsporosis nigra

111.2   *Tinea blanca*

Infection by Trichosporon (beigelii) cutaneum
White piedra

111.3   *Black piedra*

Infection by Piedraia hortai

111.8   *Other*

111.9   *Unspecified*

112   Candidiasis

Includes: infection by Candida species
            candidiosis
            moniliasis
Excludes: neonatal monilial infection (771.7)

112.0   *Of mouth*
Thrush

112.1† *Of vulva and vagina* (616.1*)
Candidal vulvovaginitis   Monilial vulvovaginitis

112.2   *Of other urogenital sites*

112.3   *Of skin and nails*
Candidal intertrigo   Candidal perionyxis [paronychia]
Candidal onychia

112.4† *Of lung* (484.7*)

112.5   *Disseminated*
Systemic candidiasis

112.8   *Of other sites*
Candidal endocarditis† (421.1*)

112.9   *Of unspecified site*

114 Coccidioidomycosis

Coccidioidal granuloma
Desert rheumatism
Infection by Coccidioides (immitis)

Posadas-Wernicke disease
San Joaquin Valley fever

115 Histoplasmosis

115.0 *Infection by Histoplasma capsulatum*

American histoplasmosis
Darling's disease

Reticuloendothelial cytomycosis
Small form histoplasmosis

115.1 *Infection by Histoplasma duboisii*

African histoplasmosis

Large form histoplasmosis

115.9 *Unspecified*

Histoplasmosis NOS

116 Blastomycotic infection

116.0 *Blastomycosis*

Blastomycetic dermatitis
Chicago disease
Cutaneous blastomycosis
Disseminated blastomycosis
Gilchrist's disease

Infection by Blastomyces
    [Ajellomyces] dermatitidis
North American blastomycosis
Primary pulmonary blastomycosis

116.1 *Paracoccidioidomycosis*

Brazilian blastomycosis
Infection by Paracoccidioides
    [Blastomyces] brasiliensis
Lutz-Splendore-Almeida disease
Mucocutaneous-lymphangitic
    paracoccidioidomycosis

Pulmonary paracoccidioido-
    mycosis
South American blastomycosis
Visceral paracoccidioidomycosis

116.2 *Lobomycosis*

Infections by Loboa [Blastomyces]
    loboi
Keloidal blastomycosis

Lobo's disease

117 Other mycoses

117.0 *Rhinosporidiosis*

Infection by Rhinosporidium seeberi

117.1 *Sporotrichosis*

Cutaneous sporotrichosis
Disseminated sporotrichosis
Infection by Sporothrix
 [Sporotrichum] schenckii

Lymphocutaneous sporotrichosis
Pulmonary sporotrichosis
Sporotrichosis of the bones

117.2 *Chromoblastomycosis*

Chromomycosis
Infection by Cladosporidium carrionii, Fonsecaea compactum, Fonsecaea pedrosoi, Phialophora verrucosa

117.3 *Aspergillosis*

Infection by Aspergillus species, mainly A. fumigatus, A. flavus group, A. terreus group

117.4 *Mycotic mycetomas*

Infection by various genera and species of Ascomycetes and Deuteromycetes such as Acremonium [Cephalosporium] falciforme, Neotestudina rosatii, Madurella grisea, Madurella mycetomii, Pyrenochaeta romeroi, Zopfia [Leptosphaeria] senegalensis
Madura foot, mycotic
Maduromycosis, mycotic

Excludes: actinomycotic mycetomas (039.–)

117.5 *Cryptococcosis*

Busse-Buschke's disease
Cryptococcal meningitis† (321.0*)
European cryptococcosis
Infection by Cryptococcus
 neoformans

Pulmonary cryptococcosis
Systemic cryptococcosis
Torula

117.6 *Allescheriosis [Petriellidosis]*

Infections by Allescheria [Petriellidium] boydii [Monosporium apiospermum]

Excludes: mycotic mycetoma (117.4)

117.7 *Zygomycosis [Phycomycosis or Mucormycosis]*

Infection by species of Absidia, Basidiobolus, Conidiobolus, Cunninghamella, Entomophthora, Mucor, Rhizopus, Saksenaea

117.8 *Infection by dematiacious fungi [Phaeohyphomycosis]*

Infection by dematiacious fungi such as Cladosporium trichoides [bantianum], Dreschlera hawaiiensis, Phialophora gougerotii, P. jeanselmei

117.9 *Other and unspecified*

118   Opportunistic mycoses

Infection of skin, subcutaneous tissues and/or organs by a wide variety of
fungi generally considered to be pathogenic to compromised hosts
only, e.g., infection by species of Alternaria, Dreschlera, Fusarium

HELMINTHIASES (120-129)

120   Schistosomiasis [bilharziasis]

120.0   *Schistosoma haematobium*

Vesical schistosomiasis NOS

120.1   *Schistosoma mansoni*

Intestinal schistosomiasis NOS

120.2   *Schistosoma japonicum*

Asiatic schistosomiasis NOS   Katayama disease or fever

120.3   *Cutaneous*

Cercarial dermatitis   Schistosome dermatitis
Infection by cercariae of Schistosoma

120.8   *Other*

Infection by Schistosoma: Infection by Schistosoma:
  bovis   mattheii
  intercalatum   spindale
                                     Schistosomiasis chestermani

120.9   *Unspecified*

Blood flukes NOS   Haemic distomiasis

121   Other trematode infections

121.0   *Opisthorchiasis*

Infection by:
  cat liver fluke
  Opisthorchis (felineus) (tenuicollis) (viverrini)

121.1   *Clonorchiasis*

Biliary cirrhosis due to clonorchiasis
Chinese liver fluke disease
Hepatic distomiasis due to Clonorchis sinensis
Oriental liver fluke disease

121.2   *Paragonimiasis*

Infection by Paragonimus   Pulmonary distomiasis
Lung fluke disease (oriental)

121.3 *Fascioliasis*

Infection by Fasciola:
  gigantica
  hepatica

Liver flukes NOS
Sheep liver fluke infection

121.4 *Fasciolopsiasis*

Infection by Fasciolopsis (buski)   Intestinal distomiasis

121.5 *Metagonimiasis*

Infection by Metagonimus yokogawai

121.6 *Heterophyiasis*

Infection by:
  Heterophyes heterophyes
  Stellantchasmus falcatus

121.8 *Other*

Infection by:
  Dicrocoelium dendriticum
  Echinostomum ilocanum

Infection by:
  Gastrodiscoides hominis

121.9 *Unspecified*

Distomiasis NOS

Fluke disease NOS

122   Echinococcosis

Includes: echinococciasis
            hydatid disease
            hydatidosis

122.0 *Echinococcus granulosus infection of liver*

122.1 *Echinococcus granulosus infection of lung*

122.2 *Echinococcus granulosus infection of thyroid*

122.3 *Echinococcus granulosus infection, other*

122.4 *Echinococcus granulosus infection, unspecified*

122.5 *Echinococcus multilocularis infection of liver*

122.6 *Echinococcus multilocularis infection, other*

122.7 *Echinococcus multilocularis infection, unspecified*

122.8 *Echinococcosis, unspecified, of liver*

122.9 *Echinococcosis, other and unspecified*

123   Other cestode infection

123.0 *Taenia solium infection, intestinal form*
Pork tapeworm (adult) (infection)

123.1 *Cysticercosis*
Cysticerciasis
Infection by:
   Cysticercus cellulosae [larval form of Taenia solium]

123.2 *Taenia saginata infection*
Beef tapeworm (infection)
Infection by Taeniarhyuchus saginatus

123.3 *Taeniasis, unspecified*

123.4 *Diphyllobothriasis, intestinal*
Diphyllobothrium (adult) (latum) (pacificum) infection
Fish tapeworm (infection)

123.5 *Sparganosis [larval diphyllobothriasis]*
Infection by:
   Diphyllobothrium larvae
   Sparganum (mansoni) (proliferum)
   Spirometra larvae

123.6 *Hymenolepiasis*
Dwarf tapeworm (infection)   Rat tapeworm (infection)
Hymenolepis (diminuta) (nana)
   infection

123.8 *Other*
Diplogonoporus (grandis) ⎤   Dog tapeworm (infection)
Dipylidium (caninum)   ⎦ infection

123.9 *Unspecified*
Tapeworm (infection) NOS

124 **Trichinosis**

Trichinella spiralis infection   Trichiniasis
Trichinellosis

125 **Filarial infection and dracontiasis**

125.0 *Bancroftian filariasis*
Chyluria ⎤
Elephantiasis ⎥
Infection   ⎥
Lymphadenitis ⎬ due to Wuchereria bancrofti
Lymphangitis   ⎥
Wuchereriasis ⎦

125.1   *Malayan filariasis*

Brugia filariasis ⎫
Chyluria   ⎪
Elephantiasis   ⎬ due to Brugia [Wuchereria] malayi
Infection   ⎪
Lymphadenitis   ⎪
Lymphangitis   ⎭

125.2   *Loiasis*

Eyeworm disease of Africa   Loa loa infection

125.3   *Onchocerciasis*

Onchocerca volvulus infection   Onchocercosis

125.4   *Dipetalonemiasis*

Infection by:
  Acanthocheilonema perstans
  Dipetalonema perstans

125.5   *Mansonella ozzardi infection*

Filariasis ozzardi

125.6   *Other specified filariusis*

Infection by: Dirofilaria infection
  Acanthocheilonema streptocerca
  Dipetalonema streptocerca

125.7   *Dracontiasis*

Guinea-worm infection   Infection by Dracunculus medi-
                                         nensis

125.9   *Unspecified filariasis*

126   Ancylostomiasis and necatoriasis

Includes: cutaneous larva migrans due to Ancylostoma
            hookworm (disease) (infection)
            uncinariasis

126.0   *Ancylostoma duodenale*

126.1   *Necator americanus*

126.2   *Ancylostoma braziliense*

126.3   *Ancylostoma ceylanicum*

126.8   *Other specified Ancylostoma*

126.9   *Unspecified*

Creeping eruption NOS   Cutaneous larva migrans NOS

127   Other intestinal helminthiases

127.0 *Ascariasis*

Ascaridiasis   Roundworm infection
Infection by Ascaris lumbricoides

127.1 *Anisakiasis*

Infection by Anisakis larva

127.2 *Strongyloidiasis*

Infection by Strongyloides stercoralis

Excludes: trichostrongyliasis (127.6)

127.3 *Trichuriasis*

Infection by Trichuris trichiura   Whipworm (disease) (infection)
Trichocephaliasis

127.4 *Enterobiasis*

Infection by Enterobius vermicularis Pinworm (disease) (infection)
Oxyuris vermicularis infection   Threadworm infection
Oxyuriasis

127.5 *Capillariasis*

Infection by Capillaria philippinensis

Excludes: infection by Capillaria hepatica (128.8)

127.6 *Trichostrongyliasis*

Infection by Trichostrongylus species

127.7 *Other intestinal helminthiasis*

Infection by:
    Oesophagostomum apiostomum and related species
    Ternidens diminutus
    other specified intestinal helminth
Physalopteriasis

127.8 *Mixed intestinal helminthiasis*

Infection by intestinal helminths classified to more than one of the cate-
    gories 120.0-127.7
Mixed helminthiasis NOS

127.9 *Intestinal helminthiasis, unspecified*

128   Other and unspecified helminthiases

128.0 *Toxocariasis*

Larva migrans visceralis   Visceral larva migrans syndrome
Toxocara (canis) (cati) infection

128.1 *Gnathostomiasis*

Infection by Gnathostoma spinigerum and related species

128.8 *Other*

Infection by:
Angiostrongylus cantonensis
Capillaria hepatica
other specified helminth

128.9 *Unspecified*

Helminthiasis NOS   Worms NOS

129   Intestinal parasitism, unspecified

OTHER INFECTIOUS AND PARASITIC DISEASES (130-136)

130   Toxoplasmosis

Infection by Toxoplasma gondii
Chorioretinitis† (363.0*) ⎫
Hepatitis† (573.2*)   ⎪
Meningoencephalitis† (323.4*) ⎬ due to acquired toxoplasmosis
Myocarditis† (422.0*)   ⎪
Pneumonitis† (484.8*)   ⎭

Excludes: congenital toxoplasmosis (771.2)

131   Trichomoniasis

131.0 *Urogenital trichomoniasis*

Fluor (vaginalis)   ⎫
Leukorrhoea (vaginalis)   ⎪
Prostatitis† (601.4*)   ⎬ trichomonal or due to Trichomonas
Urethritis† (597.8*)   ⎪   (vaginalis)
Vaginitis† (616.1*)   ⎪
Vulvovaginitis† (616.1*)   ⎭

131.8 *Other sites*

Excludes: intestinal (007.3)

131.9 *Unspecified*

132   Pediculosis and phthirus infestation

132.0 *Pediculus capitis [head louse]*

132.1 *Pediculus corporis [body louse]*

132.2 *Phthirus pubis [pubic louse]*

132.3 *Mixed*

Infestation classifiable to more than one of the categories 132.0–132.2

132.9 *Pediculosis, unspecified*

133 Acariasis

133.0 *Scabies*

Infestation by Sarcoptes scabiei   Sarcoptic itch

133.8 *Other*

Chiggers
Infestation by:
  Demodex folliculorum
  Trombiculae

133.9 *Unspecified*

Infestation by mites NOS

134 Other infestation

134.0 *Myiasis*

Infestation by: Infestation by:
  fly larvae   maggots
  Dermatobia (hominis)   Oestrus ovis
  Gasterophilus (intestinalis)

134.1 *Other arthropod infestation*

Infestation by: Jigger disease
  chigoe   Scarabiasis
  Tunga penetrans
  sand flea

134.2 *Hirudiniasis*

Hirudiniasis (external) (internal)
Leeches (aquatic) (land)

134.8 *Other*

134.9 *Unspecified*

Infestation (skin) NOS   Skin parasites NOS

135 Sarcoidosis

Besnier-Boeck-Schaumann disease   Sarcoid (any site):
Lupoid (miliary) of Boeck   NOS
Lupus pernio (Besnier)   Boeck
Lymphogranulomatosis, benign   Darier-Roussy
  (Schaumann)   Uveoparotid fever

136   Other and unspecified infectious and parasitic diseases

136.0   *Ainhum*

Dactylolysis spontanea

136.1   *Behcet's syndrome*

136.2   *Specific infections by free-living amoebae*

Meningoencephalitis due to Naegleria† (323.4*)

136.3   *Pneumocystosis*

Pneumonia due to Pneumocystis carinii† (484.8*)

136.4   *Psorospermiasis*

136.5   *Sarcosporidiosis*

136.8   *Other*

Candiru infestation

136.9   *Unspecified*

LATE EFFECTS OF INFECTIOUS AND PARASITIC DISEASES (137-139)

137   Late effects of tuberculosis

Note: This category is to be used to indicate conditions in 010-018 as
        the cause of late effects, which are themselves classified elsewhere.
        The "late effects" include those specified as such, as sequelae or
        as due to old or inactive tuberculosis, without evidence of active
        disease.   [See III Late effects, page 723].

137.0   *Late effects of respiratory or unspecified tuberculosis*

137.1   *Late effects of central nervous system tuberculosis*

137.2   *Late effects of genitourinary tuberculosis*

137.3   *Late effects of tuberculosis of bones and joints*

137.4   *Late effects of tuberculosis of other specified organs*

138   Late effects of acute poliomyelitis

Note: This category is to be used to indicate conditions in 045.– as the
        cause of late effects, which are themselves classified elsewhere.
        The "late effects" include conditions specified as such, or as
        sequelae, or those which are present one year or more after the
        onset of the acute poliomyelitis. [See III Late effects, page 723].

139   Late effects of other infectious and parasitic diseases

Note: This category is to be used to indicate conditions in categories
001-009, 020-041, 046-136 as the cause of late effects, which are
themselves classified elsewhere. The "late effects" include conditions specified as such; they also include sequela of diseases
classifiable to the above categories if there is evidence that the
disease itself is no longer present. [See III Late effects, page 723].

139.0   *Late effects of viral encephalitis*

Late effects of conditions classifiable to 049.8, 049.9, 062-064

139.1   *Late effects of trachoma*

Late effects of conditions classifiable to 076.–

139.8   *Late effects of other and unspecified infectious and parasitic diseases*

II. NEOPLASMS

Notes:

1. Content

This chapter contains the following broad groups: —

140-195 Malignant neoplasms, stated or presumed to be primary, of specified sites, except of lymphatic and haematopoietic tissue

196-198 Malignant neoplasms, stated or presumed to be secondary, of specified sites

199 Malignant neoplasm without specification of site

200-208 Malignant neoplasms, stated or presumed to be primary, of lymphatic and haematopoietic tissue

210-229 Benign neoplasms

230-234 Carcinoma in situ

235-238 Neoplasms of uncertain behaviour [see Note, page 140]

239 Neoplasms of unspecified nature

2. Functional activity

All neoplasms are classified in this chapter, whether or not functionally active. An additional code from Chapter III may be used, if desired, to identify such functional activity associated with any neoplasm, e.g.:
catecholamine-producing malignant phaeochromocytoma of adrenal
code 194.0 additional code 255.6
basophil adenoma of pituitary with Cushing's syndrome
code 227.3 additional code 255.0

3. Morphology [Histology]

For those wishing to identify the histological type of neoplasms, a comprehensive coded nomenclature, which comprises the morphology rubrics of the ICD-Oncology, is given on pages 667-690. See also Introduction, page XXX.

4. Malignant neoplasms overlapping site boundaries

Categories 140-195 are for the classification of primary malignant neoplasms according to their point of origin. A malignant neoplasm that overlaps two or more subcategories within a three-digit rubric and whose point of origin cannot be determined should be classified to the subcategory .8 "Other". For example: "carcinoma involving tip and ventral surface of tongue" should be assigned to 141.8. On the other hand, "carcinoma of tip of tongue extending to involve the ventral surface" should be coded to 141.2 as the point of origin, the tip, is known. Three subcategories, (149.8, 159.8, 165.8), have been provided for malignant neoplasms that overlap the boundaries of three-digit rubrics within certain systems. Overlapping malignant neoplasms that cannot be classified as indicated above should be assigned to the appropriate subdivision of category 195 (Malignant neoplasm of other and ill-defined sites).

MALIGNANT NEOPLASM OF LIP, ORAL CAVITY AND PHARYNX (140-149)

140   Malignant neoplasm of lip

Excludes: skin of lip (173.0)

140.0 *Upper lip, vermilion border*
Upper lip:
  NOS
  external
  lipstick area

140.1 *Lower lip, vermilion border*
Lower lip:
  NOS
  external
  lipstick area

140.3 *Upper lip, inner aspect*

Upper lip: Upper lip:
  buccal aspect   mucosa
  frenulum   oral aspect

140.4 *Lower lip, inner aspect*

Lower lip: Lower lip:
  buccal aspect   mucosa
  frenulum   oral aspect

140.5 *Lip, unspecified, inner aspect*
Lip, not specified whether upper or lower:
  buccal aspect
  frenulum
  mucosa
  oral aspect

140.6 *Commissure of lip*

140.8 *Other* [see Note 4, page 101]

140.9 *Lip, unspecified, vermilion border*
Lip not specified as upper or lower:
  NOS
  external
  lipstick area

141   Malignant neoplasm of tongue

141.0 *Base of tongue*
Dorsal surface of base of tongue   Fixed part of tongue NOS

141.1   *Dorsal surface of tongue*

Anterior two-thirds of tongue, dorsal surface

Excludes: dorsal surface of base of tongue (141.0)

141.2   *Tip and lateral border of tongue*

141.3   *Ventral surface of tongue*

Anterior two-thirds of tongue, ventral surface
Frenulum linguae

141.4   *Anterior two-thirds of tongue, part unspecified*

Mobile part of tongue NOS

141.5   *Junctional zone*

Border of tongue at junction of fixed and mobile parts at insertion of
  anterior tonsillar pillar

141.6   *Lingual tonsil*

141.8   *Other* [see Note 4, page 101]

141.9   *Tongue, unspecified*

Tongue NOS

142   Malignant neoplasm of major salivary glands

Excludes: malignant neoplasms of minor salivary glands, which are to
             be classified according to their anatomical location; if
             location is not specified, classify to 145.9

142.0   *Parotid gland*

142.1   *Submandibular gland*

Submaxillary gland

142.2   *Sublingual gland*

142.8   *Other* [see Note 4, page 101]

142.9   *Site unspecified*

Salivary gland (major) NOS

143   Malignant neoplasm of gum

Includes: alveolar (ridge) mucosa
            gingiva

Excludes: malignant odontogenic neoplasms (170.–)

143.0   *Upper gum*

143.1   *Lower gum*

143.8   *Other* [see Note 4, page 101]

143.9   *Gum, unspecified*

144   Malignant neoplasm of floor of mouth

144.0   *Anterior portion*

Anterior to the premolar-canine junction

144.1   *Lateral portion*

144.8   *Other* [see Note 4, page 101]

144.9   *Part unspecified*

145   Malignant neoplasm of other and unspecified parts of mouth

Excludes: mucosa of lips (140.–)

145.0   *Cheek mucosa*

Buccal mucosa   Internal cheek

145.1   *Vestibule of mouth*

Buccal sulcus (upper) (lower)   Labial sulcus (upper) (lower)

145.2   *Hard palate*

145.3   *Soft palate*

Excludes: nasopharyngeal [posterior] [superior] surface of soft palate
            (147.3)

145.4   *Uvula*

145.5   *Palate, unspecified*

Junction of hard and soft palate   Roof of mouth

145.6   *Retromolar area*

145.8   *Other* [see Note 4, page 101]

145.9   *Mouth, unspecified*

Minor salivary gland, unspecified site   Oral cavity NOS

146   Malignant neoplasm of oropharynx

146.0   *Tonsil*

Tonsil:
  NOS
  faucial
  palatine

Excludes: lingual tonsil (141.6)
            pharyngeal tonsil (147.1)

146.1   *Tonsillar fossa*

146.2   *Tonsillar pillars (anterior) (posterior)*

Palatoglossal arch   Palatopharyngeal arch

146.3   *Vallecula*

Anterior and medial surface of the pharyngoepiglottic fold

146.4   *Anterior aspect of epiglottis*

Epiglottis, free border [margin]   Glossoepiglottic fold(s)

Excludes: epiglottis:
                 NOS (161.1)
                 suprahyoid portion (161.1)

146.5   *Junctional region*

Junction of the free margin of the epiglottis, the aryepiglottic fold and the
     pharyngoepiglottic fold

146.6   *Lateral wall of oropharynx*

146.7   *Posterior wall of oropharynx*

146.8   *Other* [see Note 4, page 101]

146.9   *Oropharynx, unspecified*

147   Malignant neoplasm of nasopharynx

147.0   *Superior wall*

Roof of nasopharynx

147.1   *Posterior wall*

Pharyngeal tonsil   Adenoid

147.2   *Lateral wall*

Fossa of Rosenmüller   Pharyngeal recess
Opening of auditory tube

147.3   *Anterior wall*

Floor of nasopharynx
Nasopharyngeal [posterior] [superior] surface of soft palate
Posterior margin of nasal septum and choanae

147.8   *Other* [see Note 4, page 101]

147.9   *Nasopharynx, unspecified*

Nasopharyngeal wall NOS

148   Malignant neoplasm of hypopharynx

148.0   *Postcricoid region*

148.1   *Pyriform sinus*

Pyriform fossa

148.2   *Aryepiglottic fold, hypopharyngeal aspect*

Aryepiglottic fold or interarytenoid fold:
  NOS
  marginal zone

Excludes: aryepiglottic fold or interarytenoid fold, laryngeal aspect
           (161.1)

148.3   *Posterior hypopharyngeal wall*

148.8   *Other* [see Note 4, page 101]

148.9   *Hypopharynx, unspecified*

Hypopharyngeal wall NOS   Hypopharynx NOS

**149   Malignant neoplasm of other and ill-defined sites within the lip,
         oral cavity and pharynx**

149.0   *Pharynx, unspecified*

149.1   *Waldeyer's ring*

149.8   *Other* [see Note 4, page 101]

Malignant neoplasm of lip, oral cavity and pharynx whose point of origin
  cannot be assigned to any one of the categories 140-148

149.9   *Ill-defined*

MALIGNANT NEOPLASM OF DIGESTIVE ORGANS AND PERITONEUM
(150-159)

150   Malignant neoplasm of oesophagus

Note: Two alternative subclassifications are given: —
           .0-.2   by anatomical description
           .3-.5   by thirds
       This departure from the principle that categories should be
       mutually exclusive is deliberate, since both forms of terminology
       are currently encountered on medical records.

150.0   *Cervical part*

150.1   *Thoracic part*

150.2   *Abdominal part*

150.3   *Upper third*

150.4   *Middle third*

150.5   *Lower third*

150.8   *Other* [see Note 4, page 101]

150.9   *Oesophagus, unspecified*

151   Malignant neoplasm of stomach

151.0 *Cardia*

Cardiac orifice   Cardio-oesophageal junction

151.1 *Pylorus*

Pyloric canal   Prepylorus

151.2 *Pyloric antrum*

Antrum of stomach NOS

151.3 *Fundus of stomach*

151.4 *Body of stomach*

151.5 *Lesser curvature, unspecified*

Lesser curvature, not classifiable to 151.1-151.4

151.6 *Greater curvature, unspecified*

Greater curvature, not classifiable to 151.0-151.4

151.8 *Other* [see Note 4, page 101]

Anterior wall, not classifiable to 151.0-151.4
Posterior wall, not classifiable to 151.0-151.4

151.9 *Stomach, unspecified*

Carcinoma ventriculi   Gastric cancer

152   Malignant neoplasm of small intestine, including duodenum

152.0 *Duodenum*

152.1 *Jejunum*

152.2 *Ileum*

Excludes: ileocaecal valve (153.4)

152.3 *Meckel's diverticulum*

152.8 *Other* [see Note 4, page 101]

Duodenojejunal junction

152.9 *Small intestine, unspecified*

153   Malignant neoplasm of color

153.0 *Hepatic flexure*

153.1 *Transverse colon*

153.2   *Descending colon*

153.3   *Sigmoid colon*

Sigmoid (flexure)

Excludes: rectosigmoid junction (154.0)

153.4   *Caecum*

Ileocaecal valve

153.5   *Appendix*

153.6   *Ascending colon*

153.7   *Splenic flexure*

153.8   *Other* [see Note 4, page 101]

153.9   *Colon, unspecified*

Large intestine NOS

154   Malignant neoplasm of rectum, rectosigmoid junction and anus

154.0   *Rectosigmoid junction*

Rectosigmoid (colon)   Colon and rectum

154.1   *Rectum*

Rectal ampulla

154.2   *Anal canal*

Anal sphincter

154.3   *Anus, unspecified*

Excludes: anus:
            margin (172.5, 173.5)
            skin (172.5, 173.5)
            perianal skin (172.5, 173.5)

154.8   *Other* [see Note 4, page 101]

Anorectum   Cloacogenic zone

155   Malignant neoplasm of liver and intrahepatic bile ducts

155.0   *Liver, primary*

Carcinoma: Hepatoblastoma
   liver, specified as primary
   hepatocellular
   liver cell

155.1 *Intrahepatic bile ducts*

Canaliculi biliferi
Interlobular:
  bile ducts
  biliary canals

Intrahepatic:
  canaliculi
  biliary passages
  gall duct

155.2 *Liver, not specified as primary or secondary*

156 Malignant neoplasm of gallbladder and extrahepatic bile ducts

156.0 *Gallbladder*

156.1 *Extrahepatic bile ducts*

Biliary duct or passage NOS
Common bile duct

Cystic duct
Hepatic duct

156.2 *Ampulla of Vater*

156.8 *Other* [see Note 4, page 101]

156.9 *Biliary tract, part unspecified*

Malignant neoplasm involving both intrahepatic and extrahepatic bile
    ducts

157 Malignant neoplasm of pancreas

157.0 *Head of pancreas*

157.1 *Body of pancreas*

157.2 *Tail of pancreas*

157.3 *Pancreatic duct*

Duct of:
  Santorini
  Wirsung

157.4 *Islets of Langerhans*

Islets of Langerhans, any part of pancreas

157.8 *Other* [see Note 4, page 101]

157.9 *Part unspecified*

158 Malignant neoplasm of retroperitoneum and peritoneum

158.0 *Retroperitoneum*

158.8 *Specified parts of peritoneum* [see Note 4, page 101]

Mesentery
Mesocolon
Omentum

Peritoneum:
  parietal
  pelvic

158.9   *Peritoneum, unspecified*

159   Malignant neoplasm of other and ill-defined sites within the digestive organs and peritoneum

159.0   *Intestinal tract, part unspecified*

Intestine NOS

159.1   *Spleen, not elsewhere classified*

Angiosarcoma }
Fibrosarcoma } of spleen

Excludes: Hodgkin's disease (201.–)
            lymphosarcoma (200.1)
            reticulosarcoma (200.0)

159.8   *Other* [see Note 4, page 101]

Malignant neoplasm of digestive organs and peritoneum whose point of
    origin cannot be assigned to any one of the categories 150-158

Excludes: cardio-oesophageal junction (151.0)
            colon and rectum (154.0)

159.9   *Ill-defined*

Alimentary canal or tract NOS   Gastrointestinal tract NOS

MALIGNANT NEOPLASM OF RESPIRATORY AND INTRATHORACIC
ORGANS (160-165)

160   Malignant neoplasm of nasal cavities, middle ear and accessory sinuses

160.0   *Nasal cavities*

Cartilage of nose   Septum of nose
Conchae, nasal   Vestibule of nose
Internal nose

Excludes: nasal bone (170.0)
            nose NOS (195.0)
            olfactory bulb (192.0)
            posterior margin of septum and choanae (147.3)
            skin of nose (172.3, 173.3)

160.1   *Auditory tube, middle ear and mastoid air cells*

Antrum tympanicum   Tympanic cavity
Eustachian tube

Excludes: auricular canal (external) (172.2, 173.2)
            bone of ear (meatus) (170.0)
            cartilage of ear (171.0)
            ear (external) (skin) (172.2, 173.2)

160.2   *Maxillary sinus*

Antrum (Highmore) (maxillary)

160.3   *Ethmoidal sinus*

160.4   *Frontal sinus*

160.5   *Sphenoidal sinus*

160.8   *Other* [see Note 4, page 101]

160.9   *Accessory sinus, unspecified*

161   Malignant neoplasm of larynx

161.0   *Glottis*

Intrinsic larynx   True vocal cord
Laryngeal commissure (anterior)   Vocal cord NOS
  (posterior)

161.1   *Supraglottis*

Aryepiglottic fold or interarytenoid fold, laryngeal aspect
Epiglottis (suprahyoid portion) NOS
Extrinsic larynx
False vocal cords
Posterior (laryngeal) surface of epiglottis
Ventricular bands

Excludes: anterior aspect of epiglottis (146.4)
            aryepiglottic fold or interarytenoid fold:
                NOS (148.2)
                hypopharyngeal aspect (148.2)
                marginal zone (148.2)

161.2   *Subglottis*

161.3   *Laryngeal cartilages*

Cartilage: Cartilage:
  arytenoid   cuneiform
  cricoid   thyroid

161.8   *Other* [see Note 4, page 101]

161.9   *Larynx, unspecified*

162   Malignant neoplasm of trachea, bronchus and lung

162.0   *Trachea*

162.2   *Main bronchus*

Carina   Hilus

162.3 *Upper lobe, bronchus or lung*

162.4 *Middle lobe, bronchus or lung*

162.5 *Lower lobe, bronchus or lung*

162.8 *Other* [see Note 4, page 101]

162.9 *Bronchus and lung, unspecified*

163 Malignant neoplasm of pleura

163.0 *Parietal*

163.1 *Visceral*

163.8 *Other* [see Note 4, page 101]

163.9 *Pleura, unspecified*

164 Malignant neoplasm of thymus, heart and mediastinum

164.0 *Thymus*

164.1 *Heart*

Pericardium

Excludes: great vessels (171.4)

164.2 *Anterior mediastinum*

164.3 *Posterior mediastinum*

164.8 *Other* [see Note 4, page 101]

164.9 *Mediastinum, part unspecified*

165 Malignant neoplasm of other and ill-defined sites within the respiratory system and intrathoracic organs

165.0 *Upper respiratory tract, part unspecified*

165.8 *Other* [see Note 4, page 101]

Malignant neoplasms of respiratory and intrathoracic organs whose point of origin cannot be assigned to any one of the categories 160-164

165.9 *Ill-defined sites within the respiratory system*

Respiratory tract NOS

Excludes: intrathoracic NOS (195.1)
thoracic NOS (195.1)

MALIGNANT NEOPLASM OF BONE, CONNECTIVE TISSUE, SKIN AND
BREAST (170-175)

170   Malignant neoplasm of bone and articular cartilage

Excludes: bone marrow NOS (202.9)
    cartilage:
     ear (171.0)
     eyelid (171.0)
     larynx (161.3)
     nose (160.0)
     synovia (171.–)

170.0   *Bones of skull and face*

Bone:	Bone:
ethmoid	parietal
frontal	sphenoid
malar	temporal
nasal	Maxilla
occipital	Turbinate
orbital	Vomer

Excludes: carcinoma, any type other than intraosseous or odontogenic:
    maxilla, maxillary (sinus) (160.2)
    upper jaw bone (143.0)
   jaw bone (lower) (170.1)

170.1   *Lower jaw bone*

Mandible   Jaw bone NOS

Excludes: carcinoma, any type other than intraosseous or odontogenic:
    jaw bone NOS (143.9)
     lower (143.1)
    upper jaw bone (170.0)

170.2   *Vertebral column, excluding sacrum and coccyx*

Spinal column   Vertebra
Spine

170.3   *Ribs, sternum and clavicle*

Costal cartilage   Xiphoid process

170.4   *Long bones of upper limb and scapula*

Acromion process   Radius
Bone NOS of upper limb   Ulna
Humerus

170.5   *Upper limb, short bones*

Carpal   Scaphoid (of hand)
Cuneiform, wrist   Semilunar or lunate
Metacarpal   Trapezium
Phalanges of hand   Trapezoid
Pisiform   Unciform

170.6   *Pelvic bones, sacrum and coccyx*

Coccygeal vertebra   Pubic bone
Ilium   Sacral vertebra
Ischium

170.7   *Lower limb, long bones*

Bones NOS of lower limb   Fibula
Femur   Tibia

170.8   *Lower limb, short bones*

Astragalus   Navicular (of ankle)
Calcaneus   Patella
Cuboid   Phalanges of foot
Cuneiform, ankle   Tarsal
Metatarsal

170.9   *Site unspecified*

Chondrosarcoma ⎫
Chondromyxosarcoma ⎪
Ewing's sarcoma or tumour ⎬ site unspecified
Osteosarcoma ⎭

171   Malignant neoplasm of connective and other soft tissue

Includes: blood vessel   peripheral, sympathetic and para-
            bursa   sympathetic nerves and
            fascia   ganglia
            ligament, except uterine synovia
            muscle   tendon (sheath)
Excludes: cartilage (of):
                articular (170.–)
                larynx (161.3)
                nose (160.0)
            connective tissue of breast (174.–)
            heart (164.1)

171.0   *Head, face and neck*

Cartilage of:
  ear
  eyelid

171.2   *Upper limb, including shoulder*

171.3   *Lower limb, including hip*

171.4   *Thorax*

Axilla   Great vessels
Diaphragm
Excludes: thymus, heart and mediastinum (164.–)

171.5 *Abdomen*

Abdominal wall　　　　　　Hypochondrium

171.6 *Pelvis*

Buttock　　　　　　　　　Perineum
Groin

Excludes: uterine ligament, any (183.–)

171.7 *Trunk, unspecified*

Back NOS

171.8 *Other* [see Note 4, page 101]

171.9 *Site unspecified*

Fibrosarcoma
Haemangiosarcoma
Leiomysarcoma
Liposarcoma
Lymphangiosarcoma　⎰ site unspecified
Myosarcoma
Myxosarcoma
Rhabdomyosarcoma
Sarcoma
Sarcomatosis

172　Malignant melanoma of skin

Includes: melanocarcinoma
　　　　　melanoma (skin) NOS

Excludes: skin of genital organs (184.–, 187.–)

172.0 *Lip*

Excludes: vermilion border of lip (140.–)

172.1 *Eyelid, including canthus*

172.2 *Ear and external auricular canal*

Auricle (ear)　　　　　　Pinna
External meatus

172.3 *Other and unspecified parts of face*

Cheek (external)　　　　　Nose, external
Eyebrow　　　　　　　　Temple

172.4 *Scalp and neck*

172.5   *Trunk, except scrotum*

Axilla	Perianal skin
Breast	Perineum
Buttock	Umbilicus
Groin	

Excludes: anus NOS (154.3)
              scrotum (187.7)

172.6   *Upper limb including shoulder*

172.7   *Lower limb including hip*

172.8   *Other* [see Note 4, page 101]

172.9   *Site unspecified*

173   **Other malignant neoplasm of skin**

Includes: malignant neoplasm of:
              sebaceous glands
              sweat glands
Excludes: malignant melanoma of skin (172.–)
              skin of genital organs (184.–, 187.–)

173.0   *Skin of lip*
Excludes: vermilion border of lip (140.–)

173.1   *Eyelid, including canthus*
Excludes: cartilage of eyelid (171.0)

173.2   *Ear and external auricular canal*

Auricle (ear)	Pinna
External meatus	

Excludes: cartilage of ear (171.0)

173.3   *Skin of other and unspecified parts of face*

Cheek, external	Nose, external
Eyebrow	Temple

173.4   *Scalp and skin of neck*

173.5   *Skin of trunk, except scrotum*

Axillary fold	Skin of:
Perianal skin	breast
Umbilicus	buttock
Skin of:	chest wall
abdominal wall	groin
anus	perineum
back	

Excludes: anal canal (154.2)
              anus NOS (154.3)
              skin of scrotum (187.7)

173.6 *Skin of upper limb, including shoulder*

173.7 *Skin of lower limb, including hip*

173.8 *Other* [see Note 4, page 101]

173.9 *Site unspecified*

174   Malignant neoplasm of female breast

Includes: breast (female)   Paget's disease of:
             connective tissue   breast
             soft parts   nipple

Excludes: skin of breast (172.5, 173.5)

174.0 *Nipple and areola*

174.1 *Central portion*

174.2 *Upper-inner quadrant*

174.3 *Lower-inner quadrant*

174.4 *Upper-outer quadrant*

174.5 *Lower-outer quadrant*

174.6 *Axillary tail*

174.8 *Other* [see Note 4, page 101]
Ectopic sites

174.9 *Breast, unspecified*

175   Malignant neoplasm of male breast

Excludes: skin of breast (172.5, 173.5)

MALIGNANT NEOPLASM OF GENITOURINARY ORGANS (179-189)

179   Malignant neoplasm of uterus, part unspecified

180   Malignant neoplasm of cervix uteri

180.0 *Endocervix*
Cervical canal   Endocervical gland
Endocervical canal

180.1 *Exocervix*

180.8   *Other* [see Note 4, page 101]

180.9   *Cervix uteri, unspecified*

181   Malignant neoplasm of placenta

Choriocarcinoma NOS   Chorionepithelioma NOS

Excludes: chorioadenoma (destruens) (236.1)
                  hydatidiform mole (630)
                        malignant (236.1)

182   Malignant neoplasm of body of uterus

182.0   *Corpus uteri, except isthmus*

Cornu   Fundus
Endometrium   Myometrium

182.1   *Isthmus*

Lower uterine segment

182.8   *Other* [see Note 4, page 101]

183   Malignant neoplasm of ovary and other uterine adnexa

183.0   *Ovary*

183.2   *Fallopian tube*

Oviduct   Uterine tube

183.3   *Broad ligament*

183.4   *Parametrium*

Uterine ligament NOS

183.5   *Round ligament*

183.8   *Other* [see Note 4, page 101]

183.9   *Uterine adnexa, unspecified*

184   Malignant neoplasm of other and unspecified female genital organs

184.0   *Vagina*

184.1   *Labia majora*

Greater vestibular [Bartholin's] gland

184.2   *Labia minora*

184.3   *Clitoris*

184.4 *Vulva, unspecified*
External female genitalia NOS   Pudendum

184.8 *Other* [see Note 4, page 101]

184.9 *Site unspecified*
Female genitourinary tract NOS

185   Malignant neoplasm of prostate

186   Malignant neoplasm of testis

186.0 *Undescended*
Ectopic testis   Retained testis

186.9 *Other and unspecified*
Testis:
  NOS
  descended
  scrotal

187   Malignant neoplasm of penis and other male genital organs

187.1 *Prepuce*
Foreskin

187.2 *Glans penis*

187.3 *Body of penis*
Corpus cavernosum

187.4 *Penis, part unspecified*
Skin of penis NOS

187.5 *Epididymis*

187.6 *Spermatic cord*

187.7 *Scrotum*
Skin of scrotum

187.8 *Other* [see Note 4, page 101]
Seminal vesicle   Tunica vaginalis

187.9 *Site unspecified*
Male genital organ or tract NOS

188   Malignant neoplasm of bladder

188.0 *Trigone*

188.1 *Dome*

188.2 *Lateral wall*

188.3 *Anterior wall*

188.4 *Posterior wall*

188.5 *Bladder neck*
Internal urethral orifice

188.6 *Ureteric orifice*

188.7 *Urachus*

188.8 *Other* [see Note 4, page 101]

188.9 *Part unspecified*

189 Malignant neoplasm of kidney and other and unspecified urinary organs

189.0 *Kidney, except pelvis*

189.1 *Renal pelvis*
Pelviureteric junction   Renal calyces

189.2 *Ureter*
Excludes: ureteric orifice of bladder (188.6)

189.3 *Urethra*
Excludes: urethral orifice of bladder (188.5)

189.4 *Paraurethral glands*

189.8 *Other* [see Note 4, page 101]

189.9 *Site unspecified*
Urinary system NOS

MALIGNANT NEOPLASM OF OTHER AND UNSPECIFIED SITES
(190-199)

190 Malignant neoplasm of eye
Excludes: cartilage of eyelid (171.0)
eyelid (skin) (172.1, 173.1)
optic nerve (192.0)
orbital bone (170.0)

190.0 *Eyeball, except conjunctiva, cornea, retina and choroid*
Ciliary body

190.1 *Orbit*

Connective tissue of orbit   Retrobulbar
Extraocular muscle
Excludes: orbital bone (170.0)

190.2 *Lacrimal gland*

190.3 *Conjunctiva*

190.4 *Cornea*

190.5 *Retina*

190.6 *Choroid*

190.7 *Lacrimal duct*

Lacrimal sac   Nasolacrimal duct

190.8 *Other* [see Note 4, page 101]

190.9 *Part unspecified*

191   Malignant neoplasm of brain

Excludes: cranial nerves (192.–)
           retrobulbar (190.1)

191.0 *Cerebrum, except lobes and ventricles*

191.1 *Frontal lobe*

191.2 *Temporal lobe*

191.3 *Parietal lobe*

191.4 *Occipital lobe*

191.5 *Ventricle*
Floor of ventricle

191.6 *Cerebellum*

191.7 *Brain stem*

191.8 *Other* [see Note 4, page 101]

191.9 *Brain, unspecified*

Astrocytoma ⎫
Astroblastoma ⎪
Ependymoma ⎪
Glioma   ⎬ site unspecified
Medulloblastoma ⎪
Neuroepithelioma ⎪
Oligodendroblastoma ⎭

192   Malignant neoplasm of other and unspecified parts of nervous system

Excludes: peripheral, sympathetic and parasympathetic nerves and ganglia (171.–)

192.0   *Cranial nerves*

192.1   *Cerebral meninges*

Meninges NOS

192.2   *Spinal cord*

192.3   *Spinal meninges*

192.8   *Other* [see Note 4, page 101]

192.9   *Part unspecified*

Nervous system (central) NOS

Excludes: meninges NOS (192.1)

193   Malignant neoplasm of thyroid gland

194   Malignant neoplasm of other endocrine glands and related structures

Excludes: islets of Langerhans (157.4)

194.0   *Suprarenal gland*

Adrenal gland

194.1   *Parathyroid gland*

194.3   *Pituitary gland and craniopharyngeal duct*

194.4   *Pineal gland*

194.5   *Carotid body*

194.6   *Aortic body and other paraganglia*

194.8   *Other*

Pluriglandular involvement NOS

Note: If the sites of multiple involvement are known, they should be coded separately.

194.9   *Site unspecified*

Endocrine gland NOS

195 Malignant neoplasm of other and ill-defined sites

Includes: overlapping neoplasms, not elsewhere classified [see Note 4, page 101]

Excludes: malignant neoplasm:
lymphatic and haematopoietic tissue (200-208)
unspecified site (199.–)

195.0 *Head, face and neck*

Cheek NOS   Nose NOS

195.1 *Thorax*

Axilla

195.2 *Abdomen*

195.3 *Pelvis*

Groin
Sites overlapping systems within the pelvis, such as:
rectovesical (septum)
rectovaginal (septum)

195.4 *Upper limb*

195.5 *Lower limb*

195.8 *Other specified sites*

196 Secondary and unspecified malignant neoplasm of lymph nodes

Excludes: any malignant neoplasm of lymph nodes, specified as primary (200-202)
Hodgkin's disease (201.–)
lymphosarcoma (200.1)
other forms of lymphoma (202.–)
recticulosarcoma (200.0)

Note: This category should not be used for coding underlying cause of death [see page 727].

196.0 *Head, face and neck*

Cervicofacial   Supraclavicular

196.1 *Intrathoracic*

Bronchopulmonary   Tracheobronchial
Mediastinal

196.2 *Intra-abdominal*

Intestinal   Retroperitoneal
Mesenteric

196.3   *Axilla and upper limb*
Brachial   Pectoral
Epitrochlear

196.5   *Inguinal and lower limb*
Groin   Tibial
Popliteal

196.6   *Intrapelvic*
Iliac   Obturator

196.8   *Multiple sites*

196.9   *Site unspecified*
Lymph nodes NOS

197   Secondary malignant neoplasm of respiratory and digestive systems

Note: This category should not be used for coding underlying cause of
        death [see page 727].

197.0   *Lung*

197.1   *Mediastinum*

197.2   *Pleura*

197.3   *Other respiratory organs*

197.4   *Small intestine, including duodenum*

197.5   *Large intestine and rectum*

197.6   *Retroperitoneum and peritoneum*

197.7   *Liver*

197.8   *Other digestive organs*

198   Secondary malignant neoplasm of other specified sites

Note: This category should not be used for coding underlying cause of
        death [see page 727].

198.0   *Kidney*

198.1   *Other urinary organs*

198.2   *Skin*

198.3   *Brain and spinal cord*

198.4   *Other parts of nervous system*
Meninges (cerebral) (spinal)

198.5 *Bone and bone marrow*

198.6 *Ovary*

198.7 *Suprarenal gland*

198.8 *Other specified sites*

199 Malignant neoplasm without specification of site

199.0 *Disseminated*

Carcinomatosis	
Generalised:	unspecified site
cancer	(primary)
malignancy	(secondary)
Multiple cancer	

199.1 *Other*

Carcinoma	unspecified site
Cancer	(primary)
Malignancy	(secondary)

MALIGNANT NEOPLASM OF LYMPHATIC AND HAEMATOPOIETIC
TISSUE (200-208)

Excludes: secondary and unspecified neoplasm of lymph nodes (196.–)

200 Lymphosarcoma and reticulosarcoma

200.0 *Reticulosarcoma*

200.1 *Lymphosarcoma*

Excludes: lymphosarcoma-cell leukaemia (207.8)

200.2 *Burkitt's tumour*

200.8 *Other named variants*

Reticulolymphosarcoma

201 Hodgkin's disease

Note: Two alternative sub-classifications are given:
      .0-.2 Parker-Jackson
      .4-.7 Rye modification of Lukes-Butler
This departure from the principle that categories should be
mutually exclusive is deliberate, since both forms of terminology
are currently encountered on medical records.

201.0   *Hodgkin's paragranuloma*

201.1   *Hodgkin's granuloma*

201.2   *Hodgkin's sarcoma*

201.4   *Lymphocytic-histiocytic predominance*

201.5   *Nodular sclerosis*

201.6   *Mixed cellularity*

201.7   *Lymphocytic depletion*

201.9   *Unspecified*

202   Other malignant neoplasm of lymphoid and histiocytic tissue

202.0   *Nodular lymphoma*
Brill-Symmers disease   Follicular lymphoma

202.1   *Mycosis fungoides*

202.2   *Sézary's disease*

202.3   *Malignant histiocytosis*

202.4   *Leukaemic reticuloendotheliosis*
Hairy-cell leukaemia

202.5   *Letterer-Siwe disease*
Acute differentiated progressive   Acute (progressive) histiocytosis X
    histiocytosis   Acute reticulosis of infancy
Acute infantile reticuloendotheliosis
Excludes: histiocytosis (acute) (chronic) (277.8)
            histiocytosis X (chronic) (277.8)

202.6   *Malignant mast-cell tumours*
Malignant: Mast-cell sarcoma
    mastocytoma
    mastocytosis
Excludes: mast-cell leukaemia (207.8)

202.8   *Other lymphomas*
Lymphoma (malignant):
    NOS
    diffuse

202.9   *Other and unspecified*

203   Multiple myeloma and immunoproliferative neoplasms

203.0 *Multiple myeloma*

Kahler's disease   Myelomatosis

Excludes: solitary myeloma (238.6)

203.1 *Plasma cell leukaemia*

203.8 *Other immunoproliferative neoplasms*

204   Lymphoid leukaemia

Includes: leukaemia:
            lymphatic
            lymphocytic

204.0 *Acute*

Excludes: acute exacerbation of chronic lymphoid leukaemia (204.1)

204.1 *Chronic*

204.2 *Subacute*

204.8 *Other*

204.9 *Unspecified*

205   Myeloid leukaemia

Includes: leukaemia:
            granulocytic
            myelogenous

205.0 *Acute*

Excludes: acute exacerbation of chronic myeloid leukaemia (205.1)

205.1 *Chronic*

205.2 *Subacute*

205.3 *Myeloid sarcoma*

Chloroma   Granulocytic sarcoma

205.8 *Other*

205.9 *Unspecified*

206   Monocytic leukaemia

Includes: monocytoid leukaemia

206.0 *Acute*

Excludes: acute exacerbation of chronic monocytic leukaemia (206.1)

206.1 *Chronic*

206.2 *Subacute*

206.8 *Other*

206.9 *Unspecified*

207 Other specified leukaemia

Excludes: leukaemic reticuloendotheliosis (202.4)
           plasma cell leukaemia (203.1)

207.0 *Acute erythraemia and erythroleukaemia*

Acute erythraemic myelosis   Di Guglielmo's disease

207.1 *Chronic erythraemia*

Heilmeyer-Schöner disease

207.2 *Megakaryocytic leukaemia*

207.8 *Other*

Lymphosarcoma cell leukaemia

208 Leukaemia of unspecified cell type

208.0 *Acute*

Acute leukaemia NOS   Stem cell leukaemia
Blast cell leukaemia

Excludes: acute exacerbation of unspecified leukaemia (208.1)

208.1 *Chronic*

Chronic leukaemia NOS

208.2 *Subacute*

Subacute leukaemia NOS

208.8 *Other*

208.9 *Unspecified*

Leukaemia NOS

BENIGN NEOPLASMS (210-229)

210 Benign neoplasm of lip, oral cavity and pharynx

Excludes: cyst of jaw (522.–, 526.–)
           cyst of oral soft tissue (528.–)

210.0 *Lip*

Frenulum labii   Lip (inner aspect) (mucosa) (ver-
                                         milion border)

Excludes: labial commissure (210.4)
             skin of lip (216.0)

210.1 *Tongue*

Lingual tonsil

210.2 *Major salivary glands*

Gland:
  parotid
  sublingual
  submandibular

Excludes: benign neoplasms of minor salivary glands which are to be
             classified according to their anatomical location; if lo-
             cation is not specified, classify to 210.4

210.3 *Floor of mouth*

210.4 *Other and unspecified parts of mouth*

Gingiva   Oral mucosa
Labial commissure   Palate (hard) (soft)
Oral cavity NOS   Uvula

Excludes: benign odontogenic neoplasms (213.–)
             mucosa of lips (210.0)
             nasopharyngeal [posterior] [superior] surface of soft palate
             (210.7)

210.5 *Tonsil*

Tonsil (faucial) (palatine)

Excludes: lingual tonsil (210.1)
             pharyngeal tonsil (210.7)
             tonsillar:
               fossa (210.6)
               pillars (210.6)

210.6 *Other parts of oropharynx*

Epiglottis, anterior aspect   Vallecula
Tonsillar:
  fossa
  pillars

Excludes: epiglottis:
             NOS (212.1)
             suprahyoid portion (212.1)

210.7   *Nasopharynx*

210.8   *Hypopharynx*

210.9   *Pharynx, unspecified*

211   Benign neoplasm of other parts of digestive system

211.0   *Oesophagus*

211.1   *Stomach*

211.2   *Small intestine, including duodenum*
Excludes: ampulla of Vater (211.5)
            ileocaecal valve (211.3)

211.3   *Colon*
Excludes: rectosigmoid junction (211.4)

211.4   *Rectum and anal canal*
Anus NOS
Excludes: anus:
               margin (216.5)
               skin (216.5)
               perianal skin (216.5)

211.5   *Liver and biliary passages*

211.6   *Pancreas, except islets of Langerhans*

211.7   *Islets of Langerhans*
Islet cell tumour

211.8   *Retroperitoneum and peritoneum*

211.9   *Other and unspecified site*
Alimentary canal or tract NOS   Intestine NOS
Gastrointestinal tract NOS   Spleen, not elsewhere classified

212   Benign neoplasm of respiratory and intrathoracic organs

212.0   *Nasal cavities, middle ear and accessory sinuses*
Excludes: auricular canal (external) (216.2)
            bone of:
               ear (213.0)
               nose (213.0)
            cartilage of ear (215.0)
            ear (external) (skin) (216.2)

      nose NOS (229.8)
        skin (216.3)
      olfactory bulb (225.1)
      polyp of:
        accessory sinus (471.8)
        ear (387.9)
        nasal cavity (471.0)
      posterior margin of septum and choanae (210.7)

212.1 *Larynx*
Excludes: epiglottis, anterior aspect (210.6)
         polyp of vocal cord or larynx (478.4)

212.2 *Trachea*

212.3 *Bronchus and lung*

212.4 *Pleura*

212.5 *Mediastinum*

212.6 *Thymus*

212.7 *Heart*
Excludes: great vessels (215.4)

212.8 *Other specified sites*

212.9 *Site unspecified*
Respiratory organ NOS
Upper respiratory tract NOS
Excludes: intrathoracic NOS (229.8)
        thoracic NOS (229.8)

213   Benign neoplasm of bone and articular cartilage
Excludes: cartilage of:
        ear (215.0)
        eyelid (215.0)
        larynx (212.1)
        nose (212.0)
        synovia (215.–)

213.0 *Bones of skull and face*
Excludes: lower jaw bone (213.1)

213.1 *Lower jaw bone*

213.2 *Vertebral column, excluding sacrum and coccyx*

213.3 *Ribs, sternum and clavicle*

213.4 *Long bones of upper limb and scapula*

213.5 *Upper limb, short bones*

213.6 *Pelvic bones, sacrum and coccyx*

213.7 *Lower limb, long bones*

213.8 *Lower limb, short bones*

213.9 *Site unspecified*

Chondroma ⎱
Osteoma ⎰ site unspecified

214 Lipoma

Angiolipoma ⎫
Fibrolipoma ⎪
Hibernoma ⎬ any site
Lipoma (fetal) (infiltrating) (intramuscular) ⎪
Myxolipoma ⎭

215 Other benign neoplasm of connective and other soft tissue

Includes: blood vessel   peripheral, sympathetic and
           bursa   parasympathetic nerves and
           fascia   ganglia
           ligament   synovia
           muscle   tendon (sheath)

Excludes: cartilage:
               articular (213.–)
               larynx (212.1)
               nose (212.0)
           connective tissue of breast (217)

215.0 *Head, face and neck*

215.2 *Upper limb, including shoulder*

215.3 *Lower limb, including hip*

215.4 *Thorax*
Excludes: heart (212.7)
           mediastinum (212.5)
           thymus (212.6)

215.5 *Abdomen*

215.6 *Pelvis*
Excludes: uterine:
               leiomyoma (218)
               ligament, any (221.0)

215.7 *Trunk, unspecified*
Back NOS

215.8 *Other specified sites*

215.9 *Site unspecified*
Leiomyoma ⎫
Myoma ⎪
Myxofibroma ⎬ site unspecified
Myxoma ⎪
Rhabdomyoma ⎭

216   Benign neoplasm of skin

Includes: blue naevus   pigmented naevus
           dermatofibroma   syringoadenoma
           hydrocystoma   syringoma
Excludes: skin of genital organs (221.–, 222.–)

216.0 *Skin of lip*
Excludes: vermilion border of lip (210.0)

216.1 *Eyelid, including canthus*
Excludes: cartilage of eyelid (215.0)

216.2 *Ear and external auricular canal*
Auricle (ear)   Pinna
External meatus
Excludes: cartilage of ear (215.0)

216.3 *Skin of other and unspecified parts of face*
Cheek, external   Nose, external
Eyebrow   Temple

216.4 *Scalp and skin of neck*

216.5 *Skin of trunk, except scrotum*
Axillary fold   Skin of:
Perianal skin   abdominal wall
Umbilicus   anus
                              back
                              breast
                              buttock
                              chest wall
                              groin
                              perineum

Excludes: anal canal (211.4)
           anus NOS (211.4)
           skin of scrotum (222.4)

216.6   *Skin of upper limb, including shoulder*

216.7   *Skin of lower limb, including hip*

216.8   *Other*

216.9   *Site unspecified*

217   Benign neoplasm of breast

Breast (male) (female)
  connective tissue
  soft parts

Excludes: benign cyst of breast (610.–)
           skin of breast (216.5)

218   Uterine leiomyoma

Fibroid (uterus)   Fibromyoma ⎫ uterus
                                       Myoma   ⎭

219   Other benign neoplasm of uterus

219.0   *Cervix uteri*

219.1   *Corpus uteri*

219.8   *Other specified parts*

219.9   *Part unspecified*

220   Benign neoplasm of ovary

221   Benign neoplasm of other female genital organs

Includes: adenomatous polyp
           benign teratoma

221.0   *Uterine tube and ligaments*

Fallopian tube   Uterine ligament (broad) (round)
Oviduct

221.1   *Vagina*

221.2   *Vulva*

Clitoris   Labia (majora) (minora)
External female genitalia NOS   Pudendum
Greater vestibular [Bartholin's] gland

221.8   *Other specified sites*

221.9   *Site unspecified*

222   Benign neoplasm of male genital organs

222.0   *Testis*

222.1   *Penis*

Corpus cavernosum   Prepuce
Glans penis

222.2   *Prostate*

Excludes: adenomatous hyperplasia of prostate (600)
                 prostatic:
                     adenoma (600)
                     enlargement (600)
                     hypertrophy (600)

222.3   *Epididymis*

222.4   *Scrotum*

Skin of scrotum

222.8   *Other specified sites*

Seminal vesicle   Spermatic cord

222.9   *Site unspecified*

223   Benign neoplasm of kidney and other urinary organs

223.0   *Kidney, except pelvis*

Excludes: renal:
                 calyces (223.1)
                 pelvis (223.1)

223.1   *Renal pelvis*

223.2   *Ureter*

Excludes: ureteric orifice of bladder (223.3)

223.3   *Bladder*

223.8   *Other specified sites*

Paraurethral glands   Urethra
Excludes: urethral orifice of bladder (223.3)

223.9   *Site unspecified*

Urinary system NOS

224   Benign neoplasm of eye

Excludes: cartilage of eyelid (215.0)
           eyelid (skin) (216.1)
           optic nerve (225.1)
           orbital bone (213.0)

224.0 *Eyeball, except conjunctiva, cornea, retina and choroid*

224.1 *Orbit*

224.2 *Lacrimal gland*

224.3 *Conjunctiva*

224.4 *Cornea*

224.5 *Retina*

Excludes: haemangioma of retina (228.0)

224.6 *Choroid*

224.7 *Lacrimal duct*

Lacrimal sac   Nasolacrimal duct

224.8 *Other specified parts*

224.9 *Part unspecified*

225   Benign neoplasm of brain and other parts of nervous system

Excludes: haemangioma (228.0)
           peripheral, sympathetic and parasympathetic nerves and
               ganglia (215.–)
           retrobulbar (224.1)

225.0 *Brain*

225.1 *Cranial nerves*

225.2 *Cerebral meninges*

Meninges NOS   Meningioma (cerebral)

225.3 *Spinal cord*

225.4 *Spinal meninges*

Spinal meningioma

225.8 *Other*

225.9 *Part unspecified*

Nervous system (central) NOS

Excludes: meninges NOS (225.2)

226   Benign neoplasm of thyroid gland

227   Benign neoplasm of other endocrine glands and related structures

227.0   *Suprarenal gland*

Adrenal gland

227.1   *Parathyroid gland*

227.3   *Pituitary gland and craniopharyngeal duct*

227.4   *Pineal gland*

227.5   *Carotid body*

227.6   *Aortic body and other paraganglia*

227.8   *Other*

227.9   *Site unspecified*

Endocrine gland NOS

228   Haemangioma and lymphangioma, any site

Excludes: blue or pigmented naevus (216.–)

228.0   *Haemangioma, any site*

Angioma (benign) (cavernous) (congenital) NOS	Naevus: NOS
Glomus tumour	cavernous
Haemangioma (benign) (congenital)	vascular
	Systemic angiomatosis

228.1   *Lymphangioma, any site*

Congenital lymphangioma   Lymphatic naevus

229   Benign neoplasm of other and unspecified sites

229.0   *Lymph nodes*

229.8   *Other specified sites*

229.9   *Site unspecified*

CARCINOMA IN SITU   (230–234)

Includes: Bowen's disease
             erythroplasia
             Queyrat's erythroplasia

230   Carcinoma in situ of digestive organs

230.0   *Lip, oral cavity and pharynx*

Gingiva   Oropharynx
Hypopharynx   Salivary gland or duct
Mouth [any part]   Tongue
Nasopharynx

Excludes: aryepiglottic fold or interarytenoid fold, laryngeal aspect
             (231.0)
           epiglottis:
             NOS (231.0)
             suprahyoid portion (231.0)
           skin of lip (232.0)

230.1   *Oesophagus*

230.2   *Stomach*

230.3   *Colon*

Excludes: rectosigmoid junction (230.4)

230.4   *Rectum*

230.5   *Anal canal*

230.6   *Anus, unspecified*

Excludes: anus:
               margin (232.5)
               skin (232.5)
             perianal skin (232.5)

230.7   *Other and unspecified parts of intestine*

Excludes: ampulla of Vater (230.8)

230.8   *Liver and biliary system*

230.9   *Other and unspecified digestive organs*

Digestive organ NOS   Pancreas

231   Carcinoma in situ of respiratory system

231.0   *Larynx*

Excludes: aryepiglottic fold or interarytenoid fold:
               NOS (230.0)
               hypopharyngeal aspect (230.0)
               marginal zone (230.0)

231.1   *Trachea*

231.2   *Bronchus and lung*

231.8   *Other specified parts*

Accessory sinuses   Nasal cavities
Middle ear

Excludes: ear (external) (skin) (232.2)
                  nose NOS (234.8)
                      skin (232.3)

231.9   *Part unspecified*

Respiratory organ NOS

232   Carcinoma in situ of skin

Includes: pigment cells

232.0   *Skin of lip*

Excludes: vermilion border of lip (230.0)

232.1   *Eyelid, including canthus*

232.2   *Ear and external auricular canal*

232.3   *Skin of other and unspecified parts of face*

232.4   *Scalp and skin of neck*

232.5   *Skin of trunk, except scrotum*

Anus, margin   Skin of:
Axillary fold   abdominal wall
Perianal skin   anus
Umbilicus   back
                                   breast
                                   buttock
                                   chest wall
                                   groin
                                   perineum

Excludes: anal canal (230.5)
                  anus NOS (230.6)
                  skin of genital organs (233.3, 233.5, 233.6)

232.6   *Skin of upper limb, including shoulder*

232.7   *Skin of lower limb, including hip*

232.8   *Other specified sites*

232.9   *Site unspecified*

233   Carcinoma in situ of breast and genitourinary system

233.0   *Breast*

Excludes: skin of breast (232.5)

233.1 *Cervix uteri*

233.2 *Other and unspecified parts of uterus*

233.3 *Other and unspecified female genital organs*

233.4 *Prostate*

233.5 *Penis*

233.6 *Other and unspecified male genital organs*

233.7 *Bladder*

233.9 *Other and unspecified urinary organs*

234 Carcinoma in situ of other and unspecified sites

234.0 *Eye*
Excludes: eyelid (skin) (232.1)

234.8 *Other specified sites*
Endocrine gland [any]

234.9 *Site unspecified*
Carcinoma in situ NOS

NEOPLASMS OF UNCERTAIN BEHAVIOUR (235-238)

Note: Categories 235-238 classify by site certain histo-morphologically well-defined neoplasms the subsequent behaviour of which cannot be predicted from their present appearance.

235 Neoplasm of uncertain behaviour of digestive and respiratory systems

235.0 *Major salivary glands*
Gland:
  parotid
  sublingual
  submandibular

235.1 *Lip, oral cavity and pharynx*

Gingiva	Nasopharynx
Hypopharynx	Oropharynx
Mouth	Tongue

Excludes: aryepiglottic fold or interarytenoid fold, laryngeal aspect (235.6)
         epiglottis:
           NOS (235.6)
           suprahyoid portion (235.6)
         skin of lip (238.2)

235.2 *Stomach, intestines and rectum*

235.3 *Liver and biliary passages*

Ampulla of Vater   Gallbladder
Bile ducts [any]   Liver

235.4 *Retroperitoneum and peritoneum*

235.5 *Other and unspecified digestive organs*

Anal: Anus NOS
  canal   Oesophagus
  sphincter   Pancreas

Excludes: anus:
      margin (238.2)
      skin (238.2)
      perianal skin (238.2)

235.6 *Larynx*

Excludes: aryepiglottic fold or interarytenoid fold:
      NOS (235.1)
      hypopharyngeal aspect (235.1)
      marginal zone (235.1)

235.7 *Trachea, bronchus and lung*

235.8 *Pleura, thymus and mediastinum*

235.9 *Other and unspecified respiratory organs*

Accessory sinuses   Nasal cavities
Middle ear   Respiratory organ NOS

Excludes: ear (external) (skin) (238.2)
      nose (238.8)
        skin (238.2)

236 Neoplasm of uncertain behaviour of genitourinary organs

236.0 *Uterus*

236.1 *Placenta*

Chorioadenoma (destruens)   Malignant hydatid(iform) mole

236.2 *Ovary*

236.3 *Other and unspecified female genital organs*

236.4 *Testis*

236.5 *Prostate*

236.6 *Other and unspecified male genital organs*

236.7 *Bladder*

236.9 *Other and unspecified urinary organs*
Kidney   Urethra
Ureter

237   Neoplasm of uncertain behaviour of endocrine glands and nervous system

237.0 *Pituitary gland and craniopharyngeal duct*

237.1 *Pineal gland*

237.2 *Suprarenal gland*
Adrenal gland

237.3 *Paraganglia*

237.4 *Other and unspecified endocrine glands*
Parathyroid gland   Thyroid gland

237.5 *Brain and spinal cord*

237.6 *Meninges*
Meninges:
  NOS
  cerebral
  spinal

237.7 *Neurofibromatosis*
von Recklinghausen's disease

237.9 *Other and unspecified parts of nervous system*
Cranial nerves

238   Neoplasm of uncertain behaviour of other and unspecified sites and tissues

238.0 *Bone and articular cartilage*
Excludes: cartilage:
              ear (238.1)
              eyelid (238.1)
              larynx (235.6)
              nose (235.9)
            synovia (238.1)

238.1 *Connective and other soft tissue*
Excludes: cartilage (of):
        articular (238.0)
        larynx (235.6)
        nose (235.9)
        connective tissue of breast (238.3)

238.2 *Skin*
Excludes: anus NOS (235.5)
        skin of genital organs (236.3, 236.6)
        vermilion border of lip (235.1)

238.3 *Breast*
Excludes: skin of breast (238.2)

238.4 *Polycythaemia vera*

238.5 *Histiocytic and mast cells*
Mast-cell tumour NOS   Mastocytoma NOS

238.6 *Plasma cells*
Plasmacytoma NOS   Solitary myeloma

238.7 *Other lymphatic and haematopoietic tissues*
Disease:
  lymphoproliferative (chronic) NOS
  myeloproliferative (chronic) NOS
Idiopathic thrombocythaemia
Megakaryocytic myelosclerosis
Myelosclerosis with myeloid metaplasia
Panmyelosis (acute)
Excludes: myelofibrosis (298.8)
        myelosclerosis NOS (289.8)
        myelosis:
          NOS (205.9)
          megakaryocytic (207.2)

238.8 *Other specified sites*
Eye   Heart
Excludes: eyelid (skin) (238.2)
        cartilage (238.1)

238.9 *Site unspecified*

NEOPLASMS OF UNSPECIFIED NATURE (239)

Note: Category 239 classifies by site neoplasms of unspecified morphology and behaviour.

239 Neoplasm of unspecified nature

Includes: "growth" NOS
neoplasm NOS
new growth NOS
tumour NOS

239.0 *Digestive system*

Excludes: anus:
margin (239.2)
skin (239.2)
perianal skin (239.2)

239.1 *Respiratory system*

239.2 *Bone, soft tissue and skin*

Excludes: anal canal (239.0)
anus NOS (239.0)
cartilage:
larynx (239.1)
nose (239.1)
connective tissue of breast (239.3)
skin of genital organs (239.5)
vermilion border of lip (239.8)

239.3 *Breast*

Excludes: skin of breast (239.2)

239.4 *Bladder*

239.5 *Other genitourinary organs*

239.6 *Brain*

Excludes: cerebral meninges (239.7)
cranial nerves (239.7)

239.7 *Endocrine glands, and other parts of nervous system*

Excludes: peripheral, sympathetic and parasympathetic nerves and
ganglia (239.2)

239.8 *Other specified sites*

Excludes: eyelid (skin) (239.2)
cartilage (239.2)
great vessels (239.2)
optic nerve (239.7)

239.9 *Site unspecified*

III. ENDOCRINE, NUTRITIONAL AND METABOLIC DISEASES AND IMMUNITY DISORDERS

Excludes: endocrine and metabolic disturbances specific to the fetus and newborn (775.–)

Note: All neoplasms, whether functionally active or not, are classified in Chapter II. Codes in Chapter III (i.e. 242.8, 246.0, 251-253, 255-259) may be used, if desired, to identify such functional activity associated with any neoplasm, or by ectopic endocrine tissue.

DISORDERS OF THYROID GLAND (240-246)

240 Simple and unspecified goitre

240.0 *Goitre, specified as simple*

Includes: conditions in 240.9, specified as simple

240.9 *Goitre, unspecified*

Enlargement of thyroid

Goitre or struma:
 NOS
 diffuse colloid
 endemic

Goitre or struma:
 hyperplastic
 parenchymatous

Excludes: congenital (dyshormonogenic) goitre (246.1)

241 Nontoxic nodular goitre

Excludes: adenoma of thyroid (226)
 cystadenoma of thyroid (226)

241.0 *Nontoxic uninodular goitre*

Thyroid nodule

Uninodular goitre (nontoxic)

241.1 *Nontoxic multinodular goitre*

Multinodular goitre (nontoxic)

241.9 *Unspecified*

Adenomatous goitre
Nodular goitre (nontoxic) NOS

Struma nodosa (simplex)

242 Thyrotoxicosis with or without goitre

Excludes: neonatal thyrotoxicosis (775.3)

242.0 *Toxic diffuse goitre*

Exophthalmic or toxic goitre NOS

242.1   *Toxic uninodular goitre*

Thyroid nodule ⎫
Uninodular goitre ⎭ toxic or with hyperthyroidism

242.2   *Toxic multinodular goitre*

242.3   *Toxic nodular goitre, unspecified*

Any condition in 241.9 specified as toxic or with hyperthyroidism

242.4   *Thyrotoxicosis from ectopic thyroid nodule*

242.8   *Thyrotoxicosis of other specified origin*

Overproduction of thyroid-stimulating hormone
Thyrotoxicosis:
    factitia
    from ingestion of excessive thyroid material

Use additional E code, if desired, to identify cause if drug induced

242.9   *Thyrotoxicosis without mention of goitre or other cause*

Hyperthyroidism NOS

243   Congenital hypothyroidism

Congenital thyroid insufficiency   Cretinism
Use additional code, if desired, to identify associated mental retardation
Excludes: congenital (dyshormonogenic) goitre (246.1)

244   Acquired hypothyroidism

Includes: hypothyroidism (acquired)
               myxoedema (juvenile) (adult)

244.0   *Postsurgical hypothyroidism*

244.1   *Other postablative hypothyroidism*

Hypothyroidism following therapy such as irradiation

244.2   *Iodine hypothyroidism*

Hypothyroidism resulting from administration or ingestion of iodide
Use additional E code, if desired, to identify drug

244.3   *Other iatrogenic hypothyroidism*

Hypothyroidism resulting from:
    P-aminosalicylic acid [PAS]
    Phenylbutazone
    Resorcinol
Use additional E code, if desired, to identify drug

244.8   *Other*

244.9   *Unspecified hypothyroidism*

Hypothyroidism ⎱
Myxoedema   ⎰ primary or NOS

245   Thyroiditis

245.0   *Acute thyroiditis*

Abscess of thyroid
Thyroiditis:
  pyogenic
  suppurative
Use additional code, if desired, to identify organism

245.1   *Subacute thyroiditis*

Thyroiditis:
  de Quervain's
  giant-cell
  granulomatous

245.2   *Chronic lymphocytic thyroiditis*

Autoimmune thyroiditis   Lymphocytic thyroiditis (chronic)
Hashimoto's disease   Struma lymphomatosa

245.3   *Chronic fibrous thyroiditis*

Thyroiditis:
  ligneous
  Riedel's

245.4   *Iatrogenic thyroiditis*

Use additional code, if desired, to identify cause

245.8   *Other and unspecified chronic thyroiditis*

Chronic thyroiditis NOS

245.9   *Unspecified*

Thyroiditis NOS

246   Other disorders of thyroid

246.0   *Disorders of thyrocalcitonin secretion*

Hypersecretion of calcitonin or thyrocalcitonin

246.1   *Dyshormonogenic goitre*

Congenital goitre
Goitre due to enzyme defect in synthesis of thyroid hormone

246.2 *Cyst of thyroid*

Excludes: cystadenoma (226)

246.3 *Haemorrhage and infarction of thyroid*

246.8 *Other*

Abnormality of thyroid-binding   Atrophy of thyroid
     globulin

246.9 *Unspecified*

Diseases of other endocrine glands (250-259)

250   Diabetes mellitus

The following fifth-digit subclassification may be used, if desired, with category 250:

  .0   adult-onset type
  .1   juvenile type
  .9   unspecified whether adult-onset or juvenile type

Excludes: neonatal diabetes mellitus (775.1)
           nonclinical diabetes (790.2)
           when complicating pregnancy, childbirth or the puerperium (648.0)

250.0 *Diabetes mellitus without mention of complication*

Diabetes mellitus without mention of complication or manifestation classifiable to 250.1-250.9
Diabetes (mellitus) NOS

250.1 *Diabetes with ketoacidosis*

Diabetic:
   acidosis } without mention of coma
   ketosis

250.2 *Diabetes with coma*

Diabetic coma (with ketoacidosis)   Diabetes with hyperosmolar coma

250.3† *Diabetes with renal manifestations* (581.8, 582.8, 583.8*)

Diabetic nephropathy   Kimmelstiel-Wilson syndrome
Intracapillary glomerulosclerosis

250.4† *Diabetes with ophthalmic manifestations*

Diabetic:
   cataract (366.4*)
   retinopathy (362.0*)

250.5† *Diabetes with neurological manifestations* .
Diabetic:
  amyotrophy (358.1*)   Diabetic polyneuropathy (357.2*)
  mononeuropathy (354.–, 355.–*)

250.6† *Diabetes with peripheral circulatory disorders*
Diabetic:
  gangrene (785.4*)
  peripheral angiopathy (443.8*)

250.7† *Diabetes with other specified manifestations*
Excludes: intercurrent infections in diabetic patients

250.9   *Diabetes with unspecified complications*

251   Other disorders of pancreatic internal secretion

251.0   *Hypoglycaemic coma*
Iatrogenic hyperinsulinism   Insulin coma
Use additional E code, if desired, to identify cause if drug induced

251.1   *Other hyperinsulinism*
Hyperinsulinism:
  NOS
  ectopic
  functional
Hyperplasia of pancreatic islet beta cells NOS

251.2   *Hypoglycaemia, unspecified*

251.3   *Postsurgical hypoinsulinaemia*
Postpancreatectomy hyperglycaemia

251.4   *Abnormality of secretion of glucagon*
Hyperplasia of pancreatic islet alpha cells with glucagon excess

251.5   *Abnormality of secretion of gastrin*
Hyperplasia of pancreatic alpha cells with gastrin excess
Zollinger-Ellison syndrome

251.8   *Other*

251.9   *Unspecified*
Islet-cell hyperplasia NOS

252   Disorders of parathyroid gland

252.0   *Hyperparathyroidism*
Hyperplasia of parathyroid
Osteitis fibrosa cystica generalisata [von Recklinghausen's disease of bone]
Excludes: secondary hyperparathyroidism (of renal origin) (588.8)

252.1 *Hypoparathyroidism*

Parathyroiditis (autoimmune)
Tetany:
  parathyroid
  parathyroprival

Excludes: pseudohypoparathyroidism (275.4)
          pseudopseudohypoparathyroidism (275.4)
          tetany NOS (781.7)
          transitory neonatal hypoparathyroidism (775.4)

252.8 *Other*

252.9 *Unspecified*

253 Disorders of the pituitary gland and its hypothalamic control

Includes: the listed conditions whether the disorder is in the pituitary
          or the hypothalamus

Excludes: Cushing's syndrome (255.0)

253.0 *Acromegaly and gigantism*

Arthropathy associated with acromegaly† (713.0*)
Overproduction of growth hormone

253.1 *Other anterior pituitary hyperfunction*

Excludes: overproduction of:
            ACTH (255.3)
            thyroid-stimulating hormone (242.8)

253.2 *Panhypopituitarism*

Cachexia, pituitary   Sheehan's syndrome
Necrosis of pituitary   Simmonds's disease
  (post-partum)
Pituitary insufficiency NOS

Excludes: iatrogenic hypopituitarism (253.7)

253.3 *Pituitary dwarfism*

Isolated deficiency of growth hormone
Lorain-Levi dwarfism

253.4 *Other anterior pituitary disorders*

Isolated or partial deficiency of an anterior pituitary hormone, other than
  growth hormone

253.5 *Diabetes insipidus*

Excludes: nephrogenic diabetes insipidus (588.1)

253.6   *Other disorders of neurohypophysis*

Syndrome of inappropriate secretion of antidiuretic hormone

253.7   *Iatrogenic pituitary disorders*

Hypopituitarism:
  hormone-induced
  hypophysectomy-induced
  radiotherapy-induced
Use additional E code, if desired, to identify cause

253.8   *Other disorders of the pituitary and other syndromes of diencephalo-*
       hypophyseal origin

Abscess of pituitary   Cyst of Rathke's pouch
Adiposogenital dystrophy   Fröhlich's syndrome

253.9   *Unspecified*

Dyspituitarism

254   Diseases of thymus gland

Excludes: aplasia or dysplasia with immunodeficiency (279.2)
         myasthenia gravis (358.0)

254.0   *Persistent hyperplasia of thymus*

Hypertrophy of thymus

254.1   *Abscess of thymus*

254.8   *Other*

254.9   *Unspecified*

255   Disorders of adrenal glands

Includes: the listed conditions whether the basic disorder is in the
        adrenals or is pituitary induced

255.0   *Cushing's syndrome*

Cushing's syndrome: Ectopic ACTH syndrome
  NOS   Overproduction of cortisol
  iatrogenic
  idiopathic
  pituitary-dependent
Use additional E code, if desired, to identify cause if drug induced

255.1   *Hyperaldosteronism*

Conn's syndrome

255.2 *Adrenogenital disorders*

Adrenogenital syndromes, virilizing or feminizing, whether acquired or
associated with congenital adrenal hyperplasia consequent on inborn
enzyme defects in hormone synthesis

Adrenogenital syndrome
Female adrenal pseudohermaphroditism
Male:
   macrogenitosomia praecox
   sexual precocity with adrenal hyperplasia
Virilization (female)

255.3 *Other corticoadrenal overactivity*

Overproduction of ACTH

255.4 *Corticoadrenal insufficiency*

Addisonian crisis
Addison's disease:
   NOS
   tuberculous* (017.6†)

Adrenal:
   atrophy (autoimmune)
   calcification
   crisis
   haemorrhage
   infarction
   insufficiency NOS

255.5 *Other adrenal hypofunction*

Waterhouse-Friderichsen syndrome (meningoccal)* (036.3†)

255.6 *Medulloadrenal hyperfunction*

Catecholamine secretion by phaeochromocytoma

Note: Not to be used as the primary code for phaeochromocytoma.
       See note, page 145.

255.8 *Other*

Abnormality of cortisol-binding globulin

255.9 *Unspecified*

256   Ovarian dysfunction

256.0 *Hyperoestrogenism*

256.1 *Other ovarian hyperfunction*

Hypersecretion of ovarian androgens

256.2 *Postablative ovarian failure*

Ovarian failure:
   iatrogenic
   postirradiation
   postsurgical

256.3   *Other ovarian failure*

Premature menopause NOS
Primary ovarian failure

256.4   *Polycystic ovaries*

Stein-Leventhal syndrome

256.8   *Other*

256.9   *Unspecified*

257   Testicular dysfunction

257.0   *Testicular hyperfunction*

Hypersecretion of testicular hormones

257.1   *Postablative testicular hypofunction*

Testicular hypofunction:
   iatrogenic
   postirradiation
   postsurgical

257.2   *Other testicular hypofunction*

Defective biosynthesis of testicular androgen
Testicular hypogonadism

Excludes: azoospermia (606)

257.8   *Other*

Goldberg-Maxwell syndrome
Male pseudohermaphroditism with testicular feminization
Testicular feminization

257.9   *Unspecified*

258   Polyglandular dysfunction and related disorders

258.0   *Polyglandular activity in multiple endocrine adenomatosis*

Wermer's syndrome

Note: Not to be used as the primary code for multiple endocrine adeno-
        matosis.   See note, page 145.

258.1   *Other combinations of endocrine dysfunction*

Lloyd's syndrome   Schmidt's syndrome

258.8   *Other*

258.9   *Polyglandular dysfunction, unspecified*

259   Other endocrine disorders

259.0   *Delay in sexual development and puberty, not elsewhere classified*
Delayed puberty

259.1   *Precocious sexual development and puberty, not elsewhere classified*
Sexual precocity:
  NOS
  constitutional
  cryptogenic
  idiopathic

259.2   *Carcinoid syndrome*
Hormone secretion by carcinoid tumours

Note: Not to be used as the primary code for carcinoid tumour. See note, page 145.

259.3   *Ectopic hormone secretion, not elsewhere classified*

259.4   *Dwarfism, not elsewhere classified*
Dwarfism:
  NOS
  constitutional

Excludes: dwarfism:
                achondroplastic (756.4)
                intrauterine (759.7)
                nutritional (263.2)
                pituitary (253.3)
                renal (588.0)
             progeria (259.8)

259.8   *Other*

Pineal gland dysfunction   Werner's syndrome
Progeria

259.9   *Unspecified*

Disturbance: Infantilism NOS
  endocrine NOS
  hormone NOS

NUTRITIONAL DEFICIENCIES (260-269)

Excludes: deficiency anaemias (280.–, 281.–)

260   Kwashiorkor

Nutritional oedema with dyspigmentation of skin and hair

261   Nutritional marasmus

Nutritional atrophy   Severe malnutrition NOS
Severe calorie deficiency

262   Other severe protein-calorie malnutrition

Malnutrition of third degree according to Gomez classification [weight
    for age less than 60% of standard]
Nutritional oedema without mention of dyspigmentation of skin and hair

263   Other and unspecified protein-calorie malnutrition

263.0   *Malnutrition of moderate degree*

Malnutrition of second degree according to Gomez classification [weight
    for age 60% to less than 75% of standard]

263.1   *Malnutrition of mild degree*

Malnutrition of first degree according to Gomez classification [weight
    for age 75% to less than 90% of standard]

263.2   *Arrested development following protein-calorie malnutrition*

Nutritional dwarfism
Physical retardation due to malnutrition

263.8   *Other protein-calorie malnutrition*

263.9   *Unspecified*

Dystrophy due to malnutrition
Malnutrition (calorie) NOS
Excludes: nutritional deficiency NOS (269.9)

264   Vitamin A deficiency

264.0†   *With conjunctival xerosis (372.5*)*

264.1†   *With Bitot's spot and conjunctival xerosis (372.5*)*
Bitot's spot in the young child

264.2†   *With corneal xerosis (371.4*)*

264.3†   *With corneal ulceration and xerosis (370.0, 371.4*)*

264.4†   *With keratomalacia (371.4*)*

264.5†   *With night blindness (368.6*)*

264.6†   *With xerophthalmic scars of cornea (371.0*)*

264.7†   *Other ocular manifestations of vitamin A deficiency*
Xerophthalmia due to vitamin A deficiency (372.5*)

264.8 *Other manifestations of vitamin A deficiency*

Follicular keratosis
Xeroderma } due to vitamin A deficiency† (701.1*)

264.9 *Unspecified*

Hypovitaminosis A NOS

265 Thiamine and niacin deficiency states

265.0 *Beriberi*

265.1 *Other and unspecified manifestations of thiamine deficiency*

Other vitamin B_1 deficiency states

265.2 *Pellagra*

Deficiency:
  niacin(-tryptophan)
  nicotinamide
  nicotinic acid
  vitamin PP
Pellagra (alcoholic)

266 Deficiency of B-complex components

266.0 *Ariboflavinosis*

Riboflavin deficiency

266.1 *Vitamin B_6 deficiency*

Deficiency: Vitamin B_6 deficiency syndrome
  pyridoxal
  pyridoxamine
  pyridoxine

Excludes: vitamin-B_6-responsive sideroblastic anaemia (285.0)

266.2 *Other B-complex deficiencies*

Deficiency:
  cyanocobalamine
  folic acid
  vitamin B_{12}

Excludes: deficiency anaemias (281.–)

266.9 *Unspecified vitamin B deficiency*

267 Ascorbic acid deficiency

Deficiency of vitamin C   Scurvy
Excludes: scorbutic anaemia (281.3)

268   Vitamin D deficiency

Excludes: vitamin-D-resistant rickets and osteomalacia (275.3)

268.0   *Rickets, active*

Excludes: coeliac rickets (579.0)
            renal rickets (588.0)

268.1   *Rickets, late effect*

Any condition specified as rachitic or due to rickets and present one year
    or more after onset, or stated to be a late effect or sequela of rickets

268.2   *Osteomalacia*

268.9   *Unspecified*

Avitaminosis D

269   Other nutritional deficiencies

269.0   *Deficiency of vitamin K*

Excludes: deficiency of coagulation factor due to vitamin K deficiency
            (286.7)
            vitamin K deficiency of newborn (776.0)

269.1   *Deficiency of other vitamins*

Deficiency:
  vitamin E
  vitamin P

269.2   *Unspecified vitamin deficiency*

269.3   *Mineral deficiency, not elsewhere classified*

Excludes: deficiency:
                potassium (276.8)
                sodium (276.1)

269.8   *Other nutritional deficiency*

Excludes: failure to thrive (783.4)
            feeding problems (783.3)
                newborn (779.3)

269.9   *Unspecified*

OTHER METABOLIC DISORDERS AND IMMUNITY DISORDERS
(270-279)

Use additional code, if desired, to identify any associated mental retarda-
    tion

270   Disorders of amino-acid transport and metabolism

Excludes: abnormal findings without manifest disease (791-796)
            disorders of purine and pyrimidine metabolism (277.2)
            gout (274.–)

270.0   *Disturbances of amino-acid transport*

Cystinosis
Cystinuria
Fanconi (-de Toni) (-Debré) syndrome
Glycinuria (renal)
Hartnup disease

270.1   *Phenylketonuria*

Hyperphenylalaninaemia

270.2   *Other disturbances of aromatic amino-acid metabolism*

Albinism   Oast-house urine disease
Alkaptonuria   Ochronotic arthritis† (713.0*)
Disturbances of metabolism of   Tyrosinosis
    tyrosine and tryptophan   Tyrosinuria
Hydroxykynureninuria
Hypertyrosinaemia

Excludes: vitamin-B_6-deficiency syndrome (266.1)

270.3   *Disturbances of branched-chain amino-acid metabolism*

Disturbances of metabolism of leucine, isoleucine and valine
Hypervalinaemia
Leucinosis
Maple-syrup-urine disease

270.4   *Disturbances of sulphur-bearing amino-acid metabolism*

Cystathioninuria
Disturbances of metabolism of methionine, homocystine and cystathio-
    nine
Homocystinuria
Hypermethioninaemia

270.5   *Disturbances of histidine metabolism*

Histidinaemia   Imidazole amino-aciduria
Hyperhistidinaemia

270.6   *Disorders of urea cycle metabolism*

Arginosuccinic aciduria
Citrullinaemia
Disorders of metabolism of ornithine, citrulline, arginosuccinic acid,
    arginine and ammonia
Hyperammonaemia
Hyperornithinaemia

270.7 *Other disturbances of straight-chain amino-acid metabolism*

Hyperglycinaemia
Hyperlysinaemia
Pipecolic acidaemia
Saccharopinuria

Other disturbances of metabolism
  of glycine, threonine, serine,
  glutamine and lysine

270.8 *Other*

Ethanolaminuria
Hydroxyprolinaemia
Hyperprolinaemia

Iminoacidopathy
Sarcosinaemia

270.9 *Unspecified*

271   Disorders of carbohydrate transport and metabolism

Excludes: abnormality of secretion of glucagon (251.4)
           diabetes mellitus (250.–)
           hypoglycaemia NOS (251.2)
           mucopolysaccharidosis (277.5)

271.0 *Glycogenosis*

Glycogen-storage disease

271.1 *Galactosaemia*

271.2 *Hereditary fructose intolerance*

271.3 *Intestinal disaccharidase deficiencies and disaccharide malabsorption*

Intolerance or malabsorption (congenital):
  glucose-galactose
  lactose
  sucrose-isomaltose

271.4 *Renal glycosuria*

Renal diabetes

271.8 *Other*

Hyperoxaluria (primary)
Oxalosis

271.9 *Unspecified*

272   Disorders of lipid metabolism

Excludes: localized cerebral lipidoses (330.1)

272.0 *Pure hypercholesterolaemia*

Familial hypercholesterolaemia
Fredrickson Type IIa hyperlipo-
    proteinaemia
Hyper-beta-lipoproteinaemia

Hyperlipidaemia, Group A
Low-density-lipoid-type [LDL]
    hyperlipoproteinaemia

272.1   *Pure hyperglyceridaemia*

Endogenous hyperglyceridaemia
Fredrickson Type IV hyperlipo-
   proteinaemia
Hyperlipidaemia, Group B

Hyper-pre-beta lipoproteinaemia
Very-low-density-lipoid-type
   [VLDL] hyperlipoproteinae-
   mia

272.2   *Mixed hyperlipidaemia*

Broad- or floating-beta lipoproteinaemia
Fredrickson Type IIb or III hyper-
   lipoproteinaemia
Hypercholesterolaemia with
   endogenous hyperglyceridaemia

Hyper-beta-lipoproteinaemia with
   pre-beta-lipoproteinaemia
Hyperlipidaemia, Group C
Tubo-eruptive xanthoma
Xanthoma tuberosum

272.3   *Hyperchylomicronaemia*

Fredrickson's Type I or V hyper-
   lipoproteinaemia

Hyperlipidaemia, Group D
Mixed hyperglyceridaemia

272.4   *Other and unspecified hyperlipidaemia*

Alpha-lipoproteinaemia
Combined hyperlipidaemia

Hyperlipidaemia NOS

272.5   *Lipoprotein deficiencies*

A-beta-lipoproteinaemia
High-density lipoid deficiency
Hypo-alpha-lipoproteinaemia

Hypo-beta-lipoproteinaemia
   (familial)
Lecithin cholesterol acyltransfe-
   rase deficiency
Tangier disease

272.6   *Lipodystrophy*

Barraquer-Simons disease   Progressive lipodystrophy
Use additional E code, if desired, to identify cause, if iatrogenic
Excludes: intestinal lipodystrophy (040.2)

272.7   *Lipidoses*

Chemically-induced lipidosis
Disease:
   Anderson's
   Fabry's
   Gaucher's
   I-cell or mucolipidosis I
   Lipoid-storage NOS
   Niemann-Pick

Disease:
   pseudo-Hurler's or mucolipi-
      dosis III
   Sandhoff's
   triglyceride-storage, Type I or II
   Wolman's or triglyceride-
      storage, Type III
Mucolipidosis II
Primary familial xanthomatosis

272.8   *Other disorders of lipoid metabolism*

Hoffa's disease or liposynovitis prepatellaris
Launois Bensaude's lipomatosis

272.9   *Unspecified disorders of lipoid metabolism*

273   Disorders of plasma protein metabolism
Excludes: agammaglobulinaemia and hypogammaglobulinaemia (279.–)
coagulation defects (286.–)
hereditary haemolytic anaemias (282.–)

273.0   *Polyclonal hypergammaglobulinaemia*
Waldenström's hypergammaglobulinaemic purpura

273.1   *Monoclonal paraproteinaemia*
Monoclonal gammopathy:
NOS
associated with lymphoplasmacytic dyscrasias
benign
Paraproteinaemia:
benign (familial)
secondary to malignant or inflammatory disease

273.2   *Other paraproteinaemias*
Cryoglobulinaemic: Mixed cryoglobulinaemia
purpura
vasculitis

273.3   *Macroglobulinaemia*
Macroglobulinaemia (idiopathic) (primary)
Waldenström's macroglobulinaemia

273.8   *Other*
Abnormality of transport protein   Bisalbuminaemia

273.9   *Unspecified*

274   Gout
Excludes: lead gout (984.–)

274.0†   *Gouty arthropathy* (712.0*)

274.1†   *Gouty nephropathy*
Gouty nephropathy NOS (583.8*)   Uric acid nephrolithiasis (592.0*)

274.8   *Gout with other manifestations*
Gouty tophi of:
ear† (380.8*)
heart† (425.7*)

274.9   *Unspecified*

275   Disorders of mineral metabolism
Excludes: abnormal findings without clinical significance (790-796)

275.0 *Disorders of iron metabolism*

Haemochromatosis

Excludes: anaemia:
      iron deficiency (280)
      sideroblastic (285.0)

275.1 *Disorders of copper metabolism*

Hepatolenticular degeneration   Wilson's disease

275.2 *Disorders of magnesium metabolism*

Hypermagnesaemia   Hypomagnesaemia

275.3 *Disorders of phosphorus metabolism*

Familial hypophosphataemia   Vitamin-D-resistant:
Hypophosphatasia   osteomalacia
             rickets

275.4 *Disorders of calcium metabolism*

Calcinosis   Nephrocalcinosis
Hypercalcaemia   Pseudohypoparathyroidism
Hypercalcinuria   Pseudopseudohypoparathyroidism

Excludes: parathyroid disorders (252.–)
      vitamin D deficiency (268.–)

275.8 *Other*

275.9 *Unspecified*

276   **Disorders of fluid, electrolyte and acid-base balance**

Excludes: diabetes insipidus (253.5)
      familial periodic paralysis (359.3)

276.0 *Hyperosmolality and/or hypernatraemia*

Na overload   Na excess

276.1 *Hyposmolality and/or hyponatraemia*

Na deficiency

276.2 *Acidosis*

Acidosis:
  NOS
  lactic
  metabolic
  respiratory

Excludes: diabetic acidosis (250.1)

276.3   *Alkalosis*

Alkalosis:
  NOS
  metabolic
  respiratory

276.4   *Mixed acid-base balance disorder*

276.5   *Volume depletion*

Dehydration
Depletion of volume of plasma or extracellular fluid
Hypovolaemia

Excludes: hypovolaemic shock:
                  postoperative (998.0)
                  traumatic (958.4)

276.6   *Fluid overload*

Fluid retention

276.7   *Hyperpotassaemia*

K overload   K excess

276.8   *Hypopotassaemia*

K deficiency

276.9   *Electrolyte and fluid disorders, not elsewhere classified*

Electrolyte imbalance   Hypochloraemia
Hyperchloraemia

Excludes: electrolyte imbalance:
                  associated with hyperemesis gravidarum (643.1)
                  following abortion and ectopic or molar pregnancy (634-
                        638 with fourth digit .4, 639.4)

277   Other and unspecified disorders of metabolism

277.0   *Cystic fibrosis*

Fibrocystic disease of the pancreas   Mucoviscidosis

277.1   *Disorders of porphyrin metabolism*

Porphyria   Porphyrinuria

277.2   *Other disorders of purine and pyrimidine metabolism*

Hypoxanthine-guanine-phosphoribosyltransferase deficiency [HG-PRT
      deficiency]
Lesch-Nyhan syndrome

Excludes: gout (274.–)
                  orotaciduric anaemia (281.4)

277.3   Amyloidosis

Amyloidosis: Familial Mediterranean fever
  NOS   Hereditary cardiac amyloid
  inherited systemic
  nephropathic
  neuropathic (Portuguese) (Swiss)
  secondary

277.4   *Disorders of bilirubin excretion*

Syndrome: Syndrome:
  Crigler-Najjar   Gilbert's
  Dubin-Johnson   Rotor's
Excludes: hyperbilirubinaemias specific to the perinatal period (774.–)

277.5   *Mucopolysaccharidosis*

Gargoylism   Hurler's syndrome
Hunter's syndrome

277.6   *Other deficiencies of circulating enzymes*

Alpha 1-antitrypsin deficiency   Hereditary angio-oedema

277.8   *Other*

277.9   *Unspecified*

278   Obesity and other hyperalimentation

Excludes: hyperalimentation NOS (783.6)
            poisoning by vitamin preparations (963.5)

278.0   *Obesity*
Excludes: adiposogenital dystrophy (253.8)
            obesity of endocrine origin NOS (259.9)

278.1   *Localized adiposity*
Fat pad

278.2   *Hypervitaminosis A*

278.3   *Hypercarotinaemia*

278.4   *Hypervitaminosis D*

278.8   *Other*

279   Disorders involving the immune mechanism

279.0   *Deficiency of humoral immunity*
Agammaglobulinaemia: Hypogammaglobulinaemia
  NOS
  brulous type

279.1   *Deficiency of cell-mediated immunity*

Di George syndrome   Wiskott-Aldrich syndrome
Nezelof syndrome

Excludes: ataxia-telangiectasia (334.8)

279.2   *Combined immunity deficiency*

Agammaglobulinaemia, Swiss type
Combined immunity deficiency syndrome
Reticular dysgenesis
Thymic:
  alymphoplasia
  aplasia or dysplasia with immunodeficiency

279.3   *Unspecified immunity deficiency*

279.4   *Autoimmune disease, not elsewhere classified*

Autoimmune disease NOS

279.8   *Other*

279.9   *Unspecified*

IV. DISEASES OF BLOOD AND BLOOD-FORMING ORGANS

Excludes: anaemia complicating pregnancy or puerperium (648.2)

280   Iron deficiency anaemias

Anaemia:
  asiderotic
  hypochromic
  due to blood·loss (chronic)
  posthaemorrhagic

Kelly-Paterson syndrome
Plummer-Vinson syndrome
Sideropenic dysphagia

Excludes: acute posthaemorrhagic anaemia (285.1)

281   Other deficiency anaemias

281.0 *Pernicious anaemia*

Anaemia:
  Addison's
  Biermer's
  congenital pernicious

Congenital intrinsic factor
  deficiency

281.1 *Other Vitamin-B_{12}-deficiency anaemia*

Anaemia:
  vegan's
  vitamin B_{12} deficiency (dietary)
  due to selective vitamin B_{12} malabsorption with proteinuria
Syndrome:
  Imerslund's
  Imerslund-Gräsbeck

281.2 *Folate-deficiency anaemia*

Folate or folic acid deficiency anaemia:
  NOS
  dietary
  drug induced
Nutritional megaloblastic anaemia
Use additional E code, if desired, to identify drug

281.3 *Other specified megaloblastic anaemias, not elsewhere classified*

281.4 *Protein-deficiency anaemia*

Amino-acid-deficiency anaemia

281.8 *Anaemia associated with other specified nutritional deficiency*

Scorbutic anaemia

281.9   *Unspecified*

Anaemia:
  megaloblastic NOS
  nutritional NOS
  simple chronic

282   Hereditary haemolytic anaemias

282.0   *Hereditary spherocytosis*

Acholuric (familial) jaundice   Minkowski-Chauffard syndrome
Congenital spherocytosis

282.1   *Hereditary elliptocytosis*

Elliptocytosis (congenital)
Ovalocytosis (congenital) (hereditary)

282.2   *Anaemia due to disorders of glutathione metabolism*

Anaemia:
  enzyme-deficiency drug induced
  erythrocytic glutathione deficiency
  glucose-6-phosphate dehydrogenase [G-6-PD] deficiency
  glutathione-reductase deficiency
  haemolytic nonspherocytic (hereditary), type I
Favism

282.3   *Other haemolytic anaemias due to enzyme deficiency*

Anaemia:
  haemolytic nonspherocytic (hereditary), type II
  hexokinase deficiency
  pyruvate-kinase [PK] deficiency
  triose phosphate isomerase deficiency

282.4   *Thalassaemias*

Cooley's anaemia
Mediterranean anaemia (with other haemoglobinopathy)
Sickle-cell thalassaemia
Thalassaemia (alpha) (beta) (intermedia) (major) (minor) (mixed) (trait)
    (with other haemoglobinopathy)

282.5   *Sickle-cell trait*

Hb-AS genotype   Heterozygous:
Haemoglobin S [Hb-S] trait   haemoglobin S
                                    Hb-S

Excludes: with thalassaemia (282.4)
            with other haemoglobinopathy (282.6)

282.6 *Sickle-cell anaemia*

Hb-S disease
Hb-S/Hb-C disease
Hb-S/Hb-D disease
Hb-S/Hb-E disease

Sickle-cell/Hb-C disease
Sickle-cell/Hb-D disease
Sickle-cell/Hb-E disease

Excludes: sickle-cell thalassaemia (282.4)

282.7 *Other haemoglobinopathies*

Abnormal haemoglobin NOS
Congenital Heinz-body anaemia
Disease:
  Hb-C
  Hb-D
  Hb-E

Haemoglobinopathy NOS
Hereditary persistence of fetal
  haemoglobin [HPFH]
Unstable haemoglobin haemolytic
  disease

Excludes: familial polycythaemia (289.6)
         Hb-M disease (289.7)
         high-oxygen-affinity haemoglobin (289.0)

282.8 *Other*

Stomatocytosis

282.9 *Unspecified*

Hereditary haemolytic anaemia NOS

283 Acquired haemolytic anaemias

283.0 *Autoimmune haemolytic anaemias*

Autoimmune haemolytic disease (cold type) (warm type)
Chronic cold-haemagglutinin disease
Cold agglutinin disease or haemoglobinuria
Haemolytic anaemia:
  cold type (secondary) (symptomatic)
  warm type (secondary) (symptomatic)

Excludes: Evans's syndrome (287.3)
         haemolytic disease of newborn (773.–)

283.1 *Non-autoimmune haemolytic anaemias*

Haemolytic anaemia:
  mechanical
  microangiopathic
  toxic
Haemolytic-uraemic syndrome

Use additional E code, if desired, to identify cause

283.2   *Haemoglobinuria due to haemolysis from external causes*

Haemoglobinuria:
  from exertion
  march
  paroxysmal
    cold
    nocturnal
  due to other haemolysis
Marchiafava-Micheli syndrome

Use additional E code, if desired, to identify cause

283.9   *Unspecified*

Acquired haemolytic anaemia NOS
Chronic idiopathic haemolytic anaemia

284   Aplastic anaemia

284.0   *Constitutional aplastic anaemia*

Aplasia (pure) red cell: Blackfan-Diamond syndrome
  congenital   Familial hypoplastic anaemia
  of infants   Fanconi's anaemia
  primary   Pancytopenia with malformations

284.8   *Other*

Aplastic anaemia (due to):   Pancytopenia (acquired)
  drugs   Red cell aplasia (acquired) (adult)
  infection   (pure) (with thymoma)
  radiation
  toxic

Use additional E code, if desired, to identify cause

284.9   *Unspecified*

Anaemia: Medullary hypoplasia
  aplastic (idiopathic) NOS
  hypoplastic

285   Other and unspecified anaemias

285.0   *Sideroblastic anaemia*

Anaemia: Anaemia, sideroblastic
  pyridoxine-responsive   refractory
  sidero-achrestic   secondary (drug-induced) (due
  sideroblastic   to disease)
    acquired   sex-linked hypochromic
    congenital   vitamin-B_6-responsive
    hereditary
    primary

Use additional E code, if desired, to identify cause if drug induced

285.1   *Acute posthaemorrhagic anaemia*

285.8   *Other specified anaemias*

Anaemia: Infantile pseudoleukaemia
   dyserythropoietic (congenital)
   dyshaematopoietic (congenital)
   leukoerythroblastic

285.9   *Anaemia, unspecified*

286   Coagulation defects

286.0   *Congenital factor VIII disorder*

Factor VIII (functional) deficiency
Haemophilia:
   NOS
   A

Excludes: factor VIII deficiency with vascular defect (286.4)

286.1   *Congenital factor IX disorder*

Christmas disease
Deficiency:
   factor IX (functional)
   plasma thromboplastin component [PTC]
Haemophilia B

286.2   *Congenital factor XI deficiency*

Haemophilia C
Plasma thromboplastin antecedent [PTA] deficiency

286.3   *Congenital deficiency of other clotting factors*

Congenital afibrinogenaemia   Deficiency:
Deficiency of factor: AC globulin
   I or fibrinogen   proaccelerin
   II or prothrombin   Disease:
   V or labile   Owren's
   VII or stable   Stuart-Prower
   X or Stuart-Prower   Dysfibrinogenaemia (congenital)
   XII or Hageman   Hypoproconvertinaemia
   XIII or fibrin stabilizing

286.4   *von Willebrand's disease*

Angiohaemophilia   Vascular haemophilia
Factor VIII deficiency with
   vascular defect

Excludes: factor VIII deficiency:
               NOS (286.0)
               with functional defect (286.0)
            hereditary capillary fragility (287.8)

286.5   *Haemorrhagic disorder due to circulating anticoagulants*

Hyperheparinaemia
Increase in:
  antithrombin
  anti-VIIIa
  anti-IXa
  anti-Xa
  anti-XIa

Systemic lupus erythematosus
  inhibitor

Use additional E code, if desired, to identify any administered anticoagulant

286.6   *Defibrination syndrome*

Afibrinogenaemia, acquired
Consumption coagulopathy
Diffuse or disseminated intravascular coagulation
Fibrinolytic haemorrhage, acquired
Purpura:
  fibrinolytic
  fulminans

Excludes: complicating abortion, pregnancy or the puerperium (634-638 with fourth digit .1, 639.1, 641.3, 666.3)
           disseminated intravascular coagulation in newborn (776.2)

286.7   *Acquired coagulation factor deficiency*

Deficiency of coagulation factor due to:
  liver disease
  vitamin K deficiency

Excludes: vitamin K deficiency of newborn (776.0)

286.9   *Other and unspecified coagulation defects*

Defective coagulation NOS
Deficiency, coagulation factor
Delay, coagulation
Disorder, coagulation

Disorder, haemostasis
Prolongation of time of:
  bleeding
  coagulation

Excludes: complicating abortion, pregnancy or the puerperium (634-638 with fourth digit .1, 639.1, 641.3, 666.3)

287   Purpura and other haemorrhagic conditions

Excludes: haemorrhagic thrombocythaemia (238.7)
           purpura fulminans (286.6)

287.0   *Allergic purpura*

Purpura:
  anaphylactoid
  Henoch (-Schönlein)
  nonthrombocytopenic:
    haemorrhagic
    idiopathic

Vascular purpura
Vasculitis, allergic

287.1 *Qualitative platelet defects*

Thromboasthenia (haemorrhagic) (hereditary)
Thrombocytopathy

Excludes: von Willebrand's disease (286.4)

287.2 *Other nonthrombocytopenic purpuras*

Purpura:
 NOS
 senile
 simplex

287.3 *Primary thrombocytopenia*

Megakaryocytic hypoplasia
Purpura, thrombocytopenic
 congenital
 hereditary
 idiopathic

Thrombocytopenia:
 congenital
 hereditary
 primary

287.4 *Secondary thrombocytopenia*

Thrombocytopenia (due to):
 dilutional
 drugs
 extracorporeal circulation of blood
 massive blood transfusion
 platelet alloimmunization
Use additional E code, if desired, to identify cause

287.5 *Thrombocytopenia, unspecified*

287.8 *Other specified haemorrhagic conditions*

Capillary fragility (hereditary)   Vascular pseudohaemophilia

287.9 *Unspecified haemorrhagic conditions*

288 Diseases of white blood cells

288.0 *Agranulocytosis*

Agranulocytic angina
Infantile genetic agranulocytosis
Kostman's disease

Neutropenia:
 NOS
 cyclic
 drug induced
 periodic
 splenic (primary)
 toxic
Neutropenic splenomegaly

Use additional code, if desired, to identify drug

288.1 *Functional disorders of neutrophil polymorphonuclears*

Chronic (childhood) granulomatous disease
Congenital dysphagocytosis
Progressive septic granulomatosis

288.2 *Genetic anomalies of leucocytes*

Anomaly (granulation)
   (granulocyte) or syndrome:
   Alder's
   Chediak-Steinbrink
   May-Hegglin
   Pelger-Huët

Hereditary:
   hypersegmentation
   hyposegmentation
   leukomelanopathy

288.3 *Eosinophilia*

Eosinophilia
   allergic
   hereditary

Excludes: pulmonary eosinophilia (518.3)

288.8 *Other*

Leukaemoid reaction
   lymphocytic
   monocytic
   myelocytic
Leukocytosis

Lymphocytosis (symptomatic)
Lymphopenia
Monocytosis (symptomatic)
Plasmacytosis

Excludes: immunity disorders (279.–)

288.9 *Unspecified*

289 **Other diseases of blood and blood-forming organs**

289.0 *Secondary polycythaemia*

Polycythaemia:
   acquired
   due to:
      fall in plasma volume
      high altitude
   emotional

Polycythaemia:
   erythropoietin
   hypoxaemic
   nephrogenous
   relative
   stress

Excludes: polycythaemia neonatorum (776.4)
         polycythaemia vera (238.4)

289.1 *Chronic lymphadenitis*

Adenitis ⎫
Lymphadenitis ⎬ chronic, any lymph node except mesenteric

Excludes: acute lymphadenitis (683)
        mesenteric (289.2)
        enlarged glands NOS (785.6)

289.2   *Nonspecific mesenteric lymphadenitis*

Mesenteric lymphadenitis (acute) (chronic)

289.3   *Lymphadenitis, unspecified, except mesenteric*

289.4   *Hypersplenism*

289.5   *Other diseases of spleen*

Atrophy		Chronic congestive splenomegaly
Cyst	of spleen	Fibrosis of spleen:
Infarction		NOS
Rupture, nontraumatic		bilharzial* (120.–†)
		Perisplenitis

Excludes: splenomegaly NOS (789.2)

289.6   *Familial polycythaemia*

Familial:
   benign polycythaemia
   erythrocytosis

289.7   *Methaemoglobinaemia*

Congenital NADH-methaemoglobin-reductase deficiency
Haemoglobin-M disease
Methaemoglobinaemia:
   NOS
   acquired (with sulfhaemoglobinaemia)
   hereditary
   toxic
Use additional E code, if desired, to identify cause

289.8   *Other*

289.9   *Unspecified*

V. MENTAL DISORDERS

This section of the Classification differs from the others in that it includes a glossary, prepared after consultation with experts from many different countries, defining the contents of the rubrics. This difference is considered to be justified because of the special problems posed for psychiatrists by the relative lack of independent laboratory information upon which to base their diagnoses. The diagnosis of many of the most important mental disorders still relies largely upon descriptions of abnormal experience and behaviour, and without some guidance in the form of a glossary that can serve as a common frame of reference, psychiatric communications easily become unsatisfactory at both clinical and statistical levels.

Many well-known terms have different meanings in current use, and it is important for the user to use the glossary descriptions and not merely the category titles when searching for the best fit for the condition he is trying to code. This is particularly important if a separate national glossary also exists.

The instructions "Use additional code to identify..." are important because of the nature of many psychiatric conditions in which two or more codes are necessary to describe the condition and the associated or causal factors. It should be used whenever possible.

In cases where no other information is available except that a mental disorder is present, the code V40.9 (unspecified mental or behavioural problems) can be used.

Psychoses (290-299)

Mental disorders in which impairment of mental function has developed to a degree that interferes grossly with insight, ability to meet some ordinary demands of life or to maintain adequate contact with reality. It is not an exact or well defined term. Mental retardation is excluded.

Organic psychotic conditions (290-294)

Syndromes in which there is impairment of orientation, memory, comprehension, calculation, learning capacity and judgement. These are the essential features but there may also be shallowness or lability of affect, or a more persistent disturbance of mood, lowering of ethical standards and exaggeration or emergence of personality traits, and diminished capacity for independent decision.

Psychoses of the types classifiable to 295-298 and without the above features are excluded even though they may be associated with organic conditions.

The term 'dementia' in this glossary includes organic psychoses as just specified, of a chronic or progressive nature, which if untreated are usually irreversible and terminal.

The term 'delirium' in this glossary includes organic psychoses with a short course in which the above features are overshadowed by clouded consciousness, confusion, disorientation, delusions, illusions and often vivid hallucinations.

Includes: psychotic organic brain syndrome

Excludes: nonpsychotic syndromes of organic aetiology (see 310.–)
            psychoses classifiable to 295-298 and without the above
               features but associated with physical disease, injury or
               condition affecting the brain [e.g., following childbirth];
               code to 295-298 and use additional code to identify the
               associated physical condition

290   Senile and presenile organic psychotic conditions

Excludes: psychoses classifiable to 295-298.8 occurring in the senium
               without dementia or delirium (295-298)
            transient organic psychotic conditions (293.–)
            dementia not classified as senile, presenile, or arteriosclerotic
               (294.1)

290.0   *Senile dementia, simple type*

Dementia occurring usually after the age of 65 in which any cerebral pathology other
than that of senile atrophic change can be reasonably excluded.

Excludes: mild memory disturbances, not amounting to dementia,
               associated with senile brain disease (310.1)
            senile dementia:
               depressed or paranoid type (290.2)
               with confusion and/or delirium (290.3)

290.1   *Presenile dementia*

Dementia occurring usually before the age of 65 in patients with the relatively rare
forms of diffuse or lobar cerebral atrophy. Use additional code to identify the associated neurological condition.

Brain syndrome with presenile brain disease
Circumscribed atrophy of the brain
Dementia in:
   Alzheimer's disease
   Pick's disease of the brain

Excludes: arteriosclerotic dementia (290.4)
            dementia associated with other cerebral conditions (294.1)

290.2   *Senile dementia, depressed or paranoid type*

A type of senile dementia characterized by development in advanced old age, progressive
in nature, in which a variety of delusions and hallucinations of a persecutory, depressive
and somatic content are also present. Disturbance of the sleep/waking cycle and
preoccupation with dead people are often particularly prominent.

Senile psychosis NOS

Excludes: senile dementia:
               NOS (290.0)
               with confusion and/or delirium (290.3)

290.3 *Senile dementia with acute confusional state*

Senile dementia with a superimposed reversible episode of acute confusional state

Excludes: senile:
  dementia NOS (290.0)
  psychosis NOS (290.2)

290.4 *Arteriosclerotic dementia*

Dementia attributable, because of physical signs [on examination of the central nervous system] to degenerative arterial disease of the brain. Symptoms suggesting a focal lesion in the brain are common. There may be a fluctuating or patchy intellectual defect with insight, and an intermittent course is common. Clinical differentiation from senile or presenile dementia, which may coexist with it, may be very difficult or impossible. Use additional code to identify cerebral atherosclerosis (437.0).

Excludes: suspected cases with no clear evidence of arteriosclerosis
      (290.9)

290.8 *Other*

290.9 *Unspecified*

291   Alcoholic psychoses

Organic psychotic states due mainly to excessive consumption of alcohol; defects of nutrition are thought to play an important role. In some of these states, withdrawal of alcohol can be of aetiological significance.

Excludes: alcoholism without psychosis (303)

291.0 *Delirium tremens*

Acute or subacute organic psychotic states in alcoholics, characterized by clouded consciousness, disorientation, fear, illusions, delusions, hallucinations of any kind, notably visual and tactile, and restlessness, tremor and sometimes fever.

Alcoholic delirium

291.1 *Korsakov's psychosis, alcoholic*

A syndrome of prominent and lasting reduction of memory span, including striking loss of recent memory, disordered time appreciation and confabulation, occurring in alcoholics as the sequel to an acute alcoholic psychosis [especially delirium tremens] or, more rarely, in the course of chronic alcoholism. It is usually accompanied by peripheral neuritis and may be associated with Wernicke's encephalopathy.

Alcoholic polyneuritic psychosis

Excludes: Korsakov's psychosis:
      NOS (294.0)
      nonalcoholic (294.0)

291.2 *Other alcoholic dementia*

Nonhallucinatory dementias occurring in association with alcoholism but not characterized by the features of either delirium tremens or Korsakov's psychosis.

Alcoholic dementia NOS
Chronic alcoholic brain syndrome

291.3 *Other alcoholic hallucinosis*

A psychosis usually of less than six months' duration, with slight or no clouding of consciousness and much anxious restlessness in which auditory hallucinations, mostly of voices uttering insults and threats, predominate.

Excludes: schizophrenia (295.–) and paranoid states (297.–) taking the form of chronic hallucinosis with clear consciousness in an alcoholic

291.4 *Pathological drunkenness*

Acute psychotic episodes induced by relatively small amounts of alcohol. These are regarded as individual idiosyncratic reactions to alcohol, not due to excessive consumption and without conspicuous neurological signs of intoxication.

Excludes: simple drunkenness (305.0)

291.5 *Alcoholic jealousy*

Chronic paranoid psychosis characterized by delusional jealousy and associated with alcoholism.

Alcoholic paranoia

Excludes: nonalcoholic paranoid states (297.–)
schizophrenia, paranoid type (295.3)

291.8 *Other*

Alcohol withdrawal syndrome

Excludes: delirium tremens (291.0)

291.9 *Unspecified*

Alcoholic:
  mania NOS
  psychosis NOS
Alcoholism (chronic) with psychosis

292 Drug psychoses

Syndromes that do not fit the descriptions given in 295-298 (nonorganic psychoses) and which are due to consumption of drugs [notably amphetamines, barbiturates and the opiate and LSD groups] and solvents. Some of the syndromes in this group are not as severe as most conditions labelled "psychotic" but they are included here for practical reasons. Use additional E Code to identify the drug and also code drug dependence (304.—) if present.

292.0 *Drug withdrawal syndrome*

States associated with drug withdrawal ranging from severe, as specified for alcohol under 291.0 (delirium tremens) to less severe states characterized by one or more symptoms such as convulsions, tremor, anxiety, restlessness, gastrointestinal and muscular complaints, and mild disorientation and memory disturbance.

292.1 *Paranoid and/or hallucinatory states induced by drugs*

States of more than a few days but not usually of more than a few months duration, associated with large or prolonged intake of drugs, notably of the amphetamine and LSD groups. Auditory hallucinations usually predominate, and there may be anxiety and restlessness.

Excludes: the described conditions with confusion or delirium (293.–)
states following LSD or other hallucinogens, lasting only a few days or less ["bad trips"] (305.3)

292.2 *Pathological drug intoxication*

Individual idiosyncratic reactions to comparatively small quantities of a drug, which take the form of acute, brief psychotic states of any type.

Excludes: physiological side-effects of drugs [e.g., dystonias]
expected brief psychotic reactions to hallucinogens ["bad trips"] (305.3)

292.8 *Other*

292.9 *Unspecified*

293 Transient organic psychotic conditions

States characterized by clouded consciousness, confusion, disorientation, illusions and often vivid hallucinations. They are usually due to some intra- or extracerebral toxic, infectious, metabolic or other systemic disturbance and are generally reversible. Depressive and paranoid symptoms may also be present but are not the main feature. Use additional code to identify the associated physical or neurological condition.

Excludes: confusional state or delirium superimposed on senile dementia (290.3)
dementia due to:
alcohol (291.–)
arteriosclerosis (290.4)
senility (290.0)

293.0 *Acute confusional state*

Short-lived states, lasting hours or days, of the above type.

Acute:
delirium
infective psychosis
organic reaction
post-traumatic organic
psychosis

Acute:
psycho-organic syndrome
psychosis associated with endocrine, metabolic or cerebrovascular disorder
Epileptic:
confusional state
twilight state

293.1 *Subacute confusional state*

States of the above type in which the symptoms, usually less florid, last for several weeks or longer, during which they may show marked fluctuations in intensity.

Subacute:
delirium
infective psychosis
organic reaction
post-traumatic organic psychosis

Subacute:
psycho-organic syndrome
psychosis associated with endocrine or metabolic disorder

293.8 *Other*

293.9 *Unspecified*

294 Other organic psychotic conditions (chronic)

294.0 *Korsakov's psychosis or syndrome (nonalcoholic)*

Syndromes as described under 291.1 but not due to alcohol.

294.1 *Dementia in conditions classified elsewhere*

Dementia not classifiable as senile, presenile or arteriosclerotic (290.–) but associated with other underlying conditions.

Dementia in:
cerebral lipidoses
epilepsy
general paralysis of the insane
hepatolenticular degeneration
Huntington's chorea
multiple sclerosis
polyarteritis nodosa

Use additional code to identify the underlying physical condition

294.8 *Other*

States that fulfill the criteria of an organic psychosis but do not take the form of a confusional state (293.–), a nonalcoholic Korsakov's psychosis (294.0) or a dementia (294.1).

Mixed paranoid and affective
organic psychotic states

Epileptic psychosis NOS (code
also 345.–)

Excludes: mild memory disturbances, not amounting to dementia (310.1)

294.9 *Unspecified*

OTHER PSYCHOSES (295-299)

295 Schizophrenic psychoses

A group of psychoses in which there is a fundamental disturbance of personality, a characteristic distortion of thinking, often a sense of being controlled by alien forces, delusions which may be bizarre, disturbed perception, abnormal affect out of keeping with the real situation, and autism. Nevertheless, clear consciousness and intellectual capacity are usually maintained. The disturbance of personality involves its most basic functions which give the normal person his feeling of individuality, uniqueness and self-direction. The most intimate thoughts, feelings and acts are often felt to be known to or shared by others and explanatory delusions may develop, to the effect that natural or supernatural forces are at work to influence the schizophrenic person's thoughts and actions in ways that are often bizarre. He may see himself as the pivot of all that happens. Hallucinations, especially of hearing, are common and may comment on the patient or address him. Perception is frequently disturbed in other ways; there may be perplexity, irrelevant features may become all-important and, accompanied by passivity feelings, may lead the patient to believe that everyday objects and situations possess a special, usually sinister, meaning intended for him. In the characteristic schizophrenic disturbance of thinking, peripheral and irrelevant features of a total concept, which are inhibited in normal directed mental activity, are brought to the forefront and utilized in place of the elements relevant and appropriate to the situation. Thus thinking becomes vague, elliptical and obscure, and its expression in speech sometimes incomprehensible. Breaks and interpolations in the flow of consecutive thought are frequent, and the patient may be convinced that his thoughts are being withdrawn by some outside agency. Mood may be shallow, capricious or incongruous. Ambivalence and disturbance of volition may appear as inertia, negativism or stupor. Catatonia may be present. The diagnosis "schizophrenia" should not be made unless there is, or has been evident during the same illness, characteristic disturbance of thought, perception, mood, conduct, or personality—preferably in at least two of these areas. The diagnosis should not be restricted to conditions running a protracted, deteriorating, or chronic course. In addition to making the diagnosis on the criteria just given, effort should be made to specify one of the following subdivisions of schizophrenia, according to the predominant symptoms.

Includes: schizophrenia of the types described in 295.0-295.9 occurring in children

Excludes: childhood type schizophrenia (299.9)
infantile autism (299.0)

295.0 *Simple type*

A psychosis in which there is insidious development of oddities of conduct, inability to meet the demands of society, and decline in total performance. Delusions and hallucinations are not in evidence and the condition is less obviously psychotic than are the hebephrenic, catatonic and paranoid types of schizophrenia. With increasing social impoverishment vagrancy may ensue and the patient becomes self-absorbed, idle and aimless. Because the schizophrenic symptoms are not clear-cut, diagnosis of this form should be made sparingly, if at all.

Schizophrenia simplex

Excludes: latent schizophrenia (295.5)

295.1 *Hebephrenic type*

A form of schizophrenia in which affective changes are prominent, delusions and hallucinations fleeting and fragmentary, behaviour irresponsible and unpredictable and mannerisms common. The mood is shallow and inappropriate, accompanied by giggling or self-satisfied, self-absorbed smiling, or by a lofty manner, grimaces, mannerisms, pranks, hypochondriacal complaints and reiterated phrases. Thought is disorganized. There is a tendency to remain solitary, and behaviour seems empty of purpose and feeling. This form of schizophrenia usually starts between the ages of 15 and 25 years.

Hebephrenia

295.2 Catatonic type

Includes as an essential feature prominent psychomotor disturbances often alternating between extremes such as hyperkinesis and stupor, or automatic obedience and negativism. Constrained attitudes may be maintained for long periods: if the patient's limbs are put in some unnatural position they may be held there for some time after the external force has been removed. Severe excitement may be a striking feature of the condition. Depressive or hypomanic concomitants may be present.

Catatonic:
  agitation
  excitation
  stupor

Schizophrenic:
  catalepsy
  catatonia
  flexibilitas cerea

295.3 Paranoid type

The form of schizophrenia in which relatively stable delusions, which may be accompanied by hallucinations, dominate the clinical picture. The delusions are frequently of persecution but may take other forms [for example of jealousy, exalted birth, Messianic mission, or bodily change]. Hallucinations and erratic behaviour may occur; in some cases conduct is seriously disturbed from the outset, thought disorder may be gross, and affective flattening with fragmentary delusions and hallucinations may develop.

Paraphrenic schizophrenia

Excludes: paraphrenia, involutional paranoid state (297.2)
           paranoia (297.1)

295.4 Acute schizophrenic episode

Schizophrenic disorders, other than those listed above, in which there is a dream-like state with slight clouding of consciousness and perplexity. External things, people and events may become charged with personal significance for the patient. There may be ideas of reference and emotional turmoil. In many such cases remission occurs within a few weeks or months, even without treatment.

Oneirophrenia

Schizophreniform:
  attack
  psychosis, confusional type

Excludes: acute forms of schizophrenia of:
           catatonic type (295.2)
           hebephrenic type (295.1)
           paranoid type (295.3)
           simple type (295.0)

295.5 Latent schizophrenia

It has not been possible to produce a generally acceptable description for this condition. It is not recommended for general use, but a description is provided for those who believe it to be useful: a condition of eccentric or inconsequent behaviour and anomalies of affect which give the impression of schizophrenia though no definite and characteristic schizophrenic anomalies, present or past, have been manifest.

The inclusion terms indicate that this is the best place to classify some other poorly defined varieties of schizophrenia.

Latent schizophrenic reaction
Schizophrenia:
  borderline
  prepsychotic
  prodromal

Schizophrenia:
  pseudoneurotic
  pseudopsychopathic

Excludes: schizoid personality (301.2)

295.6 *Residual schizophrenia*

A chronic form of schizophrenia in which the symptoms that persist from the acute phase have mostly lost their sharpness. Emotional response is blunted and thought disorder, even when gross, does not prevent the accomplishment of routine work.

Chronic undifferentiated schizophrenia
Restzustand (schizophrenic)
Schizophrenic residual state

295.7 *Schizoaffective type*

A psychosis in which pronounced manic or depressive features are intermingled with schizophrenic features and which tends towards remission without permanent defect, but which is prone to recur. The diagnosis should be made only when both the affective and schizophrenic symptoms are pronounced.

Cyclic schizophrenia
Mixed schizophrenic and affective psychosis
Schizoaffective psychosis
Schizophreniform psychosis, affective type

295.8 *Other*

Schizophrenia of specified type not classifiable under 295.0-295.7.

Acute (undifferentiated)
  schizophrenia

Atypical schizophrenia
Coenesthopathic schizophrenia

Excludes: infantile autism (299.0)

295.9 *Unspecified*

To be used only as a last resort.

Schizophrenia NOS
Schizophrenic reaction NOS
Schizophreniform psychosis NOS

296   Affective psychoses

Mental disorders, usually recurrent, in which there is a severe disturbance of mood [mostly compounded of depression and anxiety but also manifested as elation and excitement] which is accompanied by one or more of the following: delusions, perplexity, disturbed attitude to self, disorder of perception and behaviour; these are all in keeping with the patient's prevailing mood [as are hallucinations when they occur]. There is a strong tendency to suicide. For practical reasons, mild disorders of mood may also be included here if the symptoms match closely the descriptions given; this applies particularly to mild hypomania.

Excludes: reactive depressive psychosis (298.0)
            reactive excitation (298.1)
            neurotic depression (300.4)

296.0   *Manic-depressive psychosis, manic type*

Mental disorders characterized by states of elation or excitement out of keeping with the patient's circumstances and varying from enhanced liveliness [hypomania] to violent, almost uncontrollable excitement. Aggression and anger, flight of ideas, distractibility, impaired judgement, and grandiose ideas are common.

Hypomania NOS
Hypomanic psychosis
Mania (monopolar) NOS
Manic disorder

Manic psychosis
Manic-depressive psychosis or
   reaction:
     hypomanic
     manic

Excludes: circular type if there was a previous attack of depression
            (296.2)

296.1   *Manic-depressive psychosis, depressed type*

An affective psychosis in which there is a widespread depressed mood of gloom and wretchedness with some degree of anxiety. There is often reduced activity but there may be restlessness and agitation. There is a marked tendency to recurrence; in a few cases this may be at regular intervals.

Depressive psychosis
Endogenous depression
Involutional melancholia

Manic-depressive reaction,
   depressed
Monopolar depression
Psychotic depression

Excludes: circular type if previous attack was of manic type (296.3)
            depression NOS (311)

296.2   *Manic-depressive psychosis, circular type but currently manic*

An affective psychosis which has appeared in both the depressive and the manic form, either alternating or separated by an interval of normality, but in which the manic form is currently present. [The manic phase is far less frequent than the depressive].

Bipolar disorder, now manic

Excludes: brief compensatory or rebound mood swings (296.8)

296.3   *Manic-depressive psychosis, circular type but currently depressed*

Circular type (see 296.2) in which the depressive form is currently present.

Bipolar disorder, now depressed

Excludes: brief compensatory or rebound mood swings (296.8)

296.4 *Manic-depressive psychosis, circular type, mixed*

An affective psychosis in which both manic and depressive symptoms are present at the same time.

296.5 *Manic-depressive psychosis, circular type, current condition not specified*

Circular type (see 296.2) in which the current condition is not specified as either manic or depressive.

296.6 *Manic-depressive psychosis, other and unspecified*

Use this code for cases where no other information is available, except the unspecified term, manic-depressive psychosis, or for syndromes corresponding to the descriptions of depressed (296.1) or manic (296.0) types but which for other reasons cannot be classified under 296.0-296.5.

Manic-depressive psychosis:
  NOS
  mixed type

Manic-depressive:
  reaction NOS
  syndrome NOS

296.8 *Other*

Excludes: psychogenic affective psychoses (298.–)

296.9 *Unspecified*

Affective psychosis NOS
Melancholia NOS

297 Paranoid states

Excludes: acute paranoid reaction (298.3)
  alcoholic jealousy (291.5)
  paranoid schizophrenia (295.3)

297.0 *Paranoid state, simple*

A psychosis, acute or chronic, not classifiable as schizophrenia or affective psychosis, in which delusions, especially of being influenced, persecuted or treated in some special way, are the main symptoms. The delusions are of a fairly fixed, elaborate and systematized kind.

297.1 *Paranoia*

A rare chronic psychosis in which logically constructed systematized delusions have developed gradually without concomitant hallucinations or the schizophrenic type of disordered thinking. The delusions are mostly of grandeur [the paranoiac prophet or inventor], persecution or somatic abnormality.

Excludes: paranoid personality disorder (301.0)

297.2 *Paraphrenia*

Paranoid psychosis in which there are conspicuous hallucinations, often in several modalities. Affective symptoms and disordered thinking, if present, do not dominate the clinical picture and the personality is well preserved.

Involutional paranoid state
Late paraphrenia

297.3   Induced psychosis

Mainly delusional psychosis, usually chronic and often without florid features, which appears to have developed as a result of a close, if not dependent, relationship with another person who already has an established similar psychosis. The delusions are at least partly shared. The rare cases in which several persons are affected should also be included here.

Folie à deux   Induced paranoid disorder

297.8   Other

Paranoid states which, though in many ways akin to schizophrenic or affective states, cannot readily be classified under any of the preceding rubrics, nor under 298.4.

Paranoia querulans   Sensitiver Beziehungswahn

Excludes: senile paranoid state (297.2)

297.9   Unspecified

Paranoid:
  psychosis NOS
  reaction NOS
  state NOS

298   Other nonorganic psychoses

Categories 298.0-298.8 should be restricted to the small group of psychotic conditions that are largely or entirely attributable to a recent life experience. They should not be used for the wider range of psychoses in which environmental factors play some [but not the *major*] part in aetiology.

298.0   Depressive type

A depressive psychosis which can be similar in its symptoms to manic-depressive psychosis, depressed type (296.1) but is apparently provoked by saddening stress such as a bereavement, or a severe disappointment or frustration. There may be less diurnal variation of symptoms than in 296.1, and the delusions are more often understandable in the context of the life experiences. There is usually a serious disturbance of behaviour, e.g., major suicidal attempt.

Reactive depressive psychosis
Psychogenic depressive psychosis

Excludes: manic-depressive psychosis, depressed type (296.1)
            neurotic depression (300.4)

298.1   Excitative type

An affective psychosis similar in its symptoms to manic-depressive psychosis, manic type, but apparently provoked by emotional stress.

Excludes: manic-depressive psychosis, manic type (296.0)

298.2 *Reactive confusion*

Mental disorders with clouded consciousness, disorientation [though less marked than in organic confusion] and diminished accessibility often accompanied by excessive activity and apparently provoked by emotional stress.

Psychogenic confusion
Psychogenic twilight state

Excludes: acute confusional state (293.0)

298.3 *Acute paranoid reaction*

Paranoid states apparently provoked by some emotional stress. The stress is often misconstrued as an attack or threat. Such states are particularly prone to occur in prisoners or as acute reactions to a strange and threatening environment, e.g. in immigrants.

Bouffée délirante

Excludes: paranoid states (297.–)

298.4 *Psychogenic paranoid psychosis*

Psychogenic or reactive paranoid psychosis of any type which is more protracted than the acute reactions covered in 298.3. Where there is a diagnosis of psychogenic paranoid psychosis which does not specify "acute" this coding should be made.

Protracted reactive paranoid psychosis

298.8 *Other and unspecified reactive psychosis*

Hysterical psychosis   Psychogenic stupor
Psychogenic psychosis NOS

298.9 *Unspecified psychosis*

To be used only as a last resort, when no other term can be used.

Psychosis NOS

299   Psychoses with origin specific to childhood

This category should be used only for psychoses which always begin before puberty. Adult-type psychoses such as schizophrenia or manic-depressive psychoses when occurring in childhood should be coded elsewhere under the appropriate heading—i.e., 295 and 296 for the examples given.

299.0 *Infantile autism*

A syndrome present from birth or beginning almost invariably in the first 30 months. Responses to auditory and sometimes to visual stimuli are abnormal and there are usually severe problems in the understanding of spoken language. Speech is delayed and, if it develops, is characterized by echolalia, the reversal of pronouns, immature grammatical structure and inability to use abstract terms. There is generally an impairment in the social use of both verbal and gestural language. Problems in social relationships are most severe before the age of five years and include an impairment in the development of eye-to-eye gaze, social attachments, and cooperative play. Ritualistic behaviour is usual and may include abnormal routines, resistance to change, attachment to odd objects and stereotyped patterns of play. The capacity for abstract or symbolic thought and for imaginative play is diminished. Intelligence ranges from severely subnormal to normal or above. Performance is usually better on tasks involving rote memory or visuospatial skills than on those requiring symbolic or linguistic skills.

Childhood autism   Kanner's syndrome
Infantile psychosis

Excludes: disintegrative psychosis (299.1)
            Heller's syndrome (299.1)
            schizophrenic syndrome of childhood (299.9)

299.1   Disintegrative psychosis

A disorder in which normal or near-normal development for the first few years is followed by a loss of social skills and of speech, together with a severe disorder of emotions, behaviour and relationships. Usually this loss of speech and of social competence takes place over a period of a few months and is accompanied by the emergence of overactivity and of stereotypies. In most cases there is intellectual impairment, but this is not a necessary part of the disorder. The condition may follow overt brain disease—such as measles encephalitis—but it may also occur in the absence of any known organic brain disease or damage. Use additional code to identify any associated neurological disorder.

Heller's syndrome

Excludes: infantile autism (299.0)
            schizophrenic syndrome of childhood (299.9)

299.8   Other

A variety of atypical infantile psychoses which may show some, but not all, of the features of infantile autism. Symptoms may include stereotyped repetitive movements, hyperkinesis, self-injury, retarded speech development, echolalia and impaired social relationships. Such disorders may occur in children of any level of intelligence but are particularly common in those with mental retardation.

Atypical childhood psychosis

Excludes: simple stereotypies without psychotic disturbance (307.3)

299.9   Unspecified

Child psychosis NOS
Schizophrenia, childhood type NOS
Schizophrenic syndrome of childhood NOS

Excludes: schizophrenia of adult type occurring in childhood (295.0-
            295.8)

NEUROTIC DISORDERS, PERSONALITY DISORDERS AND OTHER
NONPSYCHOTIC MENTAL DISORDERS (300-316)

300   Neurotic disorders

The distinction between neurosis and psychosis is difficult and remains subject to debate. However, it has been retained in view of its wide use.

Neurotic disorders are mental disorders without any demonstrable organic basis in which the patient may have considerable insight and has unimpaired reality testing, in that he usually does not confuse his morbid subjective experiences and fantasies with external reality. Behaviour may be greatly affected although usually remaining within socially acceptable limits, but personality is not disorganized. The principal manifestations include excessive anxiety, hysterical symptoms, phobias, obsessional and compulsive symptoms, and depression.

300.0   *Anxiety states*

Various combinations of physical and mental manifestations of anxiety, not attributable to real danger and occurring either in attacks or as a persisting state. The anxiety is usually diffuse and may extend to panic. Other neurotic features such as obsessional or hysterical symptoms may be present but do not dominate the clinical picture.

Anxiety: Panic:
  neurosis   attack
  reaction   disorder
  state (neurotic)   state

Excludes: neurasthenia (300.5)
             psychophysiological disorders (306.–)

300.1   *Hysteria*

Mental disorders in which motives, of which the patient seems unaware, produce either a restriction of the field of consciousness or disturbances of motor or sensory function which may seem to have psychological advantage or symbolic value. It may be characterized by conversion phenomena or dissociative phenomena. In the conversion form the chief or only symptoms consist of psychogenic disturbance of function in some part of the body, e.g., paralysis, tremor, blindness, deafness, seizures. In the dissociative variety, the most prominent feature is a narrowing of the field of conscious ness which seems to serve an unconscious purpose and is commonly accompanied or followed by a selective amnesia. There may be dramatic but essentially superficial changes of personality sometimes taking the form of a fugue [wandering state]. Behaviour may mimic psychosis or, rather, the patient's idea of psychosis.

Astasia-abasia, hysterical   Dissociative reaction or state
Compensation neurosis   Ganser's syndrome, hysterical
Conversion hysteria   Hysteria NOS
Conversion reaction   Multiple personality

Excludes: adjustment reaction (309.–)
             anorexia nervosa (307.1)
             gross stress reaction (308.–)
             hysterical personality (301.5)
             psychophysiological disorders (306.–)

300.2   *Phobic state*

Neurotic states with abnormally intense dread of certain objects or specific situations which would not normally have that effect.   If the anxiety tends to spread from a specified situation or object to a wider range of circumstances, it becomes akin to or identical with anxiety state, and should be classified as such (300.0).

Agoraphobia   Claustrophobia
Animal phobias   Phobia NOS
Anxiety-hysteria

Excludes: anxiety state (300.0)
            obsessional phobias (300.3)

300.3   *Obsessive-compulsive disorders*

States in which the outstanding symptom is a feeling of subjective compulsion—which must be resisted—to carry out some action, to dwell on an idea, to recall an experience, or to ruminate on an abstract topic.   Unwanted thoughts which intrude, the insistency of words or ideas, ruminations or trains of thought are perceived by the patient to be inappropriate or nonsensical.   The obsessional urge or idea is recognized as alien to the personality but as coming from within the self.   Obsessional actions may be quasi-ritual performances designed to relieve anxiety e.g., washing the hands to cope with contamination.   Attempts to dispel the unwelcome thoughts or urges may lead to a severe inner struggle, with intense anxiety.

Anankastic neurosis
Compulsive neurosis

Excludes: obsessive-compulsive symptoms occurring in:
            endogenous depression (296.1)
            schizophrenia (295.–)
            organic states, e.g., encephalitis

300.4   *Neurotic depression*

A neurotic disorder characterized by disproportionate depression which has usually recognizably ensued on a distressing experience; it does not include among its features delusions or hallucinations, and there is often preoccupation with the psychic trauma which preceded the illness, e.g., loss of a cherished person or possession.   Anxiety is also frequently present and mixed states of anxiety and depression should be included here.   The distinction between depressive neurosis and psychosis should be made not only upon the degree of depression but also on the presence or absence of other neurotic and psychotic characteristics and upon the degree of disturbance of the patient's behaviour.

Anxiety depression   Neurotic depressive state
Depressive reaction   Reactive depression

Excludes: adjustment reaction with depressive symptoms (309.0)
            depression NOS (311)
            manic-depressive psychosis, depressed type (296.1)
            reactive depressive psychosis (298.0)

300.5 *Neurasthenia*

A neurotic disorder characterized by fatigue, irritability, headache, depression, insomnia, difficulty in concentration, and lack of capacity for enjoyment [anhedonia]. It may follow or accompany an infection or exhaustion, or arise from continued emotional stress. If neurasthenia is associated with a physical disorder, the latter should also be coded.

Nervous debility

Excludes: anxiety state (300.0)
neurotic depression (300.4)
psychophysiological disorders (306.–)
specific nonpsychotic mental disorders following organic brain damage (310.–)

300.6 *Depersonalization syndrome*

A neurotic disorder with an unpleasant state of disturbed perception in which external objects or parts of one's own body are experienced as changed in their quality, unreal, remote or automatized. The patient is aware of the subjective nature of the change he experiences. Depersonalization may occur as a feature of several mental disorders including depression, obsessional neurosis, anxiety and schizophrenia; in that case the condition should not be classified here but in the corresponding major category.

Derealization (neurotic)

300.7 *Hypochondriasis*

A neurotic disorder in which the conspicuous features are excessive concern with one's health in general or the integrity and functioning of some part of one's body, or, less frequently, one's mind. It is usually associated with anxiety and depression. It may occur as a feature of severe mental disorder and in that case should not be classified here but in the corresponding major category.

Excludes: hysteria (300.1)
manic-depressive psychosis, depressed type (296.1)
neurasthenia (300.5)
obsessional disorder (300.3)
schizophrenia (295.–)

300.8 *Other neurotic disorders*

Neurotic disorders not classified elsewhere, e.g., occupational neurosis. Patients with mixed neuroses should not be classified in this category but according to the most prominent symptoms they display.

Briquet's disorder
Occupational neurosis, including writer's cramp
Psychasthenia
Psychasthenic neurosis

300.9 *Unspecified*

To be used only as a last resort.

Neurosis NOS   Psychoneurosis NOS

301   Personality disorders

Deeply ingrained maladaptive patterns of behaviour generally recognizable by the time of adolescence or earlier and continuing throughout most of adult life, although often becoming less obvious in middle or old age. The personality is abnormal either in the balance of its components, their quality and expression or in its total aspect. Because of this deviation or psychopathy the patient suffers or others have to suffer and there is an adverse effect upon the individual or on society. It includes what is sometimes called psychopathic personality, but if this is determined primarily by malfunctioning of the brain, it should not be classified here but as one of the nonpsychotic organic brain syndromes (310). When the patient exhibits an anomaly of personality directly related to his neurosis or psychosis, e.g., schizoid personality and schizophrenia or anankastic personality and obsessive compulsive neurosis, the relevant neurosis or psychosis which is in evidence should be diagnosed in addition.

Character neurosis

301.0   *Paranoid personality disorder*

Personality disorder in which there is excessive sensitiveness to setbacks or to what are taken to be humiliations and rebuffs, a tendency to distort experience by misconstruing the neutral or friendly actions of others as hostile or contemptuous, and a combative and tenacious sense of personal rights. There may be a proneness to jealousy or excessive self-importance. Such persons may feel helplessly humiliated and put upon; others, likewise excessively sensitive, are agressive and insistent. In all cases there is excessive self-reference.

Fanatic personality   Paranoid personality (disorder)
Paranoid traits

Excludes: acute paranoid reaction (298.3)
            alcoholic paranoia (291.5)
            paranoid schizophrenia (295.3)
            paranoid states (297.–)

301.1   *Affective personality disorder*

Personality disorder characterized by lifelong predominance of a pronounced mood which may be persistently depressive, persistently elated, or alternately one then the other. During periods of elation there is unshakeable optimism and an enhanced zest for life and activity, whereas periods of depression are marked by worry, pessimism, low output of energy and a sense of futility.

Cycloid personality   Depressive personality
Cyclothymic personality

Excludes: affective psychoses (296.–)
            cyclothymia (296.2–296.5)
            neurasthenia (300.5)
            neurotic depression (300.4)

301.2   *Schizoid personality disorder*

Personality disorder in which there is withdrawal from affectional, social and other contacts with autistic preference for fantasy and introspective reserve. Behaviour may be slightly eccentric or indicate avoidance of competitive situations. Apparent coolness and detachment may mask an incapacity to express feeling.

Excludes: schizophrenia (295.–)

301.3 *Explosive personality disorder*

Personality disorder characterized by instability of mood with liability to intemperate outbursts of anger, hate, violence or affection. Aggression may be expressed in words or in physical violence. The outbursts cannot readily be controlled by the affected persons, who are not otherwise prone to antisocial behaviour.

Aggressive: Emotional instability (excessive)
  personality   Pathological emotionality
  reaction   Quarrelsomeness
Aggressiveness

Excludes: dyssocial personality (301.7)
           hysterical neurosis (300.1)

301.4 *Anankastic personality disorder*

Personality disorder characterized by feelings of personal insecurity, doubt and incompleteness leading to excessive conscientiousness, checking, stubborness and caution. There may be insistent and unwelcome thoughts or impulses which do not attain the severity of an obsessional neurosis. There is perfectionism and meticulous accuracy and a need to check repeatedly in an attempt to ensure this. Rigidity and excessive doubt may be conspicuous.

Compulsive personality   Obsessional personality

Excludes: obsessive-compulsive disorder (300.3)
           phobic state (300.2)

301.5 *Hysterical personality disorder*

Personality disorder characterized by shallow, labile affectivity, dependence on others, craving for appreciation and attention, suggestibility and theatricality. There is often sexual immaturity, e.g., frigidity and over-responsiveness to stimuli. Under stress hysterical symptoms [neurosis] may develop.

Histrionic personality   Psychoinfantile personality

Excludes: hysterical neurosis (300.1)

301.6 *Asthenic personality disorder*

Personality disorder characterized by passive compliance with the wishes of elders and others and a weak inadequate response to the demands of daily life. Lack of vigour may show itself in the intellectual or emotional spheres; there is little capacity for enjoyment.

Dependent personality   Passive personality
Inadequate personality

Excludes: neurasthenia (300.5)

301.7 *Personality disorder with predominantly sociopathic or asocial manifestation*

Personality disorder characterized by disregard for social obligations, lack of feeling for others, and impetuous violence or callous unconcern. There is a gross disparity between behaviour and the prevailing social norms. Behaviour is not readily modifiable by experience, including punishment. People with this personality are often affectively cold and may be abnormally aggressive or irresponsible. Their tolerance to frustration is low; they blame others or offer plausible rationalizations for the behaviour which brings them into conflict with society.

Amoral personality   Asocial personality
Antisocial personality

Excludes: disturbance of conduct without specifiable personality disorder (312.–)
                explosive personality (301.3)

301.8 *Other personality disorders*

Personality: Personality:
  eccentric   immature
  "haltlose" type   passive-aggressive
                                              psychoneurotic

Excludes: psychoinfantile personality (301.5)

301.9 *Unspecified*

Pathological personality NOS   Psychopathic:
Personality disorder NOS   constitutional state
                                           personality (disorder)

302   Sexual deviations and disorders

Abnormal sexual inclinations or behaviour which are part of a referral problem. The limits and features of normal sexual inclination and behaviour have not been stated absolutely in different societies and cultures but are broadly such as serve approved social and biological purposes. The sexual activity of affected persons is directed primarily either towards people not of the opposite sex, or towards sexual acts not associated with coitus normally, or towards coitus performed under abnormal circumstances. If the anomalous behaviour becomes manifest only during psychosis or other mental illness the condition should be classified under the major illness. It is common for more than one anomaly to occur together in the same individual; in that case the predominant deviation is classified. It is preferable not to include in this category individuals who perform deviant sexual acts when normal sexual outlets are not available to them.

302.0 *Homosexuality*

Exclusive or predominant sexual attraction for persons of the same sex with or without physical relationship. Code homosexuality here whether or not it is considered as a mental disorder.

Lesbianism

Excludes: homosexual paedophilia (302.2)

302.1 *Bestiality*

Sexual or anal intercourse with animals.

302.2 *Paedophilia*

Sexual deviations in which an adult engages in sexual activity with a child of the same or opposite sex.

302.3 *Transvestism*

Sexual deviation in which sexual pleasure is derived from dressing in clothes of the opposite sex. There is no consistent attempt to take on the identity or behaviour of the opposite sex.

Excludes: trans-sexualism (302.5)

302.4 *Exhibitionism*

Sexual deviation in which the main sexual pleasure and gratification is derived from exposure of the genitals to a person of the opposite sex.

302.5 *Trans-sexualism*

Sexual deviation centred around fixed beliefs that the overt bodily sex is wrong. The resulting behaviour is directed towards either changing the sexual organs by operation, or completely concealing the bodily sex by adopting both the dress and behaviour of the opposite sex.

Excludes: transvestism (302.3)

302.6 *Disorders of psychosexual identity*

Behaviour occurring in preadolescents of immature psychosexuality which is similar to that shown in the sexual deviations described under transvestism (302.3) and trans-sexualism (302.5). Cross-dressing is intermittent, although it may be frequent, and identification with the behaviour and appearance of the opposite sex is not yet fixed. The commonest form is feminism in boys.

Gender-role disorder

Excludes: homosexuality (302.0)
            trans-sexualism (302.5)
            transvestism (302.3)

302.7 *Frigidity and impotence*

Frigidity—dislike of or aversion to sexual intercourse, of psychological origin, of sufficient intensity to lead, if not to active avoidance, to marked anxiety, discomfort or pain when normal sexual intercourse takes place. Less severe degrees of this disorder that also give rise to consultation should also be coded here.

Impotence—sustained inability, due to psychological causes, to maintain an erection which will allow normal heterosexual penetration and ejaculation to take place.

Dyspareunia, psychogenic

Excludes: impotence of organic origin
            normal transient symptoms from ruptured hymen
            transient or occasional failures of erection due to fatigue, anxiety, alcohol or drugs

302.8 *Other*

Fetishism   Sadism
Masochism

302.9 *Unspecified*

303   Alcohol dependence syndrome

A state, psychic and usually also physical, resulting from taking alcohol, characterized by behavioural and other responses that always include a compulsion to take alcohol on a continuous or periodic basis in order to experience its psychic effects, and sometimes to avoid the discomfort of its absence; tolerance may or may not be present. A person may be dependent on alcohol and other drugs; if so also make the appropriate 304 coding. If dependence is associated with alcoholic psychosis or with physical complications, *both* should be coded.

Acute drunkenness in alcoholism   Dipsomania
Chronic alcoholism

Excludes: alcoholic psychoses (291.–)
            drunkenness NOS (305.0)
            physical complications of alcohol, such as:
               cirrhosis of liver (571.2)
               epilepsy (345.–)
               gastritis (535.3)

304   Drug dependence

A state, psychic and sometimes also physical, resulting from taking a drug, characterized by behavioural and other responses that always include a compulsion to take a drug on a continuous or periodic basis in order to experience its psychic effects, and sometimes to avoid the discomfort of its absence. Tolerance may or may not be present. A person may be dependent on more than one drug.

Excludes: nondependent abuse of drugs (305.–)

304.0   *Morphine type*

Heroin   Opium alkaloids and their deriva-
Methadone   tives
Opium   Synthetics with morphine-like
                                  effects

304.1   *Barbiturate type*

Barbiturates
Nonbarbiturate sedatives and tranquillizers with a similar effect:
   chlordiazepoxide
   diazepam
   glutethimide
   meprobamate

304.2   *Cocaine*

Coca leaves and derivatives

304.3   *Cannabis*

Hemp   Marijuana
Hashish

304.4 *Amphetamine type and other psychostimulants*

Phenmetrazine   Methylphenidate

304.5 *Hallucinogens*

LSD and derivatives   Psilocybin
Mescaline

304.6 *Other*

Absinthe addiction   Glue sniffing

Excludes: tobacco dependence (305.1)

304.7 *Combinations of morphine type drug with any other*

304.8 *Combinations excluding morphine type drug*

304.9 *Unspecified*

Drug addiction NOS   Drug dependence NOS

305   Nondependent abuse of drugs

Includes cases where a person, for whom no other diagnosis is possible, has come under medical care because of the maladaptive effect of a drug on which he is not dependent (as defined in 304.–) and that he has taken on his own initiative to the detriment of his health or social functioning. When drug abuse is secondary to a psychiatric disorder, code the disorder.

Excludes: alcohol dependence syndrome (303)
          drug dependence (304.–)
          drug withdrawal syndrome (292.0)
          poisoning by drugs or medicaments (960-979)

305.0 *Alcohol*

Cases of acute intoxication or "hangover" effects.

Drunkenness NOS   "Hangover" (alcohol)
Excessive drinking of alcohol NOS   Inebriety NOS

Excludes: alcoholic psychoses (291.–)
          physical complications of alcohol, such as:
              cirrhosis of liver (571.2)
              epilepsy (345.–)
              gastritis (535.3)

305.1 *Tobacco*

Cases in which tobacco is used to the detriment of a person's health or social functioning or in which there is tobacco dependence. Dependence is included here rather than under 304.– because tobacco differs from other drugs of dependence in its psychotoxic effects.

Tobacco dependence

305.2 *Cannabis*

305.3 *Hallucinogens*

Cases of acute intoxication or "bad trips".

LSD reaction

305.4 *Barbiturates and tranquillizers*

Cases where a person has taken the drug to the detriment of his health or social functioning, in doses above or for periods beyond those normally regarded as therapeutic.

305.5 *Morphine type*

305.6 *Cocaine type*

305.7 *Amphetamine type*

305.8 *Antidepressants*

305.9 *Other, mixed or unspecified*

"Laxative habit"　　　　　　　　Nonprescribed use of drugs or
Misuse of drugs NOS　　　　　　　patent medicinals

306 Physiological malfunction arising from mental factors

A variety of physical symptoms or types of physiological malfunction of mental origin, not involving tissue damage and usually mediated through the autonomic nervous system. The disorders are grouped according to body system. Codes 306.0-306.9 should not be used if the physical symptom is secondary to a psychiatric disorder classifiable elsewhere. If tissue damage is involved, code under 316.

Excludes: hysteria (300.1)
psychic factors associated with physical conditions involving tissue damage classified elsewhere (316)
specific nonpsychotic mental disorders following organic brain damage (310.–)

306.0 *Musculoskeletal*

Psychogenic torticollis

Excludes: Gilles de la Tourette's syndrome (307.2)
tics (307.2)

306.1 *Respiratory*

Air hunger　　　　　　　　　　Psychogenic cough
Hiccough (psychogenic)　　　　　Yawning
Hyperventilation

Excludes: psychogenic asthma (316 and 493.9)

306.2 *Cardiovascular*

Cardiac neurosis　　　　　　　　Neurocirculatory asthenia
Cardiovascular neurosis　　　　　Psychogenic cardiovascular
　　　　　　　　　　　　　　　disorder

Excludes: psychogenic paroxysmal tachycardia (316 and 427.9)

306.3 *Skin*

Psychogenic pruritus

Excludes: psychogenic:
   alopecia (316 and 704.0)
   dermatitis (316 and 692.–)
   eczema (316 and 691.9 or 692.–)
   urticaria (316 and 708.–)

306.4 *Gastrointestinal*

Aerophagy   Cyclical vomiting, psychogenic

Excludes: cyclical vomiting NOS (536.2)
   mucous colitis (316 and 564.1)
   psychogenic:
      cardiospasm (316 and 530.0)
      duodenal ulcer (316 and 532.–)
      gastric ulcer (316 and 531.–)
      peptic ulcer (316 and 533.–)

306.5 *Genitourinary*

Psychogenic dysmenorrhoea

Excludes: dyspareunia (302.7)
   enuresis (307.6)
   frigidity (302.7)
   impotence (302.7)

306.6 *Endocrine*

306.7 *Organs of special sense*

Excludes: hysterical blindness or deafness (300.1)

306.8 *Other*

Teeth-grinding

306.9 *Unspecified*

Psychophysiologic disorder NOS   Psychosomatic disorder NOS

307 Special symptoms or syndromes not elsewhere classified

Conditions in which an outstanding symptom or group of symptoms is not manifestly part of a more fundamental classifiable condition.

Excludes: when due to mental disorders classified elsewhere
   when of organic origin

307.0 *Stammering and stuttering*

Disorders in the rhythm of speech, in which the individual knows precisely what he wishes to say, but at the time is unable to say it because of an involuntary, repetitive prolongation or cessation of a sound.

Excludes: dysphasia (784.5)
lisping or lalling (307.9)
retarded development of speech (315.3)

307.1 *Anorexia nervosa*

A disorder in which the main features are persistent active refusal to eat and marked loss of weight. The level of activity and alertness is characteristically high in relation to the degree of emaciation. Typically the disorder begins in teenage girls but it may sometimes begin before puberty and rarely it occurs in males. Amenorrhoea is usual and there may be a variety of other physiological changes including slow pulse and respiration, low body temperature and dependent oedema. Unusual eating habits and attitudes toward food are typical and sometimes starvation follows or alternates with periods of overeating. The accompanying psychiatric symptoms are diverse.

Excludes: eating disturbance NOS (307.5)
loss of appetite (783.0)
of nonorganic origin (307.5)

307.2 *Tics*

Disorders of no known organic origin in which the outstanding feature consists of quick, involuntary, apparently purposeless, and frequently repeated movements which are not due to any neurological condition. Any part of the body may be involved but the face is most frequently affected. Only one form of tic may be present, or there may be a combination of tics which are carried out simultaneously, alternatively or consecutively. Gilles de la Tourette's syndrome refers to a rare disorder occurring in individuals of any level of intelligence in which facial tics and tic-like throat noises become more marked and more generalized and in which later, whole words or short sentences [often with an obscene content] are ejaculated spasmodically and involuntarily. There is some overlap with other varieties of tic.

Excludes: nail-biting or thumb-sucking (307.9)
stereotypies occurring in isolation (307.3)
tics of organic origin (333.3)

307.3 *Stereotyped repetitive movements*

Disorders in which voluntary repetitive stereotyped movements, which are not due to any psychiatric or neurological condition, constitute the main feature. Includes head-banging, spasmus nutans, rocking, twirling, finger-flicking mannerisms and eye poking. Such movements are particularly common in cases of mental retardation with sensory impairment or with environmental monotony.

Stereotypies NOS

Excludes: tics:
NOS (307.2)
of organic origin (333.3)

307.4 *Specific disorders of sleep*

This category should only be used when a more precise medical or psychiatric diagnosis cannot be made.

Hypersomnia
Insomnia
Inversion of sleep rhythm
Nightmares
Night terrors
Sleepwalking
} of nonorganic origin

Excludes: narcolepsy (347.0)
when of unspecified cause (780.5)

307.5 *Other and unspecified disorders of eating*

This category should only be used when a more precise medical or psychiatric diagnosis cannot be made.

Infantile feeding disturbances
Loss of appetite
Overeating
Pica
} of nonorganic origin
Psychogenic vomiting

Excludes: anorexia:
nervosa (307.1)
of unspecified cause (783.0)
overeating of unspecified cause (783.6)
vomiting:
NOS (787.0)
cyclical (536.2)
psychogenic (306.4)

307.6 *Enuresis*

A disorder in which the main manifestation is a persistent involuntary voiding of urine by day or night which is considered abnormal for the age of the individual. Sometimes the child will have failed to gain bladder control and in other cases he will have gained control and then lost it. Episodic or fluctuating enuresis should be included. The disorder would not usually be diagnosed under the age of four years.

Enuresis (primary) (secondary) of nonorganic origin

Excludes: enuresis of unspecified cause (788.3)

307.7 *Encopresis*

A disorder in which the main manifestation is the persistent voluntary or involuntary passage of formed motions of normal or near-normal consistency into places not intended for that purpose in the individual's own sociocultural setting. Sometimes the child has failed to gain bowel control, and sometimes he has gained control but then later again became encopretic. There may be a variety of associated psychiatric symptoms and there may be smearing of faeces. The condition would not usually be diagnosed under the age of four years.

Encopresis (continuous) (discontinuous) of nonorganic origin

Excludes: encopresis of unspecified cause (787.6)

307.8 *Psychalgia*

Cases in which there are pains of mental origin, e.g., headache or backache, when a more precise medical or psychiatric diagnosis cannot be made.

Tension headache   Psychogenic backache

Excludes: migraine (346.–)
pains not specifically attributable to a psychological cause (in):
back (724.5)
headache (784.0)
joint (719.4)
limb (729.5)
lumbago (724.2)
rheumatic (729.0)

307.9 *Other and unspecified*

The use of this category should be discouraged. Most of the items listed in the inclusion terms are not indicative of psychiatric disorder and are included only because such terms may sometimes still appear as diagnoses.

Hair plucking   Masturbation
Lalling   Nail-biting
Lisping   Thumb-sucking

308   Acute reaction to stress

Very transient disorders of any severity and nature which occur in individuals without any apparent mental disorder in response to exceptional physical or mental stress, such as natural catastrophe or battle, and which usually subside within hours or days.

Catastrophic stress   Exhaustion delirium
Combat fatigue

Excludes: adjustment reaction (309.–)

308.0 *Predominant disturbance of emotions*

Panic states, excitability, fear, depressions and anxiety fulfilling the above criteria.

308.1 *Predominant disturbance of consciousness*

Fugues fulfilling the above criteria.

308.2 *Predominant psychomotor disturbance*

Agitation states, stupor fulfilling the above criteria.

308.3 *Other*

Acute situational disturbance

308.4 *Mixed*

Many gross stress reactions include several elements but whenever possible a specific coding under .0, .1, .2 or .3 should be made according to the *preponderant* type of disturbance. The category of mixed disorders should only be used when there is such an admixture that this cannot be done.

308.9 *Unspecified*

309 Adjustment reaction

Mild or transient disorders lasting longer than acute stress reactions (308.–) which occur in individuals of any age without any apparent pre-existing mental disorder. Such disorders are often relatively circumscribed or situation-specific, are generally reversible, and usually last only a few months. They are usually closely related in time and content to stresses such as bereavement, migration or separation experiences. Reactions to major stress that last longer than a few days are also included here. In children such disorders are associated with no significant distortion of development.

Excludes: acute reaction to major stress (308.–)
　　　　　 neurotic disorders (300.–)

309.0 *Brief depressive reaction*

States of depression, not specifiable as manic-depressive, psychotic or neurotic, generally transient, in which the depressive symptoms are usually closely related in time and content to some stressful event.

Grief reaction

Excludes: affective psychoses (296.–)
　　　　　 neurotic depression (300.4)
　　　　　 prolonged depressive reaction (309.1)
　　　　　 psychogenic depressive psychosis (298.0)

309.1 *Prolonged depressive reaction*

States of depression, not specifiable as manic-depressive, psychotic or neurotic, generally long-lasting; usually developing in association with prolonged exposure to a stressful situation.

Excludes: affective psychoses (296.–)
　　　　　 brief depressive reaction (309.0)
　　　　　 neurotic depression (300.4)
　　　　　 psychogenic depressive psychosis (298.0)

309.2 *With predominant disturbance of other emotions*

States, fulfilling the general criteria for adjustment reaction, in which the main symptoms are emotional in type [anxiety, fear, worry, etc.] but not specifically depressive.

Abnormal separation anxiety　　　　　Culture shock

309.3 *With predominant disturbance of conduct*

Mild or transient disorders, fulfilling the general criteria for adjustment reaction, in which the main disturbance predominantly involves a disturbance of conduct. For example, an adolescent grief reaction resulting in aggressive or antisocial disorder would be included here.

Excludes: disturbance of conduct NOS (312.–)
　　　　　 dyssocial behaviour without manifest psychiatric disorder (V71.0)
　　　　　 personality disorder with predominantly sociopathic or asocial manifestations (301.7)

309.4   *With mixed disturbance of emotions and conduct*

Disorders fulfilling the general definition in which both emotional disturbance and disturbance of conduct are prominent features.

309.8   *Other*

Adjustment reaction with elective mutism
Hospitalism in children NOS

309.9   *Unspecified*

Adjustment reaction NOS   Adaptation reaction NOS

310   Specific nonpsychotic mental disorders following organic brain damage

Note: This category should be used only for conditions where the *form* of the disorder is determined by the brain pathology.

Excludes: neuroses, personality disorders or other nonpsychotic conditions occurring in a form similar to that seen with functional disorders but in association with a physical condition; code to 300.–, 301.–, etc., and use additional code to identify the physical condition

310.0   *Frontal lobe syndrome*

Changes in behaviour following damage to the frontal areas of the brain or following interference with the connections of those areas. There is a general diminution of self-control, foresight, creativity and spontaneity, which may be manifest as increased irritability, selfishness, restlessness and lack of concern for others. Conscientiousness and powers of concentration are often diminished, but measurable deterioration of intellect or memory is not necessarily present. The overall picture is often one of emotional dullness, lack of drive and slowness; but, particularly in persons previously with energetic, restless or aggressive characteristics, there may be a change towards impulsiveness, boastfulness, temper outbursts, silly fatuous humour, and the development of unrealistic ambitions; the direction of change usually depends upon the previous personality. A considerable degree of recovery is possible and may continue over the course of several years.

Lobotomy syndrome
Postleucotomy syndrome (state)

Excludes: postcontusional syndrome (310.2)

310.1   *Cognitive or personality change of other type*

Chronic, mild states of memory disturbance and intellectual deterioration, often accompanied by increased irritability, querulousness, lassitude and complaints of physical weakness. These states are often associated with old age, and may precede more severe states due to brain damage classifiable under dementia of any type (290.–, and 294.–) or any condition in 293.– (Transient organic psychotic conditions).

Mild memory disturbance
Organic psychosyndrome of nonpsychotic severity

310.2 *Postconcussional syndrome*

States occurring after generalized contusion of the brain, in which the symptom picture may resemble that of the frontal lobe syndrome (310.0) or that of any of the neurotic disorders (300.0-300.9), but in which in addition, headache, giddiness, fatigue, insomnia and a subjective feeling of impaired intellectual ability are usually prominent. Mood may fluctuate, and quite ordinary stress may produce exaggerated fear and apprehension. There may be marked intolerance of mental and physical exertion, undue sensitivity to noise, and hypochondriacal preoccupation. The symptoms are more common in persons who have previously suffered from neurotic or personality disorders, or when there is a possibility of compensation. This syndrome is particularly associated with the closed type of head injury when signs of localized brain damage are slight or absent, but it may also occur in other conditions.

Postcontusional syndrome (encephalopathy)
Status post commotio cerebri
Post-traumatic brain syndrome, nonpsychotic

Excludes: frontal lobe syndrome (310.0)
postencephalitic syndrome (310.8)
any organic psychotic conditions following head injury (290.– to 294.0)

310.8 *Other*

Include here disorders resembling the postcontusional syndrome (310.2), associated with infective or other diseases of the brain or surrounding tissues.

Other focal (partial) organic psychosyndromes

310.9 *Unspecified*

311 Depressive disorder, not elsewhere classified

States of depression, usually of moderate but occasionally of marked intensity, which have no specifically manic-depressive or other psychotic depressive features and which do not appear to be associated with stressful events or other features specified under neurotic depression.

Depressive disorder NOS Depression NOS
Depressive state NOS

Excludes: acute reaction to major stress with depressive symptoms (308.0)
affective personality disorder (301.1)
affective psychoses (296.–)
brief depressive reaction (309.0)
disturbance of emotions specific to childhood and adolescence, with misery and unhappiness (313.1)
mixed adjustment reaction with depressive symptoms (309.4)
neurotic depression (300.4)
prolonged depressive adjustment reaction (309.1)
psychogenic depressive psychosis (298.0)

312   Disturbance of conduct not elsewhere classified

Disorders mainly involving aggressive and destructive behaviour and disorders involving delinquency. It should be used for abnormal behaviour, in individuals of any age, which gives rise to social disapproval but which is not part of any other psychiatric condition. Minor emotional disturbances may also be present. To be included, the behaviour—as judged by its frequency, severity and type of associations with other symptoms—must be abnormal in its context. Disturbances of conduct are distinguished from an adjustment reaction by a longer duration and by a lack of close relationship in time and content to some stress. They differ from a personality disorder by the absence of deeply ingrained maladapative patterns of behaviour present from adolescence or earlier.

Excludes: adjustment reaction with disturbance of conduct (309.3)
drug dependence (304.–)
dyssocial behaviour without manifest psychiatric disorder (V71.0)
personality disorder with predominantly sociopathic or asocial manifestations (301.7)
sexual deviations (302.–)

312.0   *Unsocialized disturbance of conduct*

Disorders characterized by behaviours such as defiance, disobedience, quarrelsomeness, aggression, destructive behaviour, tantrums, solitary stealing, lying, teasing, bullying and disturbed relationships with others. The defiance may sometimes take the form of sexual misconduct.

Unsocialized aggressive disorder

312.1   *Socialized disturbance of conduct*

Disorders in individuals who have acquired the values or behaviour of a delinquent peer group to whom they are loyal and with whom they characteristically steal, play truant, and stay out late at night. There may also be promiscuity.

Group delinquency

Excludes: gang activity without manifest psychiatric disorder (V71.0)

312.2   *Compulsive conduct disorder*

Disorder of conduct or delinquent act which is specifically compulsive in origin.

Kleptomania

312.3   *Mixed disturbance of conduct and emotions*

Disorders involving behaviours listed for 312.0 and 312.1 but in which there is also *considerable* emotional disturbance as shown for example by anxiety, misery or obsessive manifestations.

Neurotic delinquency

Excludes: compulsive conduct disorder (312.2)

312.8   *Other*

312.9   *Unspecified*

313   Disturbance of emotions specific to childhood and adolescence

Less well differentiated emotional disorders characteristic of the childhood period. Where the emotional disorder takes the form of a neurotic disorder described under 300.–, the appropriate 300.– coding should be made. This category differs from category 308.– in terms of longer duration and by the lack of close relationship in time and content to some stress.

Excludes: adjustment reaction (309.–)
           masturbation, nail-biting, thumb-sucking and other isolated symptoms (307.–)

313.0   *With anxiety and fearfulness*

Ill-defined emotional disorders characteristic of childhood in which the main symptoms involve anxiety and fearfulness. Many cases of school refusal or elective mutism might be included here.

Overanxious reaction of childhood or adolescence

Excludes: abnormal separation anxiety (309.2)
           anxiety states (300.0)
           hospitalism in children (309.8)
           phobic state (300.2)

313.1   *With misery and unhappiness*

Emotional disorders characteristic of childhood in which the main symptoms involve misery and unhappiness. There may also be eating and sleep disturbances.

Excludes: depressive neurosis (300.4)

313.2   *With sensitivity, shyness and social withdrawal*

Emotional disorders characteristic of childhood in which the main symptoms involve sensitivity, shyness, or social withdrawal. Some cases of elective mutism might be included here.

Withdrawing reaction of childhood or adolescence

Excludes: infantile autism (299.0)
           schizoid personality (301.2)
           schizophrenia (295.–)

313.3   *Relationship problems*

Emotional disorders characteristic of childhood in which the main symptoms involve relationship problems.

Sibling jealousy

Excludes: relationship problems associated with aggression, destruction or other forms of conduct disturbance (312.–)

313.8   *Other or mixed*

Many emotional disorders of childhood include several elements but whenever possible a specific coding under .0, .1, .2 or .3 should be made according to the *preponderant* type of disturbance. The category of mixed disorders should only be used when there is such an admixture that this cannot be done.

313.9 *Unspecified*

314   Hyperkinetic syndrome of childhood

Disorders in which the essential features are short attention-span and distractibility. In early childhood the most striking symptom is disinhibited, poorly organized and poorly regulated extreme overactivity but in adolescence this may be replaced by under-activity. Impulsiveness, marked mood fluctuations and aggression are also common symptoms. Delays in the development of specific skills are often present and disturbed, poor relationships are common. If the hyperkinesis is symptomatic of an underlying disorder, code the underlying disorder instead.

314.0 *Simple disturbance of activity and attention*

Cases in which short attention span, distractibility, and overactivity are the main manifestations without significant disturbance of conduct or delay in specific skills.

Overactivity NOS

314.1 *Hyperkinesis with developmental delay*

Cases in which the hyperkinetic syndrome is associated with speech delay, clumsiness, reading difficulties or other delays in specific skills.

Developmental disorder of hyperkinesis

Use additional code to identify any associated neurological disorder

314.2 *Hyperkinetic conduct disorder*

Cases in which the hyperkinetic syndrome is associated with marked conduct distur-bance but not developmental delay.

Hyperkinetic conduct disorder

Excludes: hyperkinesis with significant delays in specific skills (314.1)

314.8 *Other*

314.9 *Unspecified*

Hyperkinetic reaction of childhood   Hyperkinetic syndrome NOS
   or adolescence NOS

315   Specific delays in development

A group of disorders in which a specific delay in development is the main feature. In each case development is related to biological maturation but it is also influenced by nonbiological factors and the coding carries no aetiological implications.

Excludes: when due to a neurological disorder (320-389)

315.0 *Specific reading retardation*

Disorders in which the main feature is a serious impairment in the development of reading or spelling skills which is not explicable in terms of general intellectual retar-dation or of inadequate schooling. Speech or language difficulties, impaired right-left differentiation, perceptuo-motor problems, and coding difficulties are frequently asso-ciated. Similar problems are often present in other members of the family. Adverse psychosocial factors may be present.

Developmental dyslexia   Specific spelling difficulty

315.1   *Specific arithmetical retardation*

Disorders in which the main feature is a serious impairment in the development of arithmetical skills which is not explicable in terms of general intellectual retardation or of inadequate schooling.

Dyscalculia

315.2   *Other specific learning difficulties*

Disorders in which the main feature is a serious impairment in the development of other learning skills which are not explicable in terms of general intellectual retardation or of inadequate schooling.

Excludes: specific arithmetical retardation (315.1)
            specific reading retardation (315.0)

315.3   *Developmental speech or language disorder*

Disorders in which the main feature is a serious impairment in the development of speech or language [syntax or semantics] which is not explicable in terms of general intellectual retardation. Most commonly there is a delay in the development of normal word-sound production resulting in defects of articulation. Omissions or substitutions of consonants are most frequent. There may also be a delay in the production of spoken language. Rarely, there is also a developmental delay in the comprehension of sounds. Includes cases in which delay is largely due to environmental privation.

Developmental aphasia   Dyslalia

Excludes: acquired aphasia (784.3)
            elective mutism (309.8, 313.0 or 313.2)
            lisping and lalling (307.9)
            stammering and stuttering (307.0)

315.4   *Specific motor retardation*

Disorders in which the main feature is a serious impairment in the development of motor coordination which is not explicable in terms of general intellectual retardation. The clumsiness is commonly associated with perceptual difficulties.

Clumsiness syndrome   Dyspraxia syndrome

315.5   *Mixed development disorder*

A delay in the development of one specific skill [e.g., reading, arithmetic, speech or coordination] is frequently associated with lesser delays in other skills. When this occurs the coding should be made according to the skill most seriously impaired. The mixed category should be used only where the mixture of delayed skills is such that no one skill is preponderantly affected.

315.8   *Other*

315.9   *Unspecified*

Developmental disorder NOS

316   Psychic factors associated with diseases classified elsewhere

Mental disturbances or psychic factors of any type thought to have played a major part in the aetiology of physical conditions, usually involving tissue damage, classified elsewhere. The mental disturbance is usually mild and nonspecific and psychic factors [worry, fear, conflict, etc.] may be present without any overt psychiatric disorder. Use an additional code to identify the physical condition. In the rare instance that an overt psychiatric disorder is thought to have caused a physical condition, use a second additional code to record the psychiatric diagnosis.

Examples of the use of this category are:
  psychogenic:
      asthma 316 and 493.9
      dermatitis 316 and 692.–
      eczema 316 and 691.– or 692.–
      gastric ulcer 316 and 531.–
      mucous colitis 316 and 564.1
      ulcerative colitis 316 and 556
      urticaria 316 and 708.–
  psychosocial dwarfism 316 and 259.4

Excludes: physical symptoms and physiological malfunctions, not involving tissue damage, of mental origin (306.–)

MENTAL RETARDATION (317-319)

A condition of arrested or incomplete development of mind which is especially characterized by subnormality of intelligence. The coding should be made on the individual's *current* level of functioning *without regard to its nature* or causation—such as psychosis, cultural deprivation, Down's syndrome etc.. Where there is a specific cognitive handicap—such as in speech—the four-digit coding should be based on assessments of cognition *outside the area of specific handicap*. The assessment of intellectual level should be based on whatever information is available, including clinical evidence, adaptive behaviour and psychometric findings. The IQ levels given are based on a test with a mean of 100 and a standard deviation of 15—such as the Wechsler scales. They are provided only as a guide and should not be applied rigidly. Mental retardation often involves psychiatric disturbances and may often develop as a result of some physical disease or injury. In these cases, an additional code or codes should be used to identify any associated condition, psychiatric or physical. The Impairment and Handicap codes should also be consulted.

317   Mild mental retardation

Feeble-minded   Moron
High-grade defect   IQ 50-70
Mild mental subnormality

318   Other specified mental retardation

318.0 *Moderate mental retardation*

Imbecile   Moderate mental subnormality
IQ 35-49

318.1   *Severe mental retardation*

IQ 20-34   Severe mental subnormality

318.2   *Profound mental retardation*

Idiocy   Profound mental subnormality
IQ under 20

319   Unspecified mental retardation

Mental deficiency NOS   Mental subnormality NOS

VI.   DISEASES OF THE NERVOUS SYSTEM AND SENSE ORGANS

320   Bacterial meningitis

Includes: arachnoiditis
leptomeningitis
meningitis
meningoencephalitis } bacterial
meningomyelitis
pachymeningitis

320.0   *Haemophilus meningitis*

Meningitis due to Haemophilus influenzae [H. influenzae]

320.1   *Pneumococcal meningitis*

320.2   *Streptococcal meningitis*

320.3   *Staphylococcal meningitis*

320.4* *Tuberculous meningitis* (013.0†)

320.5* *Meningococcal meningitis* (036.0†)

320.7* *Meningitis in other bacterial diseases classified elsewhere*

Meningitis (in):
gonoccocal (098.8†)
listeriosis (027.0†)
neurosyphilis (094.2†)
salmonellosis (003.2†)
syphilis:
congenital (090.4†)
secondary (091.8†)
typhoid fever (002.0†)

320.8   *Meningitis due to other specified bacteria*

Meningitis due to:
Escherichia coli [E. coli]
Friedländer bacillus

320.9   *Meningitis due to unspecified bacterium*

Meningitis:
bacterial NOS
purulent NOS
pyogenic NOS
suppurative NOS

321* Meningitis due to other organisms

Includes: arachnoiditis
leptomeningitis
meningitis
pachymeningitis } due to organisms other than bacteria

321.0* *Fungal meningitis* (110-118†)
Cryptococcal meningitis (117.5†)

321.1* *Meningitis due to Coxsackie virus* (047.0†)

321.2* *Meningitis due to ECHO virus* (047.1†)
Meningo-eruptive syndrome

321.3* *Meningitis due to herpes zoster virus* (053.0†)

321.4* *Meningitis due to herpes simplex virus* (054.7†)

321.5* *Meningitis due to mumps virus* (072.1†)

321.6* *Meningitis due to lymphocytic choriomeningitis virus* (049.0†)

321.7* *Meningitis due to other and unspecified viruses*
Meningitis:
arbovirus (060-066†)
aseptic NOS (047.9†)
viral NOS (047.9†)

321.8* *Other*
Meningitis due to:
leptospira (100.8†)
trypanosomiasis (086.–†)

322 Meningitis of unspecified cause

Includes: arachnoiditis
leptomeningitis
meningitis
pachymeningitis } with no organism specified as cause

322.0 *Nonpyogenic meningitis*
Meningitis with clear cerebrospinal fluid

322.1 *Eosinophilic meningitis*

322.2 *Chronic meningitis*

322.9 *Meningitis, unspecified*

323 Encephalitis, myelitis and encephalomyelitis

Includes: acute disseminated encephalomyelitis
meningoencephalitis, except bacterial
meningomyelitis, except bacterial
myelitis (acute):
ascending
transverse

Excludes: bacterial:
meningoencephalitis (320.–)
meningomyelitis (320.–)

323.0* *Kuru* (046.0†)

323.1* *Subacute sclerosing panencephalitis* (046.2†)

Dawson's encephalitis
Van Bogaert's subacute sclerosing leucoencephalitis

323.2* *Poliomyelitis* (045.–†)

323.3* *Arthropod-borne viral encephalitis* (062-064†)

323.4* *Other encephalitis due to infection*

Encephalitis (in):
herpes simplex (054.3†)
meningococcal (036.1†)
mumps (072.2†)
rubella (056.0†)
syphilis (094.8†)
congenital (090.4†)

Encephalitis (in):
trypanosomiasis (086.–†)
tuberculosis (013.8†)
viral NOS (049.9†)
Meningoencephalitis due to free living amoebae [Naegleria] (136.2†)

323.5 *Encephalitis following immunization procedures*

Encephalitis ⎱
Encephalomyelitis ⎰ postimmunization or postvaccinal

Use additional E code, if desired, to identify vaccine

323.6* *Postinfectious encephalitis*

Encephalitis:
postchickenpox (052†)
postmeasles (055.0†)

323.7* *Toxic encephalitis*

Lead encephalitis (984.–†)

323.8 *Other*

323.9 *Unspecified cause*

324   Intracranial and intraspinal abscess

324.0   *Intracranial abscess*

Abscess (embolic) of brain [any part]:
  epidural
  extradural
  otogenic
  subdural
  tuberculous* (013.8†)

Abscess (embolic):
  cerebellar
  cerebral

324.1   *Intraspinal abscess*

Abscess (embolic) of spinal cord [any part]:
  epidural
  extradural
  subdural
  tuberculous* (013.8†)

324.9   *Of unspecified site*

Extradural or subdural abscess NOS

325   Phlebitis and thrombophlebitis of intracranial venous sinuses

Embolism
Endophlebitis
Phlebitis, septic or suppurative
Thrombophlebitis
Thrombosis
} of cavernous, lateral or other intracranial or unspecified intracranial venous sinus

Excludes: when specified as:
            complicating pregnancy, childbirth or the puerperium (671.5)
            of nonpyogenic origin (437.6)

326   Late effects of intracranial abscess or pyogenic infection

Note: This category is to be used to indicate conditions whose primary classification is to 320-325 [i.e. excluding those marked with an asterisk (*)] as the cause of late effects, themselves classifiable elsewhere. The "late effects" include conditions specified as such, or as sequelae, or present one year or more after the onset of the causal condition. [See III Late effects, page 723].

HEREDITARY AND DEGENERATIVE DISEASES OF THE CENTRAL
NERVOUS SYSTEM (330-337)

Excludes: hepatolenticular degeneration (275.1)
            multiple sclerosis (340)
            other demyelinating diseases of central nervous system (341.–)

330 Cerebral degenerations usually manifest in childhood

Use additional code, if desired, to identify associated mental retardation

330.0 *Leucodystrophy*

Krabbe's disease
Leucodystrophy:
 NOS
 globoid cell
 metachromatic
 sudanophilic

330.1 *Cerebral lipidoses*

Amaurotic (family) idiocy
Disease:
 Batten
 Jansky-Bielschowsky
 Kufs

Disease:
 Spielmeyer-Vogt
 Tay-Sachs
Gangliosidosis

330.2* *Cerebral degeneration in generalized lipidoses* (272.7†)

Cerebral degeneration in:
 Fabry's disease
 Gaucher's disease
 Niemann-Pick disease
 sphingolipidosis

330.3* *Cerebral degeneration of childhood in other diseases classified elsewhere*

Cerebral degeneration in:
 Hunter's disease (277.5†)
 mucopolysaccharidoses (277.5†)

330.8 *Other cerebral degenerations in childhood*

Alpers's disease or grey-matter degeneration
Leigh's disease or subacute necrotizing encephalopathy

330.9 *Unspecified*

331 Other cerebral degenerations

Use additional code, if desired, to identify associated mental disorder

331.0 *Alzheimer's disease*

331.1 *Pick's disease*

331.2 *Senile degeneration of brain*

Excludes: senility NOS (797)

331.3 *Communicating hydrocephalus*
Excludes: congenital hydrocephalus (741.0, 742.3)

331.4 *Obstructive hydrocephalus*
Acquired hydrocephalus NOS
Excludes: congenital hydrocephalus (741.0, 742.3)

331.5* *Jakob-Creutzfeldt disease* (046.1†)
Subacute spongioform encephalopathy

331.6* *Progressive multifocal leucoencephalopathy* (046.3†)

331.7* *Cerebral degeneration in other diseases classified elsewhere*
Cerebral degeneration in:
    alcoholism (303†)
    beriberi (265.0†)
    cerebrovascular disease (430-438†)
    congenital hydrocephalus (741.0, 742.3†)
    neoplastic disease (140-239†)
    myxoedema (244.–†)
    vitamin B_{12} deficiency (266.2†)

331.8 *Other cerebral degeneration*

331.9 *Unspecified*

332 **Parkinson's disease**

332.0 *Paralysis agitans*
Parkinsonism or Parkinson's disease:
    NOS
    idiopathic
    primary

332.1 *Secondary Parkinsonism*
Parkinsonism:
    due to drugs
    syphilitic* (094.8†)
Use additional E code, if desired, to identify drug, if drug-induced

333 **Other extrapyramidal disease and abnormal movement disorders**

Includes: other forms of extrapyramidal, basal ganglia or striatopalli-
dal disease

Excludes: abnormal movements of head NOS (781.0)

333.0 *Other degenerative diseases of the basal ganglia*

Hallervorden-Spatz disease or pigmentary pallidal degeneration
Olivopontocerebellar degeneration
Parkinsonian syndrome associated with:
  idiopathic orthostatic hypotension
  symptomatic orthostatic hypotension
Progressive supranuclear ophthalmoplegia
Shy-Drager syndrome
Strionigral degeneration

333.1 *Essential and other specified forms of tremor*

Benign essential tremor   Familial tremor

Use additional E code, if desired, to identify drug, if drug-induced

Excludes: tremor NOS (781.0)

333.2 *Myoclonus*

Familial essential myoclonus   Unverricht-Lundborg disease
Progressive myoclonic epilepsy

Use additional E code, if desired, to identify drug, if drug-induced

333.3 *Tics of organic origin*

Excludes: Gilles de la Tourette's syndrome (307.2)
          habit spasm (307.2)
          tic NOS (307.2)

Use additional E code, if desired, to identify drug, if drug-induced

333.4 *Huntington's chorea*

333.5 *Other choreas*

Hemiballism(us)   Paroxysmal choreo-athetosis

Excludes: Sydenham's or rheumatic chorea (392.–)

Use additional E code, if desired, to identify drug, if drug-induced

333.6 *Idiopathic torsion dystonia*

Dystonia musculorum deformans or (Schwalbe-)Ziehen-Oppenheim
    disease

333.7 *Symptomatic torsion dystonia*

Athetoid cerebral palsy or Vogt's disease
Double athetosis

Use additional E code, if desired, to identify drug, if drug-induced

333.8 *Fragments of torsion dystonia*

Blepharospasm   Orofacial dyskinesia
Organic writers' cramp   Spasmodic torticollis

Use additional E code, if desired, to identify drug, if drug-induced

333.9   *Other and unspecified*

Restless legs   Stiff man syndrome

334   Spinocerebellar disease

Excludes: olivopontocerebellar degeneration (333.0)
                    peroneal muscular atrophy (356.1)

334.0   *Friedreich's ataxia*

334.1   *Hereditary spastic paraplegia*

334.2   *Primary cerebellar degeneration*

Primary cerebellar degeneration:
   NOS
   hereditary
   sporadic

334.3   *Other cerebellar ataxia*

Cerebellar ataxia NOS

Use additional E code, if desired, to identify drug, if drug-induced

334.4*   *Cerebellar ataxia in diseases classified elsewhere*

Cerebellar ataxia in:
   alcoholism (303†)
   myxoedema (244.–†)
   neoplastic disease (140-239†)

334.8   *Other*

Ataxia telangiectasia or Louis-Bar syndrome

334.9   *Unspecified*

335   Anterior horn cell disease

335.0   *Werdnig-Hoffmann disease*

Infantile spinal muscular atrophy

335.1   *Spinal muscular atrophy*

Kugelberg-Welander disease   Adult spinal muscular atrophy

335.2   *Motor neurone disease*

Amyotrophic lateral sclerosis   Progressive muscular atrophy
Motor neurone disease (bulbar)   (pure)
   (mixed type)

335.8   *Other*

335.9   *Unspecified*

336   Other diseases of spinal cord

336.0   *Syringomyelia and syringobulbia*

336.1   *Vascular myelopathies*

Acute infarction of spinal cord (embolic) (nonembolic)
Arterial thrombosis of spinal cord
Haematomyelia
Oedema of spinal cord
Subacute necrotic myelopathy

336.2* *Subacute combined degeneration of spinal cord* (266.2, 281.0, 281.1†)

336.3* *Myelopathy in other diseases classified elsewhere*

Myelopathy (in):
   intervertebral disc disorder (722.7†)
   neoplastic disease (140-239†)
   spondylosis (721.–†)

336.8   *Other myelopathy*

Myelopathy:
   drug-induced
   radiation-induced

Use additional E code, if desired, to identify cause

336.9   *Unspecified diseases of spinal cord*

Cord compression NOS   Myelopathy NOS

Excludes: myelitis (323.–)

337   Disorders of the autonomic nervous system

Includes: disorders of peripheral autonomic, sympathetic, parasym-
                pathetic or vegetative system

Excludes: familial dysautonomia [Riley-Day syndrome] (742.8)

337.0   *Idiopathic peripheral autonomic neuropathy*

337.1* *Peripheral autonomic neuropathy in disorders classified elsewhere*

Autonomic neuropathy (peripheral) in:
   amyloidosis (277.3†)
   diabetes (250.5†)

337.9   *Unspecified*

OTHER DISORDERS OF THE CENTRAL NERVOUS SYSTEM (340-349)

340   Multiple sclerosis

Disseminated or multiple sclerosis:
  NOS
  brain stem
  cord
  generalized

341   Other demyelinating diseases of central nervous system

341.0   *Neuromyelitis optica*

341.1   *Schilder's disease*

Balo's concentric sclerosis
Encephalitis periaxialis:
  concentrica
  diffusa

341.8   *Other*

341.9   *Unspecified*

342   Hemiplegia

Note: For primary coding, this category is to be used only when hemi-
        plegia (complete) (incomplete), except of types listed in 343.1 and
        343.4, is reported without further specification, or is stated to be
        old or long standing but of unspecified cause. The category is
        also for use in multiple coding to identify these types of hemi-
        plegia resulting from any cause.

342.0   *Flaccid hemiplegia*

342.1   *Spastic hemiplegia*

342.9   *Unspecified*

343   Infantile cerebral palsy

Includes: cerebral:
              palsy NOS
              spastic infantile paralysis
            congenital spastic paralysis (cerebral)
            Little's disease
            paralysis (spastic) due to birth injury:
              intracranial
              spinal

Excludes: hereditary cerebral paralysis, such as:
              hereditary spastic paraplegia (334.1)
              Vogt's disease (333.7)

343.0   *Diplegic*

Congenital diplegia   Congenital paraplegia

343.1   *Hemiplegic*

Congenital hemiplegia

Excludes: infantile hemiplegia NOS (343.4)

343.2   *Quadriplegic*

Tetraplegic

343.3   *Monoplegic*

343.4   *Infantile hemiplegia*

Infantile hemiplegia (postnatal) NOS

343.8   *Other*

343.9   *Unspecified*

344   Other paralytic syndromes

Note: For primary coding, this category is to be used only when the
        listed conditions are reported without further specification, or
        are stated to be old or longstanding but of unspecified cause.
        The category is also for use in multiple coding to identify these
        conditions resulting from any cause.

Includes: paralysis (complete) (incomplete), except as in 342.– and 343.–

344.0   *Quadriplegia*

344.1   *Paraplegia*

Paralysis of both lower limbs   Paraplegia (lower)

344.2   *Diplegia of upper limbs*

Diplegia (upper)   Paralysis of both upper limbs

344.3   *Monoplegia of lower limb*

Paralysis of lower limb

344.4   *Monoplegia of upper limb*

Paralysis of upper limb

344.5 · *Unspecified monoplegia*

344.6   *Cauda equina syndrome*

Cord bladder   Neurogenic bladder

344.8   *Other*

344.9   *Unspecified*

345 Epilepsy

Excludes: progressive myoclonic epilepsy (333.2)

345.0 Generalized nonconvulsive epilepsy

Absences:	Seizures:
atonic	akinetic
typical	atonic
Petit mal	

345.1 Generalized convulsive epilepsy

Epileptic seizures:	Grand mal
clonic	Major epilepsy
myoclonic	
tonic	
tonic-clonic	

Excludes: infantile spasms (345.6)

345.2 Petit mal status

Epileptic absence status

345.3 Grand mal status

Status epilepticus NOS

Excludes: epilepsia partialis continua (345.7)

345.4 Partial epilepsy, with impairment of consciousness

Epilepsy:
  partial:
    with memory and ideational disturbances
    secondarily generalized
  psychomotor
  psychosensory
Epileptic automatism

345.5 Partial epilepsy, without mention of impairment of consciousness

Epilepsy:	Epilepsy:
Bravais-Jacksonian NOS	somatomotor
focal (motor) NOS	somatosensory
Jacksonian NOS	visceral
motor partial	visual
partial NOS	

345.6 Infantile spasms

Hypsarrythmia	Salaam attacks
Lighting spasms	

Excludes: salaam tic (781.0)

345.7 *Epilepsia partialis continua*
Kojevnikov's epilepsy

345.8 *Other*

345.9 *Unspecified*
Epileptic convulsions, fits or seizures NOS

346 Migraine

346.0 *Classical migraine*
Migraine preceded or accompanied by transient focal neurological phenomena
Migraine with aura

346.1 *Common migraine*

346.2 *Variants of migraine*

Cluster headache
Migraine:
  basilar
  lower-half
  retinal

Neuralgia:
  ciliary
  migrainous

346.8 *Other*
Migraine:
  hemiplegic
  ophthalmoplegic

346.9 *Unspecified*

347 Cataplexy and narcolepsy

348 Other conditions of brain

348.0 *Cerebral cysts*
Arachnoid cyst   Porencephalic cyst

348.1 *Anoxic brain damage*
Excludes: when attributable to medical care for abortion, ectopic or molar pregnancy, labour or delivery (634-638 with fourth digit .7, 639.8, 668.2, 669.4)
when of newborn (767.0, 768.–, 772.1, 772.2)
Use additional E code, if desired, to identify cause [e.g., anaesthesia]

348.2 *Benign intracranial hypertension*

348.3 *Encephalopathy, unspecified*

348.4 *Compression of brain*
Compression }
Herniation   } brain (stem)

348.5   *Cerebral oedema*

348.8   *Other*

Cerebral: Tuberculoma ⎱ of brain (active
   calcification   Tuberculosis ⎰   disease)*
   fungus   (013.8†)

348.9   *Unspecified*

349   Other and unspecified disorders of the nervous system

349.0   *Reaction to spinal or lumbar puncture*

Headache following lumbar puncture

349.1   *Nervous system complications from surgically implanted device*

Excludes: immediate postoperative complications (997.0)
            mechanical complications classifiable to 996.2 (996.2)

349.2   *Disorders of meninges, not elsewhere classified*

Meningeal adhesions (cerebral)   Tuberculoma of meninges (cere-
   (spinal)   bral) (spinal)* (013.1†)

349.8   *Other*

349.9   *Unspecified*

DISORDERS OF THE PERIPHERAL NERVOUS SYSTEM (350-359)

Excludes: diseases of:
            acoustic [8th] nerve (388.5)
            oculomotor [3rd, 4th, 6th] nerves (378.–)
            optic [2nd] nerve (377.–)
            neuralgia ⎫
            neuritis   ⎬ NOS or "rheumatic" (729.2)
            radiculitis ⎭
            peripheral neuritis in pregnancy (646.4)

350   Trigeminal nerve disorders

Includes: disorders of 5th cranial nerve

350.0* *Post-herpetic trigeminal neuralgia* (053.1†)

350.1   *Other trigeminal neuralgia*

Trigeminal neuralgia NOS

350.2   *Atypical face pain*

350.8   *Other*

350.9   *Unspecified*

351   Facial nerve disorders

Includes: disorders of 7th cranial nerve

351.0   *Bell's palsy*

Facial palsy

351.1   *Geniculate ganglionitis*

Geniculate ganglionitis:
  NOS
  herpetic* (053.1†)

351.8   *Other*

351.9   *Unspecified*

352   Disorders of other cranial nerves

352.0   *Disorders of olfactory [1st] nerve*

352.1   *Glossopharyngeal neuralgia*

352.2   *Other disorders of glossopharyngeal [9th] nerve*

352.3   *Disorders of pneumogastric [10th] nerve*

352.4   *Disorders of accessory [11th] nerve*

352.5   *Disorders of hypoglossal [12th] nerve*

352.6   *Multiple cranial nerve palsies*

Polyneuritis cranialis

352.9   *Unspecified*

353   Nerve root and plexus disorders

Excludes: conditions due to:
              intervertebral disc disorders (722.–)
              spondylosis (720.–, 721.–)
              vertebrogenic disorders (723.–, 724.–)

353.0   *Brachial plexus lesions*

Excludes: brachial neuritis or radiculitis NOS (723.4)

353.1   *Lumbosacral plexus lesions*

353.2   *Cervical root lesions, not elsewhere classified*

353.3   *Thoracic root lesions, not elsewhere classified*

353.4   *Lumbosacral root lesions, not elsewhere classified*

353.5   *Neuralgic amyotrophy*
Parsonage-Aldren-Turner syndrome

353.6   *Phantom limb syndrome*

353.8   *Other*

353.9   *Unspecified*

354   Mononeuritis of upper limb and mononeuritis multiplex

354.0   *Carpal tunnel syndrome*

354.1   *Other lesion of median nerve*

354.2   *Lesion of ulnar nerve*
Tardy ulnar nerve palsy

354.3   *Lesion of radial nerve*

354.4   *Causalgia*

354.5   *Mononeuritis multiplex*
Combinations of single conditions classifiable to 354.– or to 355.-

354.8   *Other*

354.9   *Unspecified*

355   Mononeuritis of lower limb

355.0   *Lesion of sciatic nerve*
Excludes: sciatica NOS (724.3)

355.1   *Meralgia paraesthetica*
Lateral cutaneous nerve of thigh syndrome

355.2   *Lesion of femoral nerve*

355.3   *Lesion of lateral popliteal nerve*

355.4   *Lesion of medial popliteal nerve*

355.5   *Tarsal tunnel syndrome*

355.6   *Lesion of plantar nerve*
Morton's metatarsalgia

355.7   *Other*

355.8   *Unspecified mononeuritis of lower limb*

355.9   *Mononeuritis of unspecified site*
Diabetic mononeuropathy NOS* (250.5†)

356 Hereditary and idiopathic peripheral neuropathy

356.0 *Hereditary peripheral neuropathy*
Dejerine-Sottas disease

356.1 *Peroneal muscular atrophy*
Charcot-Marie-Tooth disease

356.2 *Hereditary sensory neuropathy*

356.3 *Refsum's disease*

356.4 *Idiopathic progressive polyneuropathy*

356.8 *Other*

356.9 *Unspecified*

357 Inflammatory and toxic neuropathy

357.0 *Acute infective polyneuritis*
Guillain-Barré syndrome

357.1* *Polyneuropathy in collagen vascular disease*
Polyneuropathy in:
  disseminated lupus erythematosus (710.0†)
  polyarteritis nodosa (446.0†)
  rheumatoid arthritis (714.0†)

357.2* *Polyneuropathy in diabetes* (250.5†)

357.3* *Polyneuropathy in malignant disease* (140-208†)

357.4* *Polyneuropathy in other diseases classified elsewhere*
Polyneuropathy in:
  amyloidosis (277.3†)
  beriberi (265.0†)
  deficiency of B vitamins (266.–†)
  diphtheria (032.–†)
  herpes zoster (053.1†)
  hypoglycaemia (251.2†)

Polyneuropathy in:
  mumps (072.7†)
  pellagra (265.2†)
  porphyria (277.1†)
  sarcoidosis (135†)
  uraemia (585†)

357.5 *Alcoholic polyneuropathy*

357.6 *Polyneuropathy due to drugs*
Use additional E code, if desired, to identify drug

357.7 *Polyneuropathy due to other toxic agents*
Use additional E code, if desired, to identify toxic agent

357.8 *Other*

357.9 *Unspecified*

358   Myoneural disorders

358.0   *Myasthenia gravis*

358.1*   *Myasthenic syndromes in diseases classified elsewhere*

Diabetic amyotrophy (250.5†)

Myasthenic syndromes in:
    malignant disease (140-208†)
    thyrotoxicosis (242.–†)

358.2   *Toxic myoneural disorders*

Use additional E code, if desired, to identify toxic agent

358.8   *Other*

358.9   *Unspecified*

359   Muscular dystrophies and other myopathies

Excludes: idiopathic polymyositis (710.4)

359.0   *Congenital hereditary muscular dystrophy*

Benign congenital myopathy
Central core disease

Myotubular myopathy
Nemaline body disease

Excludes: arthrogryposis multiplex congenita (755.8)

359.1   *Hereditary progressive muscular dystrophy*

Muscular dystrophy:
   NOS
   distal
   Duchenne
   Erb's
   facioscapulohumeral

Muscular dystrophy:
   Landouzy-Dejerine
   limb-girdle
   ocular
   oculopharyngeal

359.2   *Myotonic disorders*

Dystrophia myotonica
Myotonia congenita

Paramyotonia congenita
Steinert's disease

359.3   *Familial periodic paralysis*

Hypokalaemic familial periodic paralysis

359.4   *Toxic myopathy*

Use additional E code, if desired, to identify toxic agent

359.5*   *Endocrine myopathy*

Myopathy in:
   Addison's disease (255.4†)
   Cushing's syndrome (255.0†)
   hypopituitarism (253.2†)

Myopathy in:
   myxoedema (244.–†)
   thyrotoxicosis (242.–†)

359.6* *Symptomatic inflammatory myopathy*

Myopathy in:
amyloidosis (277.3†)
disseminated lupus erythematosus (710.0†)
malignant neoplasm (140-208†)
polyarteritis nodosa (446.0†)
rheumatoid arthritis (714.0†)
sarcoidosis (135†)
scleroderma (710.1†)
Sjögren's disease (710.2†)

359.8 *Other*

359.9 *Unspecified*

DISORDERS OF THE EYE AND ADNEXA (360-379)

360 Disorders of the globe

Includes: disorders affecting multiple structures of eye

360.0 *Purulent endophthalmitis*

Panophthalmitis   Vitreous abscess

360.1 *Other endophthalmitis*

Ophthalmia nodosa   Sympathetic uveitis
Parasitic endophthalmitis NOS

360.2 *Degenerative disorders of globe*

Chalcosis   Siderosis of eye
Malignant myopia

360.3 *Hypotony of eye*

360.4 *Degenerated conditions of globe*

Absolute glaucoma   Haemophthalmos
Atrophy of globe   Phthisis bulbi

360.5 *Retained (old) intraocular foreign body, magnetic*

Retained (old) magnetic foreign body (in):
anterior chamber
ciliary body
iris
lens
posterior wall of globe
vitreous

360.6 *Retained (old) intraocular foreign body, nonmagnetic*

Retained (old) foreign body in sites listed in 360.5:
  NOS
  nonmagnetic

360.8 *Other disorders of globe*

Luxation of globe

360.9 *Unspecified*

361　Retinal detachments and defects

361.0 *Retinal detachment with retinal defect*

Giant tear of retina (with　　　　Rhegmatogenous retinal
  detachment)　　　　　　　　　detachment

361.1 *Retinoschisis and retinal cysts*

Cyst of ora serrata　　　　　　Pseudocyst of retina

Excludes:　microcystoid degeneration of retina (362.6)
　　　　　　parasitic cyst of retina (360.1)

361.2 *Serous retinal detachment*

Retinal detachment without retinal defect

361.3 *Retinal defects without detachment*

Horseshoe tear ⎫
Round hole　　　⎬ of retina, without mention of detachment
Operculum　　　⎭

Excludes:　chorioretinal scars after surgery for detachment (363.3)
　　　　　　peripheral retinal degeneration without defect (362.6)

361.8 *Other forms of retinal detachment*

Traction detachment of retina

361.9 *Unspecified*

362　Other retinal disorders

Excludes:　chorioretinitis (363.–)
　　　　　　chorioretinal scars (363.3)

362.0* *Diabetic retinopathy* (250.4†)

Diabetic:　　　　　　　　　　Diabetic:
  retinal microaneurysms　　　　retinopathy (background)
　　　　　　　　　　　　　　　(proliferative)

362.1 *Other background retinopathy and retinal vascular changes*

Changes in retinal vascular
  appearance
Retinal:
  micro-aneurysms NOS
  neovascularization NOS
  perivasculitis
  varices
  vascular sheathing
  vasculitis

Retinopathy:
  NOS
  atherosclerotic* (440.8†)
  background NOS
  Coat's
  exudative
  hypertensive

362.2 *Other proliferative retinopathy*

Retrolental fibroplasia

Proliferative sickle-cell
  retinopathy* (282.6†)

362.3 *Retinal vascular occlusion*

Microembolism, retinal
Occlusion (partial) (total) (transient):
  retinal artery (branch) (central)
  retinal vein (central) (tributary)

Venous engorgement, retina

362.4 *Separation of retinal layers*

Central serous chorioretinopathy

Detachment of retinal pigment
  epithelium

Excludes: serous retinal detachment (361.2)

362.5 *Degeneration of macula and posterior pole*

Cyst ⎤
Hole ⎬ of macula
Puckering ⎦

Drusen (degenerative)
Kuhnt-Junius degeneration
Senile macular degeneration
  (atrophic) (exudative)
Toxic maculopathy

Use additional E code, if desired, to identify drug, if drug-induced

362.6 *Peripheral retinal degenerations*

Degeneration, retina:
  lattice
  microcystoid
  palisade

Degeneration, retina:
  paving stone
  peripheral
  reticular

362.7 *Hereditary retinal dystrophies*

Dystrophy:
  retinal (albipunctate)
    (pigmentary) (vitelliform)
  tapetoretinal
  vitreoretinal
Retinitis pigmentosa
Stargardt's disease

Hereditary retinal dystrophy in:
  cerebroretinal lipidoses*
    (330.1†)
  systemic lipidoses* (272.7†)

362.8   *Other retinal disorders*

Haemorrhage:
  preretinal
  retinal (deep) (superficial)
  subretinal

Retinal:
  cotton wool spots
  exudates
  ischaemia
  oedema

Excludes: chorioretinal inflammations and scars (363.–)

362.9   *Unspecified*

363   Chorioretinal inflammations and scars and other disorders of choroid

363.0   *Focal chorioretinitis and focal retinochoroiditis*

Focal:
  chorioretinitis or choroiditis
  retinochoroiditis or retinitis:
    NOS
    in:
      histoplasmosis* (115.–†)
      toxoplasmosis:
        acquired* (130†)
        congenital* (771.2†)

363.1   *Disseminated chorioretinitis and disseminated retinochoroiditis*

Disseminated:
  chorioretinitis or choroiditis:
    NOS
    syphilitic* (091.5†)
    tuberculous* (017.3†)
  retinochoroiditis or retinitis:
    NOS
    in neurosyphilis* (094.8†)

Excludes: retinal:
              perivasculitis (362.1)
              vasculitis (362.1)

363.2   *Other and unspecified forms of chorioretinitis and retinochoroiditis*

Pars planitis   Posterior cyclitis

Excludes: panophthalmitis (360.0)
            sympathetic uveitis (360.1)

363.3   *Chorioretinal scars*

Scar (postinflammatory) (postsurgical) (post-traumatic):
  choroid
  macula
  posterior pole
  retina
Solar retinopathy

363.4   *Choroidal degenerations*

Angioid streaks ⎫
Atrophy   ⎬ of choroid
Sclerosis   ⎭

363.5   *Hereditary choroidal dystrophies*

Choroideremia
Dystrophy, choroidal (central areolar) (generalized) (gyrate) (peripapil-
    lary)
Gyrate atrophy, choroid

363.6   *Choroidal haemorrhage and rupture*

Choroidal haemorrhage:
    NOS
    expulsive

363.7   *Choroidal detachment*

363.8   *Other disorders of choroid*

363.9   *Unspecified*

364   Disorders of iris and ciliary body

364.0   *Acute and subacute iridocyclitis*

Anterior uveitis ⎫ acute
Cyclitis   ⎪ recurrent
Iridocyclitis   ⎬ subacute
Iritis   ⎪ in herpes simplex* (054.4†)
                     ⎭ in herpes zoster* (053.2†)
                       with hypopyon

364.1   *Chronic iridocyclitis*

Iridocyclitis:
    chronic
    syphilitic* (091.5†)
    tuberculous* (017.3†)

364.2   *Certain types of iridocyclitis*

Fuchs's heterochromic cyclitis   Lens-induced iridocyclitis
Glaucomatocyclitic crises

364.3   *Unspecified iridocyclitis*

364.4   *Vascular disorders of iris and ciliary body*

Haemorrhage   ⎫
Neovascularization ⎬ of iris or ciliary body
Hyphaema
Rubeosis of iris

364.5 *Degenerations of iris and ciliary body*

Degeneration:
    iris (pigmentary)
    pupillary margin
Iris atrophy (essential) (progressive)

Iridoschisis
Miotic pupillary cyst
Translucency of iris

364.6 *Cysts of iris, ciliary body and anterior chamber*

Cyst of iris, ciliary body or anterior chamber:
    NOS
    exudative
    implantation

Excludes: miotic pupillary cyst (364.5)
            parasitic cyst (360.1)

364.7 *Adhesions and disruptions of iris and ciliary body*

Ectopic pupil
Goniosynechiae
Iridodialysis
Pupillary:
    membranes
    occlusion
    seclusion

Recession, chamber angle
Synechiae (iris):
    NOS
    anterior
    posterior

364.8 *Other disorders of iris and ciliary body*

364.9 *Unspecified*

365   Glaucoma

Excludes: glaucoma:
                absolute (360.4)
                congenital (743.2)

365.0 *Borderline glaucoma*

Anatomical narrow angle
    Ocular hypertension
    Steroid responder

Open-angle with:
    borderline intraocular pressure
    cupping of discs

365.1 *Open-angle glaucoma*

Glaucoma (primary) (residual
    stage):
    chronic simple
    low tension

Glaucoma (primary) (residual
    stage):
    open angle
    pigmentary

365.2 *Primary angle-closure glaucoma*

Angle-closure glaucoma (primary) (residual stage):
  acute
  chronic
  intermittent

365.3 *Corticosteroid-induced glaucoma*

Corticosteroid-induced glaucoma (glaucomatous stage) (residual stage)
Use additional E code, if desired, to identify drug

365.4 *Glaucoma associated with congenital anomalies, with dystrophies and with systemic syndromes*

Glaucoma in:
  aniridia* (743.4†)
  Axenfeld's anomaly* (743.4†)

Glaucoma in:
  Rieger's anomaly* (743.4†)
  Sturge-Weber(-Dimitri)
    syndrome* (759.6†)

365.5 *Glaucoma associated with disorders of the lens*

Glaucoma (in):
  hypermature cataract
  postdislocation of lens
  pseudoexfoliation of capsule

Phacolytic glaucoma

365.6 *Glaucoma associated with other ocular disorders*

Glaucoma in:
  concussion of globe
  iridocyclitis
  retinal vein occlusion

Glaucoma in:
  rubeosis of iris
  tumours of globe

365.8 *Other glaucoma*

Hypersecretion glaucoma

365.9 *Unspecified*

366 **Cataract**

Excludes: congenital cataract (743.3)

366.0 *Infantile, juvenile and presenile cataract*

366.1 *Senile cataract*

Pseudoexfoliation of (lens) capsule

Senile cataract (hypermature)
  (incipient) (mature)

366.2 *Traumatic cataract*

366.3 *Cataract secondary to ocular disorders*

Cataracta complicata
Cataract in chronic iridocyclitis

Glaucomatous flecks (subcapsular)

366.4   *Cataract associated with other disorders*

Cataract: Cataract:
  diabetic* (250.4†)   tetanic* (275.4†)
  drug-induced   in hypoparathyroidism*
  myotonic* (359.2†)   (252.1†)

Use additional E code, if desired, to identify cause if due to drug or other
  toxic substance

366.5   *After-cataract*

Soemering's ring   Secondary cataract

366.8   *Other cataract*

366.9   *Unspecified*

367   Disorders of refraction and accommodation

367.0   *Hypermetropia*

367.1   *Myopia*

367.2   *Astigmatism*

367.3   *Anisometropia and aniseikonia*

367.4   *Presbyopia*

367.5   *Disorders of accommodation*

Internal ophthalmoplegia (complete) (total)

Paresis ⎫
     ⎬ of accommodation
Spasm ⎭

367.8   *Other*

367.9   *Unspecified*

368   Visual disturbances

Excludes: electrophysiological disturbances (794.1)

368.0   *Amblyopia ex anopsia*

Amblyopia:
  deprivation
  strabismic
  suppression

368.1   *Subjective visual disturbances*

Asthenopia   Visual:
Metamorphopsia   hallucinations
Photophobia   halos
Scintillating scotoma
Sudden visual loss

368.2 *Diplopia*

Double vision

368.3 *Other disorders of binocular vision*

Abnormal retinal correspondence
Fusion with defective stereopsis
Simultaneous visual perception without fusion
Suppression of binocular vision

368.4 *Visual field defects*

Enlarged blind spot
Generalized contraction of visual
 field
Hemianop(s)ia (heteronymous)
 (homonymous)
Quadrant anop(s)ia

Scotoma:
 arcuate
 Bjerrum
 central
 ring

368.5 *Colour vision deficiencies*

Achromatopsia
Deuteranomaly
Deuteranopia
Protanomaly

Protanopia
Tritanomaly
Tritanopia

368.6 *Night blindness*

Night blindness:
 NOS
 due to vitamin A deficiency* (264.5†)

368.8 *Other visual disturbances*

368.9 *Unspecified*

369 **Blindness and low vision**

369.0 *Blindness, both eyes*

369.1 *Blindness, one eye, low vision other eye*

369.2 *Low vision, both eyes*

369.3 *Unqualified visual loss, both eyes*

369.6 *Blindness, one eye*

369.7 *Low vision, one eye*

369.8 *Unqualified visual loss, one eye*

369.9 *Unspecified visual loss*

Note: The table below gives a classification of severity of visual impairment recommended by a WHO Study Group on the Prevention of Blindness, Geneva, 6-10 November 1972.[1] The term "low vision" in the above category comprises categories 1 and 2 of the table below, the term "blindness" categories 3, 4 and 5 and the term "unqualified visual loss" category 9.

Category of visual impairment	Visual acuity with best possible correction	
	maximum less than	minimum equal to or better than
1	6/18 3/10 (0.3) 20/70	6/60 1/10 (0.1) 20/200
2	6/60 1/10 (0.1) 20/200	3/60 1/20 (0.05) 20/400
3	3/60 1/20 (0.05) 20/400	1/60 (finger counting at 1 metre) 1/50 (0.02) 5/300 (20/1200)
4	1/60 (finger counting at 1 metre) 1/50 (0.02) 5/300	Light perception
5	No light perception	
9	Undetermined or unspecified	

If the extent of the visual field is taken into account, patients with a field no greater than 10° but greater than 5° around central fixation should be placed in category 3 and patients with a field no greater than 5° around central fixation should be placed in category 4, even if the central acuity is not impaired.

1. WHO Technical Report Series 518

370 Keratitis

370.0 *Corneal ulcer*

Ulcer:
  cornea (central) (marginal)
    (perforated) (ring)
  hypopyon

Ulcer:
  Mooren's

370.1* *Dendritic keratitis* (054.4†)

370.2 *Other superficial keratitis without conjunctivitis*

Keratitis:
  areolar
  filamentary
  nummular

Keratitis:
  stellate
  striate
  superficial punctate
Photokeratitis
Snow blindness

370.3 *Certain types of keratoconjunctivitis*

Keratoconjunctivitis:
  exposure
  neurotrophic
  phlyctenular

Keratoconjunctivitis:
  sicca* (710.2†)
  tuberculous (phlyctenular)*
    (017.3†)

370.4 *Other and unspecified keratoconjunctivitis*

Keratitis or keratoconjunctivitis:
  herpes zoster* (053.2†)
  herpes simplex* (054.4†)
  measles* (055.7†)
  in other exanthemata

Keratoconjunctivitis:
  NOS
  epidemic* (077.1†)
Superficial keratitis with
  conjunctivitis

370.5 *Interstitial and deep keratitis*

Corneal abscess
Interstitial keratitis:
  NOS
  nonsyphilitic
  syphilitic* (090.3†)
  tuberculous* (017.3†)

Keratitis:
  disciform* (054.4†)
  sclerosing

370.6 *Corneal neovascularization*

Ghost vessels (corneal)

Pannus (corneal)

370.8 *Other forms of keratitis*

370.9 *Unspecified*

371 Corneal opacity and other disorders of cornea

371.0 *Corneal scars and opacities*

Corneal:
  leucoma (adherent)
  macula
  nebula

371.1 *Corneal pigmentations and deposits*

Haematocornea   Krukenberg spindle
Kayser-Fleischer ring   Staehli's line

371.2 *Corneal oedema*

Bullous keratopathy

371.3 *Changes of corneal membranes*

Fold
Rupture } in Descemet's membrane

371.4 *Corneal degenerations*

Arcus senilis   Recurrent corneal erosion
Band-shaped keratopathy
Keratomalacia
  due to Vitamin A deficiency* (264.4†)

Excludes: Mooren's ulcer (370.0)

371.5 *Hereditary corneal dystrophies*

Corneal dystrophy (epithelial) (granular) (lattice) (macular)
Fuchs's endothelial dystrophy

371.6 *Keratoconus*

371.7 *Other corneal deformities*

Corneal ectasia   Descemetocele
Corneal staphyloma

371.8 *Other corneal disorders*

Anaesthesia
Hypaesthesia } of cornea

371.9 *Unspecified*

372 Disorders of conjunctiva

Excludes: keratoconjunctivitis (370.3, 370.4)

372.0 *Acute conjunctivitis*

Conjunctivitis:
  adenoviral follicular (acute)* (077.3†)
  epidemic haemorrhagic* (077.4†)
  inclusion* (077.0†)
  mucopurulent
  Newcastle* (077.8†)
  pseudomembranous
    diphtheritic* (032.8†)
  serous
  viral NOS* (077.9†)
Neonatal gonococcal blennorrhoea* (098.4†)
Pharyngoconjunctival fever* (077.2†)

Excludes: ophthalmia neonatorum NOS (771.6)

372.1 *Chronic conjunctivitis*

Vernal conjunctivitis

Filarial infestation of
  conjunctiva* (125.–†)

372.2 *Blepharoconjunctivitis*

372.3 *Other and unspecified conjunctivitis*

Ocular pemphigoid* (694.6†)

Reiter's conjunctivitis* (099.3†)

372.4 *Pterygium*

Excludes: pseudopterygium (372.5)

372.5 *Conjunctival degenerations and deposits*

Conjunctival:
  argyrosis
  concretions
  pigmentation

Conjunctival xerosis:
  NOS
  in vitamin A deficiency*
    (264.0†)
  Pseudopterygium

372.6 *Conjunctival scars*

Symblepharon

372.7 *Conjunctival vascular disorders and cysts*

Aneurysm ⎤
         ⎬ of conjunctiva
Chemosis ⎦

Hyposphagma
Subconjunctival haemorrhage

372.8 *Other disorders of conjunctiva*

372.9 *Unspecified*

373 Inflammation of eyelids

373.0 *Blepharitis*

Excludes: blepharoconjunctivitis (372.2)

373.1 *Hordeolum and other deep inflammation of eyelid*

Abscess ⎫
Furuncle ⎬ of eyelid   Stye

373.2 *Chalazion*

373.3 *Noninfectious dermatoses of eyelid*

Dermatitis: ⎫
  allergic ⎪
  contact ⎪
  eczematous ⎬ of eyelid
Discoid lupus erythematosus ⎪
Xeroderma ⎭

373.4* *Infective dermatitis of eyelid of types resulting in deformity*

Leprosy (030.–†) ⎫
Lupus vulgaris (tuberculous) (017.0†) ⎬ involving eyelid
Yaws (102.–†) ⎭

373.5* *Other infective dermatitis of eyelid*

Herpes simplex (054.4†) ⎫
Herpes zoster (053.2†) ⎪
Impetigo (684†) ⎬ involving eyelid
Vaccinia (051.0†) ⎪
  postvaccination (999.0†) ⎭

373.6* *Parasitic infestation of eyelid*

Leishmaniasis (085.–†) ⎫
Loiasis (125.2†) ⎬ involving eyelid
Onchocerciasis (125.3†) ⎭

373.8 *Other*

373.9 *Unspecified*

374   Other disorders of eyelids

374.0 *Entropion and trichiasis of eyelid*

374.1 *Ectropion*

374.2 *Lagophthalmos*

374.3 *Ptosis of eyelid*

Blepharochalasis

374.4 *Other disorders affecting eyelid function*

Ankyloblepharon   Lid retraction
Blepharophimosis

Excludes: blepharospasm (333.8)
           tic (psychogenic) (307.2)
               organic (333.3)

374.5 *Degenerative disorders of eyelids and periocular area*

Chloasma   ⎫   Madarosis
Hypertrichosis ⎬ of eyelid   Xanthelasma* (272.–†)
Vitiligo   ⎭

374.8 *Other disorders of eyelid*

Retained foreign body in eyelid

374.9 *Unspecified*

375   **Disorders of lacrimal system**

375.0 *Dacryoadenitis*

Chronic enlargement of lacrimal gland

375.1 *Other disorders of lacrimal gland*

Dacryops   Lacrimal:
Dry eye syndrome   atrophy
                                     cyst

375.2 *Epiphora*

375.3 *Acute and unspecified inflammation of lacrimal passages*

Canaliculitis, lacrimal   ⎫ NOS
Dacryocystitis (phlegmonous)   ⎬ acute
Dacryopericystitis   ⎭ subacute

Excludes: neonatal dacryocystitis (771.6)

375.4 *Chronic inflammation of lacrimal passages*

Canaliculitis, lacrimal ⎫
Dacryocystitis   ⎬ chronic
Mucocele, lacrimal   ⎭

375.5 *Stenosis and insufficiency of lacrimal passages*

Dacryolith   Stenosis:
Eversion of lacrimal punctum   lacrimal
                                        canaliculi
                                        punctum
                                        sac
                                     nasolacrimal duct

375.6 *Other changes of lacrimal passages*
Lacrimal fistula

375.8 *Other disorders of lacrimal system*

375.9 *Unspecified*

376   Disorders of the orbit

376.0 *Acute inflammation of orbit*

Abscess ⎤
Cellulitis ⎥ of orbit   Tenonitis
Osteomyelitis ⎥
Periostitis ⎦

376.1 *Chronic inflammatory disorders of orbit*

Granuloma ⎤
Myositis ⎥ of orbit   Hydatid infestation of orbit*
Pseudotumour ⎦   (122.9†)
                           Myiasis of orbit* (134.0†)

376.2* *Endocrine exophthalmos*
Thyrotoxic exophthalmos (242.–†)

376.3 *Other exophthalmic conditions*

Displacement of globe (lateral) NOS Haemorrhage ⎤
Exophthalmos, except endocrine   Oedema ⎦ of orbit

376.4 *Deformity of orbit*

Atrophy ⎤ of orbit
Exostosis ⎦

376.5 *Enophthalmos*

376.6 *Retained (old) foreign body following penetrating wound of orbit*
Retrobulbar foreign body

376.8 *Other disorders of orbit*
Cyst of orbit   Myopathy of extraocular muscles

376.9 *Unspecified*

377   Disorders of optic nerve and visual pathways

377.0 *Papilloedema*

377.1 *Optic atrophy*

Optic atrophy:
  NOS
  syphilitic* (094.8†)

Temporal pallor, optic disc

377.2 *Other disorders of optic disc*

Coloboma ⎱
Drusen ⎰ of optic disc

Pseudopapilloedema

377.3 *Optic neuritis*

Meningococcal optic neuritis*
  (036.8†)
Optic neuropathy, except ischaemic
Optic papillitis

Retrobulbar neuritis:
  NOS
  syphilitic* (094.8†)

377.4 *Other disorders of optic nerve*

Compression of optic nerve
Haemorrhage in optic nerve sheath

Optic neuropathy, ischaemic

377.5 *Disorders of optic chiasm*

377.6 *Disorders of other visual pathways*

Disorders of optic tracts, geniculate nuclei and optic radiations

377.7 *Disorders of visual cortex*

377.9 *Unspecified*

378   Strabismus and other disorders of binocular eye movements

Excludes: nystagmus and other irregular eye movements (379.5)

378.0 *Convergent concomitant strabismus*

Esotropia (alternating) (monocular), except intermittent

378.1 *Divergent concomitant strabismus*

Exotropia (alternating) (monocular), except intermittent

378.2 *Intermittent heterotropia*

Intermittent:
  esotropia ⎱
  exotropia ⎰ (alternating) (monocular)

378.3 *Other and unspecified heterotropia*

Concomitant strabismus NOS
Cyclotropia
Hypertropia
Hypotropia

Microtropia
Monofixation syndrome
Vertical heterotropia

378.4 *Heterophoria*

Alternating hyperphoria

Esophoria

Exophoria

378.5 *Paralytic strabismus*

Strabismus due to palsy:
  third or oculomotor nerve
  fourth or trochlear nerve
  sixth or abducent nerve

Total (external) ophthalmoplegia

378.6 *Mechanical strabismus*

Brown's sheath syndrome
Strabismus due to adhesions

Traumatic limitation of duction of
  eye muscle

378.7 *Other strabismus*

Duane's syndrome

Progressive external ophthalmoplegia

378.8 *Other disorders of binocular eye movements*

Conjugate gaze palsy or spasm
Convergence:
  excess
  insufficiency

Dissociated deviation of eye movements
Internuclear ophthalmoplegia

378.9 *Unspecified*

Ophthalmoplegia NOS

Strabismus NOS

379 Other disorders of eye

379.0 *Scleritis and episcleritis*

Episcleritis:
  NOS
  syphilitic* (095†)
Scleromalacia perforans

Sclerotenonitis

379.1 *Other disorders of sclera*

Equatorial staphyloma

Scleral ectasia

379.2 *Disorders of vitreous body*

Asteroid hyalitis
Synchysis scintillans

Vitreous:
  detachment
  floaters
  haemorrhage
  opacities
  prolapse

379.3 *Aphakia and other disorders of lens*

Dislocation of lens

Subluxation of lens

379.4   *Anomalies of pupillary function*

Adie pupil
Anisocoria
Argyll Robertson phenomenon or pupil (syphilitic)* (094.8†)
    atypical (nonsyphilitic)
Hippus
Miosis (persistent), not due to miotics
Mydriasis (persistent), not due to mydriatics
Pupillary reaction:
    abnormal
    tonic
    unequal

379.5   *Nystagmus and other irregular eye movements*

Nystagmus: Nystagmus:
    NOS   dissociated
    congenital   latent
    deprivation

379.8   *Other disorders of eye and adnexa*

379.9   *Unspecified*

DISEASES OF THE EAR AND MASTOID PROCESS (380-389)

380   Disorders of external ear

380.0   *Perichondritis of pinna*

Perichondritis of auricle

380.1   *Infective otitis externa*

Erysipelas* (035†)   ⎤
Herpes simplex* (054.7†)   ⎥
Herpes zoster* (053.7†)   ⎬ of external ear
Impetigo* (684†)   ⎦
Furunculosis of external auditory meatus* (680.0†)
Otitis externa:
    NOS
    diffuse
    haemorrhagica
    malignant
Otomycosis (in):
    NOS* (111.9†)
    aspergillosis* (117.3†)
    moniliasis* (112.8†)
Swimmer's ear

380.2   *Other otitis externa*

Cholesteatoma ⎫
Eczema   ⎬ of external ear (canal)
Keratosis obturans ⎭

380.3   *Noninfective disorders of pinna*

Acquired deformity: Haematoma:
  auricle   auricle
  pinna   pinna

380.4   *Impacted cerumen*

Wax in ear

380.5   *Acquired stenosis of external ear canal*

Collapse of external ear canal

380.8   *Other disorders of external ear*

Exostosis of external ear canal   Gouty tophi of ear* (274.8†)

380.9   *Unspecified*

381   Nonsuppurative otitis media and Eustachian tube disorders

381.0   *Acute nonsuppurative otitis media*

Acute tubotympanal catarrh   Otitis media, acute:
Otitic barotrauma* (993.0†)   mucoid
Otitis media, acute: secretory
  allergic   seromucinous
  catarrhal   serous
  exudative   transudative
                                          with effusion

381.1   *Chronic serous otitis media*

Chronic tubotympanal catarrh

381.2   *Chronic mucoid otitis media*

Glue ear   Otitis media, chronic mucinous
Excludes: adhesive middle ear disease (385.1)

381.3   *Other and unspecified chronic nonsuppurative otitis media*

Otitis media, chronic: Otitis media, chronic:
  allergic   seromucinous
  exudative   transudative
  secretory   with effusion

381.4 *Nonsuppurative otitis media, not specified as acute or chronic*

Otitis media:
  allergic
  catarrhal
  exudative
  mucoid

Otitis media:
  secretory
  seromucinous
  serous
  transudative
  with effusion

381.5 *Eustachian salpingitis*

381.6 *Obstruction of Eustachian tube*

Compression ⎫
Stenosis ⎬ of Eustachian tube
Stricture ⎭

381.7 *Patulous Eustachian tube*

381.8 *Other disorders of Eustachian tube*

381.9 *Unspecified Eustachian tube disorder*

382 Suppurative and unspecified otitis media

382.0 *Acute suppurative otitis media*

Otitis media, acute necrotizing (in): Otitis media, acute purulent
  NOS
  influenza* (487.8†)
  measles* (055.2†)
  scarlet fever* (034.1†)

382.1 *Chronic tubotympanic suppurative otitis media*

Benign chronic suppurative otitis   Chronic tubotympanic disease
  media

382.2 *Chronic atticoantral suppurative otitis media*

Chronic atticoantral disease

382.3 *Unspecified chronic suppurative otitis media*

Chronic purulent otitis media   Tuberculosis of ear* (017.4†)

382.4 *Unspecified suppurative otitis media*

Purulent otitis media NOS

382.9 *Unspecified otitis media*

Otitis media:
  NOS
  acute NOS
  chronic NOS

383 Mastoiditis and related conditions

383.0 *Acute mastoiditis*
Abscess of mastoid   Empyema of mastoid

383.1 *Chronic mastoiditis*
Caries of mastoid   Tuberculous mastoiditis* (015.7†)
Fistula of mastoid

383.2 *Petrositis*
Inflammation of petrous bone (acute) (chronic)

383.3 *Complications following mastoidectomy*
Cyst
Granulations } of postmastoidectomy cavity
Inflammation

383.8 *Other*

383.9 *Unspecified mastoiditis*

384 Other disorders of tympanic membrane

384.0 *Acute myringitis without mention of otitis media*
Acute tympanitis   Bullous myringitis

384.1 *Chronic myringitis without mention of otitis media*
Chronic tympanitis

384.2 *Perforation of tympanic membrane*
Perforation of ear drum:
   NOS
   persistent post-traumatic
   postinflammatory

384.8 *Other*

384.9 *Unspecified*

385 Other disorders of middle ear and mastoid

385.0 *Tympanosclerosis*

385.1 *Adhesive middle ear disease*
Adhesive otitis
Excludes: glue ear (381.2)

385.2 *Other acquired abnormality of ear ossicles*
Ankylosis
Impaired mobility } of ear ossicles
Partial loss

385.3   *Cholesteatoma of middle ear and mastoid*
Polyp of (middle) ear

385.8   *Other*

385.9   *Unspecified*

386   Vertiginous syndromes and other disorders of vestibular system

Excludes: vertigo NOS (780.4)

386.0   *Ménière's disease*
Endolymphatic hydrops   Ménière's syndrome or vertigo
Lermoyez's syndrome

386.1   *Other and unspecified peripheral vertigo*
Aural vertigo   Otogenic vertigo
Benign paroxysmal vertigo or   Vestibular neuronitis
   nystagmus
Epidemic vertigo* (078.8†)

386.2   *Vertigo of central origin*
Central positional nystagmus

386.3   *Labyrinthitis*

386.4   *Labyrinthine fistula*

386.5   *Labyrinthine dysfunction*
Hypofunction   ⎫
Hypersensitivity   ⎬ of labyrinth
Loss of function   ⎭

386.8   *Other disorders of labyrinth*

386.9   *Unspecified vertiginous syndromes and labyrinthine disorders*

387   Otosclerosis

Includes: otospongiosis

387.0   *Otosclerosis involving oval window, nonobliterative*

387.1   *Otosclerosis involving oval window, obliterative*

387.2   *Cochlear otosclerosis*
Otosclerosis involving:
   otic capsule
   round window

387.8   *Other*

387.9   *Unspecified*

388   Other disorders of ear

388.0   *Degenerative and vascular disorders of ear*

Presbyacusis   Transient ischaemic deafness

388.1   *Noise effects on inner ear*

Acoustic trauma (explosive) to ear   Noise-induced hearing loss

388.2   *Sudden hearing loss, unspecified*

388.3   *Tinnitus*

388.4   *Other abnormal auditory perception*

Auditory recruitment   Hyperacusis
Diplacusis   Impairment of auditory discrimi-
                                            nation

388.5   *Disorders of acoustic nerve*

Acoustic neuritis: Degeneration ⎫ of acoustic or
  NOS   Disorder   ⎭   eighth nerve
  syphilitic* (094.8†)

388.6   *Otorrhoea*

Discharging ear

388.7   *Otalgia*

Earache

388.8   *Other*

388.9   *Unspecified*

389   Deafness

389.0   *Conductive deafness*

Conductive hearing loss

389.1   *Sensorineural deafness*

Deafness: Hearing loss:
  central   central
  neural   neural
  perceptive   perceptive
  sensory   sensorineural
                                              sensory

Excludes: abnormal auditory perception (388.4)
           psychogenic deafness (306.7)

389.2   *Mixed conductive and sensorineural deafness*

Deafness or hearing loss of type in 389.0 with type in 389.1

389.7   *Deaf mutism, not elsewhere classifiable*

389.8   *Other specified forms of deafness*

389.9   *Unspecified deafness*

Hearing loss NOS

VII. DISEASES OF THE CIRCULATORY SYSTEM

ACUTE RHEUMATIC FEVER (390-392)

390 Rheumatic fever without mention of heart involvement

Arthritis, rheumatic, acute or subacute
Rheumatic fever (active) (acute)
Rheumatism, articular, acute or subacute

391 Rheumatic fever with heart involvement

Excludes: chronic heart diseases of rheumatic origin (393-398) unless
rheumatic fever is also present or there is evidence of
recrudescence or activity of the rheumatic process. In
cases where there is doubt as to rheumatic activity at the
time of death see Rules for Classification

391.0 *Acute rheumatic pericarditis*

Rheumatic pericarditis (acute)
Any condition in 390 with pericarditis

Excludes: when not specified as rheumatic (420.–)

391.1 *Acute rheumatic endocarditis*

Rheumatic:
  endocarditis, acute
  valvulitis, acute
Any condition in 390 with endocarditis or valvulitis

391.2 *Acute rheumatic myocarditis*

Any condition in 390 with myocarditis

391.8 *Other acute rheumatic heart disease*

Rheumatic pancarditis, acute
Any condition in 390 with other or multiple types of heart involvement

391.9 *Acute rheumatic heart disease, unspecified*

Rheumatic:
  carditis, acute
  heart disease, active or acute
Any condition in 390 with unspecified type of heart involvement

392 Rheumatic chorea

Includes: Sydenham's chorea

Excludes: chorea:
          NOS (333.5)
          Huntington's (333.4)

— 259 —

392.0 *With heart involvement*

Rheumatic chorea with heart involvement of any type classifiable under 391.–

392.9 *Without mention of heart involvement*

CHRONIC RHEUMATIC HEART DISEASE (393-398)

393 Chronic rheumatic pericarditis

Chronic rheumatic:
  mediastinopericarditis
  myopericarditis

Adherent pericardium, rheumatic

Excludes: when not specified as rheumatic (423.9)

394 Diseases of mitral valve

394.0 *Mitral stenosis*

Mitral (valve) obstruction (rheumatic)

394.1 *Rheumatic mitral insufficiency*

Rheumatic mitral:
  incompetence
  regurgitation

Excludes: when not specified as rheumatic (424.0)

394.2 *Mitral stenosis with insufficiency*

Mitral stenosis with incompetence or regurgitation

394.9 *Other and unspecified*

Mitral (valve):
  disease (chronic)
  failure

395 Diseases of aortic valve

Excludes: when not specified as rheumatic (424.1)

395.0 *Rheumatic aortic stenosis*

Rheumatic aortic (valve) obstruction

395.1 *Rheumatic aortic insufficiency*

Rheumatic aortic:
  incompetence
  regurgitation

395.2 *Rheumatic aortic stenosis with insufficiency*

Rheumatic aortic stenosis with incompetence or regurgitation

395.9 *Other and unspecified*
Rheumatic aortic (valve) disease

396   Diseases of mitral and aortic valves

Involvement of both mitral and aortic valves whether specified as rheumatic or not

397   Diseases of other endocardial structures

397.0 *Diseases of tricuspid valve*
Tricuspid (valve) (rheumatic):
   disease
   obstruction
   stenosis

397.1 *Rheumatic diseases of pulmonary valve*
Excludes: when not specified as rheumatic (424.3)

397.9 *Rheumatic diseases of endocardium, valve unspecified*
Rheumatic:
   endocarditis (chronic)
   valvulitis (chronic)
Excludes: when not specified as rheumatic (424.9)

398   Other rheumatic heart disease

398.0 *Rheumatic myocarditis*
Excludes: myocarditis not specified as rheumatic (429.0)

398.9 *Other and unspecified*
Rheumatic:
   carditis
   heart disease NOS

Excludes: carditis not specified as rheumatic (429.8)
           heart disease NOS not specified as rheumatic (429.9)

HYPERTENSIVE DISEASE (401-405)

The following fourth-digit subdivisions are for use with categories
   401-405:
   .0 Specified as malignant
   .1 Specified as benign
   .9 Not specified as malignant or benign

Excludes: when complicating pregnancy, childbirth or the puerperium
           (642.–)
           when involving coronary vessels (410-414)

401   Essential hypertension

[See page 261 for fourth-digit subdivisions]

Includes: high blood pressure
             hyperpiesia
             hyperpiesis
             hypertension (arterial) (essential) (primary) (systemic)

Excludes: when involving vessels of:
             brain (430-438)
             eye (362.1)

402   Hypertensive heart disease

[See page 261 for fourth-digit subdivisions]

Includes: hypertensive heart (disease) (failure)
             any condition in 428, 429.0-429.3, 429.8, 429.9 due to hyper-
             tension

403   Hypertensive renal disease

[See page 261 for fourth-digit subdivisions]

Includes: arteriolar nephritis
             arteriosclerosis of kidney
             arteriosclerotic nephritis (chronic) (interstitial)
             hypertensive:
               nephropathy
               renal failure
             nephrosclerosis
             any condition in 585, 586 or 587 with any condition in 401

404   Hypertensive heart and renal disease

[See page 261 for fourth-digit subdivisions]

Includes: disease:
               cardiorenal
               cardiovascular renal
             any condition in 402.– with any condition in 403.–

405   Secondary hypertension

[See page 261 for fourth-digit subdivisions]

Excludes: when involving vessels of:
             brain (430-438)
             eye (362.1)

ISCHAEMIC HEART DISEASE (410-414)

Includes: with mention of hypertension (conditions in 401-405)

Use additional code, if desired, to identify presence of hypertension

410   Acute myocardial infarction

Cardiac infarction
Coronary (artery):
  embolism
  occlusion
  rupture
  thrombosis
Infarction:
  heart
  myocardium
  ventricle

Rupture:
  heart
  myocardium
Subendocardial infarction
Any condition in 414.1-414.9 specified as acute or with a stated duration of 8 weeks or less

411   Other acute and subacute forms of ischaemic heart disease

Coronary:
  failure
  insufficiency (acute)
Intermediate coronary syndrome

Microinfarct of heart
Preinfarction syndrome
Postmyocardial infarction or
  Dressler's syndrome

412   Old myocardial infarction

Healed myocardial infarct
Past myocardial infarction diagnosed on ECG or other special investigation, but currently presenting no symptoms

413   Angina pectoris

Angina:
  NOS
  cardiac
  decubitus
  of effort

Anginal syndrome
Stenocardia

414   Other forms of chronic ischaemic heart disease

Excludes: cardiovascular arteriosclerosis, degeneration, disease or sclerosis (429.2)

414.0 *Coronary atherosclerosis*

Atherosclerotic heart disease
Coronary atheroma

Coronary (artery) sclerosis

414.1 *Aneurysm of heart*

Aneurysm: Ventricular aneurysm
  coronary
  mural

414.8 *Other*

Ischaemia, myocardial (chronic)
Any condition in 410 specified as chronic or with a stated duration of
  over 8 weeks

414.9 *Unspecified*

Ischaemic heart disease NOS

DISEASES OF PULMONARY CIRCULATION (415-417)

415   **Acute pulmonary heart disease**

415.0 *Acute cor pulmonale*

415.1 *Pulmonary embolism*

Pulmonary (artery) (vein):
  apoplexy
  infarction (haemorrhagic)
  thrombosis

Excludes: when complicating:
          abortion (634-638 with fourth digit .6, 639.6)
          ectopic or molar pregnancy (639.6)
          pregnancy, childbirth or the puerperium (673.–)

416   **Chronic pulmonary heart disease**

416.0 *Primary pulmonary hypertension*

Pulmonary hypertension (primary) (idiopathic)

416.1 *Kyphoscoliotic heart disease*

416.8 *Other*

416.9 *Pulmonary heart disease, unspecified*

Chronic cardiopulmonary disease   Cor pulmonale (chronic) NOS

417   **Other diseases of pulmonary circulation**

417.0 *Arteriovenous fistula of pulmonary vessels*

417.1 *Aneurysm of pulmonary artery*

417.8 *Other*

Rupture }
Stricture } of pulmonary vessel

417.9 *Unspecified*

OTHER FORMS OF HEART DISEASE (420-429)

420   Acute pericarditis

Includes: acute:
   mediastinopericarditis
   myopericarditis
   pericardial effusion
   pleuropericarditis
   pneumopericarditis

420.0* *Pericarditis in diseases classified elsewhere*

Pericarditis (acute):
   Coxsackie (074.2†)
   meningococcal (036.4†)
   syphilitic (093.8†)

Pericarditis (acute):
   tuberculous (017.8†)
   uraemic (585†)

Excludes: acute rheumatic pericarditis (391.0)

420.9   *Other and unspecified acute pericarditis*

Pericarditis:
   infective
   pneumococcal
   purulent
   staphylococcal

Pericarditis:
   streptococcal
   viral
Pyopericarditis

421   Acute and subacute endocarditis

421.0   *Acute and subacute bacterial endocarditis*

Endocarditis (acute) (chronic)
   (subacute):
   bacterial
   infective NOS
   lenta
   malignant

Endocarditis (acute) (chronic)
   (subacute):
   septic
   ulcerative
   vegetative
Infective aneurysm

Use additional code, if desired, to identify infectious organism [e.g., streptococcus 041.0; staphylococcus 041.1]

421.1* *Acute and subacute infective endocarditis in diseases classified elsewhere*

Endocarditis:
   candidal (112.8†)
   Coxsackie (074.2†)
   gonococcal (098.8†)
   meningococcal (036.4†)
   monilial (112.8†)
   typhoid (002.0†)

421.9 *Acute endocarditis, unspecified*

Endocarditis ⎤
Myoendocarditis ⎬ acute or subacute
Periendocarditis ⎦

Excludes: acute rheumatic endocarditis (391.1)

422 Acute myocarditis

422.0* *Acute myocarditis in diseases classified elsewhere*

Aseptic myocarditis of newborn (074.2†)
Myocarditis (acute):
  Coxsackie (074.2†)
  diphtheritic (032.8†)
Myocarditis (acute):
  influenzal (487.8†)
  syphilitic (093.8†)
  toxoplasmosis (130†)
  tuberculous (017.8†)

422.9 *Other and unspecified acute myocarditis*

Acute or subacute (interstitial) myocarditis
Septic myocarditis
Toxic myocarditis

423 Other diseases of pericardium

Excludes: when specified as rheumatic (393)

423.0 *Haemopericardium*

423.1 *Adhesive pericarditis*
Adherent pericardium

423.2 *Constrictive pericarditis*

423.8 *Other*

423.9 *Unspecified*

424 Other diseases of endocardium

424.0 *Mitral valve disorders*

Mitral (valve): ⎤
  incompetence ⎥ NOS
  insufficiency ⎬ of specified cause, except rheumatic
  regurgitation ⎦

Excludes: mitral (valve):
    disease (394.9)
    failure (394.9)
    stenosis (394.0)
   the listed conditions:
    when specified as rheumatic (394.1)
    when of unspecified cause but with mention of:
      diseases of aortic valve (396)
      mitral stenosis or obstruction (394.2)

424.1 *Aortic valve disorders*

Aortic (valve):
  incompetence
  insufficiency
  regurgitation
  stenosis
} NOS
of specified cause,
      except rheumatic
syphilitic* (093.2†)

Excludes: when specified as rheumatic (395.–)
      when of unspecified cause but with mention of diseases of
        mitral valve (396)
      hypertrophic subaortic stenosis (425.1)

424.2 *Tricuspid valve disorders, specified as nonrheumatic*

Tricuspid valve:
  incompetence
  insufficiency
  regurgitation
  stenosis
} of specified cause, except rheumatic

Excludes: when of unspecified cause (397.0)

424.3 *Pulmonary valve disorders*

Pulmonic regurgitation:
  NOS
  syphilitic* (093.2†)

Excludes: when specified as rheumatic (397.1)

424.9 *Endocarditis, valve unspecified*

Atypical veruccous endocarditis [Libman-Sacks]* (710.0†)
Endocarditis (chronic)
Valvular:
  incompetence
  insufficiency
  regurgitation
  stenosis
Valvulitis (chronic)
} of un-
specified
valve
{ specified cause, except rheumatic
  tuberculous* (017.8†)
  unspecified cause

Excludes: when specified as rheumatic (397.9)
      endocardial fibroelastosis (425.3)

425 Cardiomyopathy

Includes: myocardiopathy
Excludes: cardiomyopathy arising during pregnancy or the puerperium
      (674.8)

425.0 *Endomyocardial fibrosis*

425.1 *Hypertrophic obstructive cardiomyopathy*
Hypertrophic subaortic stenosis

425.2   *Obscure cardiomyopathy of Africa*

Becker's disease

425.3   *Endocardial fibroelastosis*

425.4   *Other primary cardiomyopathies*

Cardiovascular collagenosis

Cardiomyopathy:
  NOS
  constrictive
  familial

Cardiomyopathy:
  hypertrophic nonobstructive
  idiopathic
  obstructive

425.5   *Alcoholic cardiomyopathy*

425.6*   *Cardiomyopathy in Chagas's disease* (086.0†)

425.7*   *Nutritional and metabolic cardiomyopathies*

Amyloid heart (disease) (277.3†)
Beriberi heart (disease) (265.0†)
Cardiac glycogenosis (271.0†)

Gouty tophi of heart (274.8†)
Mucopolysaccharidosis
  cardiopathy (277.5†)
Thyrotoxic heart disease (242.–†)

425.8*   *Cardiomyopathy in other diseases classified elsewhere*

Cardiac sarcoidosis (135†)

425.9   *Secondary cardiomyopathy, unspecified*

426   Conduction disorders

426.0   *Atrioventricular block, complete*

426.1   *Atrioventricular block, other and unspecified*

Atrioventricular block:
  NOS
  incomplete
  partial

Wenkebach's phenomenon

426.2   *Left bundle branch hemiblock*

426.3   *Other left bundle branch block*

426.4   *Right bundle branch block*

426.5   *Bundle branch block, unspecified*

426.6   *Other heart block*

Sinoatrial block

Sinoauricular block

426.7   *Anomalous atrioventricular excitation*
Atrioventricular conduction: Wolff-Parkinson-White syndrome
  accelerated
  accessory
  pre-excitation

426.8   *Other*
Atrioventricular [AV] dissociation   Lown-Ganong-Levine syndrome
Interference dissociation

426.9   *Unspecified*
Heart block NOS   Stokes-Adams syndrome

427   Cardiac dysrhythmias
Excludes: postoperative (997.1)
      when attributable to medical care for abortion, ectopic or
      molar pregnancy, labour or delivery (634-638 with fourth
      digit .7, 639.8, 668.1, 669.4)

427.0   *Paroxysmal supraventricular tachycardia*
Paroxysmal tachycardia:
  atrial
  atrioventricular [AV]
  junctional
  nodal

427.1   *Paroxysmal ventricular tachycardia*

427.2   *Paroxysmal tachycardia, unspecified*
Bouveret-Hoffman syndrome

427.3   *Atrial fibrillation and flutter*

427.4   *Ventricular fibrillation and flutter*

427.5   *Cardiac arrest*

427.6   *Premature beats*
Ectopic beats   Premature:
Extrasystoles   beats
Extrasystolic arrhythmia   atrial
                    nodal
                    supraventricular
                    ventricular
                    contractions
427.8   *Other*
Rhythm disorder: Syndrome:
  coronary sinus   sick sinus
  ectopic   tachycardia-bradycardia
  nodal   Wandering pacemaker

427.9   *Unspecified*

Arrhythmia (cardiac) NOS

428   Heart failure

Excludes: postoperative (997.1)
when attributable to medical care for abortion, ectopic or
molar pregnancy, labour or delivery (634-638 with fourth
digit .7, 639.8, 668.1, 669.4)
when due to hypertension (402.–)

428.0   *Congestive heart failure*

Congestive heart disease   Right heart failure (secondary
to left heart failure)

428.1   *Left heart failure*

Acute oedema of lung   ⎫ with mention of heart disease
Acute pulmonary oedema ⎬   NOS or heart failure
Cardiac asthma   ⎭
Left ventricular failure

428.9   *Unspecified*

Cardiac, heart or myocardial   Weak heart
failure NOS

429   Ill-defined descriptions and complications of heart disease

Excludes: any condition in 429.0-429.3, 429.8, 429.9 due to hypertension (402.–)

429.0   Myocarditis, unspecified

Myocarditis: ⎫
NOS   ⎪
chronic (interstitial) ⎬ (with mention of arteriosclerosis)
fibroid   ⎪
senile   ⎭

Use additional code, if desired, to identify presence of arteriosclerosis

429.1   *Myocardial degeneration*

Degeneration of heart or myocardium: ⎫
fatty   ⎪
mural   ⎪
muscular   ⎬ (with mention of
Myocardial: ⎪ arteriosclerosis)
degeneration   ⎪
disease   ⎭

Use additional code, if desired, to identify presence of arteriosclerosis

429.2   *Cardiovascular disease, unspecified*

Cardiovascular arteriosclerosis
Cardiovascular:
  degeneration
  disease   } (with mention of arteriosclerosis)
  sclerosis

Use additional code, if desired, to identify presence of arteriosclerosis

429.3   *Cardiomegaly*

Cardiac: Ventricular dilatation
  dilatation
  hypertrophy

429.4   *Functional disturbances following cardiac surgery*

Cardiac insufficiency] following cardiac surgery or due to presence
Heart failure   ∫   of prosthesis
Postcardiotomy syndrome

Excludes: cardiac failure in the immediate postoperative period (997.1)

429.5   *Rupture of chordae tendinae*

429.6   *Rupture of papillary muscle*

429.8   *Other*

Carditis

429.9   *Unspecified*

Heart disease (organic) NOS   Morbus cordis NOS

CEREBROVASCULAR DISEASE (430-438)

Includes: with mention of hypertension (conditions in 401 and 405)

Use additional code, if desired, to identify presence of hypertension

Excludes: any condition in 430-434, 436, 437 occurring during preg-
            nancy, childbirth or the puerperium, or specified as
            puerperal (674.0)

430   Subarachnoid haemorrhage

Meningeal haemorrhage   Ruptured (congenital) cerebral
                                      aneurysm:
                                      NOS
                                      syphilitic* (094.8†)

431 Intracerebral haemorrhage

Haemorrhage (of):
basilar
bulbar
cerebral
cerebromeningeal
cerebellar
cortical
internal capsule

Haemorrhage:
intrapontine
pontine
subcortical
ventricular
Rupture of blood vessel in brain

432 Other and unspecified intracranial haemorrhage

432.0 *Nontraumatic extradural haemorrhage*
Nontraumatic epidural haemorrhage

432.1 *Subdural haemorrhage*
Subdural haemorrhage (nontraumatic)

432.9 *Unspecified intracranial haemorrhage*

433 Occlusion and stenosis of precerebral arteries

Includes: embolism
narrowing
obstruction (complete)
(partial)
thrombosis
} of basilar, carotid and vertebral arteries

Excludes: insufficiency NOS of precerebral arteries (435)

433.0 *Basilar artery*

433.1 *Carotid artery*

433.2 *Vertebral artery*

433.3 *Multiple and bilateral*

433.8 *Other*

433.9 *Unspecified*
Precerebral artery NOS

434 Occlusion of cerebral arteries

434.0 *Cerebral thrombosis*
Thrombosis of cerebral arteries

434.1 *Cerebral embolism*

434.9 *Unspecified*
Cerebral infarction NOS

435   Transient cerebral ischaemia

Basilar artery syndrome
Cerebrovascular insufficiency
    (acute) with transient
    focal neurological
    signs and symptoms
Insufficiency:
    basilar
    carotid   } artery
    vertebral

Intermittent cerebral ischaemia
Spasm of cerebral arteries
Subclavian steal syndrome
Transient ischaemic attack [TIA]
Vertebral artery syndrome

Excludes: acute cerebrovascular insufficiency NOS (437.1)
            when due to conditions in 433.– (433.–)

436   Acute but ill-defined cerebrovascular disease

Apoplexy, apoplectic:
    NOS
    attack
    seizure

Cerebrovascular accident NOS
Stroke

437   Other and ill-defined cerebrovascular disease

437.0   *Cerebral atherosclerosis*

Atheroma of cerebral arteries

437.1   *Other generalized ischaemic cerebrovascular disease*

Acute cerebrovascular insufficiency NOS
Cerebral ischaemia (chronic)

437.2   *Hypertensive encephalopathy*

437.3   *Cerebral aneurysm, nonruptured*

437.4   *Cerebral arteritis*

437.5   *Moyamoya disease*

437.6   *Nonpyogenic thrombosis of intracranial venous sinus*

437.8   *Other*

437.9   *Unspecified*

438   Late effects of cerebrovascular disease

Note: This category is to be used to indicate conditions in 430-437 as the
       cause of late effects, themselves classifiable elsewhere. The "late
       effects" include conditions specified as such, as sequelae, or present
       one year or more after the onset of the causal condition.   [See
       III Latte effect, page 723].

DISEASES OF ARTERIES, ARTERIOLES AND CAPILLARIES
(440-448)

440   Atherosclerosis

Includes: arteriolosclerosis
arteriosclerosis
arteriosclerotic vascular disease
atheroma
degeneration:
arterial
arteriovascular
vascular
endarteritis deformans or obliterans
senile:
arteritis
endarteritis

440.0   *Of aorta*

440.1   *Of renal artery*

Excludes: atherosclerosis of renal arterioles (403.–)

440.2   *Of arteries of the extremities*

Atherosclerotic gangrene† (785.4*)
Mönckeberg's (medial) sclerosis

440.8   *Of other specified arteries*

Excludes: cerebral (437.0)
coronary (414.0)
mesenteric (557.1)
pulmonary (416.0)

440.9   *Generalized and unspecified*

441   Aortic aneurysm

441.0   *Dissecting aneurysm [any part]*

441.1   *Thoracic aneurysm, ruptured*

441.2   *Thoracic aneurysm without mention of rupture*

441.3   *Abdominal aneurysm, ruptured*

441.4   *Abdominal aneurysm without mention of rupture*

441.5   *Aortic aneurysm of unspecified site, ruptured*

Rupture of aorta NOS

441.6 *Aortic aneurysm of unspecified site without mention of rupture*

Aneurysm ⎫
Dilatation ⎬ of aorta
Hyaline necrosis ⎭

441.7* *Syphilitic aneurysm of aorta* (093.0†)

442   Other aneurysm

Includes: aneurysm (rupture) (cirsoid) (false) (varicose)
            aneurysmal varix

Excludes: arteriovenous aneurysm, acquired (447.0)

442.0 *Of artery of upper extremity*

442.1 *Of renal artery*

442.2 *Of iliac artery*

442.3 *Of artery of lower extremity*

442.8 *Of other specified artery*

Excludes: cerebral (nonruptured) (437.3)
                ruptured (430)
            coronary (414.1)
            heart (414.1)
            pulmonary (417.1)

442.9 *Of unspecified site*

443   Other peripheral vascular disease

443.0 *Raynaud's syndrome*
Raynaud's:
  disease
  gangrene† (785.4*)
  phenomenon (secondary)

443.1 *Thromboangiitis obliterans [Buerger's disease]*

443.8 *Other*

Acrocyanosis
Acroparaesthesia:
  simple [Schulze's type]
  vasomotor [Nothnagel's type]

Diabetic peripheral angiopathy*
  (250.6†)
Erythrocyanosis
Erythromelalgia

Excludes: chilblains (991.5)
            frostbite (991.0 – 991.3, E901.–)
            immersion foot (991.4, E901.0)

443.9 *Unspecified*

Intermittent claudication   Spasm of artery
Peripheral vascular disease NOS

Excludes: spasm of cerebral artery (435)

444   **Arterial embolism and thrombosis**

Includes: infarction:
              embolic
              thrombotic
              occlusion

Excludes: when complicating:
              abortion (634-638 with fourth digit .6, 639.6)
              ectopic or molar pregnancy (639.6)
              pregnancy, childbirth or the puerperium (673.–)

444.0 *Of abdominal aorta*

Aortic bifurcation syndrome   Leriche's syndrome

444.1 *Of other aorta*

444.2 *Of arteries of the extremities*

Peripheral arterial embolism

444.8 *Of other specified artery*

Excludes: basilar (433.0)
              carotid (433.1)
              cerebral (434.–)
              coronary (410)
              mesenteric (557.0)
              ophthalmic (362.3)
              precerebral (433.–)
              pulmonary (415.1)
              renal (593.8)
              retinal (362.3)
              vertebral (433.2)

444.9 *Of unspecified artery*

446   **Polyarteritis nodosa and allied conditions**

446.0 *Polyarteritis nodosa*

Disseminated necrotizing   Periarteritis (nodosa)
  periarteritis
Panarteritis

446.1 *Acute febrile mucocutaneous lymphnode syndrome [MCLS]*

446.2 *Hypersensitivity angiitis*
Goodpasture's syndrome

446.3 *Lethal midline granuloma*

446.4 *Wegener's granulomatosis*

446.5 *Giant cell arteritis*
Cranial arteritis   Temporal arteritis
Horton's disease

446.6 *Thrombotic microangiopathy*
Thrombotic thrombocytopenic purpura

446.7 *Takayasu disease*
Aortic arch arteritis   Pulseless disease

447   Other disorders of arteries and arterioles

447.0 *Arteriovenous fistula, acquired*
Arteriovenous aneurysm, acquired
Excludes: cerebral (437.3)
            coronary (414.1)
            pulmonary (417.0)
            traumatic (900-904)

447.1 *Stricture of artery*

447.2 *Rupture of artery*
Erosion ⎫
Fistula ⎬ of artery
Ulcer   ⎭
Excludes: traumatic rupture of artery (900.– to 904.–)

447.3 *Hyperplasia of renal artery*

447.4 *Coeliac artery compression syndrome*

447.5 *Necrosis of artery*

447.6 *Arteritis, unspecified*
Aortitis NOS
Endarteritis NOS
Excludes: arteritis, endarteritis:
            aortic arch (446.7)
            cerebral (437.4)
            coronary (414.8)
            deformans (440.–)
            obliterans (440.–)
            senile (440.–)

447.7* *Syphilitic aortitis* (093.1†)

447.8 *Other*
Fibromuscular hyperplasia of arteries

447.9 *Unspecified*

448 Diseases of capillaries

448.0 *Hereditary haemorrhagic telangiectasia*
Rendu-Osler-Weber disease

448.1 *Naevus, non-neoplastic*

Naevus: Naevus:
  araneus   spider
  senile   stellar

448.9 *Other and unspecified*

DISEASES OF VEINS AND LYMPHATICS, AND OTHER DISEASES
OF CIRCULATORY SYSTEM (451-459)

451 Phlebitis and thrombophlebitis

Includes: endophlebitis
     inflammation, vein
     periphlebitis
     suppurative phlebitis

Excludes: when complicating:
     abortion (634-638 with fourth digit .7, 639.8)
     ectopic or molar pregnancy (639.8)
     pregnancy, childbirth or the puerperium (671.–)

451.0 *Of superficial vessels of lower extremities*

451.1 *Of deep vessels of lower extremities*

451.2 *Of lower extremities, unspecified*

451.8 *Of other sites*
Use additional E code, if desired, to identify drug, if drug-induced
Excludes: intracranial venous sinuses (325)
     nonpyogenic (437.6)
     portal (vein) (572.1)

451.9 *Of unspecified site*

452 Portal vein thrombosis
Portal (vein) obstruction
Excludes: phlebitis of portal vein (572.1)

453 Other venous embolism and thrombosis

Excludes: when complicating:
        abortion (634-638 with fourth digit .7, 639.8)
        ectopic or molar pregnancy (639.8)
        pregnancy, chilbirth or the puerperium (671.–)

453.0 *Budd-Chiari syndrome*

453.1 *Thrombophlebitis migrans*

453.2 *Of vena cava*

453.3 *Of renal vein*

453.8 *Of other specified veins*

Excludes: cerebral (434.–)
        coronary (410)
        intracranial venous sinuses (325)
          nonpyogenic (437.6)
        lower extremities (451.0–451.2)
        mesenteric (557.0)
        portal (452)
        precerebral (433.–)
        pulmonary (415.1)

453.9 *Of unspecified site*

Embolism of vein   Thrombosis (vein)

454 Varicose veins of lower extremities

Excludes: when complicating pregnancy or the puerperium (671.0)

454.0 *With ulcer*

Varicose ulcer (lower extremity, any part)
Any condition in 454.9 with ulcer or specified as ulcerated

454.1 *With inflammation*

Any condition in 454.9 with inflammation or specified as inflamed

454.2 *With ulcer and inflammation*

Any condition in 454.9 with ulcer and inflammation

454.9 *Without mention of ulcer or inflammation*

Phlebectasia ⎫
Varicose veins ⎬ of lower extremity [any part] or of unspecified site
Varix ⎭

455 Haemorrhoids

Includes: haemorrhoids (rectum)
        piles
        varicose veins, anus or rectum

Excludes: when complicating pregnancy, childbirth or the puerperium
        (671.8)

455.0   *Internal haemorrhoids, without mention of complication*

455.1   *Internal thrombosed haemorrhoids*

455.2   *Internal haemorrhoids with other complication*

Internal haemorrhoids:	Internal haemorrhoids:
bleeding	strangulated
prolapsed	ulcerated

455.3   *External haemorrhoids without mention of complication*

455.4   *External thrombosed haemorrhoids*

455.5   *External haemorrhoids with other complication*

External haemorrhoids:	External haemorrhoids:
bleeding	strangulated
prolapsed	ulcerated

455.6   *Unspecified haemorrhoids, without mention of complication*

Haemorrhoids NOS

455.7   *Unspecified thrombosed haemorrhoids*

Thrombosed haemorrhoids, unspecified whether internal or external

455.8   *Unspecified haemorrhoids with other complication*

Haemorrhoids, unspecified whether internal or external:	Haemorrhoids, unspecified whether internal or external:
bleeding	strangulated
prolapsed	ulcerated

455.9   *Residual haemorrhoidal skin tags*

Skin tags, anus or rectum

456   **Varicose veins of other sites**

456.0   *Oesophageal varices with bleeding*

456.1   *Oesophageal varices without mention of bleeding*

456.2*   *Oesophageal varices in cirrhosis of liver (571.–†)*

456.3   *Sublingual varices*

456.4   *Scrotal varices*

Varicocele

456.5   *Pelvic varices*

456.6   *Vulval varices*

Excludes: when complicating pregnancy, childbirth or the puerperium (671.1)

456.8 *Other*

Excludes: retinal varices (362.1)
              varicose veins of unspecified site (454.9)

457   Noninfective disorders of lymphatic channels

457.0 *Postmastectomy lymphoedema syndrome*

Elephantiasis
Obliteration of lymphatic vessel } due to mastectomy operation

457.1 *Other lymphoedema*

Elephantiasis (nonfilarial) NOS   Obliteration, lymphatic vessel
Lymphangiectasis

Excludes: elephantiasis (nonfilarial):
              congenital (757.0)
              eyelid (374.8)
              vulva (628.4)

457.2 *Lymphangitis*

Lymphangitis:
  NOS
  chronic
  subacute

Excludes: acute lymphangitis (682.–)

457.8 *Other noninfective disorders of lymphatic channels*

Chylocele (nonfilarial)

Excludes: chylocele:
              filarial (125.–)
              tunica vaginalis (nonfilarial) (608.8)

457.9 *Unspecified*

458   Hypotension

Includes: hypopiesis

Excludes: cardiovascular collapse (785.5)
              maternal hypotension syndrome (669.2)
              syndrome Shy-Drager (333.0)

458.0 *Orthostatic hypotension*

Hypotension:
  orthostatic (chronic)
  postural

458.1 *Chronic hypotension*

Permanent idiopathic hypotension

458.9 *Unspecified*

Hypotension (arterial) NOS

459 Other disorders of circulatory system

459.0 *Haemorrhage, unspecified*

Excludes: haemorrhage:
      gastrointestinal (578.9)
      in newborn NOS (772.9)

459.1 *Post-phlebitic syndrome*

459.2 *Compression of vein*

Stricture of vein
Vena cava syndrome (inferior) (superior)

459.8 *Other*

Collateral circulation (venous), any site
Phlebosclerosis

459.9 *Unspecified*

VIII. DISEASES OF THE RESPIRATORY SYSTEM

Use additional code, if desired, to identify infectious organism

ACUTE RESPIRATORY INFECTIONS (460-466)

Excludes: pneumonia and influenza (480-487)

460   Acute nasopharyngitis [common cold]

Coryza (acute)
Nasal catarrh, acute
Nasopharyngitis:
  NOS
  acute
  infective NOS

Rhinitis:
  acute
  infective

Excludes: nasopharyngitis, chronic (472.2)
            pharyngitis:
              acute or unspecified (462)
              chronic (472.1)
            rhinitis:
              allergic (477.–)
              chronic or unspecified (472.0)
            sore throat:
              acute or unspecified (462)
              chronic (472.1)

461   Acute sinusitis

Includes: abscess
            empyema
            infection   } acute, of sinus (accessory) (nasal)
            inflammation
            suppuration

Excludes: chronic or unspecified (473.–)

461.0 *Maxillary*
Acute antritis

461.1 *Frontal*

461.2 *Ethmoidal*

461.3 *Sphenoidal*

461.8 *Other*
Acute pansinusitis

461.9 *Unspecified*
Acute sinusitis NOS

462   Acute pharyngitis

Acute sore throat NOS
Pharyngitis (acute):
  NOS
  gangrenous
  infective
  phlegmonous
  pneumococcal

Pharyngitis (acute):
  staphylococcal
  suppurative
  ulcerative
Sore throat (viral) NOS
Viral pharyngitis

Excludes: abscess:
    peritonsillar [quinsy] (475)
    pharyngeal (478.2)
    retropharyngeal.(478.2)
   chronic pharyngitis (472.1)
   the conditions if specified as (due to):
    Coxsackie virus (074.0)
    herpes simplex (054.7)
    influenzal (487.1)
    septic (034.0)
    streptococcal (034.0)

463   Acute tonsillitis

Tonsillitis (acute):
  NOS
  follicular
  gangrenous
  infective
  pneumococcal

Tonsillitis (acute):
  septic
  staphylococcal
  suppurative
  ulcerative
  viral

Excludes: peritonsillar abscess [quinsy] (475)
     sore throat:
      acute or NOS (462)
      septic (034.0)
     streptococcal tonsillitis (034.0)

464   Acute laryngitis and tracheitis

Excludes: when specified as due to streptococcus (034.0)

464.0   *Acute laryngitis*

Laryngitis (acute):
  NOS
  Haemophilus influenzae
    [H. influenzae]
  oedematous
  pneumococcal

Laryngitis (acute):
  septic
  suppurative
  ulcerative

Excludes: chronic laryngitis (476.–)
     influenzal laryngitis (487.1)

464.1   *Acute tracheitis*

Tracheitis (acute):
  NOS
  catarrhal
  viral

Excludes: chronic tracheitis (491.8)

464.2   *Acute laryngotracheitis*

Laryngotracheitis (acute)
Tracheitis (acute) with laryngitis (acute)

464.3   *Acute epiglottitis*

464.4   *Croup*

465   Acute upper respiratory infections of multiple or unspecified site

465.0   *Acute laryngopharyngitis*

465.8   *Other multiple sites*

465.9   *Unspecified site*

Upper respiratory:
  disease (acute)
  infection (acute)

Excludes: upper respiratory infection due to:
                 influenza (487.1)
                 streptococcus (034.0)

466   Acute bronchitis and bronchiolitis

Includes: the listed conditions with or without mention of obstruction
                 or bronchospasm

Excludes: for single-condition coding, acute exacerbation of chronic
                 bronchitis (491.–)

466.0   *Acute bronchitis*

Bronchitis, acute or subacute: Bronchitis, acute or subacute:
  fibrinous   viral
  membranous   with tracheitis
  pneumococcal   Croupous bronchitis
  purulent   Tracheobronchitis, acute
  septic

466.1   *Acute bronchiolitis*

Bronchiolitis (acute)   Capillary pneumonia

OTHER DISEASES OF UPPER RESPIRATORY TRACT (470-478)

470　　Deflected nasal septum

Deflection or deviation of septum (nasal) (acquired)

471　　Nasal polyps

Excludes: adenomatous polyps (212.0)

471.0　*Polyp of nasal cavity*

Polyp:
  choanal
  nasopharyngeal

471.1　*Polypoid sinus degeneration*

Woakes's syndrome or ethmoiditis

471.8　*Other polyp of sinus*

Polyp of sinus:　　　　　　　Polyp of sinus:
  accessory　　　　　　　 maxillary
  ethmoidal　　　　　　　 sphenoidal

471.9　*Unspecified*

Nasal polyp NOS

472　　Chronic pharyngitis and nasopharyngitis

472.0　*Chronic rhinitis*

Ozena　　　　　　　　　　　Rhinitis:
Rhinitis:　　　　　　　　　 obstructive
  NOS　　　　　　　　　　 purulent
  atrophic　　　　　　　　 ulcerative
  granulomatous
  hypertrophic

Excludes: allergic rhinitis (477.–)

472.1　*Chronic pharyngitis*

Chronic sore throat
Pharyngitis:
  atrophic
  granular (chronic)
  hypertrophic

472.2　*Chronic nasopharyngitis*

Excludes: acute or unspecified nasopharyngitis (460)

473   Chronic sinusitis

Includes: abscess
empyema
infection   } (chronic) of sinus (accessory) (nasal)
suppuration

Excludes: acute sinusitis (461.–)

473.0   *Maxillary*
Antritis (chronic)

473.1   *Frontal*

473.2   *Ethmoidal*

473.3   *Sphenoidal*

473.8   *Other*
Pansinusitis (chronic)

473.9   *Unspecified*
Sinusitis (chronic) NOS

474   Chronic disease of tonsils and adenoids

474.0   *Chronic tonsillitis*
Excludes: acute or unspecified tonsillitis (463)

474.1   *Hypertrophy of tonsils and adenoids*
Enlargement
Hyperplasia   } of tonsils (and adenoids)
Hypertrophy

474.2   *Adenoid vegetations*

474.8   *Other chronic disease of tonsils and adenoids*
Amygdalolith   Tonsillar tag
Calculus, tonsil   Ulcer, tonsil
Cicatrix of tonsil (and adenoid)

474.9   *Unspecified*

Disease (chronic) of tonsils (and adenoids)

475   Peritonsillar abscess

Abscess of tonsil   Quinsy
Peritonsillar cellulitis
Excludes: tonsillitis:
acute or NOS (463)
chronic (474.0)

476 Chronic laryngitis and laryngotracheitis

476.0 *Chronic laryngitis*

Laryngitis:
  catarrhal
  hypertrophic
  sicca

476.1 *Chronic laryngotracheitis*

Laryngitis, chronic, with tracheitis (chronic)
Tracheitis, chronic, with laryngitis

Excludes: chronic tracheitis (491.8)
　　　　　laryngitis and tracheitis, acute or unspecified (464.–)

477 Allergic rhinitis

Includes: allergic rhinitis (nonseasonal) (seasonal)
　　　　　hay fever
　　　　　pollinosis
　　　　　spasmodic rhinorrhoea

Excludes: allergic rhinitis with asthma (bronchial) (493.0)

477.0 *Due to pollen*

477.8 *Due to other allergen*

477.9 *Cause unspecified*

478 Other diseases of upper respiratory tract

478.0 *Hypertrophy of nasal turbinates*

478.1 *Other diseases of nasal cavity and sinuses*

Abscess ⎫
Necrosis ⎬ of nose (septum)
Ulceration ⎭

Cyst or mucocele of sinus (nasal)
Rhinolith

Excludes: varicose ulcer of nasal septum (456.8)

478.2 *Other diseases of pharynx, not elsewhere classified*

Abscess ⎫
Cellulitis ⎬ of pharynx or nasopharynx
Cyst ⎬
Oedema ⎭
Retropharyngeal abscess

Excludes: ulcerative pharyngitis (462)

478.3 *Paralysis of vocal cords or larynx*

Laryngoplegia　　　　　　　　　　　Paralysis of glottis

478.4   *Polyp of vocal cord or larynx*
Excludes: adenomatous polyps (212.1)

478.5   *Other diseases of vocal cords*

Abscess ⎱
Cellulitis ⎰ of vocal cords
Granuloma
Leukoplakia

Chorditis (fibrinous) (nodosa)
    (tuberosa)
Singers' nodes

478.6   *Oedema of larynx*
Oedema:
  glottis
  subglottic
  supraglottic

478.7   *Other diseases of larynx, not elsewhere classified*

Abscess ⎱
Cellulitis
Necrosis ⎰ of larynx
Obstruction
Pachyderma

Perichondritis ⎱
Spasm
Stenosis ⎰ of larynx
Ulcer
Laryngismus (stridulus)

Excludes: ulcerative laryngitis (464.0)

478.8   *Upper respiratory tract hypersensitivity reaction, site unspecified*

478.9   *Other and unspecified diseases of upper respiratory tract*

Abscess ⎱
Cicatrix ⎰ of trachea

PNEUMONIA AND INFLUENZA (480-487)

Excludes: pneumonia:
          allergic or eosinophilic (518.3)
          aspiration:
            NOS (507.0)
            newborn (770.1)
            solids and liquids (507.–)
          congenital (770.0)
          lipoid (507.1)
          passive (514)
          postoperative (997.3)
          rheumatic (390†, 517.1*)

480   Viral pneumonia

480.0   *Pneumonia due to adenovirus*

480.1   *Pneumonia due to respiratory syncytial virus*

480.2   *Pneumonia due to parainfluenza virus*

480.8 *Pneumonia due to other virus, not elsewhere classified*

Excludes: congenital rubella pneumonitis (771.0)
influenza with pneumonia, any form (487.0)
pneumonia complicating viral diseases classified elsewhere
(045-079†, 484.–*)

480.9 *Viral pneumonia, unspecified*

481 Pneumococcal pneumonia

Lobar pneumonia, organism unspecified

482 Other bacterial pneumonia

482.0 *Pneumonia due to Klebsiella pneumoniae*

482.1 *Pneumonia due to Pseudomonas*

482.2 *Pneumonia due to Haemophilus influenzae [H. influenzae]*

482.3 *Pneumonia due to Streptococcus*

482.4 *Pneumonia due to Staphylococcus*

482.8 *Pneumonia due to other specified bacteria*

Pneumonia due to:
Escherichia coli [E. coli]
Proteus

Excludes: pneumonia complicating infectious diseases classified elsewhere (001-136†, 484.–*)

482.9 *Bacterial pneumonia, unspecified*

483 Pneumonia due to other specified organism

Pneumonia due to:
Eaton's agent
Mycoplasma (pneumoniae)
Pleuropneumonia-like organisms [PPLO]

484* Pneumonia in infectious diseases classified elsewhere

Excludes: influenza with pneumonia, any form (487.0)

484.0* *Measles (055.1†)*

484.1* *Cytomegalic inclusion disease (078.5†)*

484.2* *Ornithosis (073†)*

484.3* *Whooping cough (033.–†)*

484.4* *Tularaemia (021†)*

484.5* *Anthrax* (022.1†)

484.6* *Aspergillosis* (117.3†)

484.7* *Pneumonia in other systemic mycoses*
Candidiasis (112.4†)   Histoplasmosis (115.–†)
Coccidioidomycosis (114†)

484.8* *Pneumonia in other infectious diseases*
Pneumonia in: Pneumonia in:
  actinomycosis (039.1†)   salmonellosis (003.2†)
  nocardiasis (039.1†)   toxoplasmosis (130†)
  pneumocystosis (136.3†)   typhoid fever (002.0†)
  Q-fever (083.0†)   varicella (052†)

485   Bronchopneumonia, organism unspecified

Excludes: bronchiolitis (466.1)
            lipoid pneumonia (507.1)

486   Pneumonia, organism unspecified

Excludes: hypostatic or passive pneumonia (514)
            influenza with pneumonia, any form (487.0)
            inhalation or inspiration pneumonia due to foreign material
               (507.–)
            pneumonitis due to fumes and vapours (506.0)

487   Influenza

Excludes: Haemophilus influenzae [H. influenzae]:
               infection NOS (041.5)
               meningitis (320.0)
               pneumonia (482.2)

487.0   *With pneumonia*
Influenza with pneumonia, any form
Influenzal:
  bronchopneumonia
  pneumonia

487.1   *With other respiratory manifestations*
Influenzal: Influenza NOS
  laryngitis
  pharyngitis
  respiratory infection (upper) (acute)

487.8   *With other manifestations*
Encephalopathy due to influenza
Influenza with involvement of gastrointestinal tract

CHRONIC OBSTRUCTIVE PULMONARY DISEASE AND ALLIED
CONDITIONS (490-496)

490 Bronchitis, not specified as acute or chronic

Bronchitis NOS: Tracheobronchitis NOS
  catarrhal
  with tracheitis NOS

Excludes: bronchitis:
        allergic NOS (493.9)
        asthmatic NOS (493.9)
        due to fumes and vapours (506.0)

491 Chronic bronchitis

Includes: in single-condition coding, acute exacerbation of chronic
        bronchitis

491.0 *Simple chronic bronchitis*

Catarrhal bronchitis, chronic   Smokers' cough

491.1 *Mucopurulent chronic bronchitis*

Bronchitis (chronic) (recurrent):
  mucopurulent
  purulent

491.2 *Obstructive chronic bronchitis*

Bronchitis: Bronchitis:
  asthmatic, chronic   obstructive (chronic) (diffuse)
  emphysematous   with airways obstruction

491.8 *Other chronic bronchitis*

Chronic:
  tracheitis
  tracheobronchitis

491.9 *Unspecified*

492 Emphysema

Emphysema (lung or pulmonary):   Emphysematous bleb
  bullous   MacLeod's syndrome or unilateral
  centriacinar   emphysema
  centrilobular
  obstructive
  panacinar
  panlobular
  vesicular

Excludes: emphysema:
   compensatory (518.2)
   due to fumes and vapours (506.4)
   interstitial (518.1)
    newborn (770.2)
   mediastinal (518.1)
   surgical (subcutaneous) (998.8)
   traumatic (958.7)

493 Asthma

493.0 *Extrinsic asthma*

Asthma: Hayfever with asthma
 atopic
 allergic, stated cause
 childhood
 hay
 platinum

Excludes: asthma:
   allergic NOS (493.9)
   detergent (507.8)
   miners' (500)
   wood (495.8)

493.1 *Intrinsic asthma*

Asthma due to internal immunological process
Late-onset asthma

493.9 *Asthma, unspecified*

Asthma (bronchial) (allergic NOS) Status asthmaticus
Bronchitis:
 allergic
 asthmatic

494 Bronchiectasis

Bronchiectasis (fusiform) (postinfectional) (recurrent)
Bronchiolectasis

Excludes: tuberculous bronchiectasis (current disease) (011.5)

495 Extrinsic allergic alveolitis

Includes: allergic alveolitis and pneumonitis due to inhaled organic
   dust particles of fungal, thermophilic actinomycete or
   other origin

495.0 *Farmers' lung*

495.1 *Bagassosis*

495.2 *Bird fanciers' lung*

Budgerigar fanciers' disease or lung
Pigeon fanciers' disease or lung

495.3 *Suberosis*

Corkhandlers' disease or lung

495.4 *Maltworkers' lung*

Alveolitis due to Aspergillus clavatus

495.5 *Mushroom-workers' lung*

495.6 *Maple-bark-strippers' lung*

Alveolitis due to Cryptostroma corticale

495.7 *"Ventilation" pneumonitis*

Allergic alveolitis due to fungal, thermophilic actinomycete and other
organisms growing in ventilation [air conditioning] systems

495.8 *Other allergic pneumonitis*

Cheese-washers' lung
Coffee-workers' lung
Fish-meal workers' lung
Furriers' lung

Grain-handlers' disease or lung
Pituitary-snuff-takers' disease
Sequoiosis or red-cedar asthma

495.9 *Unspecified allergic alveolitis*

Alveolitis, allergic (extrinsic)   Hypersensitivity pneumonitis

496   Chronic airways obstruction, not elsewhere classified

Chronic:
  nonspecific lung disease
  obstructive lung disease

Excludes: that with mention of:
            allergic alveolitis (495.–)
            asthma (493.–)
            bronchiectasis (494)
            bronchitis (491.2)
            emphysema (492)

PNEUMOCONIOSES AND OTHER LUNG DISEASES DUE TO EXTERNAL
AGENTS (500-508)

500   Coalworkers' pneumoconiosis

Anthracosilicosis
Anthracosis

Coalworkers' lung
Miners' asthma

501   Asbestosis

502   Pneumoconiosis due to other silica or silicates

Pneumoconiosis due to talc
Silicotic fibrosis (massive) of lung
Silicosis (simple) (complicated)

503   Pneumoconiosis due to other inorganic dust

Aluminosis (of lung)   Graphite fibrosis (of lung)
Bauxite fibrosis (of lung)   Siderosis
Berylliosis   Stannosis

504   Pneumopathy due to inhalation of other dust

Byssinosis   Cannabinosis
Flax-dressers' disease

Excludes: allergic alveolitis (495.–)
            asbestosis (501)
            bagassosis (495.1)
            farmers' lung (495.0)

505   Pneumoconiosis, unspecified

506   Respiratory conditions due to chemical fumes and vapours

Use additional E code, if desired, to identify cause

506.0   *Bronchitis and pneumonitis due to fumes and vapours*

Chemical bronchitis (acute)

506.1   *Acute pulmonary oedema due to fumes and vapours*

Chemical pulmonary oedema (acute)

506.2   *Upper respiratory inflammation due to fumes and vapours*

506.3   *Other acute and subacute respiratory conditions due to fumes and
        vapours*

506.4   *Chronic respiratory conditions due to fumes and vapours*

Emphysema (diffuse) (chronic)   ⎫ due to inhalation
Obliterative bronchiolitis (chronic) (subacute)   ⎬   of chemical fumes
Pulmonary fibrosis (chronic)   ⎭   and vapours

506.9   *Unspecified*

Silo-fillers' disease

507   Pneumonitis due to solids and liquids

Excludes: fetal aspiration pneumonitis (770.1)

507.0   *Due to inhalation of food or vomit*

Aspiration pneumonia (due to):   Aspiration pneumonia (due to):
  NOS   milk
  food (regurgitated)   vomit
  gastric secretions

Excludes: pneumonia due to aspiration of microorganisms (480.–)
             postoperative [Mendelson's syndrome] (997.3)

507.1   *Due to inhalation of oils and essences*

Lipoid pneumonia (exogenous)

Excludes: endogenous lipoid pneumonia (516.8)

507.8   *Other*

Detergent asthma

508   Respiratory conditions due to other and unspecified external agents

Use additional E code, if desired, to identify cause

508.0   *Acute pulmonary manifestations due to radiation*

Radiation pneumonitis

508.1   *Chronic and other pulmonary manifestations due to radiation*

Fibrosis of lung following radiation

508.8   *Other*

508.9   *Unspecified*

OTHER DISEASES OF RESPIRATORY SYSTEM (510-519)

510   Empyema

Use additional code, if desired, to identify infectious organism

510.0   *With fistula*

Any condition in 510.9 with fistula   Fistula:
Fistula: mediastinal
  bronchocutaneous   pleural
  hepatopleural   thoracic

510.9   *Without mention of fistula*

Abscess:
  pleura
  thorax
Empyema (chest) (lung) (pleura)
Pyopneumothorax
Pyothorax

Pleurisy:
  fibrinopurulent
  purulent
  septic
  seropurulent
  suppurative

511   Pleurisy

Excludes: pleurisy with mention of tuberculosis, current disease (012.0)

511.0   *Without mention of effusion or current tuberculosis*

Adhesion, lung or pleura
Calcification of pleura
Pleurisy (acute) (sterile):
  diaphragmatic
  fibrinous
  interlobar

Pleurisy:
  NOS
  pneumococcal
  staphylococcal
  streptococcal
Thickening of pleura

511.1   *With effusion, with mention of a bacterial cause other than tuber-culosis*

Pleurisy:
  with effusion ⎤   ⎰ pneumococcal
  exudative   ⎢   ⎱ staphylococcal
  serofibrinous ⎢   streptococcal
  serous   ⎦   other specified nontuberculous bacterial cause

511.8   *Other specified forms of effusion, except tuberculous*

Encysted pleurisy
Haemopneumothorax
Haemothorax

Hydropneumothorax
Hydrothorax

511.9   *Unspecified pleural effusion*

Pleural effusion NOS
Pleurisy:
  with effusion NOS
  exudative

Pleurisy:
  serofibrinous
  serous

512   Pneumothorax

Pneumothorax:
  NOS
  acute
  chronic

Pneumothorax:
  spontaneous
  tension

Excludes: pneumothorax:
               congenital (770.2)
               traumatic (860.–)
               tuberculous, current disease (011.7)

513 Abscess of lung and mediastinum

513.0 *Abscess of lung*

Abscess (multiple) of lung
Gangrenous or necrotic pneumonia
Pulmonary gangrene or necrosis

513.1 *Abscess of mediastinum*

514 Pulmonary congestion and hypostasis

Hypostatic: Pulmonary oedema:
  bronchopneumonia   NOS
  pneumonia   chronic
Passive pneumonia
Pulmonary congestion (passive)

Excludes: acute pulmonary oedema:
      NOS (518.4)
      with mention of heart disease or failure (428.1)

515 Postinflammatory pulmonary fibrosis

Cirrhosis of lung
Fibrosis of lung (atrophic) (confluent) (massive) | chronic or
    (perialveolar) (peribronchial) | unspecified
Induration of lung |

516 Other alveolar and parietoalveolar pneumopathy

516.0 *Pulmonary alveolar proteinosis*

516.1* *Idiopathic pulmonary haemosiderosis* (275.0†)

Essential brown induration of lung

516.2 *Pulmonary alveolar microlithiasis*

516.3 *Idiopathic fibrosing alveolitis*

Alveolocapillary block
Diffuse (idiopathic) (interstitial) pulmonary fibrosis
Hamman-Rich syndrome

516.8 *Other*

516.9 *Unspecified*

517* Lung involvement in conditions classified elsewhere

517.0* *Rheumatoid lung* (714.8†)

Diffuse interstitial rheumatoid disease of the lung
Fibrosing alveolitis, rheumatoid

517.1* *Rheumatic pneumonia* (390†)

517.2* *Lung involvement in systemic sclerosis* (710.1†)

517.8* *Other*

Lung involvement in: Pulmonary amyloidosis (277.3†)
    polymyositis (710.4†)
    sarcoidosis (135†)
    Sjögren's disease (710.2†)
    syphilis (095†)
    systemic lupus erythematosus (710.0†)

518   Other diseases of lung

518.0 *Pulmonary collapse*

Atelectasis Collapse of lung

Excludes: congenital atelectasis (770.4)
        partial (770.5)
        tuberculous atelectasis, current disease (011.8)

518.1 *Interstitial emphysema*

Mediastinal emphysema

Excludes: in fetus or newborn (770.2)
        surgical (subcutaneous) emphysema (998.8)
        traumatic emphysema (958.7)

518.2 *Compensatory emphysema*

518.3 *Pulmonary eosinophilia*

Eosinophilic asthma Tropical eosinophilia
Loeffler's syndrome
Pneumonia:
    allergic
    eosinophilic

518.4 *Acute oedema of lung, unspecified*

Excludes: pulmonary oedema:
        acute with mention of heart disease or failure (428.1)
        chronic or unspecified (514)
        due to external agents (506-508)

518.5 *Pulmonary insufficiency following trauma and surgery*

Adult respiratory distress syndrome   Shock lung
Pulmonary insufficiency following:
    shock
    surgery
    trauma

518.8　*Other diseases of lung, not elsewhere classified*

Broncholithiasis　　　　　　　　　　Pulmolithiasis
Calcification of lung

519　　Other diseases of respiratory system

519.0　*Tracheostomy malfunction*

Haemorrhage from ⎱ tracheostomy　Obstruction of tracheostomy
Sepsis of　　　　　⎰　　stoma　　　airway
　　　　　　　　　　　　　　　　Tracheo-oesophageal fistula
　　　　　　　　　　　　　　　　　following tracheostomy

519.1　*Other diseases of trachea and bronchus, not elsewhere classified*

Calcification ⎱
Stenosis　　⎰ of bronchus or trachea
Ulcer

519.2　*Mediastinitis*

519.3　*Other diseases of mediastinum, not elsewhere classified*

Fibrosis　　⎱
Hernia　　 ⎰ of mediastinum
Retraction

519.4　*Disorders of diaphragm*

Diaphragmatitis　　　　　　　　Relaxation of diaphragm
Paralysis of diaphragm

Excludes:　congenital defect of diaphragm (756.6)
　　　　　diaphragmatic hernia (553.3)
　　　　　　congenital (756.6)

519.8　*Other diseases of respiratory system, not elsewhere classified*

519.9　*Unspecified*

Respiratory disease (chronic) NOS

IX. DISEASES OF THE DIGESTIVE SYSTEM

DISEASES OF ORAL CAVITY, SALIVARY GLANDS AND JAWS (520-529)

520   Disorders of tooth development and eruption

520.0   *Anodontia*

Hypodontia   Oligodontia

520.1   *Supernumerary teeth*

Distomolar   Paramolar
Fourth molar   Supplemental teeth
Mesiodens

520.2   *Abnormalities of size and form*

Concrescence ⎤   Enamel pearls
Fusion   ⎬ of teeth   Macrodontia
Gemination   ⎦   Microdontia
Dens evaginatus   Peg-shaped [conical] teeth
Dens in dente   Taurodontism
Dens invaginatus   Tuberculum paramolare

Excludes: tuberculum Carabelli, which is regarded as a normal variation

520.3   *Mottled teeth*

Dental fluorosis   Nonfluoride enamel opacities
Mottling of enamel

520.4   *Disturbances of tooth formation*

Aplasia and hypoplasia of   Regional odontodysplasia
   cementum   Turner tooth
Dilaceration of tooth
Enamel hypoplasia (neonatal)
   (postnatal) (prenatal)

Excludes: Hutchinson's teeth and mulberry molars in congenital syphilis
            (090.5)
            mottled teeth (520.3)

520.5   *Hereditary disturbances in tooth structure, not elsewhere classified*

Amelogenesis   ⎤   Dentinal dysplasia
Dentinogenesis ⎬ imperfecta   Shell teeth
Odontogenesis ⎦

520.6   *Disturbances in tooth eruption*

Teeth: Tooth eruption:
  embedded   late
  impacted   premature
  natal
  neonatal
  primary [deciduous]:
    persistent
    shedding, premature

Excludes: exfoliation of teeth (attributable to disease of surrounding
            tissues) (525.0, 525,1)
            impacted or embedded teeth with abnormal position of such
            teeth or adjacent teeth (524.3)

520.7   *Teething syndrome*

520.8   *Other disorders of tooth development*

Colour changes during tooth formation

520.9   *Unspecified*

521   Diseases of hard tissues of teeth

521.0   *Dental caries*

Caries (of):   Infantile melanodontia
  arrested   Odontoclasia
  cementum   White spot lesions of teeth
  dentine (acute) (chronic)
  enamel (acute) (chronic) (incipient)

521.1   *Excessive attrition*

Approximal wear   Occlusal wear

521.2   *Abrasion*

Abrasion: Abrasion:
  dentifrice   ritual
  habitual   } of teeth   traditional   } of teeth
  occupational   Wedge defect NOS

521.3   *Erosion*

Erosion of teeth: Erosion of teeth:
  NOS   idiopathic
  due to: occupational
    medicine
    persistent vomiting

521.4   *Pathological resorption*

Internal granuloma of pulp   Resorption of teeth (external)

521.5   *Hypercementosis*
Cementation hyperplasia

521.6   *Ankylosis of teeth*

521.7   *Posteruptive colour changes*
Staining of teeth
Excludes: accretions [deposits] on teeth (523.6)

521.8   *Other diseases of hard tissues of teeth*
Irradiated enamel   Sensitive dentine

521.9   *Unspecified*

522   Diseases of pulp and periapical tissues

522.0   *Pulpitis*
Pulpal: Pulpitis:
  abscess   acute
  polyp   chronic (hyperplastic)
                                         (ulcerative)
                                       suppurative

522.1   *Necrosis of the pulp*
Pulp gangrene

522.2   *Pulp degeneration*
Denticles   Pulp stones
Pulp calcifications

522.3   *Abnormal hard tissue formation in pulp*
Secondary or irregular dentine

522.4   *Acute apical periodontitis of pulpal origin*

522.5   *Periapical abscess without sinus*
Dental abscess   Dentoalveolar abscess

522.6   *Chronic apical periodontitis*
Apical or periapical granuloma   Apical periodontitis NOS

522.7   *Periapical abscess with sinus*

522.8   *Radicular cyst*
Cyst: Residual radicular cyst
  apical (periodontal)
  periapical
Excludes: lateral developmental cyst (526.0)

522.9   *Other and unspecified*

523   Gingival and periodontal diseases

523.0   *Acute gingivitis*

Excludes: acute necrotizing ulcerative gingivitis (101)
            herpetic gingivostomatitis (054.2)

523.1   *Chronic gingivitis*

Gingivitis (chronic):   Gingivitis (chronic):
  NOS   simple marginal
  desquamative   ulcerative
  hyperplastic

523.2   *Gingival recession*

Gingival recession (generalized) (localized) (postinfective) (postoperative)

523.3   *Acute periodontitis*

Acute pericoronitis   Periodontal abscess
Paradontal abscess

Excludes: acute apical periodontitis (522.4)
            periapical abscess (522.5, 522.7)

523.4   *Chronic periodontitis*

Chronic pericoronitis   Periodontitis:
Periodontitis NOS   complex
                                 simplex

523.5   *Periodontosis*

523.6   *Accretions on teeth*

Dental calculus: Deposit on teeth:
  subgingival   betel
  supragingival   black
                                 green
                                 materia alba
                                 orange
                                 tobacco

523.8   *Other periodontal diseases*

Giant cell: Gingival:
  epulis   fibromatosis
  peripheral granuloma   polyp
Gingival: Periodontal lesions due to
  cysts   traumatic occlusion
  enlargement NOS

523.9   *Unspecified*

524   Dentofacial anomalies, including malocclusion

524.0 *Major anomalies of jaw size*

Hyperplasia, hypoplasia:
  mandibular
  maxillary

Macrognathism (mandibular)
  (maxillary)
Micrognathism (mandibular)
  (maxillary)

Excludes: hemifacial atrophy or hypertrophy (754.0)
  unilateral condylar hyperplasia (526.8)

524.1 *Anomalies of relationship of jaw to cranial base*

Asymmetry of jaw
Prognathism (mandibular)
  (maxillary)

Retrognathism (mandibular)
  (maxillary)

524.2 *Anomalies of dental arch relationship*

Crossbite (anterior) (posterior)
Disto-occlusion
Mesio-occlusion
Midline deviation
Openbite (anterior) (posterior)
Overbite (excessive)
  deep
  horizontal
  vertical

Overjet
Posterior lingual occlusion of
  mandibular teeth
Soft tissue impingement

Excludes: hemifacial atrophy or hypertrophy (754.0)
  unilateral condylar hyperplasia (526.8)

524.3 *Anomalies of tooth position*

Crowding ⎫
Diastema ⎬ of tooth, teeth
Displacement ⎭

Rotation ⎫
Spacing, abnormal ⎬ of tooth,
Transposition ⎭   teeth

Impacted or embedded teeth with abnormal position of such teeth or
  adjacent teeth

524.4 *Malocclusion, unspecified*

524.5 *Dentofacial functional abnormalities*

Abnormal jaw closure
Malocclusion due to:
  abnormal swallowing
  tongue, lip or finger habits

Malocclusion due to mouth
  breathing

524.6 *Temporomandibular joint disorders*
Costen's complex or syndrome
Derangement of temporomandibular joint
Snapping jaw
Temporomandibular joint-pain-dysfunction syndrome
Excludes: current temporomandibular joint:
dislocation (830.–)
strain (848.1)

524.8 *Other dentofacial anomalies*

524.9 *Unspecified*

525 Other diseases and conditions of the teeth and supporting structures

525.0 *Exfoliation of teeth due to systemic causes*

525.1 *Loss of teeth due to accident, extraction or local periodontal disease*

525.2 *Atrophy of edentulous alveolar ridge*

525.3 *Retained dental root*

525.8 *Other*
Enlargement of alveolar ridge NOS   Irregular alveolar process

525.9 *Unspecified*

526 Diseases of the jaws

526.0 *Developmental odontogenic cysts*
Cyst:
  dentigerous
  eruption
  follicular
Cyst:
  lateral periodontal
  primordial
  Keratocyst
Excludes: radicular cyst (522.8)

526.1 *Fissural cysts of jaw*
Cyst:
  globulomaxillary
  incisor canal
  median palatal
Cyst:
  nasopalatine
  palatine of papilla

526.2 *Other cysts of jaws*
Cyst of jaw:
  NOS
  aneurysmal
Cyst of jaw:
  haemorrhagic
  traumatic

526.3 *Central giant cell (reparative) granuloma*
Excludes: peripheral giant cell granuloma (523.8)

526.4 *Inflammatory conditions*

Osteitis
Osteomyelitis (neonatal) } of jaw (acute) (chronic) (suppurative)
Periostitis
Sequestrum of jaw bone

526.5 *Alveolitis of jaw*

Alveolar osteitis Dry socket

526.8 *Other diseases of the jaws*

Cherubism
Exostosis of jaw
Fibrous dysplasia of jaws
Latent bone cyst of jaw
Osteoradionecrosis of jaw

Torus:
  mandibularis
  palatinus
Unilateral condylar hyperplasia or
  hypoplasia of mandible

526.9 *Unspecified*

527 Diseases of the salivary glands

527.0 *Atrophy*

527.1 *Hypertrophy*

527.2 *Sialoadenitis*

Excludes: epidemic parotitis (072.9)
         uveoparotid fever (135)

527.3 *Abscess*

527.4 *Fistula*

Excludes: congenital fistula of salivary gland (750.2)

527.5 *Sialolithiasis*

Calculus } of salivary gland or duct
Stone

527.6 *Mucocele*

Mucous: Ranula
  extravasation cyst of salivary gland
  retention cyst of salivary gland

527.7 *Disturbance of salivary secretion*

Hyposecretion Xerostomia
Ptyalism

527.8 *Other*

Benign lymphoepithelial lesion of
  salivary gland
Sialectasia

Sialosis
Stenosis } of salivary duct
Stricture

527.9   *Unspecified*

528   Diseases of the oral soft tissues, excluding lesions specific for gingiva and tongue

528.0   *Stomatitis*

Stomatitis: Stomatitis, vesicular
   NOS
   ulcerative

Excludes: stomatitis:
              aphthous (528.2)
              acute necrotizing ulcerative (101)
              gangrenous (528.1)
              herpetic (054.2)

528.1   *Cancrum oris*

Gangrenous stomatitis   Noma

528.2   *Oral aphthae*

Aphthous stomatitis   Recurrent aphthous ulcer
Periadenitis mucosa necrotica   Stomatitis herpetiformis
   recurrens

528.3   *Cellulitis and abscess*

Cellulitis of mouth (floor)

528.4   *Cysts*

Dermoid cyst   ⎫   Nasoalveolar cyst ⎫
Epidermoid cyst   ⎬ of mouth   Nasolabial cyst   ⎬ of mouth
Epstein's pearl   ⎪   Palatal papilla cyst ⎭
Lymphoepithelial cyst ⎭

528.5   *Diseases of lips*

Cheilitis: Cheilodynia
   NOS   Cheilosis
   angular

Excludes: actinic cheilitis (692.8)

528.6   *Leukoplakia of oral mucosa, including tongue*
Excludes: leukokeratosis nicotina palati (528.7)

528.7   *Other disturbances of oral epithelium, including tongue*

Erythroplakia   ⎫ of mouth or   Leukoedema of mouth or tongue
Focal epithelial   ⎬ tongue   Leukokeratosis nicotina palati
   hyperplasia   ⎭

Excludes: white sponge naevus (750.2)

528.8   *Oral submucous fibrosis, including of tongue*

528.9 *Other and unspecified*

Cheek and lip biting
Denture sore mouth
Denture stomatitis
Melanoplakia
Papillary hyperplasia of palate

Eosinophilic granuloma ⎱
Irritative hyperplasia   of oral
Pyogenic granuloma   mu-
Ulcer (traumatic) ⎰   cosa

529   Diseases and other conditions of the tongue

529.0 *Glossitis*

Abscess ⎱
Ulceration (traumatic) ⎰ of tongue

529.1 *Geographic tongue*

Glossitis areata exfoliativa   Benign migratory glossitis

529.2 *Median rhomboid glossitis*

529.3 *Hypertrophy of tongue papillae*

Black hairy tongue
Coated tongue

Hypertrophy of foliate papillae
Lingua villosa nigra

529.4 *Atrophy of tongue papillae*

529.5 *Plicated tongue*

Fissured ⎱
Furrowed ⎰ tongue
Scrotal

Excludes: fissure of tongue, congenital (750.1)

529.6 *Glossodynia*

Glossopyrosis   Painful tongue

529.8 *Other conditions of the tongue*

Atrophy ⎱
Crenated ⎰ (of) tongue

Enlargement ⎱
Hypertrophy ⎰ of tongue

Excludes: congenital macroglossia (750.1)

529.9 *Unspecified*

DISEASES OF OESOPHAGUS, STOMACH AND DUODENUM (530-537)

530   Diseases of oesophagus

Excludes: oesophageal varices (456.0, 456.1)

530.0 *Achalasia and cardiospasm*

Achalasia (of cardia)
Excludes: congenital cardiospasm (750.7)

530.1   *Oesophagitis*

Abscess of oesophagus
Oesophagitis:
  NOS
  chemical
  peptic

Oesophagitis:
  postoperative
  reflux
  tuberculous* (017.8†)
Oesophageal reflux

Use additional E code, if desired, to identify cause, if induced by chemical

530.2   *Ulcer of oesophagus*

Ulcer of oesophagus
  fungal
  peptic

Ulcer of oesophagus due to ingestion of:
  aspirin
  chemicals
  medicaments

Use additional E code, if desired, to identify cause, if induced by chemical
  or drug

530.3   *Stricture and stenosis of oesophagus*

Compression of oesophagus   Obstruction of oesophagus

Excludes: congenital stricture of oesophagus (750.3)

530.4   *Perforation of oesophagus*

Rupture of oesophagus

Excludes: traumatic perforation of oesophagus (862.–, 874.4)

530.5   *Dyskinesia of oesophagus*

Corkscrew oesophagus   Spasm of oesophagus
Diffuse oesophageal spasm

Excludes: cardiospasm (530.0)

530.6   *Diverticulum of oesophagus, acquired*

Oesophageal pouch, acquired

Excludes: congenital diverticulum of oesophagus (750.4)

530.7   *Gastro-oesophageal laceration-haemorrhage syndrome*

Mallory-Weiss syndrome

530.8   *Other disorders of oesophagus*

Haemorrhage of oesophagus

530.9   *Unspecified*

The following fourth-digit subdivisions are for use with categories
  531-534:
  .0   Acute with haemorrhage
  .1   Acute with perforation
  .2   Acute with haemorrhage and perforation

.3 Acute without mention of haemorrhage or perforation
.4 Chronic or unspecified with haemorrhage
.5 Chronic or unspecified with perforation
.6 Chronic or unspecified with haemorrhage and perforation
.7 Chronic without mention of haemorrhage or perforation
.9 Unspecified as acute or chronic, without mention of haemorrhage or perforation

531 Gastric ulcer

[See page 310 for fourth-digit subdivisions]

Includes: erosion (acute) of stomach
ulcer (peptic):
pylorus
stomach

Excludes: peptic ulcer NOS (533.–)

Use additional E code, if desired, to identify drug, if drug-induced

532 Duodenal ulcer

[See page 310 for fourth-digit subdivisions]

Includes: erosion (acute) of duodenum
ulcer (peptic):
duodenum
postpyloric

Excludes: peptic ulcer NOS (533.–)

Use additional E code, if desired, to identify drug, if drug-induced

533 Peptic ulcer, site unspecified

[See page 310 for fourth-digit subdivisions]

Includes: gastroduodenal ulcer NOS
peptic ulcer NOS

534 Gastrojejunal ulcer

[See page 310 for fourth-digit subdivisions]

Includes: ulcer (peptic) or erosion:
anastomotic
gastrocolic
gastrointestinal
gastrojejunal
jejunal
marginal
stomal

Excludes: primary ulcer of small intestine (569.8)

535   Gastritis and duodenitis

535.0   *Acute gastritis*

Use additional code, if desired, to identify any associated haemorrhage (578.–)

535.1   *Atrophic gastritis*

Chronic (atrophic) gastritis

535.2   *Gastric mucosal hypertrophy*

535.3   *Alcoholic gastritis*

535.4   *Other gastritis*

Superficial gastritis

535.5   *Unspecified gastritis and gastroduodenitis*

535.6   *Duodenitis*

536   Disorders of function of stomach

Excludes: functional disorders of stomach specified as psychogenic (306.4)

536.0   *Achlorhydria*

536.1   *Acute dilatation of stomach*

Acute distention of stomach

536.2   *Habit vomiting*

Persistent vomiting [not of pregnancy]

Excludes: excessive vomiting in pregnancy (643.–)

536.8   *Dyspepsia and other disorders of function of stomach*

Achylia gastrica   Hyperchlorhydria
Hourglass contraction of stomach   Hypochlorhydria
Hyperacidity   Indigestion

536.9   *Unspecified*

Functional gastrointestinal: Functional gastrointestinal
  disorder   irritation
  disturbance

537   Other disorders of stomach and duodenum

537.0   *Adult hypertrophic pyloric stenosis*

Excludes: congenital or infantile pyloric stenosis (750.5)

537.1 *Gastric diverticulum*

Excludes: congenital diverticulum of stomach (750.7)

537.2 *Chronic duodenal ileus*

537.3 *Other obstruction of duodenum*

537.4 *Fistula of stomach or duodenum*

Gastrocolic fistula   Gastrojejunocolic fistula

537.5 *Gastroptosis*

537.6 *Hourglass stricture or stenosis of stomach*

Excludes: congenital hourglass stomach (750.7)
          hourglass contraction of stomach (536.8)

537.8 *Other*

Intestinal metaplasia of gastric mucosa

Excludes: diverticula of duodenum (562.0)
          gastrointestinal haemorrhage (578.–)

537.9 *Unspecified*

APPENDICITIS (540-543)

540   Acute appendicitis

540.0 *With generalized peritonitis*

Appendicitis (acute) ⎤ with:
Caecitis (acute)   ⎬   perforation
                     ⎭   peritonitis (generalized)
                           rupture
Rupture of appendix

540.1 *With peritoneal abscess*

Abscess, appendix

540.9 *Without mention of peritonitis*

Acute: ⎤
  appendicitis   ⎬ without mention of perforation, peritonitis or rupture
  caecitis   ⎦

541   Appendicitis, unqualified

542   Other appendicitis

Chronic appendicitis   Recurrent appendicitis

543   Other diseases of appendix

Appendicular or appendiceal: Diverticulum ⎫
   colic   Hyperplasia ⎪
   concretion   Intussusception ⎬ of appendix
   fistula   Mucocele ⎪
                            Stercolith ⎭

HERNIA OF ABDOMINAL CAVITY (550-553)

Includes: hernia: hernia:
          acquired   recurrent
          bilateral   unilateral
          congenital (except
             diaphragmatic or hiatal)

550   Inguinal hernia

Includes: bubonocele   inguinal hernia:
          inguinal hernia: indirect
             NOS   oblique
             direct   scrotal hernia
             double

550.0   *Inguinal hernia, with gangrene*

550.1   *Inguinal hernia, with obstruction, without mention of gangrene*

Inguinal hernia with mention of incarceration, irreducibility or strangulation

550.9   *Inguinal hernia, without mention of obstruction or gangrene*

551   Other hernia of abdominal cavity, with gangrene

551.0   *Femoral, with gangrene*

551.1   *Umbilical, with gangrene*

Umbilical hernia as defined in 553.1 if specified as gangrenous

551.2   *Ventral [incisional], with gangrene*

Ventral hernia as defined in 553.2 if specified as gangrenous

551.3   *Diaphragmatic, with gangrene*

Diaphragmatic hernia as defined in 553.3 if specified as gangrenous

551.8   *Of other specified sites, with gangrene*

Any condition in 553.8 if specified as gangrenous

551.9   *Of unspecified site, with gangrene*

Any condition in 553.9 if specified as gangrenous

552 Other hernia of abdominal cavity with obstruction, without mention of gangrene

Excludes: with mention of gangrene (551.–)

552.0 *Femoral, with obstruction*

Femoral hernia specified as incarcerated, irreducible, strangulated or causing obstruction

552.1 *Umbilical, with obstruction*

Umbilical hernia as defined in 553.1 if specified as incarcerated, irreducible, strangulated or causing obstruction

552.2 *Ventral [incisional], with obstruction*

Ventral hernia as defined in 553.2 if specified as incarcerated, irreducible, strangulated or causing obstruction

552.3 *Diaphragmatic, with obstruction*

Diaphragmatic hernia as defined in 553.3 if specified as incarcerated, irreducible, strangulated or causing obstruction

552.8 *Of other specified sites, with obstruction*

Any condition in 553.8 if specified as incarcerated, irreducible, strangulated or causing obstruction

552.9 *Of unspecified site, with obstruction*

Any condition in 553.9 if specified as incarcerated, irreducible, strangulated or causing obstruction

553 Other hernia of abdominal cavity without mention of obstruction or gangrene

Excludes: the listed conditions with mention of:
gangrene (551.–)
obstruction (552.–)

553.0 *Femoral*

553.1 *Umbilical*

Omphalocele   Paraumbilical hernia

553.2 *Ventral [incisional]*

Epigastric hernia

553.3 *Diaphragmatic*

Hiatal hernia (oesophageal) (sliding) Paraoesophageal hernia

Excludes: congenital hernia:
diaphragmatic (756.6)
hiatus (750.6)

553.8   *Of other specified sites*

Hernia:
  lumbar
  obturator
  pudendal

Hernia:
  retroperitoneal
  sciatic
Other abdominal hernia of
  specified site

Excludes: vaginal enterocele (618.6)

553.9   *Of unspecified site*

Enterocele
Epiplocele
Hernia:
  NOS
  interstitial

Hernia:
  intestinal
  intra-abdominal
Rupture (nontraumatic)
Sarcoepiplocele

NONINFECTIVE ENTERITIS AND COLITIS (555-558)

555   Regional enteritis

Includes: Crohn's disease

555.0   *Small intestine*

Ileitis:
  regional
  terminal

Regional enteritis or Crohn's
  disease of:
  duodenum
  ileum
  jejunum

555.1   *Large intestine*

Colitis:
  granulomatous
  regional

Regional enteritis or Crohn's
  disease of:
  colon
  large bowel
  large intestine
  rectum

555.2   *Small intestine with large intestine*

555.9   *Unspecified site*

Crohn's disease NOS

Regional enteritis NOS

556   Idiopathic proctocolitis

Pseudopolyposis of colon
Toxic megacolon
Ulcerative (chronic):
  colitis
  enteritis

Ulcerative (chronic):
  enterocolitis
  ileocolitis
  proctitis
  rectosigmoiditis

557   Vascular insufficiency of intestine

Excludes: necrotizing enterocolitis of the newborn (777.5)

557.0   *Acute*

Acute:
  haemorrhagic enterocolitis
  ischaemic colitis, enteritis or
    enterocolitis
  massive necrosis of intestine
Embolism of mesenteric artery
Fulminant enterocolitis
Haemorrhagic necrosis of
  intestine
Intestinal gangrene

Intestinal infarction
  acute
  agnogenic
  haemorrhagic
  nonocclusive
Mesenteric infarction
  embolic
  thrombotic
Terminal haemorrhagic
  enteropathy
Thrombosis of mesenteric artery

557.1   *Chronic*

Chronic ischaemic colitis, enteritis or enterocolitis
Ischaemic stricture of intestine
Mesenteric:
  angina
  artery syndrome (superior)
  vascular insufficiency

557.9   *Unspecified*

Alimentary pain due to vascular insufficiency
Ischaemic colitis, enteritis or enterocolitis NOS

558   Other noninfective gastroenteritis and colitis

Colitis
Diarrhoea
Enteritis
Enterocolitis   specified as allergic, dietetic, noninfectious
Gastroenteritis   or toxic
Ileitis   unspecified, in countries where the conditions can be
Jejunitis   presumed to be of noninfectious origin
Sigmoiditis

Excludes: colitis, diarrhoea, enteritis, gastroenteritis:
        infectious (009.0, 009.2)
        unspecified, in countries where presumed to be of infectious
          origin (009.1, 009.3)
      functional diarrhoea (564.5)
      psychogenic diarrhoea (306.4)

OTHER DISEASES OF INTESTINES AND PERITONEUM (560-569)

560   Intestinal obstruction without mention of hernia

Excludes: inguinal hernia with obstruction (550.1)
             intestinal obstruction complicating hernia (552.–)
             mesenteric:
                 embolism (557.0)
                 infarction (557.0)
                 thrombosis (557.0)
             neonatal intestinal obstruction (777.–)

560.0   *Intussusception*

Intussusception (intestine) (colon) (rectum)
Invagination of intestine or colon

Excludes: intussusception of appendix (543)

560.1   *Paralytic ileus*

Ileus (of intestine) (of bowel) (of colon)
Paralysis of intestine or colon

560.2   *Volvulus*

Strangulation ⎫
Torsion   ⎬ of intestine, bowel or colon
Twist   ⎭

560.3   *Impaction of intestine*

Enterolith   Impaction of colon
Faecal impaction   Obstruction of intestine by
                                        gallstone

560.8   *Other intestinal obstruction*

Intestinal adhesions with obstruction

560.9   *Unspecified intestinal obstruction*

Enterostenosis
Obstruction ⎫
Occlusion   ⎪
Stenosis   ⎬ of intestine or colon
Stricture   ⎭

Excludes: congenital stricture or stenosis of intestine (751.1, 751.2)
             ischaemic stricture of intestine (557.1)
             postoperative intestinal obstruction NOS (997.4)

562   Diverticula of intestine

Excludes: congenital diverticulum of colon (751.5)
             Meckel's diverticulum (751.0)

562.0   *Small intestine*

Diverticulitis, diverticulosis:
  duodenum
  jejunum

562.1   *Colon*

Diverticular disease, diverticulitis, diverticulosis:
  NOS
  colon
  large intestine

Use additional code, if desired, to identify any associated haemorrhage
  (578.–) or peritonitis (567.–)

564   Functional digestive disorders, not elsewhere classified

Excludes: functional disorders of stomach (536.–)
            when specified as psychogenic (306.4)

564.0   *Constipation*

564.1   *Irritable colon*

Enterospasm   Mucous colitis
Irritable bowel syndrome   Spastic colon

564.2   *Postgastric surgery syndromes*

Dumping syndrome   Postvagotomy syndrome
Postgastrectomy syndrome

Excludes: postgastrojejunostomy ulcer (534.–)

564.3   *Vomiting following gastrointestinal surgery*

Vomiting (bilious) following gastrointestinal surgery

564.4   *Other postoperative functional disorders*

Diarrhoea following gastrointestinal surgery

564.5   *Functional diarrhoea*

Excludes: psychogenic diarrhoea (306.4)

564.6   *Anal spasm*

Proctalgia fugax

564.7   *Megacolon, other than Hirschsprung's*

Dilatation of colon

Excludes: megacolon:
              congenital (751.3)
              toxic (556)

564.8   *Other functional disorders of intestine*
Atony of colon
Excludes: malabsorption (579.–)

564.9   *Unspecified*

565   Anal fissure and fistula

565.0   *Anal fissure*
Tear of anus, nontraumatic

565.1   *Anal fistula*
Fistula of rectum to skin

566   Abscess of anal and rectal regions
Cellulitis of anus or rectum   Perianal abscess
Ischiorectal abscess or fistula   Perirectal abscess or cellulitis

567   Peritonitis
Excludes: peritonitis:
                     benign paroxysmal (277.3)
                     chronic proliferative (567.8)
                     pelvic, female (614.5, 614.7)
                     periodic familial (277.3)
                     puerperal (670)
                     with or following:
                        abortion (634–638 with fourth digit .0, 639.0)
                        appendicitis (540.0, 540.1)
                        ectopic or molar pregnancy (639.0)

567.0*   *Peritonitis in infectious diseases classified elsewhere*
Peritonitis:
    gonococcal (098.8†)
    syphilitic (095†)
    tuberculous (014†)

567.1   *Pneumococcal peritonitis*

567.2   *Other suppurative peritonitis*
Abscess (of):   Peritonitis (acute):
    abdominopelvic   general
    mesenteric   pelvic, male
    omentum   subphrenic
    peritoneum   suppurative
    retrocaecal
    retroperitoneal
    subdiaphragmatic
    subhepatic
    subphrenic

567.8 *Other peritonitis*

Chronic proliferative peritonitis
Fat necrosis of peritoneum
Mesenteric saponification

Peritonitis due to:
  bile
  urine

Excludes: peritonitis (postoperative):
      chemical (998.7)
      due to talc (998.7)

567.9 *Unspecified*

Peritonitis:
  NOS
  of unspecified cause

568   Other disorders of peritoneum

568.0 *Peritoneal adhesions*

Adhesions (of):
  abdominal (wall)
  diaphragm
  intestine
  male pelvis

Adhesions (of):
  mesenteric
  omentum
  stomach
Adhesive bands

Excludes: adhesions:
      female pelvis (614.6)
      with intestinal obstruction (560.8)

568.8 *Other*

568.9 *Unspecified*

569   Other disorders of intestine

569.0 *Anal and rectal polyp*

569.1 *Rectal prolapse*

Prolapse:
  anal canal
  rectal mucosa

569.2 *Stenosis of rectum and anus*

Stricture of anus (sphincter)

569.3 *Haemorrhage of rectum and anus*

569.4   *Other disorders of rectum and anus*

Solitary ulcer ⎫
Stercoral ulcer ⎭ of anus (sphincter) or rectum (sphincter)

Excludes: fistula of rectum to:
                    skin (565.1)
                    internal organs – see Alphabetical Index
                    haemorrhoids (455.–)
                    incontinence of sphincter ani (787.6)

569.5   *Abscess of intestine*

Excludes: appendiceal abscess (540.9)

569.6   *Colostomy or enterostomy malfunction*

569.8   *Other*

Pericolitis   Ulcer of colon
Perisigmoiditis   Visceroptosis

Excludes: gangrene of intestine, mesentery or omentum (557.0)
                    haemorrhage of intestine NOS (578.9)

569.9   *Unspecified*

OTHER DISEASES OF DIGESTIVE SYSTEM (570-579)

570   Acute and subacute necrosis of liver

Acute hepatic failure
Acute or subacute hepatitis, not specified as infective
Necrosis of liver (acute) (subacute) (diffuse) (massive)
Yellow atrophy (liver) (acute) (subacute)

Excludes: the listed conditions complicating:
                    abortion (634-638 with fourth digit .7, 639.8)
                    ectopic or molar pregnancy (639.8)
                    pregnancy, childbirth or the puerperium (646.7)
                    icterus gravis of newborn (773.–)
                    postoperative (997.4)
                    serum hepatitis (070.–, E875.–)
                    viral hepatitis (070.–)

571   Chronic liver disease and cirrhosis

571.0   *Alcoholic fatty liver*

571.1   *Acute alcoholic hepatitis*

571.2   *Alcoholic cirrhosis of liver*

Laënnec's cirrhosis

571.3   *Alcoholic liver damage, unspecified*

571.4 *Chronic hepatitis*

Chronic hepatitis:
  NOS
  active

Chronic hepatitis:
  aggressive
  persistent
Recurrent hepatitis

571.5 *Cirrhosis of liver without mention of alcohol*

Cirrhosis of liver:
  NOS
  cryptogenic
  macronodular

Cirrhosis of liver:
  micronodular
  postnecrotic
Portal cirrhosis

571.6 *Biliary cirrhosis*

Chronic nonsuppurative destructive cholangitis

571.8 *Other chronic nonalcoholic liver disease*

Chronic yellow atrophy (liver)
Fatty liver, without mention of alcohol

571.9 *Unspecified chronic liver disease without mention of alcohol*

572 Liver abscess and sequelae of chronic liver disease

572.0 *Abscess of liver*

Excludes: amoebic liver abscess (006.3)

572.1 *Portal pyaemia*

Phlebitis of portal vein   Pylephlebitis

572.2 *Hepatic coma*

Portosystemic encephalopathy

572.3 *Portal hypertension*

572.4 *Hepatorenal syndrome*

Excludes: postoperative (997.4)

572.8 *Other sequelae of chronic liver disease*

573 Other disorders of liver

Excludes: amyloid or lardaceous degeneration of liver (277.3)
           congenital cystic disease of liver (751.6)
           glycogen infiltration of liver (271.0)
           hepatomegaly NOS (789.1)
           portal vein obstruction (452)

573.0 *Chronic passive congestion of liver*

573.1* *Hepatitis in viral diseases classified elsewhere*

Hepatitis (in):　　　　　　　　　　Viral hepatitis (070.–†)
  Coxsackie (074.8†)
  cytomegalic inclusion virus (078.5†)
  infectious mononucleosis (075†)
  mumps (072.7†)
  yellow fever (060.–†)

573.2* *Hepatitis in other infectious diseases classified elsewhere*

Hepatitis in:　　　　　　　　　　　Hepatitis in toxoplasmosis (130†)
  malaria (084.9†)
  syphilis:
    late (095†)
    secondary (091.6†)

573.3　*Hepatitis unspecified*

Toxic (noninfectious) hepatitis

573.4　*Hepatic infarction*

573.8　*Other*

Hepatoptosis

573.9　*Unspecified*

574　　Cholelithiasis

574.0　*Calculus of gallbladder with acute cholecystitis*

Any condition listed in 574.2 with acute cholecystitis

574.1　*Calculus of gallbladder with other cholecystitis*

Cholecystitis with cholelithiasis NOS
Any condition listed in 574.2 with cholecystitis (chronic)

574.2　*Calculus of gallbladder without mention of cholecystitis*

Biliary:　　　　　　　　　　　Cholelithiasis NOS
  calculus NOS　　　　　　　　Colic (recurrent) of gallbladder
  colic NOS　　　　　　　　　Gallstone (impacted)
Calculus of cystic duct

574.3　*Calculus of bile duct with acute cholecystitis*

Any condition listed in 574.5 with acute cholecystitis

574.4　*Calculus of bile duct with other cholecystitis*

Any condition listed in 574.5 with cholecystitis (chronic)

574.5 *Calculus of bile duct without mention of cholecystitis*

Calculus of:
  bile duct [any]
  common duct
  hepatic duct

Choledocholithiasis
Hepatic:
  colic (recurrent)
  lithiasis

575   Other disorders of gallbladder

575.0 *Acute cholecystitis*

Abscess of gallbladder
Angiocholecystitis
Cholecystitis:
  emphysematous (acute)
  gangrenous
  suppurative
Empyema of gallbladder
Gangrene of gallbladder
} without mention of calculus

Excludes: with cholelithiasis (574.–)

575.1 *Other cholecystitis*

Cholecystitis:
  NOS
  chronic
} without mention of calculus

Excludes: with cholelithiasis (574.–)

575.2 *Obstruction of gallbladder*

Occlusion
Stenosis
Stricture
} of cystic duct or gallbladder without mention of calculus

Excludes: with cholelithiasis (574.–)

575.3 *Hydrops of gallbladder*

Mucocele of gallbladder

575.4 *Perforation of gallbladder*

Rupture of cystic duct or gallbladder

575.5 *Fistula of gallbladder*

Cholecystoduodenal fistula

575.6 *Cholesterolosis of gallbladder*

Strawberry gallbladder

575.8 *Other*

Adhesions
Atrophy
Cyst   (of) { cystic duct
Hypertrophy   gallbladder
Nonfunctioning
Ulcer

Biliary dyskinesia

Excludes: nonvisualization of gallbladder (793.3)

575.9 *Unspecified*

576   **Other disorders of biliary tract**

Excludes: the listed conditions involving the:
          cystic duct (575.–)
          gallbladder (575.–)

576.0 *Postcholecystectomy syndrome*

576.1 *Cholangitis*

Cholangitis:
  NOS
  ascending
  primary
  recurrent

Cholangitis:
  sclerosing
  secondary
  stenosing
  suppurative

576.2 *Obstruction of bile duct*

Occlusion
Stenosis } of bile duct [any] without mention of calculus
Stricture

Excludes: with cholelithiasis (574.–)

576.3 *Perforation of bile duct*

Rupture of [any] bile duct

576.4 *Fistula of bile duct*

Choledochoduodenal fistula

576.5 *Spasm of sphincter of Oddi*

576.8 *Other*

Adhesions
Atrophy } of [any] bile duct
Cyst

Hypertrophy } of [any] bile duct
Ulcer

576.9 *Unspecified*

577   Diseases of pancreas

577.0   *Acute pancreatitis*

Abscess of pancreas
Mumps pancreatitis* (072.3†)
Necrosis of pancreas:
　acute
　infective

Pancreatitis:
　NOS
　acute (recurrent)
　haemorrhagic
　subacute
　suppurative

577.1   *Chronic pancreatitis*

Chronic pancreatitis:
　NOS
　infectious

Pancreatitis:
　recurrent
　relapsing

577.2   *Cyst and pseudocyst of pancreas*

577.8   *Other diseases of pancreas*

Atrophy ⎤
Calculus ⎥ of pancreas
Cirrhosis ⎥
Fibrosis ⎦

Pancreatic:
　infantilism
　necrosis:
　　NOS
　　aseptic
　　fat

Excludes: fibrocystic disease of pancreas (277.0)
　　　　　　 islet cell tumour of pancreas (211.7)
　　　　　　 pancreatic steatorrhoea (579.4)

577.9   *Unspecified*

578   Gastrointestinal haemorrhage

Excludes: with mention of duodenal, gastric, gastrojejunal or peptic
　　　　　　 ulcer (531-534)

578.0   *Haematemesis*

578.1   *Melaena*

Excludes: melaena of the newborn (772.4, 777.3)

578.9   *Haemorrhage of gastrointestinal tract, unspecified*

Gastric haemorrhage   Intestinal haemorrhage

579   Intestinal malabsorption

579.0   *Coeliac disease*

Gluten enteropathy   Nontropical sprue
Idiopathic steatorrhoea

579.1 *Tropical sprue*

Sprue: Tropical steatorrhoea
  NOS
  tropical

579.2 *Blind loop syndrome*

Postoperative blind loop syndrome

579.3 *Other and unspecified postsurgical nonabsorption*

Hypoglycaemia ⎤
Malnutrition ⎦ following gastrointestinal surgery

579.4 *Pancreatic steatorrhoea*

579.8 *Other*

579.9 *Unspecified*

X. DISEASES OF THE GENITOURINARY SYSTEM

NEPHRITIS, NEPHROTIC SYNDROME AND NEPHROSIS (580-589)

Excludes: hypertensive renal disease (403.–)

Note: The fourth-digit subdivisions which indicate the pathological lesion in categories 580-584 have been standardized, but they do not all apply to each three-digit category.

580 Acute glomerulonephritis

Includes: acute nephritis

580.0 *With lesion of proliferative glomerulonephritis*
Acute (diffuse) proliferative glomerulonephritis

580.4 *With lesion of rapidly progressive glomerulonephritis*
Acute nephritis with lesion of necrotizing glomerulitis

580.8 *With other specified pathological lesion in kidney*

580.9 *Unspecified*

581 Nephrotic syndrome

581.0 *With lesion of proliferative glomerulonephritis*

581.1 *With lesion of membranous glomerulonephritis*
Idiopathic membranous glomerular disease

581.2 *With lesion of membranoproliferative glomerulonephritis*
Nephrotic syndrome with lesion of:
hypocomplementaemic persistent
lobular
mesangiocapillary
mixed membranous and proliferative
} glomerulonephritis

581.3 *With lesion of minimal change glomerulonephritis*

Lipoid nephrosis	Minimal change:
Minimal change:	glomerulitis
glomerular disease	nephrotic syndrome

581.8   *With other specified pathological lesion in kidney*

Haemorrhagic nephrosonephritis* (078.6†)
Nephrotic syndrome in:
  amyloidosis* (277.3†)
  diabetes mellitus* (250.3†)
  epidemic haemorrhagic fever* (078.6†)
  malaria* (084.9†)
  systemic lupus erythematosus* (710.0†)

581.9   *Unspecified*

Nephrosis NOS

582   **Chronic glomerulonephritis**

Includes: chronic nephritis

582.0   *With lesion of proliferative glomerulonephritis*

Chronic (diffuse) proliferative glomerulonephritis

582.1   *With lesion of membranous glomerulonephritis*

Chronic membranous glomerulonephritis

582.2   *With lesion of membranoproliferative glomerulonephritis*

Chronic glomerulonephritis:
  hypocomplementaemic persistent
  lobular
  membranoproliferative
  mesangiocapillary
  mixed membranous and proliferative

582.4   *With lesion of rapidly progressive glomerulonephritis*

Chronic nephritis with lesion of necrotizing glomerulitis

582.8   *With other specified pathological lesion in kidney*

Chronic nephritis in:
  amyloidosis* (277.3†)
  systemic lupus erythematosus* (710.0†)

582.9   *Unspecified*

583   **Nephritis and nephropathy, not specified as acute or chronic**

Includes: "renal disease" so described, not specified as acute or chronic
              but with stated pathology or cause

583.0   *With lesion of proliferative glomerulonephritis*
Proliferative: Proliferative nephropathy NOS
  glomerulonephritis NOS
  nephritis NOS

583.1   *With lesion of membranous glomerulonephritis*
Membranous: Membranous nephropathy NOS
  glomerulonephritis NOS
  nephritis NOS

583.2   *With lesion of membranoproliferative glomerulonephritis*
Membranoproliferative:
  glomerulonephritis NOS
  nephritis NOS
  nephropathy NOS
Nephritis NOS, with lesion of:
  hypocomplementaemic persistent
  lobular
  mesangiocapillary   } glomerulonephritis
  mixed membranous and proliferative

583.4   *With lesion of rapidly progressive glomerulonephritis*
Necrotizing or rapidly progressive:
  glomerulitis NOS
  glomerulonephritis NOS
  nephritis NOS
  nephropathy NOS
Nephritis, unspecified, with lesion of necrotizing glomerulitis

583.6   *With lesion of renal cortical necrosis*
Nephritis NOS   } with (renal) cortical necrosis
Nephropathy NOS }
Renal cortical necrosis NOS

583.7   *With lesion of renal medullary necrosis*
Nephritis NOS   } with (renal) medullary [papillary] necrosis
Nephropathy NOS }

583.8   *With other specified pathological lesion in kidney*
Glomerulitis   } with:
Glomerulonephritis | lesion of interstitial nephritis
Nephritis   } stated cause classified elsewhere:
Nephropathy | amyloidosis* (277.3†)
Renal disease   }   diabetes mellitus* (250.3†)
                    gonococcal infection* (098.1†)
                    gout* (274.1†)
                    systemic lupus erythematosus* (710.0†)
                    syphilis* (095†)
                    tuberculosis* (016.0†)

583.9   *With unspecified pathological lesion in kidney*
Glomerulitis ⎤
Glomerulonephritis ⎟ NOS
Nephritis ⎟
Nephropathy ⎦
Excludes: nephropathy complicating pregnancy, labour or the puer-
                  perium (642.–, 646.2)
              renal disease NOS with no stated cause (593.9)

584   Acute renal failure
Excludes: when complicating:
                  abortion (634-638 with fourth digit .3, 639.3)
                    ectopic or molar pregnancy (639.3)
                  following labour and delivery (669.3)
                  postoperative (997.5)

584.5   *With lesion of tubular necrosis*
Renal failure with (acute) tubular necrosis
Tubular necrosis:
  NOS
  acute

584.6   *With lesion of renal cortical necrosis*

584.7   *With lesion of renal medullary [papillary] necrosis*

584.8   *With other specified pathological lesion in kidney*

584.9   *Unspecified*

585   Chronic renal failure
Chronic uraemia
Uraemic:
  neuropathy† (357.4*)
  pericarditis† (420.0*)
Excludes: with any condition in 401.– (403.–)

586   Renal failure, unspecified
Uraemia NOS
Excludes: when complicating:
                  abortion (634-638 with fourth digit .3, 639.3)
                    ectopic or molar pregnancy (639.3)
                  following labour and delivery (669.3)
                  postoperative renal failure (997.5)
                  uraemia:
                    extrarenal (788.9)
                    prerenal (788.9)
                  with any condition in 401.– (403.–)

587   Renal sclerosis, unspecified

Atrophy of kidney   Contracted kidney

Excludes: nephrosclerosis (arteriolar) (arteriosclerotic) (403.–)
                     with hypertension (403.–)

588   Disorders resulting from impaired renal function

588.0   *Renal osteodystrophy*

Azotaemic osteodystrophy   Renal:
Phosphate-losing tubular disorders   dwarfism
                                                                    rickets

588.1   *Nephrogenic diabetes insipidus*

588.8   *Other*

Secondary hyperparathyroidism (of renal origin)

Excludes: secondary hypertension (405.–)

588.9   *Unspecified*

589   Small kidney of unknown cause

589.0   *Unilateral*

589.1   *Bilateral*

589.9   *Unspecified*

OTHER DISEASES OF URINARY SYSTEM (590-599)

Excludes: urinary infections (conditions in 590, 595, 597, 599.0)
                     complicating:
                     abortion (634-638 with fourth digit .7, 639.8)
                     ectopic or molar pregnancy (639.8)
                     pregnancy, childbirth and the puerperium (646.6)

590   Infections of kidney

Use additional code, if desired, to identify organism, such as Escherichia
     coli (041.4)

590.0   *Chronic pyelonephritis and chronic pyonephrosis*

590.1   *Acute pyelonephritis and acute pyonephrosis*

Acute pyelitis

590.2   *Renal and perinephric abscess*

590.3   *Pyeloureteritis cystica*

Infection of renal pelvis and ureter

590.8   *Pyelonephritis or pyonephrosis, not specified as acute or chronic*

Pyelitis: Pyelonephritis:
  NOS   NOS
  tuberculous* (016.0†)   tuberculous* (016.0†)

Excludes: calculous pyelonephritis (592.9)

590.9   *Infection of kidney, unspecified*

Excludes: urinary tract infection NOS (599.0)

591   Hydronephrosis

592   Calculus of kidney and ureter

Excludes: nephrocalcinosis (275.4)

592.0   *Calculus of kidney*

Nephrolithiasis: Staghorn calculus
  NOS   Stone in kidney
  uric acid* (274.1†)
Renal calculus or stone

592.1   *Calculus of ureter*

Ureteric stone

592.9   *Urinary calculus, unspecified*

Calculous pyelonephritis

593   Other disorders of kidney and ureter

593.0   *Nephroptosis*

Mobile kidney

593.1   *Hypertrophy of kidney*

593.2   *Cyst of kidney, acquired*

Cyst (multiple) (solitary) of kidney, not congenital

Excludes: congenital cyst of kidney (753.1)

593.3   *Stricture or kinking of ureter*

Stricture of pelviureteric junction

593.4   *Other ureteric obstruction*

593.5   *Hydroureter*

Excludes: congenital (753.2)

593.6   *Postural proteinuria*

593.7   *Vesicoureteric reflux*

593.8   *Other*

Intestinoureteric fistula   Tuberculosis of ureter* (016.1†)
Renal infarction

Excludes: fistula between ureter and female genital tract (619.0)

593.9   *Unspecified*

Renal disease NOS

Excludes: cystic kidney disease (753.1)
            nephropathy, so described (583.–)
            renal disease:
              acute (580.–)
              arising in pregnancy or the puerperium (642.–, 646.2)
              chronic (582.–)
              not specified as acute or chronic but with stated pathology
                or cause (583.–)

594   Calculus of lower urinary tract

594.0   *Calculus in diverticulum of bladder*

594.1   *Other calculus in bladder*

Urinary bladder stone

Excludes: staghorn calculus (592.0)

594.2   *Calculus in urethra*

594.8   *Other lower urinary tract calculus*

594.9   *Unspecified*

595   Cystitis

Excludes: prostatocystitis (601.3)

Use additional code, if desired, to identify organism, such as Escherichia
    coli (041.4)

595.0   *Acute cystitis*

Excludes: trigonitis (595.3)

595.1   *Chronic interstitial cystitis*

595.2   *Other chronic cystitis*

595.3   *Trigonitis*

Urethrotrigonitis

595.4* *Cystitis in diseases classified elsewhere*

Cystitis:
  gonococcal (098.1†)
  tuberculous (016.1†)

Ulceration of bladder:
  bilharzial (120.–†)

595.8 *Other*

Abscess of bladder   Irradiation cystitis

Use additional E code, if desired, to identify any external cause

595.9 *Unspecified*

596   **Other disorders of bladder**

596.0 *Bladder-neck obstruction*

Bladder-neck obstruction or stenosis (acquired)

596.1 *Intestinovesical fistula*

596.2 *Vesical fistula, not elsewhere classified*

Excludes: fistula between bladder and female genital tract (619.0)

596.3 *Diverticulum of bladder*

Diverticulitis of bladder

596.4 *Atony of bladder*

596.5 *Other functional disorders of bladder*

Relaxation of bladder sphincter

596.6 *Rupture of bladder, nontraumatic*

596.7 *Haemorrhage into bladder wall*

Hyperaemia of bladder

596.8 *Other*

Bladder:
  calcified
  contracted

Excludes: cystocele, female (618.–)
          hernia or prolapse of bladder, female (618.–)

596.9 *Unspecified*

597   **Urethritis, not sexually transmitted, and urethral syndrome**

Excludes: nonspecific urethritis so stated (099.4)

597.0 *Urethral abscess*

Abscess of:
  Cowper's gland
  Littré's gland

Abscess (of):
  periurethral
  urethral (gland)

Excludes: urethral caruncle (599.3)

597.8 *Other urethritis*

Adenitis, Skene's gland
Cowperitis
Meatitis, urethral
Ulcer, urethra (meatus)

Urethral syndrome NOS
Urethritis:
  NOS
  nonvenereal
  trichomonal* (131.0†)

598   Urethral stricture

Includes: pinhole meatus
            stricture of urinary meatus

Excludes: congenital stricture of urethra and urinary meatus (753.6)

598.0 *Infective*

Stricture of urethra:
  associated with schistosomiasis* (120.–†)
  gonococcal* (098.2†)

598.1 *Traumatic*

Stricture of urethra:
  late effect of injury
  postobstetric

598.2 *Postoperative*

Postcatheterization

598.8 *Other*

598.9 *Unspecified*

599   Other disorders of urethra and urinary tract

599.0 *Urinary tract infection, site not specified*

Use additional code, if desired, to identify organism

599.1 *Urethral fistula*

Fistula:
  urethroperineal
  urethrorectal

Urinary fistula NOS

Excludes: fistula:
            urethroscrotal (608.8)
            urethrovaginal (619.0)

599.2   *Urethral diverticulum*

599.3   *Urethral caruncle*

599.4   *Urethral false passage*

599.5   *Prolapsed urethral mucosa*

Prolapse of urethra   Urethrocele, male

Excludes: urethrocele, female (618.–)

599.6   *Urinary obstruction, unspecified*

Urinary (tract) obstruction NOS

599.7   *Haematuria*

599.8   *Other*

599.9   *Unspecified*

DISEASES OF MALE GENITAL ORGANS (600-608)

600   Hyperplasia of prostate

Adenofibromatous hypertrophy of   Fibroadenoma of prostate
   prostate   Hypertrophy of prostate (benign)
Adenoma (benign) of prostate   Median bar (prostate)
Enlargement of prostate (benign)   Myoma of prostate
Fibroma of prostate   Prostatic obstruction NOS

Excludes: benign neoplasms of prostate (222.2)

601   Inflammatory diseases of prostate

Use additional code, if desired, to identify infectious organism

601.0   *Acute prostatitis*

601.1   *Chronic prostatitis*

601.2   *Abscess of prostate*

601.3   *Prostatocystitis*

601.4*   *Prostatitis in diseases classified elsewhere*

Prostatitis:
  gonococcal (098.1†)
  trichomonal (131.0†)
  tuberculous (016.3†)

601.8   *Other*

601.9   *Unspecified*

Prostatitis NOS

602 Other disorders of prostate

602.0 *Calculus of prostate*

Prostatic stone

602.1 *Congestion or haemorrhage of prostate*

602.2 *Atrophy of prostate*

602.8 *Other*

602.9 *Unspecified*

603 Hydrocele

Includes: hydrocele of spermatic cord, testis or tunica vaginalis

Excludes: congenital (778.6)

603.0 *Encysted hydrocele*

603.1 *Infected hydrocele*

Use additional code, if desired, to identify organism

603.8 *Other*

603.9 *Unspecified*

604 Orchitis and epididymitis

Use additional code, if desired, to identify organism, such as Escherichia coli (041.4), Streptococcus (041.0) or Staphylococcus (041.1)

604.0 *Orchitis, epididymitis and epididymo-orchitis, with abscess*

Abscess of epididymis or testis

604.9 *Orchitis, epididymitis and epididymo-orchitis, without mention of abscess*

Orchitis:
  NOS
  gonococcal* (098.1†)

Mumps orchitis* (072.0†)
Tuberculous epididymitis*
  (016.2†)

605 Redundant prepuce and phimosis

Adherent prepuce
Paraphimosis

Phimosis (congenital)
Tight foreskin

606 Infertility, male

Azoospermia

Oligospermia

607   Disorders of penis

607.0   *Leukoplakia of penis*

Kraurosis of penis

Excludes: carcinoma in situ of penis (233.5)

607.1   *Balanoposthitis*

Balanitis

Use additional code, if desired, to identify organism

607.2   *Other inflammatory disorders of penis*

Abscess ⎤
Boil   ⎥
Carbuncle ⎬ of corpus cavernosum or penis
Cellulitis ⎦
Cavernitis (penis)

Use additional code, if desired, to identify organism

607.3   *Priapism*

Painful erection

607.8   *Other*

Atrophy ⎤   Balanitis xerotica obliterans
Fibrosis ⎥   Induratio penis plastica
Haematoma ⎬ of corpus cavernosum
Hypertrophy ⎥   or penis
Thrombosis ⎥
Ulcer ⎦

607.9   *Unspecified*

608   Other disorders of male genital organs

608.0   *Seminal vesiculitis*

Vesiculitis (seminal)

Use additional code, if desired, to identify organism

608.1   *Spermatocele*

608.2   *Torsion of testis*

Torsion of:
   epididymis
   spermatic cord
   testicle

608.3   *Atrophy of testis*

608.4 *Other inflammatory disorders of male genital organs*

Abscess
Boil
Carbuncle } of scrotum, spermatic cord, testis [except abscess], tunica
Cellulitis   vaginalis, or vas deferens
Vasitis

Use additional code, if desired, to identify organism

Excludes: abscess of testis (604.0)

608.8 *Other*

Atrophy
Fibrosis
Haematoma
Haemorrhage } of seminal vesicle, spermatic cord, testis [except atrophy],
Hypertrophy   scrotum, tunica vaginalis or vas deferens
Oedema
Thrombosis
Ulcer

Chylocele, tunica vaginalis: Tuberculosis of:
  NOS   seminal vesicle* (016.3†)
  filarial* (125.–†)   testis* (016.3†)
Haematocele NOS, male
Stricture of:
  spermatic cord
  tunica vaginalis
  vas deferens

608.9 *Unspecified*

DISORDERS OF BREAST (610-611)

610   Benign mammary dysplasias

610.0 *Solitary cyst of breast*

Cyst (solitary) of breast

610.1 *Diffuse cystic mastopathy*

Cystic breast

610.2 *Fibroadenosis of breast*

Fibroadenosis of breast: Fibroadenosis of breast:
  NOS   diffuse
  chronic   periodic
  cystic   segmental

610.3 *Fibrosclerosis of breast*

610.4 *Mammary duct ectasia*

Duct ectasia

610.8 *Other*

610.9 *Mammary dysplasia, unspecified*

611 Other disorders of breast

Excludes: when associated with lactation or the puerperium (675.–, 676.–)

611.0 *Inflammatory disease of breast*

Abscess (acute) (chronic) (nonpuerperal) of:
  areola
  breast
Antibioma of breast
Mammillary fistula
Mastitis (acute) (subacute) (nonpuerperal):
  NOS
  infective

Excludes: carbuncle of breast (680.2)
  neonatal infective mastitis (771.5)
  thrombophlebitis of breast, or Mondor's disease (451.8)

611.1 *Hypertrophy of breast*

Gynaecomastia

Hypertrophy of breast:
  NOS
  massive pubertal

611.2 *Fissure of nipple*

611.3 *Fat necrosis of breast*

Fat necrosis (segmental) of breast

611.4 *Atrophy of breast*

611.5 *Galactocele*

611.6 *Galactorrhoea not associated with childbirth*

611.7 *Signs and symptoms in breast*

Induration of breast
Lump in breast

Mastodynia
Nipple discharge
Retraction of nipple

611.8 *Other*

Subinvolution of breast (postlactational) (postpartum)

611.9 *Unspecified*

INFLAMMATORY DISEASE OF FEMALE PELVIC ORGANS (614-616)

Excludes: when associated with pregnancy, abortion, childbirth or the
           puerperium (630-676)

**614   Inflammatory disease of ovary, fallopian tube, pelvic cellular tissue
         and peritoneum**

Excludes: endometritis (615.–)
           major infection following delivery (670)
           when complicating:
             abortion (634-638 with fourth digit .0, 639.0)
             ectopic or molar pregnancy (639.0)
             pregnancy or labour (646.6)

614.0 *Acute salpingitis and oophoritis*

Any condition in 614.2 specified as acute or subacute

614.1 *Chronic salpingitis and oophoritis*

Any condition in 614.2 specified as chronic
Hydrosalpinx

614.2 *Salpingitis and oophoritis, not specified as acute, subacute or chronic*

Abscess (of):   Salpingitis and oophoritis:
  fallopian tube   gonococcal* (098.3†)
  ovary   tuberculous* (016.4†)
  tubo-ovarian   Salpingo-oophoritis
Oophoritis   Tubo-ovarian inflammatory
Pyosalpinx   disease
Salpingitis

Use additional code, if desired, to identify organism, such as Staphylo-
    coccus (041.1) or Streptococcus (041.0)

614.3 *Acute parametritis and pelvic cellulitis*

Any condition in 614.4, specified as acute

614.4 *Chronic or unspecified parametritis and pelvic cellulitis*

Abscess (of): ⎫
  broad ligament   ⎬ chronic or NOS
  pouch of Douglas ⎪
  parametrium   ⎭
Pelvic cellulitis, female

Use additional code, if desired, to identify organism, such as Staphylo-
    coccus (041.1) or Streptococcus (041.0)

614.5 *Acute or unspecified pelvic peritonitis, female*

614.6 *Pelvic peritoneal adhesions, female*

Infertility associated with peritubal adhesions† (628.2*)

614.7 *Other chronic pelvic peritonitis, female*

614.8 *Other specified inflammatory disease of female pelvic organs and tissues*

614.9 *Unspecified inflammatory disease of female pelvic organs and tissues*

Pelvic infection or inflammation, female, NOS

615 Inflammatory diseases of uterus, except cervix

Excludes: when complicating:
  abortion (634-638 with fourth digit .0, 639.0)
  ectopic or molar pregnancy (639.0)
  pregnancy or labour (646.6)
  following delivery (670)

615.0 *Acute*

Any condition in 615.9 specified as acute or subacute

615.1 *Chronic*

Any condition in 615.9 specified as chronic

615.9 *Unspecified*

Endometritis	Myometritis
gonococcal* (098.1†)	Perimetritis
Endomyometritis	Pyometra
Metritis	Uterine abscess

616 Inflammatory disease of cervix, vagina and vulva

Excludes: when complicating:
  abortion (634-638 with fourth digit .0, 639.0)
  ectopic or molar pregnancy (639.0)
  pregnancy, childbirth or the puerperium (646.6)

616.0 *Cervicitis and endocervicitis*

Cervicitis ⎫
Endocervicitis ⎬ with or without mention of erosion or ectropion

Gonococcal infection (acute) of cervix* (098.1†)

Excludes: erosion or ectropion of cervix without mention of cervicitis
  (622.0)

616.1 *Vaginitis and vulvovaginitis*

Vaginitis, vulvitis or vulvovaginitis:
  NOS
  herpetic* (054.1†)
  pinworm* (127.4†)
  trichomonal* (131.0†)
Vulvovaginal candidiasis* (112.1†)

Use additional code, if desired, to identify organism, such as Escherichia
  coli (041.4), Staphylococcus (041.1) or Streptococcus (041.0)

Excludes: noninfective leukorrhoea (623.5)
           postmenopausal or senile vaginitis (627.3)

616.2 *Cyst of Bartholin's gland*

616.3 *Abscess of Bartholin's gland*

616.4 *Other abscess of vulva*

Abscess }
Furuncle } of vulva

616.5 *Ulceration of vulva*

Ulceration of vulva:
  NOS
  in Behcet's syndrome* (136.1†)
  herpes simplex* (054.1†)

Excludes: gonococcal (098.0)
           syphilitic (091.0)
           tuberculous (016.4)

616.8 *Other*

Excludes: noninflammatory disorders of:
           cervix (622.–)
           vagina (623.–)
           vulva (624.–)

616.9 *Unspecified*

OTHER DISORDERS OF FEMALE GENITAL TRACT (617–629)

617   Endometriosis

617.0 *Uterus*
Adenomyosis

617.1 *Ovary*

617.2 *Fallopian tube*

617.3 *Pelvic peritoneum*

617.4 *Rectovaginal septum and vagina*

617.5 *Intestine*

617.6 *Endometriosis in scar or skin*

617.8 *Other specified sites*

617.9 *Site unspecified*

618   Genital prolapse

Excludes: when complicating pregnancy, labour or delivery (654.4)

618.0 *Prolapse of vaginal walls, without mention of uterine prolapse*

Cystocele ⎫
Rectocele ⎪
Urethrocele ⎬ without mention of uterine prolapse
Vaginal prolapse ⎭

618.1 *Uterine prolapse without mention of vaginal wall prolapse*

618.2 *Uterovaginal prolapse, incomplete*

618.3 *Uterovaginal prolapse, complete*

618.4 *Uterovaginal prolapse, unspecified*

618.5 *Prolapse of vaginal vault after hysterectomy*

618.6 *Vaginal enterocele, congenital or acquired*

618.7 *Old laceration of muscles of pelvic floor*

618.8 *Other*

Incompetence or weakening of pelvic fundus

618.9 *Unspecified*

619   Fistulae involving female genital tract

Excludes: vesicorectal and intestinovesical fistulae (596.–)

619.0 *Urinary - genital tract fistulae, female*

Fistula:
    cervicovesical
    ureterovaginal
    urethrovaginal

Fistula:
    uteroureteric
    uterovesical
    vesicovaginal

619.1 *Digestive - genital tract fistulae, female*

Fistula: Fistula, rectovaginal
  intestinouterine
  intestinovaginal

619.2 *Genital tract - skin fistulae, female*

Fistula, uterus to abdominal wall   Fistula, vaginoperineal

619.8 *Other*

619.9 *Unspecified fistula involving female genital tract*

620   Noninflammatory disorders of ovary, fallopian tube and broad ligament

Excludes: hydrosalpinx (614.1)

620.0 *Follicular cyst of ovary*

Cyst of graafian follicle

620.1 *Corpus luteum cyst or haematoma*

620.2 *Other and unspecified ovarian cyst*

Retention cyst of ovary NOS   Serous cyst of ovary

Excludes: developmental cysts (752.0)
           neoplastic cysts (220.–)
           polycystic ovaries (256.4)
           Stein-Leventhal syndrome (256.4)

620.3 *Acquired atrophy of ovary and fallopian tube*

620.4 *Prolapse or hernia of ovary and fallopian tube*

620.5 *Torsion of ovary, ovarian pedicle or fallopian tube*

Torsion:
  accessory tube
  hydatid of Morgagni

620.6 *Broad ligament laceration syndrome*

Masters-Allen syndrome

620.7 *Haematoma of broad ligament*

Haematosalpinx

Excludes: in ectopic pregnancy (639.2)

620.8 *Other*

620.9 *Unspecified*

621   Disorders of uterus, not elsewhere classified

621.0   *Polyp of corpus uteri*

Polyp:
  endometrium
  uterus NOS

621.1   *Chronic subinvolution of uterus*

Excludes: puerperal (674.8)

621.2   *Hypertrophy of uterus*

Bulky or enlarged uterus

Excludes: puerperal (674.8)

621.3   *Endometrial cystic hyperplasia*

Hyperplasia (cystic) (glandular) of endometrium

621.4   *Haematometra*

Excludes: in congenital anomaly (752.–)

621.5   *Intrauterine synechiae*

Adhesions of uterus   Band(s) of uterus

621.6   *Malposition of uterus*

Anteversion ⎫
Retroflexion ⎬ of uterus
Retroversion ⎭

Excludes: malposition complicating pregnancy, labour or delivery
            (654.3, 654.4)
            prolapse of uterus (618.–)

621.7   *Chronic inversion of uterus*

Excludes: current obstetrical trauma (665.2)
            prolapse of uterus (618.–)

621.8   *Other*

Atrophy of uterus, acquired   Fibrosis of uterus:
                                              NOS
                                              bilharzial* (120.–†)

Excludes: inflammatory diseases (615.–)
            endometriosis (617.0)

621.9   *Unspecified disorders of uterus*

622   Noninflammatory disorders of cervix

Excludes: abnormality of cervix complicating pregnancy, labour or
            delivery (654.5, 654.6)
            fistulae (619.–)

622.0 *Erosion and ectropion of cervix*
Eversion of cervix
Excludes: in chronic cervicitis (616.0)

622.1 *Dysplasia of cervix (uteri)*
Excludes: carcinoma in situ of cervix (233.1)

622.2 *Leukoplakia of cervix (uteri)*
Excludes: carcinoma in situ of cervix uteri (233.1)

622.3 *Old laceration of cervix*
Adhesions of cervix
Excludes: current obstetrical trauma (665.3)

622.4 *Stricture and stenosis of cervix*
Excludes: complicating labour (654.6)

622.5 *Incompetence of cervix*
Excludes: affecting fetus or newborn (761.0)
           complicating pregnancy (654.5)

622.6 *Hypertrophic elongation of cervix*

622.7 *Mucous polyp of cervix*
Polyp NOS of cervix
Excludes: adenomatous polyp of cervix (219.0)

622.8 *Other*
Excludes: inflammatory diseases (616.0)

622.9 *Unspecified*

623 Noninflammatory disorders of vagina
Excludes: abnormality of vagina complicating pregnancy, labour or
           delivery (654.7)
           congenital absence of vagina (752.4)
           congenital diaphragm or bands (752.4)
           fistulae involving vagina (619.–)

623.0 *Dysplasia of vagina*
Excludes: carcinoma in situ of vagina (233.3)

623.1 *Leukoplakia of vagina*

623.2 *Stricture or atresia of vagina*
Adhesions (postoperative) (postradiation) of vagina
Stenosis, vagina
Use additional E code, if desired, to identify any external cause

623.3 *Tight hymenal ring*

Rigid hymen
Tight hymenal ring ⎱ acquired or congenital
Tight introitus ⎰

Excludes: imperforate hymen (752.4)

623.4 *Old vaginal laceration*

Excludes: old laceration involving muscles of pelvic floor (618.7)

623.5 *Leukorrhoea, not specified as infective*

Excludes: trichomonal (131.0)

623.6 *Vaginal haematoma*

Excludes: current obstetrical trauma (665.7)

623.7 *Polyp of vagina*

623.8 *Other*

623.9 *Unspecified*

624 **Noninflammatory disorders of vulva and perineum**

Excludes: abnormality of vulva and perineum complicating pregnancy,
labour or delivery (654.8)
condyloma acuminatum (078.1)
fistulae involving:
perineum - see Alphabetical Index
vulva (619.–)
vulval involvement in skin conditions (690-709)

624.0 *Dystrophy of vulva*

Kraurosis ⎱ of vulva
Leukoplakia ⎰

Excludes: carcinoma in situ of vulva (233.3)

624.1 *Atrophy of vulva*

624.2 *Hypertrophy of clitoris*

Excludes: in endocrine disorders (255.2, 256.1)

624.3 *Hypertrophy of labia*

Hypertrophy of vulva NOS

624.4 *Old laceration or scarring of vulva*

624.5 *Haematoma of vulva*

Excludes: complication of delivery (664.5)

624.6 *Polyp of labia and vulva*

624.8 *Other*

624.9 *Unspecified*

625 Pain and other symptoms associated with female genital organs

625.0 *Dyspareunia*
Excludes: when associated with frigidity (302.7)

625.1 *Vaginismus*
Excludes: psychogenic vaginismus (306.5)

625.2 *Mittelschmerz*

625.3 *Dysmenorrhoea*
Excludes: psychogenic dysmenorrhoea (306.5)

625.4 *Premenstrual tension syndromes*
Menstrual migraine

625.5 *Pelvic congestion syndrome*

625.6 *Stress incontinence, female*

625.8 *Other*

625.9 *Unspecified*

626 Disorders of menstruation and other abnormal bleeding from female genital tract
Excludes: menopausal and premenopausal bleeding (627.0)
    pain and other symptoms associated with menstrual cycle
        (625.–)
    postmenopausal bleeding (627.1)

626.0 *Absence of menstruation*
Amenorrhoea (primary) (secondary)

626.1 *Scanty or infrequent menstruation*
Hypomenorrhoea   Oligomenorrhoea

626.2 *Excessive or frequent menstruation*
Heavy periods   Menorrhagia
Menometrorrhagia   Polymenorrhoea
Excludes: in puberty (626.3)
    premenopausal (627.0)

626.3 *Puberty bleeding*
Excessive bleeding associated with onset of menstrual periods
Puberal menorrhagia

626.4   *Irregular menstrual cycle*

Irregular:
  bleeding NOS
  menstruation
  periods

626.5   *Ovulation bleeding*

Regular intermenstrual bleeding

626.6   *Metrorrhagia*

Bleeding unrelated to menstrual cycle
Irregular intermenstrual bleeding

626.7   *Postcoital bleeding*

626.8   *Other*

Dysfunctional or functional uterine haemorrhage NOS

626.9   *Unspecified*

627   Menopausal and postmenopausal disorders

627.0   *Premenopausal menorrhagia*

Menorrhagia: Menorrhagia:
  climacteric   preclimacteric
  menopausal

627.1   *Postmenopausal bleeding*

627.2   *Menopausal or female climacteric states*

Symptoms such as flushing, sleeplessness, headache, lack of concentration, associated with the menopause

627.3   *Postmenopausal atrophic vaginitis*

Senile (atrophic) vaginitis

627.4   *States associated with artificial menopause*

Any condition in 627.1, .2 or .3 which follows induced menopause
Post-artificial-menopause syndromes

627.8   *Other*

Excludes: premature menopause NOS (256.3)

627.9   *Unspecified*

628   Infertility, female

Includes: primary and secondary sterility

628.0 *Associated with anovulation*

Associated with Stein-Leventhal syndrome* (256.4†)

628.1* *Of pituitary-hypothalamic origin* (253.–†)

628.2 *Of tubal origin*

Associated with:	Tubal:
congenital anomaly of tube	block
peritubal adhesions* (614.6†)	occlusion
	stenosis

628.3 *Of uterine origin*

Associated with:	Nonimplantation
congenital anomaly of uterus	
tuberculous endometritis* (016.4†)	

628.4 *Of cervical or vaginal origin*

Associated with:
anomaly of cervical mucus
congenital structural anomaly

628.8 *Of other specified origin*

628.9 *Of unspecified origin*

629 Other disorders of female genital organs

629.0 *Haematocele, female*

Excludes: when associated with ectopic pregnancy (633.–)

629.1 *Hydrocele, canal of Nuck*

Cyst of canal of Nuck

629.8 *Other*

629.9 *Unspecified*

XI. COMPLICATIONS OF PREGNANCY, CHILDBIRTH AND THE PUERPERIUM

PREGNANCY WITH ABORTIVE OUTCOME (630-639)

630 Hydatidiform mole

Trophoblastic disease NOS
Vesicular mole

Excludes: chorionepithelioma (181)

631 Other abnormal product of conception

Blighted ovum
Mole:
  NOS
  carneous
  fleshy

Excludes: with mention of conditions in 630 (630)

632 Missed abortion

Early fetal death with retention of dead fetus
Retained products of conception, not following spontaneous or induced
    abortion or delivery

Excludes: failed induced abortion (638)
    missed delivery (656.4)
    with abnormal product of conception (630, 631)

633 Ectopic pregnancy

Includes: ruptured ectopic pregnancy

633.0 *Abdominal pregnancy*

633.1 *Tubal pregnancy*

Fallopian pregnancy
Rupture of (fallopian) tube due to pregnancy
Tubal abortion

633.2 *Ovarian pregnancy*

633.8 *Other ectopic pregnancy*

Pregnancy:
  cervical
  combined
  cornual

Pregnancy:
  intraligamentous
  mesometric
  mural

— 355 —

633.9 *Unspecified*

The following fourth-digit subdivisions are for use with categories 634-638:

.0 Complicated by genital tract and pelvic infection [any condition listed in 639.0]
.1 Complicated by delayed or excessive haemorrhage [any condition listed in 639.1]
.2 Complicated by damage to pelvic organs and tissues [any condition listed in 639.2]
.3 Complicated by renal failure [any condition listed in 639.3]
.4 Complicated by metabolic disorder [any condition listed in 639.4]
.5 Complicated by shock [any condition listed in 639.5]
.6 Complicated by embolism [any condition listed in 639.6]
.7 With other specified complications [any condition listed in 639.8]
.8 With unspecified complications
.9 Without mention of complication

634 Spontaneous abortion

[See above for fourth-digit subdivisions]

Includes: spontaneous abortion (complete) (incomplete)

635 Legally induced abortion

[See above for fourth-digit subdivisions]

Includes: abortion:
legal
therapeutic
termination of pregnancy:
legal
therapeutic

Excludes: menstrual extraction or regulation (V25.3)

636 Illegally induced abortion

[See above for fourth-digit subdivisions]

Includes: abortion (complete) (incomplete):
criminal
illegal

637 Unspecified abortion

[See above for fourth-digit subdivisions]

Includes: abortion (complete) (incomplete) NOS
retained products of conception following abortion, not classifiable elsewhere

638   Failed attempted abortion

[See page 356 for fourth-digit subdivisions]

Includes: failure of attempted induction of (legal) abortion

Excludes: incomplete abortion (634-637)

639   Complications following abortion and ectopic and molar pregnancies

Note: This category is provided for use when it is required to classify separately the complications listed at fourth-digit level in categories 634-638; for example:

a) when the complication itself was responsible for an episode of medical care, the abortion, ectopic or molar pregnancy itself having been dealt with at a previous episode

b) when these conditions are immediate complications of ectopic or molar pregnancies classifiable to 630-633 where they cannot be identified at fourth-digit level.

639.0   *Genital tract and pelvic infection*

Endometritis
Parametritis
Pelvic peritonitis
Salpingitis   } following conditions classifiable to 630-638
Salpingo-oophoritis
Sepsis NOS
Septicaemia NOS

Excludes: urinary tract infection (639.8)

639.1   *Delayed or excessive haemorrhage*

Afibrinogenaemia
Defibrination syndrome   } following conditions classifiable to 630-638
Intravascular haemolysis

639.2   *Damage to pelvic organs and tissues*

Laceration, perforation or tear of:
  bladder
  bowel
  broad ligament   } following conditions classifiable to 630-638
  cervix
  periurethral tissue
  uterus

639.3   *Renal failure*

Oliguria
Renal:
  failure (acute)
  shutdown   } following conditions classifiable to 630-638
  tubular necrosis
Uraemia

639.4 *Metabolic disorders*

Electrolyte imbalance following conditions classifiable to 630-638

639.5 *Shock*

Circulatory collapse ⎱ following conditions
Shock (postoperative) (septic) ⎰   classifiable to 630-638

639.6 *Embolism*

Embolism:
  NOS
  air
  amniotic fluid
  blood-clot   ⎰ following conditions classifiable to 630-638
  pulmonary
  pyaemic
  septic
  soap

639.8 *Other specified complications*

Cardiac arrest or failure ⎱ following conditions classifiable to 630-638
Cerebral anoxia   ⎰

639.9 *Unspecified complications following conditions classifiable to 630-638*

COMPLICATIONS MAINLY RELATED TO PREGNANCY (640-648)

Includes: the listed conditions even if they arose or were present during labour, delivery or the puerperium

640 Haemorrhage in early pregnancy

Includes: haemorrhage before completion of 22 weeks' gestation

640.0 *Threatened abortion*

640.8 *Other*

640.9 *Unspecified*

641 Antepartum haemorrhage, abruptio placentae, and placenta praevia

641.0 *Placenta praevia without·haemorrhage*

Low implantation of placenta without haemorrhage
Placenta praevia noted:
  during pregnancy
  before labour and delivered by caesarean section, without mention of haemorrhage

641.1   *Haemorrhage from placenta praevia*

Low-lying placenta
Placenta praevia:
  marginal   } NOS or with haemorrhage (intrapartum)
  partial
  total

Excludes: haemorrhage from vasa praevia (663.5)

641.2   *Premature separation of placenta*

Ablatio placentae   Accidental   antepartum haemor-
Abruptio placentae   rhage
                                 Premature separation of normally
                                   implanted placenta

641.3   *Antepartum haemorrhage associated with coagulation defects*

Antepartum or intrapartum haemorrhage associated with:
  afibrinogenaemia
  hypofibrinogenaemia
  hyperfibrinolysis

641.8   *Other antepartum haemorrhage*

Antepartum or intrapartum haemorrhage associated with:
  trauma
  uterine leiomyoma

641.9   *Unspecified antepartum haemorrhage*

Haemorrhage:
  antepartum NOS
  intrapartum NOS
  of pregnancy NOS

642   Hypertension complicating pregnancy, childbirth and the puerperium

642.0   *Benign essential hypertension complicating pregnancy, childbirth and the puerperium*

Hypertension:
  benign essential   } specified as complicating, or as a reason for
  chronic NOS   obstetric care during, pregnancy, childbirth
  essential   or the puerperium
  pre-existing NOS

642.1   *Hypertension secondary to renal disease, complicating pregnancy, childbirth and the puerperium*

Hypertension secondary to renal disease, specified as complicating, or as
  a reason for obstetric care during, pregnancy, childbirth or the
  puerperium

642.2　*Other pre-existing hypertension complicating pregnancy, childbirth and the puerperium*

Malignant hypertension
Hypertensive:　　　　　　　　　　specified as complicating, or as a reason for
　heart disease　　　　　　　　　　obstetric care during, pregnancy, child-
　heart and renal disease　　　　　birth or the puerperium
　renal disease

642.3　*Transient hypertension of pregnancy*

Transient hypertension, so described, in pregnancy, childbirth or the puerperium

642.4　*Mild or unspecified pre-eclampsia*

Hypertension in pregnancy, childbirth or the puerperium, not specified as pre-existing, with either albuminuria or oedema, or both; mild or unspecified

Pre-eclampsia:　　　　　　　　　Toxaemia (pre-eclamptic):
　NOS　　　　　　　　　　　　　　NOS
　mild　　　　　　　　　　　　　　mild

Excludes:　albuminuria in pregnancy, without mention of hypertension (646.2)
　　　　　　oedema in pregnancy, without mention of hypertension (646.1)

642.5　*Severe pre-eclampsia*

Hypertension in pregnancy, childbirth or the puerperium, not specified as pre-existing, with either albuminuria or oedema, or both; specified as severe

Pre-eclampsia, severe　　　　　　Toxaemia (pre-eclamptic), severe

642.6　*Eclampsia*

Toxaemia:
　eclamptic
　with convulsions

642.7　*Pre-eclampsia or eclampsia superimposed on pre-existing hypertension*

Conditions in 642.4-642.6, with conditions in 642.0-642.2

642.9　*Unspecified hypertention complicating pregnancy, childbirth and the puerperium*

Hypertension NOS, without mention of albuminuria or oedema, complicating pregnancy, childbirth or the puerperium

643　Excessive vomiting in pregnancy

643.0 *Mild hyperemesis gravidarum*

Hyperemesis gravidarum, mild or unspecified, starting before the end of the 22nd week

643.1 *Hyperemesis gravidarum with metabolic disturbance*

Hyperemesis gravidarum, starting before the end of the 22nd week, with metabolic disturbance such as:
carbohydrate depletion
dehydration
electrolyte imbalance

643.2 *Late vomiting of pregnancy*

Excessive vomiting starting after 22 completed weeks of gestation

643.8 *Other vomiting complicating pregnancy*

Vomiting due to organic disease or other cause, specified as complicating pregnancy, or as a reason for obstetric care during pregnancy

Use additional code, if desired, to identify cause

643.9 *Unspecified vomiting of pregnancy*

Vomiting as a reason for care during pregnancy, length of gestation unspecified

644 Early or threatened labour

644.0 *Threatened labour*

False labour

644.1 *Early onset of delivery*

Onset (spontaneous) of delivery before 37 weeks gestation

645 Prolonged pregnancy

Post-dates   Post-term

646 Other complications of pregnancy, not elsewhere classified

646.0 *Papyraceous fetus*

646.1 *Oedema or excessive weight gain in pregnancy, without mention of hypertension*

Gestational oedema

Excludes: with mention of hypertension (642.–)

646.2 *Unspecified renal disease in pregnancy, without mention of hypertension*

Albuminuria
Nephropathy NOS   } in pregnancy, without mention of hypertension
Renal disease NOS
Gestational proteinuria

Excludes: with mention of hypertension (642.–)

646.3   *Habitual aborter*

Excludes: with current abortion (634.–)
            without current pregnancy (629.9)

646.4   *Peripheral neuritis in pregnancy*

646.5   *Asymptomatic bacteriuria in pregnancy*

646.6   *Infections of genitourinary tract in pregnancy*

Conditions in 590, 595, 597, 599.0, 614-616 complicating pregnancy or labour

Excludes: major puerperal infection (670)

646.7   *Liver disorders in pregnancy*

Excludes: hepatorenal syndrome following delivery (674.8)

646.8   *Other specified complications of pregnancy*

Fatigue during pregnancy   Herpes gestationis

646.9   *Unspecified complication of pregnancy*

647   Infective and parasitic conditions in the mother classifiable else-where but complicating pregnancy, childbirth and the puerperium

Includes: the listed conditions when complicating the pregnant state, aggravated by the pregnancy, or when a main reason for obstetric care

Excludes: when the reason for the mother's medical care is that the condition is known or suspected to have affected the fetus (655.–)

647.0   *Syphilis*

Conditions in 090-097

647.1   *Gonorrhoea*

Conditions in 098

647.2   *Other venereal diseases*

Conditions in 099

647.3   *Tuberculosis*

Conditions in 010-018

647.4   *Malaria*

Conditions in 084

647.5   *Rubella*

Conditions in 056

647.6   *Other viral diseases*
Conditions in 050-079, except 056

647.8   *Other specified infective and parasitic diseases*

647.9   *Unspecified infection or infestation*

648   Other current conditions in the mother classifiable elsewhere but complicating pregnancy, childbirth and the puerperium

Includes: the listed conditions when complicating the pregnant state, aggravated by the pregnancy or when a main reason for obstetric care

Excludes: when the main reason for the mother's medical care is that the condition is known or suspected to have affected the fetus (655.–)

648.0   *Diabetes mellitus*
Conditions in 250

648.1   *Thyroid dysfunction*
Conditions in 240-246

648.2   *Anaemia*
Conditions in 280-285

648.3   *Drug dependence*
Conditions in 304.–

648.4   *Mental disorders*
Conditions in 290-303, 305-316, 317-319

648.5   *Congenital cardiovascular disorders*
Conditions in 745-747

648.6   *Other cardiovascular diseases*
Conditions in 390-398, 410-459

Excludes: cerebral haemorrhage in the puerperium (674.0)
                venous complications (671.–)

648.7   *Bone and joint disorders of back, pelvis and lower limbs*
Conditions in 720-724 and those classifiable to 711-719 or 725-738 specified as affecting the lower limbs

648.8   *Abnormal glucose tolerance*
Conditions in 790.2

648.9   *Other*
Nutritional deficiencies (conditions in 260-269)

NORMAL DELIVERY, AND OTHER INDICATIONS FOR CARE IN
PREGNANCY, LABOUR AND DELIVERY (650-659)

650   Delivery in a completely normal case

Delivery without abnormality or complication classifiable elsewhere in
  categories 630-676, and with spontaneous cephalic delivery, without
  mention of manipulation or instrumentation

Excludes: delivery by vacuum extractor, forceps, caesarean section or
             breech extraction, without specified complication (669.5-
             669.7)
           breech delivery (assisted) (spontaneous) NOS (652.2)

651   Multiple gestation

651.0   *Twin pregnancy*

651.1   *Triplet pregnancy*

651.2   *Quadruplet pregnancy*

651.8   *Other*

651.9   *Unspecified*

652   Malposition and malpresentation of fetus

Excludes: with obstructed labour (660.0)

652.0   *Unstable lie*

652.1   *Breech or other malpresentation successfully converted to cephalic
         presentation*

Cephalic version NOS

652.2   *Breech presentation without mention of version*

652.3   *Transverse or oblique presentation*

Oblique lie   Transverse lie

Excludes: transverse arrest of fetal head (660.3)

652.4   *Face or brow presentation*

Mentum presentation

652.5   *High head at term*

Failure of head to enter pelvic brim

652.6   *Multiple gestation with malpresentation of one fetus or more*

652.7   *Prolapsed arm*

652.8   *Other*

652.9   *Unspecified*

653   Disproportion
Excludes: with obstructed labour (660.1)

653.0   *Major abnormality of bony pelvis, not further specified*
Pelvic deformity NOS

653.1   *Generally contracted pelvis*
Contracted pelvis NOS

653.2   *Inlet contraction of pelvis*
Inlet contraction (pelvis)

653.3   *Outlet contraction of pelvis*
Outlet contraction (pelvis)

653.4   *Fetopelvic disproportion*
Disproportion of mixed maternal and fetal origin, with normally formed
    fetus
Cephalopelvic disproportion NOS

653.5   *Unusually large fetus causing disproportion*
Disproportion of fetal origin with normally formed fetus
Fetal disproportion NOS
Excludes: when the reason for medical care was concern for the fetus
                 (656.6)

653.6   *Hydrocephalic fetus causing disproportion*
Excludes: when the reason for medical care was concern for the fetus
                 (655.0)

653.7   *Other fetal abnormality causing disproportion*

Conjoined twins	Fetal:
Fetal:	myelomeningocele
ascites	sacral teratoma
hydrops	tumour

653.8   *Disproportion of other origin*

653.9   *Unspecified*

654   Abnormality of organs and soft tissues of pelvis
Includes: the listed conditions during pregnancy, childbirth or the
                 puerperium
Excludes: with obstructed labour (660.2)

654.0   *Congenital abnormalities of uterus*

Double uterus   Uterus bicornis

654.1   *Tumours of body of uterus*

Uterine fibroids

654.2   *Uterine scar from previous surgery*

Previous caesarean section NOS

654.3   *Retroverted and incarcerated gravid uterus*

654.4   *Other abnormalities in shape or position of gravid uterus and of neighbouring structures*

Cystocele   Prolapse of gravid uterus
Pelvic floor repair   Rectocele
Pendulous abdomen   Rigid pelvic floor

654.5   *Cervical incompetence*

Shirodkar suture with or without mention of cervical incompetence

654.6   *Other congenital or acquired abnormality of cervix*

Polyp of cervix   Tumour of cervix
Previous surgery to cervix

654.7   *Congenital or acquired abnormality of vagina*

Previous surgery to vagina   Stricture of vagina
Septate vagina   Tumour of vagina
Stenosis of vagina (acquired)
   (congenital)

654.8   *Congenital or acquired abnormality of vulva*

Fibrosis of perineum   Rigid perineum
Persistent hymen   Tumour of vulva
Previous surgery to perineum or
   vulva

Excludes: varicose veins of vulva (671.1)

654.9   *Unspecified*

655   Known or suspected fetal abnormality affecting management of mother

Includes: the listed conditions in the fetus as a reason for observation, or obstetrical care to the mother, or for termination of pregnancy

655.0 *Central nervous system malformation in fetus*

Fetal or suspected fetal:
  anencephaly
  hydrocephalus
  spina bifida

655.1 *Chromosomal abnormality in fetus*

655.2 *Hereditary disease in family possibly affecting fetus*

655.3 *Suspected damage to fetus from viral disease in the mother*

Suspected damage to fetus from maternal rubella

655.4 *Suspected damage to fetus from other disease in the mother*

Suspected damage to fetus from maternal:
  alcohol addiction
  listeriosis
  toxoplasmosis

655.5 *Suspected damage to fetus from drugs*

Excludes: fetal distress in labour and delivery due to drug administration (656.3)

655.6 *Suspected damage to fetus from radiation*

655.8 *Other known or suspected fetal abnormality, not elsewhere classified*

Suspected damage to fetus from intrauterine contraceptive device

655.9 *Unspecified*

656 **Other fetal and placental problems affecting management of mother**

656.0 *Fetal-maternal haemorrhage*

Leakage (microscopic) of fetal blood into maternal circulation

656.1 *Rhesus isoimmunization*

Anti-D [Rh] antibodies
Rh incompatibility

656.2 *Isoimmunization from other and unspecified blood-group incompatibility*

ABO isoimmunization

656.3 *Fetal distress*

Abnormal fetal:
  acid-base balance
  heart-rate or rhythm

Fetal:
  acidaemia
  bradycardia
Meconium in liquor

656.4   *Intrauterine death*

656.5   *Poor fetal growth*
"Light-for-dates"   "Small-for-dates"
"Placental insufficiency"

656.6   *Excessive fetal growth*
"Large-for-dates"

656.7   *Other placental conditions*
Abnormal placenta   Placental infarct

656.8   *Other*

656.9   *Unspecified*

657   Polyhydramnios
Hydramnios

658   Other problems associated with amniotic cavity and membranes
Excludes: amniotic fluid embolism (673.1)

658.0   *Oligohydramnios*
Oligohydramnios without mention of rupture of membranes

658.1   *Premature rupture of membranes*

658.2   *Delayed delivery after spontaneous or unspecified rupture of membranes*

658.3   *Delayed delivery after artificial rupture of membranes*

658.4   *Infection of amniotic cavity*
Amnionitis   Membranitis
Chorioamnionitis   Placentitis

658.8   *Other*

658.9   *Unspecified*

659   Other indications for care or intervention related to labour and delivery and not elsewhere classified

659.0   *Failed mechanical induction*
Failure of induction of labour by surgical or other instrumental methods

659.1   *Failed medical or unspecified induction*
Failed induction NOS
Failure of induction of labour by medical methods, such as oxytocic
    drugs

659.2   *Maternal pyrexia during labour, unspecified*

659.3   *Generalized infection during labour*

Septicaemia during labour

659.4   *Grand multiparity*

Excludes: supervision only, in pregnancy (V23.3)
           without current pregnancy (V61.5)

659.5   *Elderly primigravida*

659.8   *Other*

659.9   *Unspecified*

COMPLICATIONS OCCURING MAINLY IN THE COURSE OF LABOUR AND DELIVERY (660-669)

660   Obstructed labour

660.0   *Obstruction caused by malposition of fetus at onset of labour*

Any condition in 652.– causing obstruction during labour

Use additional code from 652.–, if desired, to identify condition

660.1   *Obstruction by bony pelvis*

Any condition in 653.– causing obstruction during labour

Use additional code from 653.–, if desired, to identify condition

660.2   *Obstruction by abnormal pelvic soft tissues*

Any condition in 654.– causing obstruction during labour
Prolapse of anterior lip of cervix

Use additional code from 654.–, if desired, to identify condition

660.3   *Deep transverse arrest and persistent occipitoposterior or occipito-anterior position*

660.4   *Shoulder dystocia*

Impacted shoulders

660.5   *Locked twins*

660.6   *Failed trial of labour, unspecified*

Failed trial of labour, without mention of condition or suspected condition, and with subsequent delivery by caesarean section

660.7   *Failed forceps or ventouse, unspecified*

Application of ventouse or forceps, without mention of condition, with subsequent delivery by forceps or caesarean section respectively

660.8   *Other*

660.9   *Unspecified*

Dystocia:
  NOS
  fetal NOS
  maternal NOS

661   Abnormality of forces of labour

661.0   *Primary uterine inertia*

Failure of cervical dilatation
Hypotonic uterine dysfunction, primary

661.1   *Secondary uterine inertia*

Arrested active phase of labour
Hypotonic uterine dysfunction, secondary

661.2   *Other and unspecified uterine inertia*

Atony of uterus   Irregular labour
Desultory labour   Poor contractions

661.3   *Precipitate labour*

661.4   *Hypertonic, incoordinate, or prolonged uterine contractions*

Cervical spasm   Incoordinate uterine action
Contraction ring (dystocia)   Retraction ring (pathological)
Dyscoordinate labour   (Bandl's)
Hour-glass contraction of uterus   Tetanic contractions
Hypertonic uterine dysfunction   Uterine dystocia NOS
                                    Uterine spasm

661.9   *Unspecified*

662   Long labour

662.0   *Prolonged first stage*

662.1   *Prolonged labour, unspecified*

662.2   *Prolonged second stage*

662.3   *Delayed delivery of second twin, triplet, etc.*

663   Umbilical cord complications

663.0   *Prolapse of cord*

Presentation of cord

663.1   *Cord around neck, with compression*

Cord tightly around neck

663.2 *Other and unspecified cord entanglement, with compression*

Entanglement of cords of twins in mono-amniotic sac
Knot in cord

663.3 *Other and unspecified cord entanglement, without mention of compression*

663.4 *Short cord*

663.5 *Vasa praevia*

663.6 *Vascular lesions of cord*

Bruising of cord   Thrombosis of vessels of cord
Haematoma of cord

663.8 *Other*

663.9 *Unspecified*

664   Trauma to perineum and vulva during delivery

664.0 *First-degree perineal laceration*

Perineal laceration, rupture or tear (involving):
  fourchette
  hymen
  labia
  skin
  slight
  vagina
  vulva

664.1 *Second-degree perineal laceration*

Perineal laceration, rupture or tear (following episiotomy) involving:
  pelvic floor
  perineal muscles
  vaginal muscles
Excludes: involving anal sphincter (664.2)

664.2 *Third-degree perineal laceration*

Perineal laceration, rupture or tear (following episiotomy) involving:
  anal sphincter
  rectovaginal septum
  sphincter NOS
Excludes: with anal or rectal mucosa (664.3)

664.3 *Fourth-degree perineal laceration*

Perineal laceration, rupture or tear as in 664.2 and involving also:
  anal mucosa
  rectal mucosa

664.4   *Unspecified perineal laceration*

Central laceration

664.5   *Vulval and perineal haematoma*

664.8   *Other*

664.9   *Unspecified*

665   Other obstetrical trauma

Includes: damage from instruments

665.0   *Rupture of uterus before onset of labour*

665.1   *Rupture of uterus during and after labour*

Rupture of uterus NOS

665.2   *Inversion of uterus*

665.3   *Laceration of cervix*

665.4   *High vaginal laceration*

Laceration of vaginal wall without mention of perineal laceration

665.5   *Other injury to pelvic organs*

Injury to:
  bladder
  urethra

665.6   *Damage to pelvic joints and ligaments*

Avulsion of inner symphyseal cartilage
Damage to coccyx
Separation of symphysis (pubis)

665.7   *Pelvic haematoma*

Haematoma of vagina

665.8   *Other*

665.9   *Unspecified*

666   Postpartum haemorrhage

666.0   *Third-stage haemorrhage*

Haemorrhage associated with retained, trapped or adherent placenta
Retained placenta NOS

666.1   *Other immediate postpartum haemorrhage*

Haemorrhage following delivery of placenta
Postpartum haemorrhage (atonic) NOS

666.2 *Delayed and secondary postpartum haemorrhage*

Haemorrhage associated with retained portions of placenta or membranes
Postpartum haemorrhage specified as delayed or secondary
Retained products of conception, NOS, following delivery

666.3 *Postpartum coagulation defects*

Postpartum:
  afibrinogenaemia
  fibrinolysis

667 Retained placenta or membranes, without haemorrhage

667.0 *Retained placenta without haemorrhage*

Placenta accreta
Retained placenta: }
  NOS   } without haemorrhage
  total

667.1 *Retained portions of placenta or membranes, without haemorrhage*

Retained products of conception following delivery, without haemorrhage

668 Complications of the administration of anaesthetic or other sedation in labour and delivery

Includes: complications arising from the administration of a general
           or local anaesthetic, analgesic or other sedation in labour
           and delivery

668.0 *Pulmonary complications*

Inhalation of stomach contents or secretions
Mendelson's syndrome
Pressure collapse of lung

668.1 *Cardiac complications*

Cardiac:
  arrest
  failure

668.2 *Central nervous system complications*

Cerebral anoxia

668.8 *Other*

668.9 *Unspecified*

669 Other complications of labour and delivery, not elsewhere classified

669.0 *Maternal distress*

669.1 *Shock during or following labour and delivery*
Obstetric shock

669.2 *Maternal hypotension syndrome*

669.3 *Acute renal failure following labour and delivery*

669.4 *Other complications of obstetrical surgery and procedures*
Cardiac:
  arrest   following caesarean or other obstetrical surgery or
  failure   procedure, including delivery NOS
Cerebral anoxia
Excludes: complications of obstetrical surgical wounds (674.3)

669.5 *Forceps or ventouse delivery without mention of indication*
Delivery by vacuum extractor, without mention of indication

669.6 *Breech extraction, without mention of indication*
Excludes: breech delivery NOS (652.2)

669.7 *Caesarean delivery, without mention of indication*

669.8 *Other*

669.9 *Unspecified*

METHOD OF DELIVERY

If a full classification of surgical and other procedures is not being used
to identify the method of delivery, the following classification is
recommended:

.0 Normal, spontaneous vertex vaginal delivery, occipitoanterior

.1 Cephalic vaginal delivery with abnormal presentation of head at
    delivery, without instruments, with or without manipulation

.2 Forceps, low application, without manipulation
    Forceps delivery NOS

.3 Other forceps delivery
    Forceps with manipulation
    High forceps
    Mid forceps

.4 Vacuum extraction
    Ventouse

.5 Breech delivery, spontaneous, assisted or unspecified
    Partial breech extraction

.6 Breech extraction
Breech extraction:
    NOS
    total
Version with breech extraction

.7 Elective caesarean section
Caesarean section before, or at onset of, labour

.8 Other and unspecified caesarean section

.9 Other and unspecified method of delivery
Application of weight to leg in breech delivery
Destructive operation to facilitate delivery
Other surgical or instrumental delivery

COMPLICATIONS OF THE PUERPERIUM (670-676)

Note: Categories 671 and 673-676 include the listed conditions even if they occur during pregnancy or childbirth.

670 Major puerperal infection

Puerperal:
    endometritis
    fever
    pelvic cellulitis

Puerperal:
    pelvic sepsis
    peritonitis

Excludes: infection following abortion (639.0)
minor genital tract infection following delivery (646.6)
urinary tract infection following delivery (646.6)

671 Venous complications in pregnancy and the puerperium

671.0 *Varicose veins of legs*

Varicose veins NOS

671.1 *Varicose veins of vulva and perineum*

671.2 *Superficial thrombophlebitis*

Thrombophlebitis (superficial)

671.3 *Deep phlebothrombosis, antepartum*

Deep-vein thrombosis, antepartum

671.4 *Deep phlebothrombosis, postpartum*

Deep-vein thrombosis, postpartum
Pelvic thrombophlebitis, postpartum

671.5 *Other phlebitis and thrombosis*

Cerebral venous thrombosis

671.8 *Other*

Haemorrhoids

671.9 *Unspecified*

Phlebitis NOS
Thrombosis NOS

672 Pyrexia of unknown origin during the puerperium

Puerperal pyrexia NOS

673 Obstetrical pulmonary embolism

Includes: pulmonary emboli in pregnancy, childbirth or the puerperium, or specified as puerperal

Excludes: embolism following abortion (639.6)

673.0 *Obstetrical air embolism*

673.1 *Amniotic fluid embolism*

673.2 *Obstetrical blood-clot embolism*

Puerperal pulmonary embolism NOS

673.3 *Obstetrical pyaemic and septic embolism*

673.8 *Other*

Fat embolism

674 Other and unspecified complications of the puerperium, not elsewhere classified

674.0 *Cerebrovascular disorders in the puerperium*

Any condition in 430-434, 436-437 occurring during pregnancy, childbirth or the puerperium, or specified as puerperal

674.1 *Disruption of caesarean wound*

674.2 *Disruption of perineal wound*

Breakdown of perineum   Secondary perineal tear
Disruption of wound of:
  episiotomy
  perineal laceration

674.3   *Other complications of obstetrical surgical wounds*

Haematoma ⎫
Haemorrhage ⎬ of caesarean section, or perineal, wound
Infection ⎭

Excludes: damage from instruments in delivery (664.–, 665.–)

674.4   *Placental polyp*

674.8   *Other*

Hepatorenal syndrome following   Postpartum:
   delivery   cardiomyopathy
                                                      subinvolution of uterus

674.9   *Unspecified*

Sudden death of unknown cause during the puerperium

675   Infections of the breast and nipple associated with childbirth

675.0   *Infections of nipple*

Abscess of nipple

675.1   *Abscess of breast*

Mammary abscess   Subareolar abscess
Purulent mastitis

675.2   *Nonpurulent mastitis*

Lymphangitis of breast   Mastitis:
Mastitis: interstitial
   NOS   parenchymatous

675.8   *Other*

675.9   *Unspecified*

676   Other disorders of the breast associated with childbirth, and disorders of lactation

Includes: the listed conditions during pregnancy, the puerperium or
                  lactation

676.0   *Retracted nipple*

676.1   *Cracked nipple*

Fissure of nipple

676.2   *Engorgement of breasts*

676.3   *Other and unspecified disorder of breast*

676.4 *Failure of lactation*

Agalactia

676.5 *Suppressed lactation*

676.6 *Galactorrhoea*

Excludes: galactorrhoea not associated with childbirth (611.6)

676.8 *Other disorders of lactation*

Galactocele

676.9 *Unspecified disorder of lactation*

XII. DISEASES OF THE SKIN AND SUBCUTANEOUS TISSUE

INFECTIONS OF SKIN AND SUBCUTANEOUS TISSUE (680-686)

Excludes: certain local infections of skin classified under "Infectious and Parasitic Diseases", such as:
  erysipelas (035)
  erysipeloid of Rosenbach (027.1)
  herpes:
    simplex (054.–)
    zoster (053.–)
  molluscum contagiosum (078.0)
  viral warts (078.1)

680 Carbuncle and furuncle

Includes: boil
  furunculosis

680.0 *Face*

Ear [any part]
Face [any part, except eye]
Nose (septum)
Temple (region)

Excludes: eyelid (373.1)
  lacrimal glands or sac (375.3)
  orbit (376.0)

680.1 *Neck*

680.2 *Trunk*

Abdominal wall
Back [any part, except buttock]
Breast
Chest wall
Groin
Perineum
Umbilicus

680.3 *Upper arm and forearm*

Arm [any part, except hand]
Axilla
Shoulder

680.4 *Hand*

Finger
Thumb
Wrist

680.5 *Buttock*

Anus
Gluteal region

680.6 *Leg, except foot*

Ankle   Knee
Hip   Thigh

680.7 *Foot*

Heel   Toe

680.8 *Other specified site*

Head [any part, except face]   Scalp

Excludes: genital organs (external) (607.2, 608.4, 616.4)

680.9 *Unspecified site*

Boil NOS   Furuncle NOS

681   Cellulitis and abscess of finger and toe

Includes: cellulitis of finger or toe ⎤
             felon   ⎥
             infection, nail   ⎥
             onychia   ⎬ (with lymphangitis)
             panaritium   ⎥
             paronychia   ⎥
             perionychia   ⎦

Use additional code, if desired, to identify infectious organism

681.0 *Finger*

681.1 *Toe*

681.9 *Unspecified digit*

682   Other cellulitis and abscess

Includes: abscess (acute)   ⎤
             cellulitis (diffuse)   ⎬ (with lymphangitis) except of finger or
             lymphangitis, acute   ⎦   toe

Excludes: cellulitis or abscess of:
                 anal and rectal region (566)
                 external auditory canal (380.1)
                 external genital organs:
                     female (616.4)
                     male (607.2, 608.4)
                 eyelid (373.1)
                 lacrimal apparatus (375.3)
                 nose, except external (478.1)
             lymphangitis (chronic) (subacute) (457.2)

Use additional code, if desired, to identify infectious organism

682.0 *Face*

Cheek
Chin
Forehead

Nose
Submandibular
Temple (region)

Excludes: ear (380.1)

682.1 *Neck*

682.2 *Trunk*

Abdominal wall
Back [any part, except buttock]
Chest wall
Groin

Pectoral region
Perineum
Umbilicus

Excludes: of umbilicus in newborn (771.4)

682.3 *Upper arm and forearm*

Arm [any part, except hand]
Axilla

Shoulder

Excludes: hand (682.4)

682.4 *Hand, except fingers*

Hand [except finger or thumb]

Wrist

Excludes: finger and thumb (681.0)

682.5 *Buttock*

Gluteal region

682.6 *Leg, except foot*

Ankle
Hip

Knee
Thigh

682.7 *Foot, except toes*

Heel

Excludes: toe (681.1)

682.8 *Other specified site*

Head [except face]

Scalp

682.9 *Unspecified site*

Abscess NOS

Cellulitis NOS

683   Acute lymphadenitis

Abscess (acute)
Adenitis, acute ⎱ any lymph node except mesenteric
Lymphadenitis, acute ⎰

Excludes: enlarged glands NOS (785.6)
            lymphadenitis:
                chronic or subacute, except mesenteric (289.1)
                mesenteric (acute) (chronic) (subacute) (289.2)
                unspecified (289.3)
Use additional code, if desired, to identify infectious organism

684   Impetigo

Impetiginization of other dermatoses
Impetigo (contagiosa) [any site] [any organism]:
    bullous
    circinate
    neonatorum
    simplex
Pemphigus neonatorum

Excludes: impetigo herpetiformis (694.3)

685   Pilonidal cyst

Includes: fistula ⎱ coccygeal or pilonidal
            sinus ⎰

685.0   *With abscess*
685.1   *Without mention of abscess*

686   Other local infections of skin and subcutaneous tissue

Use additional code, if desired, to identify infectious organism

686.0   *Pyoderma*

Dermatitis: Dermatitis, suppurative
    purulent
    septic

686.1   *Pyogenic granuloma*

Granuloma: Granuloma telangiectaticum
    septic
    suppurative

686.8   *Other local infections of skin and subcutaneous tissue*

Dermatitis vegetans   Perleche
Ecthyma

Excludes: dermatitis infectiosa eczematoides (690)
            panniculitis (729.3)

686.9   *Unspecified local infections of skin and subcutaneous tissue*

OTHER INFLAMMATORY CONDITIONS OF SKIN AND SUBCUTANEOUS
TISSUE (690-698)

Excludes: panniculitis (729.3)

690   Erythematosquamous dermatosis

Dermatitis infectiosa eczematoides   Seborrhoeic:
Parakeratosis   dermatitis
Pityriasis: eczema
  capitis
  simplex

Excludes: eczematous dermatitis of eyelid (373.3)
           psoriasis (696.–)

691   Atopic dermatitis and related conditions

691.0 *Diaper or napkin rash*

Diaper or napkin: Psoriasiform napkin eruption
  dermatitis
  erythema
  rash

691.8 *Other*

Atopic dermatitis
Eczema: Neurodermatitis:
  atopic   atopic
  flexural   diffuse (Brocq)
  infantile (acute) (chronic)
  intrinsic (allergic)

692   Contact dermatitis and other eczema

Includes: dermatitis: eczema (acute) (chronic):
       NOS   NOS
       contact   allergic
       occupational   erythematous
       venenata   occupational

Excludes: allergy NOS (995.3)
           contact dermatitis of eyelids (373.3)
           dermatitis due to ingested substances (693.–)
           eczema of external ear (380.2)
           perioral dermatitis (695.3)

692.0 *Due to detergents*

692.1 *Due to oils and greases*

692.2 *Due to solvents*

Solvents of:
  chlorocompound ⎫
  cyclohexane   ⎬ group
  ester   ⎭

Solvents of:
  glycol   ⎫
  hydrocarbon ⎬ group
  ketone   ⎭

692.3 *Due to drugs and medicaments in contact with skin*

Arnica
Fungicides
Iodine
Keratolytics
Mercury

Neomycin
Phenol
Scabicides
Any drug causing contact
  dermatitis

Excludes: allergy NOS due to drugs (995.2, E930-E949)
          dermatitis due to ingested drugs (693.0)

Use additional E code, if desired, to identify drug

692.4 *Due to other chemical products*

Acids
Adhesive plaster
Alkalis
Caustics
Dichromate

Insecticide
Nylon
Plastic
Rubber

692.5 *Due to food in contact with skin*

Cereals
Fish
Flour

Fruit
Meat
Milk

Excludes: dermatitis due to:
          dyes (692.8)
          ingested food (693.1)
          preservatives (692.8)

692.6 *Due to plants [except food]*

Lacquer tree [Rhus verniciflua]
Poison:
  ivy [Rhus toxicodendron]
  oak [Rhus diversiloba]
  sumac [Rhus venenata]
  vine [Rhus radicans]

Primrose [Primula]
Ragweed [Senecio jacobaea]

Excludes: allergy NOS due to pollen (477.0)

692.7 *Due to solar radiation*

Hydroa (aestivale) Sunburn

692.8 *Due to other specified agents*

Due to:
cold weather
cosmetics
dyes
furs
hot weather
infra-red rays

Due to:
light
preservatives
radiation NOS
ultraviolet rays
X-rays

Excludes: allergy NOS due to animal hair, dander (animal) or dust (477.8)

692.9 *Unspecified cause*

Dermatitis:
NOS
contact NOS
venenata NOS

Eczema NOS

693 Dermatitis due to substances taken internally

Excludes: adverse effect NOS of drugs and medicaments (995.2)
allergy NOS (995.3)
contact dermatitis (692.–)
urticarial reactions (708.0)

693.0 *Due to drugs and medicaments*

Use additional E code, if desired, to identify drug

693.1 *Due to food*

693.8 *Due to other specified substance*

693.9 *Due to unspecified substance*

Excludes: dermatitis NOS (692.9)

694 Bullous dermatoses

694.0 *Dermatitis herpetiformis*

Dermatosis herpetiformis
Duhring's disease

Hydroa herpetiformis

Excludes: senile dermatitis herpetiformis (694.5)

694.1 *Subcorneal pustular dermatosis*

Sneddon-Wilkinson disease or syndrome

694.2 *Juvenile dermatitis herpetiformis*

694.3 *Impetigo herpetiformis*

694.4 *Pemphigus*

Pemphigus:
  erythematodes
  foliaceous
  malignant

Pemphigus:
  vegetans
  vulgaris
Pemphigus NOS

Excludes: pemphigus neonatorum (684)

694.5 *Pemphigoid*

Benign pemphigus NOS
Bullous pemphigoid

Herpes circinatus bullosus
Senile dermatitis herpetiformis

694.6 *Benign mucous membrane pemphigoid*

Mucosynechial atrophic bullous
  dermatitis

Ocular pemphigoid † (372.3*)

694.8 *Other bullous dermatoses*

Excludes: herpes gestationis (646.8)

694.9 *Unspecified*

695 Erythematous conditions

695.0 *Toxic erythema*

695.1 *Erythema multiforme*

Erythema iris
Herpes iris

Stevens-Johnson syndrome
Toxic epidermal necrolysis

695.2 *Erythema nodosum*

Excludes: tuberculous erythema nodosum (017.1)

695.3 *Rosacea*

Acne rosacea
Perioral dermatitis

Rhinophyma

695.4 *Lupus erythematosus*

Lupus:
  erythematodes (discoid)
  erythematosus (discoid), not disseminated

Excludes: lupus NOS or vulgaris (017.0)
          disseminated lupus erythematosus (710.0)

695.8 *Other erythematous conditions*

Erythema intertrigo
Intertrigo

Pityriasis rubra (Hebra)
Ritter's disease

Excludes: mycotic intertrigo (111.–)

695.9   *Unspecified*

Erythema NOS   Erythroderma (secondary)

696   Psoriasis and similar disorders

696.0† *Psoriatic arthropathy (713.3*)*

696.1   *Other psoriasis*

Acrodermatitis continua   Psoriasis, any type, except
                                         arthropathic

696.2   *Parapsoriasis*

Pityriasis lichenoides et varioliformis

696.3   *Pityriasis rosea*

Pityriasis circinata (et maculata)

696.4   *Pityriasis rubra pilaris*

Devergie's disease

Excludes: pityriasis rubra (Hebra) (695.8)

696.5   *Other and unspecified pityriasis*

Excludes: pityriasis:
                 simplex (690)
                 versicolor (111.0)

696.8   *Other*

697   Lichen

Excludes: lichen:
                 pilaris (757.3)
                 sclerosus et atrophicus (701.0)
                 scrofulosus (017.0)
                 simplex chronicus (698.3)
                 spinulosus (757.3)

697.0   *Lichen planus*

Lichen ruber planus

697.1   *Lichen nitidus*

697.8   *Other lichen, not elsewhere classified*

Lichen:
  ruber moniliforme
  striata

697.9   *Unspecified*

698 Pruritus and related conditions

Excludes: pruritus specified as psychogenic (306.3)

698.0 *Pruritis ani*

698.1 *Pruritis of genital organs*

698.2 *Prurigo*

Prurigo: Prurigo mitis
  NOS
  Hebra's

698.3 *Lichenification and lichen simplex chronicus*

Neurodermatitis (local)   Prurigo nodularis
  (circumscripta)
Hyde's disease

Excludes: neurodermatitis diffuse (Brocq) (691.8)

698.4 *Dermatitis factitia [artefacta]*

Neurotic excoriation

Use additional code, if desired, to identify any associated mental disorder

698.8 *Other pruritic conditions*

Pruritis senilis

698.9 *Unspecified*

Itch NOS

OTHER DISEASES OF SKIN AND SUBCUTANEOUS TISSUE (700-709)

Excludes: congenital conditions of skin, hair and nails (757.–)

700 Corns and callosities

Callus   Clavus

701 Other hypertrophic and atrophic conditions of skin

Excludes: dermatomyositis (710.3)
         hereditary oedema of legs (757.0)
         scleroderma (generalized) (710.1)

701.0 *Circumscribed scleroderma*

Dermatosclerosis, localized   Morphoea
Lichen sclerosus et atrophicus   Scleroderma, localized

701.1 Keratoderma, acquired

Acquired:
  ichthyosis
  keratodermia palmaris et plantaris
Elastosis perforans serpiginosa
Hyperkeratosis:
  NOS
  follicularis in cutem penetrans
  palmoplantaris climacterica

Keratoderma:
  climactericum
  tylodes progressive
Keratosis (blennorrhagica):
  NOS
  gonococcal* (098.8†)

Excludes: Darier's disease (757.3)
  dyskeratosis follicularis (757.3)
  keratosis:
    arsenical (692.4)
    follicularis (757.3)

701.2 Acquired acanthosis nigricans

Keratosis nigricans

701.3 Striae atrophicae

Atrophic spots of skin
Atrophoderma maculatum
Atrophy blanche (of Milian)

Degenerative colloid atrophy
Senile degenerative atrophy
Striae distensae

701.4 Keloid scar

Cheloid
Hypertrophic scar

Keloid

701.5 Other abnormal granulation tissue

Excessive granulation

701.8 Other hypertrophic and atrophic conditions of skin

Acrodermatitis atrophicans
  chronica
Atrophia cutis senilis
Atrophoderma neuriticum
Confluent and reticulate
  papillomatosis

Cutis laxa senilis
Elastosis senilis
Folliculitis ulerythematosa
  reticulata
Gougerot-Carteaud syndrome
  or disease

701.9 Unspecified

702 Other dermatoses

Cutaneous horn
Hyperkeratosis, senile
Keratoma, senile

Leukokeratosis
Leukoplakia

Excludes: carcinoma in situ (232.–)

703   Diseases of nail

703.0   *Ingrowing nail*

703.8   *Other diseases of nail*

Dystrophia unguium
Hypertrophy of nail
Leukonychia (punctata) (striata)

Onychogryposis
Onycholysis

703.9   *Unspecified*

Excludes: onychia and paronychia (681.–)

704   Diseases of hair and hair follicles

704.0   *Alopecia*

Baldness
Folliculitis decalvans

Hypotrichosis:
  NOS
  postinfectional NOS
Ophiasis
Pseudopelade

Excludes: madarosis (374.5)
            syphilitic alopecia (091.8)

704.1   *Hirsutism*

Hypertrichosis:
  NOS
  lanuginosa, acquired

Polytrichia

704.2   *Abnormalities of the hair*

Atrophic hair
Clastothrix
Fragilitas crinium

Trichiasis:
  NOS
  cicatricial
Trichorrhexis (nodosa)

Excludes: trichiasis of eyelid (374.0)

704.3   *Variations in hair colour*

Canities (premature)
Greyness, hair (premature)
Heterochromia of hair

Poliosis:
  NOS
  circumscripta, acquired

704.8 *Other diseases of hair and hair follicles*

Folliculitis:
  NOS
  abscedens et suffodiens
  pustular
Perifolliculitis:
  NOS
  capitis abscedens et suffodiens
  scalp

Sycosis:
  NOS
  barbae [not parasitic]
  lipoides
  vulgaris

704.9 *Unspecified*

705   Disorders of sweat glands

705.0 *Anhidrosis*

Hypohidrosis   Oligohidrosis

705.1 *Prickly heat*

Heat rash   Sudamina
Miliaria rubra (tropicalis)

705.8 *Other disorders of sweat glands*

Bromhidrosis   Pompholyx
Cheiropompholyx   Urhidrosis
Chromhidrosis

Excludes: hidrocystoma (216.–)
            hyperhidrosis (780.8)

705.9 *Unspecified*

706   Diseases of sebaceous glands

706.0 *Acne varioliformis*

Acne necrotica

706.1 *Other acne*

Acne: Acne:
  NOS   pustular
  conglobata   vulgaris
  cystic   Comedo

Excludes: acne rosacea (695.3)

706.2 *Sebaceous cyst*

Atheroma, skin   Wen

706.3 *Seborrhoea*

Excludes: seborrhoea:
  capilitii (704.8)
  sicca (690)
  seborrhoeic keratosis (702)

706.8 *Other disorders of sebaceous glands*

Xerosis cutis

706.9 *Unspecified*

707   Chronic ulcer of skin

Excludes: gangrene (785.4)
  skin infections (680-686)
  specific infections classified under "Infectious and Parasitic
    Diseases" (001-136)
  varicose ulcer (454.–)

707.0 *Decubitus ulcer*

Decubitus ulcer, any site   Pressure ulcer
Plaster ulcer

707.1 *Ulcer of lower limbs, except decubitus*

707.8 *Chronic ulcer of other specified sites*

707.9 *Chronic ulcer of unspecified site*

Chronic ulcer NOS   Ulcer of skin NOS
Tropical ulcer NOS

708   Urticaria

Excludes: angioneurotic oedema (995.1)
  hereditary angio-oedema (277.6)
  Quincke's oedema (995.1)
  urticaria:
    giant (995.1)
    papulosa (Hebra) (698.2)
    pigmentosa (757.3)

708.0 *Allergic urticaria*

708.1 *Idiopathic urticaria*

708.2 *Urticaria due to cold and heat*

Thermal urticaria

708.3   *Dermatographic urticaria*

Factitial urticaria

708.4   *Vibratory urticaria*

708.5   *Cholinergic urticaria*

708.8   *Other specified urticaria*

Urticaria:
  chronic
  recurrent periodic

708.9   *Unspecified*

709   Other disorders of skin and subcutaneous tissue

709.0   *Dyschromia*

Café au lait spots   Anomalous pigmentation NOS
Chloasma: Hyperpigmentation
  NOS   Tattoo
  idiopathic   Vitiligo
  symptomatic

709.1   *Vascular disorders of skin*

Angioma serpiginosum   Purpura (primary) annularis
                                        telangiectodes

709.2   *Scar conditions and fibrosis of skin*

Adherent scar (skin)   Fibrosis, skin NOS
Cicatrix   Scar NOS
Disfigurement (due to scar)

709.3   *Degenerative skin disorders*

Calcinosis: Degeneration, skin
  circumscripta   Deposits, skin
  cutis   Senile dermatosis NOS
Colloid milium   Subcutaneous calcification

709.4   *Foreign body granuloma of skin and subcutaneous tissue*

709.8   *Other diseases of skin*

Epithelial hyperplasia   Vesicular eruption
Menstrual dermatosis

709.9   *Unspecified*

XIII. DISEASES OF THE MUSCULOSKELETAL SYSTEM AND CONNECTIVE TISSUE

The following fifth-digit subclassification may be used, if desired, with appropriate categories in Chapter XIII:

.0 *Multiple sites*

.1 *Shoulder region*
clavicle
scapula

acromioclavicular ⎫
glenohumeral   ⎬ joints
sternoclavicular ⎭

.2 *Upper arm*
humerus

elbow joint

.3 *Forearm*
radius
ulna

wrist joint

.4 *Hand*
carpus
metacarpus
phalanges [fingers]

joints between these bones

.5 *Pelvic region and thigh*
buttock
femur

hip (joint)

.6 *Lower leg*
fibula
tibia

knee joint

.7 *Ankle and foot*
digits [toes]
metatarsus
tarsus

ankle joint
other joints in foot

.8 *Other*
ribs
skull
vertebral column

head
neck
trunk

.9 *Site unspecified*

ARTHROPATHIES AND RELATED DISORDERS (710-719)

Excludes: disorders of spine (720-724)

710   Diffuse diseases of connective tissue
Includes: all collagen diseases whose effects are not mainly confined to a single system
Excludes: those affecting mainly the cardiovascular system, i.e., polyarteritis nodosa and allied conditions (446)

710.0 *Systemic lupus erythematosus*

Disseminated lupus erythematosus

Excludes: lupus erythematosus (discoid) NOS (695.4)

710.1 *Systemic sclerosis*

Scleroderma

Excludes: circumscribed scleroderma (701.0)

710.2 *Sicca syndrome*

Keratoconjunctivitis sicca† (370.3*)
Sjögren's disease

710.3 *Dermatomyositis*

Polymyositis with skin involvement

710.4 *Polymyositis*

710.8 *Other*

710.9 *Unspecified*

Collagen disease NOS

711   Arthropathy associated with infections

Excludes: rheumatic fever (390)

711.0 *Pyogenic arthritis*

Arthritis or polyarthritis (due to):
    coliform [Escherichia coli]
    Haemophilus influenzae
        [H. influenzae]
    pneumococcal

Arthritis or polyarthritis (due to):
    Pseudomonas
    staphylococcal
    streptococcal

Use additional code, if desired, to identify infectious organism

711.1* *Arthropathy in Reiter's disease and allied conditions* (099.3, 099.4†)

Arthritis or polyarthritis associated with nonspecific urethritis

711.2* *Arthropathy in Behcet's syndrome* (136.1†)

711.3* *Postdysenteric arthropathy*

Arthritis or polyarthritis associated with:
    dysentery (009.0†)
    enteritis (008.–, 009.–†)
    paratyphoid (002.–†)
    salmonellosis (003.2†)
    typhoid (002.0†)

711.4* *Arthropathy associated with other bacterial diseases*

Arthritis or polyarthritis (associated with):
  diseases classifiable to 010-040, 090-099 except as in 711.1*, 711.3*
    and 713.5*
  gonococcal (098.5†)
  leprosy (030.–†)
  meningococcal (036.8†)
  tuberculous (015.–†)

711.5* *Arthropathy associated with other viral diseases*

Arthritis or polyarthritis associated with:
  diseases classifiable to 045-049, 050-079, 480, 487
  O'nyong nyong (066.3†)
  rubella (056.7†)

711.6* *Arthropathy associated with mycoses* (110-118†)

711.7* *Arthropathy associated with helminthiasis*

Arthritis in dracontiasis (125.7†)
Chylous arthritis (125.9†)

711.8* *Arthropathy associated with other infectious and parasitic diseases*
    (080-088, 100-104, 130-136†)

Excludes: arthropathy associated with sarcoidosis (135†, 713.7*)

711.9 *Unspecified infective arthritis*

Infective arthritis or polyarthritis (acute) (chronic) (subacute) NOS

712   **Crystal arthropathies**

Includes: crystal-induced arthritis and synovitis

712.0* *Gouty arthritis* (274.0†)

712.1* *Chondrocalcinosis due to dicalcium phosphate crystals* (275.4†)

Chondrocalcinosis due to dicalcium phosphate crystals (with other
  crystals)

712.2* *Chondrocalcinosis due to pyrophosphate crystals* (275.4†)

712.3* *Chondrocalcinosis, unspecified* (275.4†)

712.8 *Other crystal arthropathies*

712.9 *Unspecified crystal arthropathy*

713* **Arthropathy associated with other disorders classified elsewhere**

Includes: arthritis
arthropathy
polyarthritis
polyarthropathy } associated with conditions listed below

713.0* *Arthropathy associated with other endocrine and metabolic disorders*

Associated with:
  acromegaly (253.0†)
  haemochromatosis (275.0†)
  hyperparathyroidism (252.0†)
  hypogammaglobulinaemia (279.0†)
  hypothyroidism (243, 244.–†)
  lipoid dermatoarthritis (272.8†)
  ochronosis (270.2†)

Excludes: arthropathy associated with amyloidosis (713.7*)
  arthropathy associated with diabetic neuropathy (713.5*)
  arthropathy in gout and other crystal deposition disorders
  (712.–*)

713.1* *Arthropathy associated with gastrointestinal conditions other than infections*

Associated with:
  regional enteritis (555.–†)
  ulcerative colitis (556†)

713.2* *Arthropathy associated with haematological disorders*

Associated with:
  haemoglobinopathy (282.4-282.7†)
  haemophilia (286.0-286.2†)
  leukaemia (204-208†)
  malignant reticulosis (202.3†)
  multiple myelomatosis (203.0†)

Excludes: arthropathy associated with Henoch-Schönlein purpura
  (713.6*)

713.3* *Arthropathy associated with dermatological disorders*

Associated with:
  erythema multiforme (695.1†)
  erythema nodosum (695.2†)
  psoriasis (696.0†)

713.4* *Arthropathy associated with respiratory disorders* (490-519†)

Excludes: arthropathy associated with respiratory infections (711.–*)

713.5* *Arthropathy associated with neurological disorders*

Charcot's arthropathy: Neuropathic arthritis (094.0†)
  NOS (094.0†)
  diabetic (250.5†)
  syringomyelic (336.0†)
  tabetic (094.0†)

713.6* *Arthropathy associated with hypersensitivity reaction*

Arthropathy associated with: Serum arthritis (999.5†)
  Henoch(-Schönlein) purpura (287.0†)
  serum sickness (999.5†)

Excludes: allergic arthritis NOS (716.2)

713.7* *Other general diseases with articular involvement*

Arthropathy associated with:
  amyloidosis (277.3†)
  familial Mediterranean fever (277.3†)
  sarcoidosis (135†)

713.8* *Arthropathy associated with other conditions classified elsewhere*

Arthropathy associated with conditions classified elsewhere, except as in
  711.1* to 711.8*, 712.–* and 713.0* to 713.7*

714   Rheumatoid arthritis and other inflammatory polyarthropathies

Excludes: rheumatic fever (390)
          rheumatoid arthritis of spine (720.–)

714.0 *Rheumatoid arthritis*

714.1 *Felty's syndrome*

Rheumatoid arthritis with splenoadenomegaly and leukopenia

714.2 *Other rheumatoid arthritis with visceral or systemic involvement*

714.3 *Juvenile chronic polyarthritis*

Juvenile rheumatoid arthritis   Still's disease

714.4 *Chronic postrheumatic arthropathy*

Jaccoud's syndrome

714.8 *Other*

714.9 *Unspecified*

Inflammatory polyarthropathy or polyarthritis NOS

715   Osteoarthrosis and allied disorders

Note: Localized, in the subcategories below, includes bilateral involvement of the same site.

Excludes: osteoarthrosis of spine (721.–)

715.0   *Generalized*

715.1   *Localized, primary*

715.2   *Localized, secondary*

715.3   *Localized, not specified whether primary or secondary*

715.8   *Involving or with mention of more than one site but not specified as generalized*

715.9   *Unspecified whether generalized or localized*

716   Other and unspecified arthropathies

Excludes: cricoarytenoid arthropathy (478.7)

716.0   *Kaschin-Beck disease*

716.1   *Traumatic arthropathy*

716.2   *Allergic arthritis*

Excludes: arthritis associated with Henoch-Schönlein purpura or serum sickness (713.6*)

716.3   *Climacteric arthritis*

716.4   *Transient arthropathy*

Excludes: palindromic rheumatism (719.3)

716.5   *Unspecified polyarthropathy or polyarthritis*

716.6   *Unspecified monoarthritis*

716.8   *Other specified arthropathy*

716.9   *Unspecified*

717   Internal derangement of knee

Excludes: ankylosis (718.5)
            contracture (718.4)
            current injury (836.–)
            deformity (736.6)
            recurrent dislocation (718.3)

717.0   *Old bucket handle tear of medial meniscus*

Old bucket handle tear of unspecified cartilage

717.1   *Derangement of anterior horn of medial meniscus*

717.2   *Derangement of posterior horn of medial meniscus*

717.3   *Other and unspecified derangement of medial meniscus*

717.4   *Derangement of lateral meniscus*

717.5   *Derangement of meniscus, not elsewhere classified*
Congenital discoid meniscus

717.6   *Loose body in knee*

717.7   *Chondromalacia patellae*

717.8   *Other*
Old disruption of ligament(s) of knee

717.9   *Unspecified*
Derangement NOS of knee

718   Other derangement of joint
Excludes: current injury (830.– to 848.–)

718.0   *Articular cartilage disorder*
Meniscus disorder
Excludes: chondrocalcinosis (275.4†, 712.–*)
in ochronosis (270.2)
knee (717.–)
metastatic calcification (275.4)

718.1   *Loose body in joint*
Excludes: knee (717.6)

718.2   *Pathological dislocation*
Dislocation or displacement of joint, not recurrent and not current injury
Spontaneous dislocation (joint)

718.3   *Recurrent dislocation of joint*

718.4   *Contracture of joint*

718.5   *Ankylosis of joint*
Excludes: spine (724.9)
stiffness of joint without mention of ankylosis (719.5)

718.6   *Unspecified protrusio acetabuli*

718.8   *Other joint derangement not elsewhere classified*
Excludes: deformities classifiable to 736.– (736.–)

718.9   *Unspecified*

719 Other and unspecified disorder of joint

719.0 *Effusion of joint*

Swelling of joint, with or without pain

719.1 *Haemarthrosis*

Excludes: current injury (840-848)
in haemophilia (286.0-286.2)

719.2 *Villonodular synovitis*

719.3 *Palindromic rheumatism*

719.4 *Pain in joint*

719.5 *Stiffness of joint, not elsewhere classified*

719.6 *Other symptoms referable to joint*

719.7 *Difficulty in walking*

719.8 *Other*

Excludes: temporomandibular joint-pain-dysfunction syndrome [Costen's syndrome] (524.6)

719.9 *Unspecified*

DORSOPATHIES (720-724)

Excludes: curvature of spine (737.–)
osteochondrosis of spine (732.–)

720 Ankylosing spondylitis and other inflammatory spondylopathies

720.0 *Ankylosing spondylitis*

Rheumatoid arthritis of spine NOS

720.1 *Spinal enthesopathy*

Disorder of peripheral ligamentous or muscular attachments of spine
Romanus lesion

720.2 *Sacroiliitis, not elsewhere classified*

720.8 *Other inflammatory spondylopathies*

Tuberculous spondylitis* (015.0†)

720.9 *Unspecified inflammatory spondylopathy*

721 Spondylosis and allied disorders

721.0 *Cervical spondylosis without myelopathy*

721.1† *Cervical spondylosis with myelopathy* (336.3*)

Anterior spinal artery compression syndrome
Spondylogenic compression of cervical spinal cord
Vertebral artery compression syndrome

721.2   *Thoracic spondylosis without myelopathy*

721.3   *Lumbosacral spondylosis without myelopathy*

721.4† *Thoracic or lumbar spondylosis with myelopathy* (336.3*)

Spondylogenic compression of thoracic or lumbar spinal cord

721.5   *Kissing spine*

Baastrup's syndrome

721.6   *Ankylosing vertebral hyperostosis*

721.7   *Traumatic spondylopathy*

Kümmell's disease or spondylitis

721.8   *Other*

721.9   *Spondylosis of unspecified site*

Spondylogenic compression of spinal cord NOS† (336.3*)

722   Intervertebral disc disorders

722.0   *Displacement of cervical intervertebral disc without myelopathy*

Neuritis (brachial) or radiculitis due to displacement or rupture of cervical
    intervertebral disc

722.1   *Displacement of thoracic or lumbar intervertebral disc without
    myelopathy*

Lumbago or sciatica due to displacement of intervertebral disc
Neuritis or radiculitis due to displacement or rupture of thoracolumbar
    intervertebral disc

722.2   *Displacement of intervertebral disc, site unspecified, without
    myelopathy*

Neuritis or radiculitis due to displacement or rupture of intervertebral disc

722.3   *Schmorl's nodes*

722.4   *Degeneration of cervical intervertebral disc*

Degeneration of cervicothoracic intervertebral disc

722.5   *Degeneration of thoracic or lumbar intervertebral disc*

Degeneration of thoracolumbar or lumbosacral intervertebral disc

722.6 *Degeneration of intervertebral disc, site unspecified*

722.7† *Intervertebral disc disorder with myelopathy (336.3*)*

722.8 *Postlaminectomy syndrome*

722.9 *Other and unspecified disc disorder*

723 Other disorders of cervical region

Excludes: conditions due to:
   intervertebral disc disorders (722.–)
   spondylosis (721.–)

723.0 *Spinal stenosis in cervical region*

723.1 *Cervicalgia*

723.2 *Cervicocranial syndrome*
Posterior cervical sympathetic syndrome

723.3 *Cervicobrachial syndrome (diffuse)*

723.4 *Brachial neuritis or radiculitis NOS*

723.5 *Torticollis, unspecified*
Excludes: congenital (756.8)
   due to birth injury (767.8)
   hysterical (300.1)
   psychogenic (306.0)
   spasmodic (333.8)
   traumatic, current (847.0)

723.6 *Panniculitis specified as affecting neck*

723.7 *Ossification of posterior longitudinal ligament in cervical region*

723.8 *Other syndromes affecting cervical region*

723.9 *Unspecified disorders and symptoms referable to neck*

724 Other and unspecified disorders of back

Excludes: collapsed vertebra (code to cause, e.g., osteoporosis, 733.0)
   conditions due to:
    intervertebral disc disorders (722.–)
    spondylosis (721.–)

724.0 *Spinal stenosis, other than cervical*

724.1 *Pain in thoracic spine*

724.2 *Lumbago*

724.3 *Sciatica*

Excludes: specified lesion of sciatic nerve (355.0)

724.4 *Thoracic or lumbosacral neuritis or radiculitis NOS*

724.5 *Backache, unspecified*

724.6 *Disorders of sacrum*

724.7 *Disorders of coccyx*

724.8 *Other symptoms referable to back*

Ossification of posterior longitudinal ligament NOS
Panniculitis specified as sacral or affecting back

724.9 *Unspecified back disorders*

Affection of sacroiliac joint NOS   Ankylosis of spine NOS

Excludes: sacroiliitis (720.2)

RHEUMATISM, EXCLUDING THE BACK (725-729)

Includes: disorders of muscles and tendons and their attachments, and
of other soft tissues

725   Polymyalgia rheumatica

726   Peripheral enthesopathies and allied syndromes

Note: Enthesopathies are disorders of peripheral ligamentous or muscular attachments.

Excludes: spinal enthesopathy (720.1)

726.0 *Adhesive capsulitis of shoulder*

726.1 *Rotator cuff syndrome of shoulder, and allied disorders*

Disorders of bursae and tendons in shoulder region

726.2 *Other affections of shoulder region, not elsewhere classified*

Periarthritis of shoulder   Scapulohumeral fibrositis

726.3 *Enthesopathy of elbow region*

Epicondylitis   Tennis elbow

726.4 *Enthesopathy of wrist and carpus*

Periarthritis of wrist

726.5   *Enthesopathy of hip region*

Gluteal tendinitis
Iliac crest spur

Psoas tendinitis
Trochanteric tendinitis

726.6   *Enthesopathy of knee*

Patellar tendinitis

Pellegrini-Stieda syndrome

726.7   *Enthesopathy of ankle and tarsus*

Achilles bursitis or tendinitis
Calcaneal spur

Metatarsalgia NOS
Tibialis anterior tendinitis

Excludes: Morton's metatarsalgia (355.6)

726.8   *Other peripheral enthesopathies*

726.9   *Unspecified enthesopathy*

Bone spur NOS
Capsulitis NOS

Periarthritis NOS
Tendinitis NOS

727   Other disorders of synovium, tendon and bursa

727.0   *Synovitis and tenosynovitis*

Synovitis:
  NOS
  gonococcal* (098.5†)

Synovitis:
  syphilitic* (095†)
  tuberculous* (015.–†)

Excludes: crystal-induced (275.4†, 712.–*)
            gouty (274.0†, 712.0*)

727.1   *Bunion*

727.2   *Specific bursitides often of occupational origin*

Beat:
  elbow
  hand
  knee

Chronic crepitant synovitis of wrist
Miners':
  elbow
  knee

727.3   *Other bursitis*

Bursitis:
  NOS
  gonococcal* (098.5†)
  syphilitic* (095†)

Excludes: bursitis:
            subacromial (726.1)
            subcoracoid (726.1)
            subdeltoid (726.1)
            "frozen shoulder" (726.0)

727.4 *Ganglion and cyst of synovium, tendon and bursa*

Cyst, bursal or synovial
Ganglion of joint or tendon

727.5 *Rupture of synovium*

727.6 *Rupture of tendon, nontraumatic*

727.8 *Other*

Abscess of bursa or tendon   Calcium deposits in bursa
Calcification of tendon NOS   Contracture of tendon (sheath)
Calcific tendinitis NOS   Short tendon

Excludes: xanthomatosis localized to tendons (272.7)

727.9 *Unspecified*

728   **Disorders of muscle, ligament and fascia**

Excludes: disruption of ligaments of knee (717.8)
            muscular dystrophies (359.–)
            myoneural disorders (358.–)
            myopathies (359.–)

728.0 *Infective myositis*

Myositis:
  purulent
  suppurative
  tropical* (040.8†)

Excludes: epidemic myositis (074.1)

728.1 *Muscular calcification and ossification*

Massive calcification (paraplegic)   Polymyositis ossificans
Myositis ossificans

728.2 *Muscular wasting and disuse atrophy, not elsewhere classified*

Myofibrosis

Excludes: neuralgic amyotrophy (353.5)
            progressive muscular atrophy (335.–)

728.3 *Other specific muscle disorders*

Arthrogryposis   Immobility syndrome (paraplegic)

Excludes: arthrogryposis multiplex congenita (755.8)
            stiff man syndrome (333.9)

728.4 *Laxity of ligament*

728.5 *Hypermobility syndrome*

728.6 *Contracture of palmar fascia*
Dupuytren's contracture

728.7 *Other fibromatoses*

Garrod's or knuckle pads
Nodular fasciitis

Plantar fasciitis (traumatic)
Pseudosarcomatous fibromatosis
(proliferative) (subcutaneous)

728.8 *Other disorders of muscle, ligament and fascia*

Foreign-body granuloma
Interstitial myositis

Talc granuloma

728.9 *Unspecified*

729 Other disorders of soft tissues
Excludes: acroparaesthesia (443.8)
carpal tunnel syndrome (354.0)
disorders of the back (720-724)
entrapment syndromes (354.–, 355.–)
palindromic rheumatism (719.3)
periarthritis (726.–)
psychogenic rheumatism (306.0)

729.0 *Rheumatism, unspecified, and fibrositis*

729.1 *Myalgia and myositis, unspecified*

729.2 *Neuralgia, neuritis and radiculitis, unspecified*
Excludes: brachial radiculitis (723.4)
lumbosacral radiculitis (724.4)
mononeuritis (354.–, 355.–)
sciatica (724.3)

729.3 *Panniculitis, unspecified*
Excludes: panniculitis specified as (affecting):
back (724.8)
neck (723.6)
sacral (724.8)

729.4 *Fasciitis, unspecified*
Excludes: nodular fasciitis (728.7)

729.5 *Pain in limb*

729.6 *Residual foreign body in soft tissue*

729.8 *Other symptoms referable to limbs*
Cramp   Swelling of limb

729.9 *Other and unspecified disorders of soft tissue*
Polyalgia

OSTEOPATHIES, CHONDROPATHIES AND ACQUIRED MUSCULOSKELETAL
DEFORMITIES (730-739)

730   Osteomyelitis, periostitis and other infections involving bone

Excludes: jaw (526.4, 526.5)
             petrous bone, i.e., mastoiditis (383.–)

Use additional code, if desired, to identify infectious organism, e.g.,
    Staphylococcus (041.1)

730.0 *Acute osteomyelitis*

Abscess of any bone except accessory sinus or mastoid
Acute or subacute osteomyelitis, with or without mention of periostitis

730.1 *Chronic osteomyelitis*

Chronic or old osteomyelitis, with or without mention of periostitis

730.2 *Unspecified osteomyelitis*

Osteitis or osteomyelitis NOS, with or without mention of periostitis

730.3 *Periostitis without mention of osteomyelitis*

Secondary syphilitic periostitis* (091.6†)

730.4* *Tuberculosis of spine* (015.0†)

Pott's disease

730.5* *Tuberculosis of limb bones* (015.1, 015.2, 015.7†)

730.6* *Tuberculosis of other bones* (015.7†)

730.7* *Osteopathy resulting from poliomyelitis* (045.–†)

730.8* *Other infections involving bone*

Syphilis of bone NOS (095†)

730.9 *Unspecified infection of bone*

**731   Osteitis deformans and osteopathies associated with other disorders
classified elsewhere**

731.0 *Osteitis deformans without mention of bone tumour*

Paget's disease of bone

731.1* *Osteitis deformans in diseases classified elsewhere*

731.2 *Hypertrophic pulmonary osteoarthropathy*

Bamberger-Marie disease

731.8* *Other bone involvement in diseases classified elsewhere*

732 Osteochondropathies

732.0 *Juvenile osteochondrosis of spine*
Juvenile osteochondrosis:
  marginal or vertebral epiphysis (of Schuermann)
  spine NOS
  vertebral body (of Calvé)
Excludes: adolescent postural kyphosis (737.0)

732.1 *Juvenile osteochondrosis of hip and pelvis*
Osteochondrosis (juvenile):
  acetabulum
  head of femur (of Legg-Calvé-Perthes)
  iliac crest (of Buchanan)
  ischiopubic synchondrosis (of van Neck)
  symphysis pubis (of Pierson)

732.2 *Nontraumatic slipped upper femoral epiphysis*
Slipped upper femoral epiphysis NOS

732.3 *Juvenile osteochondrosis of upper extremity*
Osteochondrosis (juvenile):
  capitulum of humerus (of Panner)
  carpal lunate (of Kienbock)
  hand NOS
  head of humerus (of Hass)
  heads of metacarpals (of Mauclaire)
  lower ulna (of Burns)
  upper extremity NOS

732.4 *Juvenile osteochondrosis of lower extremity, excluding foot*
Osteochondrosis (juvenile):
  lower extremity NOS
  primary patellar centre (of Köhler)
  proximal tibia (of Blount)
  secondary patellar centre (of Sinding-Larsen)
  tibial tubercle (of Osgood-Schlatter)

732.5 *Juvenile osteochondrosis of foot*
Calcaneal apophysitis
Osteochondrosis (juvenile):
  astragalus (of Diaz)
  calcaneum (of Sever)
  foot NOS
  metatarsal
    fifth (of Iselin)
    second (of Freiberg)
  os tibiale externum (of Haglund)
  tarsal navicular (of Köhler)

732.6   *Other juvenile osteochondrosis*

Apophysitis ⎫
Epiphysitis ⎪
Osteochondritis ⎬ specified as juvenile, of other site, or site NOS
Osteochondrosis ⎭

732.7   *Osteochondritis dissecans*

732.8   *Other specified forms of osteochondropathy*

Adult osteochondrosis of spine

732.9   *Unspecified osteochondropathy*

Apophysitis ⎫
Epiphysitis ⎪
Osteochondritis ⎬ not specified as adult or juvenile, of unspecified site
Osteochondrosis ⎭

733   Other disorders of bone and cartilage

Excludes: bone spur (726.9)
            cartilage or loose body in joint (717.–, 718.–)
            giant cell granuloma of jaw (526.3)
            osteitis fibrosa cystica generalisata (252.0)
            osteomalacia (268.2)
            polyostotic fibrous dysplasia of bone (756.5)
            prognathism, retrognathism (524.1)
            xanthomatosis localized to bone (272.7)

733.0   *Osteoporosis*

733.1   *Pathological fracture*

Spontaneous fracture

733.2   *Cyst of bone*

Cyst of bone (localized)

Excludes: cyst of jaw (526.–)
            osteitis fibrosa cystica (252.0)

733.3   *Hyperostosis of skull*

733.4   *Aseptic necrosis of bone*

Excludes: necrosis of bone, NOS (730.1)
            osteochondropathies (732.–)

733.5   *Osteitis condensans*

733.6   *Tietze's disease*

733.7   *Algoneurodystrophy*

733.8   *Malunion and nonunion of fracture*

Pseudoarthrosis

733.9   *Other and unspecified*

Diaphysitis   Relapsing polychondritis

734   Flat foot

Pes planus (acquired)

Excludes: congenital (754.6)
              rigid flat foot (754.6)
              spastic (everted) flat foot (754.6)

735   Acquired deformities of toe

Excludes: congenital (754.6, 755.6)

735.0   *Hallux valgus (acquired)*

735.1   *Hallux varus (acquired)*

735.2   *Hallux rigidus*

735.3   *Hallux malleus*

735.4   *Other hammer toe (acquired)*

735.5   *Clawtoe (acquired)*

735.8   *Other*

735.9   *Unspecified*

736   Other acquired deformities of limbs

Excludes: congenital (754.–, 755.–)

736.0   *Acquired deformities of forearm, excluding fingers*

Clawhand   Deformity of elbow, forearm, hand
Clubhand, acquired   or wrist (acquired) NOS
Cubitus valgus or varus (acquired)

Excludes: lobster-claw hand (755.5)

736.1   *Mallet finger*

736.2   *Other acquired deformities of finger*

Deformity of finger (acquired) NOS
              clubbing of fingers (781.5)

Excludes: trigger finger (727.0)

736.3   *Acquired deformities of hip*

Coxa valga or vara (acquired)   Deformity of hip (acquired) NOS

736.4   *Genu valgum or varum (acquired)*

736.5   *Genu recurvatum (acquired)*

736.6   *Other acquired deformities of knee*

Genu extrorsum   Deformity of knee (acquired) NOS

736.7   *Other acquired deformities of ankle and foot*

Acquired: Acquired:
  clawfoot   equinovarus
  clubfoot   pes, except planus
  deformity of ankle or foot   talipes, except planus

Excludes: clubfoot not specified as acquired (754.–)
            deformities of toe (acquired) (735.–)
            pes planus (acquired) (734)

736.8   *Acquired deformities of other parts of limbs*

Deformity (acquired):
  arm or leg, not elsewhere classified
  shoulder

736.9   *Acquired deformity of limb, site unspecified*

737   Curvature of spine

Excludes: congenital (754.2)

737.0   *Adolescent postural kyphosis*

Excludes: osteochondrosis of spine (732.0, 732.8)

737.1   *Kyphosis (acquired)*

737.2   *Lordosis (acquired) (postural)*

737.3   *Kyphoscoliosis and scoliosis*

Excludes: in kyphoscoliotic heart disease (416.1)

737.4* *Curvature of spine associated with other conditions*

Associated with:
  Charcot-Marie-Tooth disease (356.1†)
  osteitis deformans (731.0†)
  osteitis fibrosa cystica (252.0†)
  tuberculosis [Pott's curvature] (015.0†)

737.8   *Other*

737.9   *Unspecified*

Curvature of spine (acquired) (idiopathic) NOS
Hunchback, acquired

Excludes: deformity of spine NOS (738.5)

738 Other acquired deformity

Excludes: congenital (754-756 and 758-759)
dentofacial anomalies (524.-)

738.0 *Acquired deformity of nose*

Deformity of nose (acquired)   Overdevelopment of nasal bones

Excludes: deflected nasal septum (470)

738.1 *Other acquired deformity of head*

738.2 *Acquired deformity of neck*

738.3 *Acquired deformity of chest and rib*

Deformity:
  chest (acquired)
  rib (acquired)

738.4 *Acquired spondylolisthesis*

Degenerative spondylolisthesis

Excludes: congenital (756.1)

738.5 *Other acquired deformity of back or spine*

Excludes: curvature of spine (737.-)

738.6 *Acquired deformity of pelvis*

Excludes: in relation to labour and delivery (653.-)

738.7 *Cauliflower ear*

738.8 *Acquired deformity of other specified site*

738.9 *Acquired deformity of unspecified site*

739 Nonallopathic lesions, not elsewhere classified

Includes: segmental dysfunction
somatic dysfunction

739.0 *Head region*

739.1 *Cervical region*

Cervicothoracic region

739.2 *Thoracic region*

Thoracolumbar region

739.3 *Lumbar region*

Lumbosacral region

739.4   *Sacral region*

Sacrococcygeal region   Sacroiliac region

739.5   *Pelvic region*

Hip region   Pubic region

739.6   *Lower extremities*

739.7   *Upper extremities*

Acromioclavicular   Sternoclavicular

739.8   *Rib cage*

Costochondral   Sternochondral
Costovertebral

739.9   *Abdomen and other*

XIV. CONGENITAL ANOMALIES

740   Anencephalus and similar anomalies

740.0   *Anencephalus*

Acrania
Amyelencephalus

Hemianencephaly
Hemicephaly

740.1   *Craniorachischisis*

740.2   *Iniencephaly*

741   Spina bifida

Excludes: spina bifida occulta (756.1)

741.0   *With hydrocephalus*

Arnold-Chiari syndrome
Any condition in 741.9 with any condition in 742.3

741.9   *Without mention of hydrocephalus*

Hydromeningocele (spinal)
Meningocele (spinal)
Meningomyelocele
Myelocele

Myelocystocele
Rachischisis
Spina bifida (aperta)
Syringomyelocele

742   Other congenital anomalies of nervous system

742.0   *Encephalocele*

Encephalomyelocele
Hydroencephalocele
Hydromeningocele, cranial

Meningocele, cerebral
Meningoencephalocele

742.1   *Microcephalus*

Hydromicrocephaly

Micrencephalon

742.2   *Reduction deformities of brain*

Absence ⎫
Agenesis ⎬ of part of brain
Aplasia ⎪
Hypoplasia ⎭

Agyria
Arhinencephaly
Microgyria

742.3   *Congenital hydrocephalus*

Aqueduct of Sylvius:
   anomaly
   obstruction, congenital
   stenosis

Atresia of foramina of Magendie
   and Luschka
Hydrocephalus in newborn

Excludes: hydrocephalus:
            acquired (331.4)
            due to congenital toxoplasmosis (771.2†, 331.4*)
            with any condition in 741.9 (741.0)

742.4 *Other specified anomalies of brain*

Congenital cerebral cyst
Lissencephaly
Macrogyria
Megalencephaly

Porencephaly
Ulegyria
Multiple anomalies of brain NOS

742.5 *Other specified anomalies of spinal cord*

Amyelia
Atelomyelia
Congenital anomaly of spinal
   meninges
Defective development of cauda
   equina

Hydromyelia
Hydrorhachis
Hypoplasia of spinal cord
Myelatelia

742.8 *Other specified anomalies of nervous system*

Agenesis of nerve
Displacement of brachial plexus

Familial dysautonomia

Excludes: neurofibromatosis (237.7)

742.9 *Unspecified anomalies of brain, spinal cord and nervous system*

Anomaly
Congenital disease or lesion } of { brain
Deformity   { nervous system
                                                    { spinal cord

743   **Congenital anomalies of eye**

743.0 *Anophthalmos*

Agenesis of eye

Cryptophthalmos

743.1 *Microphthalmos*

Aplasia of eye
Dysplasia of eye

Hypoplasia of eye
Rudimentary eye

743.2 *Buphthalmos*

Glaucoma:
  congenital
  newborn

Hydrophthalmos
Keratoglobus, congenital
Megalocornea

743.3 *Congenital cataract and lens anomalies*

Congenital aphakia

Spherophakia

743.4 *Coloboma and other anomalies of anterior segments*

Aniridia
Anisocoria, congenital
Atresia of pupil
Coloboma of iris
Corectopia

Corneal opacity, congenital
Microcornea
Peter's anomaly
Rieger's anomaly

743.5 *Congenital anomalies of posterior segment*

Coloboma: Congenital:
  fundus   retinal aneurysm
  optic disc   vitreous opacity

743.6 *Congenital anomalies of eyelids, lacrimal system and orbit*

Ablepharon   Accessory:
Absence, agenesis of   eyelid
  cilia   eye muscles
  eyelid   Congenital:
  lacrimal apparatus   entropion
  punctum lacrimale   ptosis

743.8 *Other specified anomalies of eye*

Ocular albinism* (270.2)

Excludes: congenital nystagmus (379.5)
          retinitis pigmentosa (362.7)

743.9 *Unspecified anomalies of eye*

Congenital:
  anomaly NOS } of eye [any part]
  deformity NOS

744 **Congenital anomalies of ear, face and neck**

Excludes: anomaly of:
          cervical spine (754.2, 756.1)
          larynx (748.2, 748.3)
          parathyroid gland (759.2)
          thyroid gland (759.2)
        cleft lip (749.1)

744.0 *Anomalies of ear causing impairment of hearing*

Absence of: Congenital anomaly of:
  auditory canal (external)   membranous labyrinth
  auricle (ear)   middle ear
  ear, congenital   organ of Corti
Atresia or stricture of: Fusion, ear ossicles
  auditory canal (external)
  osseous meatus (ear)

Excludes: congenital deafness without mention of cause (389.–)

744.1 *Accessory auricle*

Accessory tragus   Supernumerary:
Polyotia   ear
Preauricular appendage   lobule

744.2   *Other specified anomalies of ear*

Absence: Darwin's tubercle
    Eustachian tube   Macrotia
    lobe, congenital   Microtia
Bat ear   Pointed ear

Excludes: preauricular sinus (744.4)

744.3   *Unspecified anomalies of ear*

Congenital: ⎫
    anomaly NOS   ⎬ of ear [any part]
    deformity NOS . ⎭

744.4   *Branchial cleft, cyst or fistula; preauricular sinus*

Branchial: Fistula of:
    sinus (internal) (external)   auricle, congenital
    vestige   cervicoaural
Cervical auricle   Preauricular cyst

744.5   *Webbing of neck*

Pterygium colli

744.8   *Other specified anomalies of face and neck*

Hypertrophy of lip, congenital   Microcheilia
Macrocheilia   Microstomia
Macrostomia

Excludes: those conditions classified to 754.–

744.9   *Unspecified anomalies of face and neck*
Congenital: ⎫
    anomaly NOS   ⎬ of face [any part] or neck [any part]
    deformity NOS   ⎭

745   Bulbus cordis anomalies and anomalies of cardiac septal closure

745.0   *Common truncus*

Absent septum   ⎫
Communication (abnormal)   ⎬ between aorta and pulmonary artery
Aortic septal defect
Persistent truncus arteriosus

745.1   *Transposition of great vessels*

Dextra transposition of aorta
Origin of both great vessels from right ventricle
Taussig-Bing syndrome
Transposition of great vessels (complete) (corrected) (incomplete)

745.2 *Tetralogy of Fallot*

Ventricular septal defect with pulmonary stenosis or atresia, dextraposition of aorta and hypertrophy of right ventricle

745.3 *Common ventricle*

Cor triloculare biatriatum   Single ventricle

745.4 *Ventricular septal defect*

Eisenmenger defect   Left ventricular-right atrial com-
Gerbode defect   munication
Interventricular septal defect   Roger's disease

Excludes: common atrioventricular canal type (745.6)

745.5 *Ostium secundum type atrial septal defect*

Patent or persistent:
   foramen ovale
   ostium secundum

745.6 *Endocardial cushion defects*

Atrioventricular canal type   Common atrium
   ventricular septal defect   Persistent ostium primum
Common atrioventricular canal

745.7 *Cor biloculare*

745.8 *Other*

745.9 *Unspecified defect of septal closure*

Septal defect NOS

746   **Other congenital anomalies of heart**

Excludes: endocardial fibroelastosis (425.3)

746.0 *Anomalies of pulmonary valve*

Congenital:
   atresia
   insufficiency   } of pulmonary valve
   stenosis

746.1 *Tricuspid atresia and stenosis, congenital*

746.2 *Ebstein's anomaly*

746.3 *Congenital stenosis of aortic valve*

Congenital aortic stenosis

746.4 *Congenital insufficiency of aortic valve*

Bicuspid aortic valve   Congenital aortic insufficiency

746.5   *Congenital mitral stenosis*

746.6   *Congenital mitral insufficiency*

746.7   *Hypoplastic left heart syndrome*

Atresia, or marked hypoplasia, of aortic orifice or valve, with hypoplasia
of ascending aorta and defective development of left ventricle (with
mitral valve atresia)

746.8   *Other specified anomalies of heart*

Congenital: Dextrocardia
  heart block   Ectopia cordis
  diverticulum, left ventricle Levocardia (isolated)
  pericardial defect   Malposition of heart
Cor triatriatum   Pulmonary infundibular stenosis
Coronary artery anomaly   Uhl's disease

746.9   *Unspecified anomalies of heart*

Congenital:
  anomaly, heart NOS
  heart disease NOS

747   Other congenital anomalies of circulatory system

747.0   *Patent ductus arteriosus*

Patent ductus Botalli   Persistent ductus arteriosus

747.1   *Coarctation of aorta*

Coarctation of aorta (preductal) (postductal)
Interruption of aortic arch

747.2   *Other anomalies of aorta*

Absence ⎫   Hypoplasia of aorta
Aplasia ⎪   Overriding aorta
Atresia ⎬ of aorta   Persistent:
Congenital: ⎪   convolutions, aortic arch
  aneurysm ⎪   right aortic arch
  dilatation ⎭   Stenosis ⎫
Aneurysm of sinus of Valsalva   Stricture ⎬ of aorta (ascending)
Dextraposition of aorta   Supra-aortic stenosis

Excludes: congenital aortic stenosis or stricture, so described (746.3)
          hypoplasia of aorta in hypoplastic left heart syndrome (746.7)

747.3   *Anomalies of pulmonary artery*

Agenesis   ⎫
Anomaly   ⎪
Atresia   ⎬ of pulmonary artery
Hypoplasia ⎪
Stenosis   ⎭
Pulmonary arteriovenous aneurysm

747.4 *Anomalies of great veins*

Absence
Anomaly } of vena cava (inferior) (superior)
Congenital stenosis
Persistent:
   left posterior cardinal vein
   left superior vena cava
Total anomalous pulmonary venous connection

747.5 *Absence or hypoplasia of umbilical artery*

Single umbilical artery

747.6 *Other anomalies of peripheral vascular system*

Absence   Congenital:
Anomaly } of artery or vein, not   aneurysm (peripheral)
Atresia   elsewhere classified   phlebectasia
Arteriovenous aneurysm (peripheral)   stricture, artery
Multiple renal arteries   varix

Excludes: anomalies of:
               cerebral vessels (747.8)
               pulmonary artery (747.3)
               congenital retinal aneurysm (743.8)
               haemangioma and lymphangioma (228.–)

747.8 *Other specified anomalies of circulatory system*

Aneurysm:
   arteriovenous, congenital of brain
   congenital, specified site not elsewhere classified
Congenital anomalies of cerebral vessels

Excludes: congenital aneurysm:
               coronary (746.8)
               peripheral (747.6)
               pulmonary (747.3)
               retinal (743.8)
               ruptured:
                   cerebral arteriovenous aneurysm (430)
                   congenital cerebral aneurysm (430)

747.9 *Unspecified anomalies of circulatory system*

748   Congenital anomalies of respiratory system

Excludes: congenital defect of diaphragm (756.6)

748.0 *Choanal atresia*

Atresia
Congenital stenosis } of nares (anterior) (posterior)

748.1 Other anomalies of nose

Absent nose
Accessory nose
Cleft nose
Deformity of wall of nasal sinus

Congenital:
deformity of nose
notching of tip of nose
perforation of wall of nasal sinus

Excludes: congenital deviation, nasal septum (754.0)

748.2 Web of larynx

Web of larynx:
NOS
glottic
subglottic

748.3 Other anomalies of larynx, trachea and bronchus

Absence ⎱ of bronchus, larynx or
Agenesis ⎰ trachea
Anomaly (of):
cricoid cartilage
epiglottis
thyroid cartilage
tracheal cartilage
Atresia (of):
epiglottis
glottis
larynx
trachea
Cleft thyroid, cartilage, congenital

Congenital:
dilatation, trachea
stenosis:
larynx
trachea
tracheocele
Diverticulum, bronchus
Fissure of epiglottis
Laryngocele
Posterior cleft of cricoid cartilage
(congenital)
Rudimentary tracheal bronchus
Stridor, laryngeal, congenital

748.4 Congenital cystic lung

Disease, lung:
cystic, congenital
polycystic, congenital

Honeycomb lung, congenital

Excludes: acquired or unspecified (518.8)

748.5 Agenesis, hypoplasia and dysplasia of lung

Absence of lung (lobe)
Aplasia of lung

Hypoplasia of lung (lobe)
Sequestration of lung

748.6 Other anomalies of lung

Congenital bronchiectasis

748.8 Other specified anomalies of respiratory system

Anomaly, pleural folds
Atresia of nasopharynx

Congenital cyst of mediastinum

748.9   *Unspecified anomalies of respiratory system*

Absence of respiratory organ NOS   Anomaly of respiratory system
                                                      NOS

749   Cleft palate and cleft lip

749.0   *Cleft palate*

Cleft uvula   Palatoschisis
Fissure, palate

749.1   *Cleft lip*

Cheiloschisis   Harelip
Congenital fissure of lip   Labium leporinum

749.2   *Cleft palate with cleft lip*

750   Other congenital anomalies of upper alimentary tract

750.0   *Tongue tie*

Ankyloglossia

750.1   *Other anomalies of tongue*

Aglossia   Fissure of tongue
Congenital: Hypoplasia of tongue
  adhesion of tongue   Macroglossia
  hypertrophy of tongue   Microglossia

750.2   *Other specified anomalies of mouth and pharynx*

Absence: Congenital fistula of:
  salivary gland   lip
  uvula   salivary gland
Accessory salivary gland   Diverticulum of pharynx
Atresia, salivary duct   Pharyngeal pouch

750.3   *Tracheo-oesophageal fistula, oesophageal atresia and stenosis*

Absent oesophagus   Congenital:
Atresia of oesophagus   stenosis of oesophagus
Congenital fistula: stricture of oesophagus
  oesophagobronchial   Imperforate oesophagus
  oesophagotracheal   Webbed oesophagus

750.4 *Other specified anomalies of oesophagus*

Dilatation, congenital
Displacement, congenital
Diverticulum } (of) oesophagus
Duplication
Giant
Oesophageal pouch

750.5 *Congenital hypertrophic pyloric stenosis*

Congenital or infantile:
  constriction
  hypertrophy
  spasm } of pylorus
  stenosis
  stricture

750.6 *Congenital hiatus hernia*

Displacement of cardia through oesophageal hiatus

Excludes: congenital diaphragmatic hernia (756.6)

750.7 *Other specified anomalies of stomach*

Congenital:
  cardiospasm
  hourglass stomach
Displacement of stomach
Diverticulum of stomach, congenital

Duplication of stomach
Megalogastria
Microgastria
Transposition of stomach

750.8 *Other specified anomalies of upper alimentary tract*

750.9 *Unspecified anomalies of upper alimentary tract*

Congenital:
  anomaly NOS } of upper alimentary tract [any part, except tongue]
  deformity NOS

751 Other congenital anomalies of digestive system

751.0 *Meckel's diverticulum*

Meckel's diverticulum (displaced) (hypertrophic)
Persistent:
  omphalomesenteric duct
  vitelline duct

751.1 *Atresia and stenosis of small intestine*

Atresia of:
  duodenum
  ileum
  intestine NOS
Imperforate jejunum

Congenital:
  absence
  obstruction } of small intestine
  stenosis   or intestine
  stricture   NOS

751.2 Atresia and stenosis of large intestine, rectum and anal canal

Absence:
  anus (congenital)
  appendix, congenital
  large intestine, congenital
  rectum
Atresia of:
  anus
  colon
  rectum

Congenital or infantile:
  obstruction of large intestine
  occlusion of anus
  stricture of anus
Imperforate:
  anus
  rectum
Stricture of rectum, congenital

751.3 Hirschsprung's disease and other congenital functional disorders of colon

Anganglionosis
Congenital dilatation of colon

Congenital megacolon
Macrocolon

751.4 Anomalies of intestinal fixation

Congenital adhesions:
  omental, anomalous
  peritoneal
Jackson's membrane
Malrotation of colon

Rotation:
  failure of ⎫
  incomplete ⎬ of caecum or
  insufficient ⎭ colon
Universal mesentery

751.5 Other anomalies of intestine

Congenital diverticulitis, colon
Dolichocolon
Duplication of:
  anus
  appendix
  caecum
  intestine
Ectopic anus

Megaloappendix
Megaloduodenum
Microcolon
Persistent cloaca
Transposition of:
  appendix
  colon
  intestine

Excludes: congenital pilonidal cyst or sinus (685)

751.6 Anomalies of gallbladder, bile ducts and liver

Absence of:
  bile duct, congenital
  gallbladder, congenital
  liver
Accessory:
  hepatic ducts
  liver
Atresia of bile duct
Congenital:
  cystic disease of liver
  hepatomegaly
  obstruction, bile duct or passage†
    (774.5*)

Congenital:
  polycystic disease of liver
  stricture of:
    bile duct
    common duct
Duplication of:
  biliary duct
  cystic duct
  gallbladder
  liver
Fibrocystic disease of liver
Intrahepatic gallbladder

751.7   *Anomalies of pancreas*

Absence ⎫
Agenesis ⎬ of pancreas   Accessory pancreas
Hypoplasia ⎭   Annular pancreas

Excludes: diabetes mellitus:
                congenital (250.–)
                neonatal (775.1)
            fibrocystic disease of pancreas (277.0)

751.8   *Other specified anomalies of digestive system*

Absence (complete) (partial) of alimentary tract NOS
Duplication ⎫
Malposition, congenital ⎬ of digestive organs NOS

Excludes: congenital diaphragmatic hernia (756.6)
            congenital hiatus hernia (750.6)

751.9   *Unspecified anomalies of digestive system*

Congenital: ⎫
    anomaly NOS ⎬ of digestive system NOS
    deformity NOS ⎭

752   Congenital anomalies of genital organs

Excludes: syndromes associated with anomalies in the number and form
                of chromosomes (758.–)
            testicular feminization syndrome (251.8)

752.0   *Anomalies of ovaries*

Absence ⎫
Agenesis ⎬ (of) ovary
Streak ⎭

752.1   *Anomalies of fallopian tubes and broad ligaments*

Absence ⎫
Accessory ⎬ (of) fallopian tube or broad ligament
Atresia ⎭
Cyst:
    epoophoron
    fimbrial
    Gartner's duct
    parovarian

752.2   *Doubling of uterus*

Doubling of uterus [any degree] (associated with doubling of cervix and
    vagina)

752.3   Other anomalies of uterus

Absence ⎤
Agenesis ⎬ of uterus
Aplasia ⎦

Bicornuate uterus
Uterus unicornis
Uterus with only one functioning
    horn

752.4   Anomalies of cervix, vagina and external female genitalia

Absence ⎤
Agenesis ⎬ of cervix, clitoris, vagina or vulva
Anomalous development ⎦
Cyst of:
    canal of Nuck, congenital
    vagina, embryonal
    vulva, congenital
Imperforate hymen

Excludes: double vagina associated with total duplication (752.2)

752.5   Undescended testicle

Cryptorchism   Ectopic testis

752.6   Hypospadias and epispadias

Anaspadias   Congenital chordee

752.7   Indeterminate sex and pseudohermaphroditism

Gynandrism   Pseudohermaphroditism (male)
Hermaphroditism   (female)
Ovotestis   Pure gonadal dysgenesis

Excludes: pseudohermaphroditism:
                female, with adrenocortical disorder (255.2)
                male, with gonadal disorder (257.9)
                with specified chromosomal anomaly (758.–)

752.8   Other specified anomalies of genital organs

Absence of:
    penis
    prostate
    spermatic cord
Aplasia (congenital) of:
    prostate
    round ligament
    testicle
Atresia of:
    ejaculatory duct
    vas deferens

Curvature of penis (lateral)
Fusion of testes
Hypoplasia of:
    penis
    testis
Monorchism
Paraspadias
Polyorchism

Excludes: congenital hydrocele (778.6)

752.9   *Unspecified anomalies of genital organs*

Congenital: ⎫
   anomaly NOS ⎬ of genital organ, not else-
   deformity NOS ⎭ where classified

753   Congenital anomalies of urinary system

753.0   *Renal agenesis and dysgenesis*

Atrophy of kidney: Congenital absence of kidney(s)
   congenital   Hypoplasia of kidney(s)
   infantile

753.1   *Cystic kidney disease*

Cyst of kidney (congenital) (multiple)   Renal degeneration or disease:
Fibrocystic kidney   fibrocystic
Polycystic (disease of) kidney   polycystic

Excludes: acquired cyst of kidney (593.2)

753.2   *Obstructive defects of renal pelvis and ureter*

Atresia of ureter   Congenital:
Congenital: stricture of:
   dilatation of ureter   ureter
   hydronephrosis   ureteropelvic junction
   megaloureter   ureterovesical orifice
   occlusion of ureter   ureterocele
                                        Impervious ureter

753.3   *Other specified anomalies of kidney*

Accessory kidney   Fusion of kidneys
Congenital: Giant kidney
   calculus of kidney   Horseshoe kidney
   displaced kidney   Hyperplasia of kidney
Double kidney with double pelvis   Lobulation of kidney, foetal
Ectopic kidney   Malrotation of kidney

753.4   *Other specified anomalies of ureter*

Absent ureter   Double ureter
Accessory ureter   Ectopic ureter
Deviation of ureter   Implantation, anomalous of
Displaced ureteric orifice   ureter

753.5   *Exstrophy of urinary bladder*

Ectopia vesicae   Extroversion of bladder

753.6   *Atresia and stenosis of urethra and bladder neck*

Congenital bladder neck obstruction   Impervious urethra
Congenital stricture of:
   urethra (valvular)
   urinary meatus
   vesicourethral orifice

753.7   *Anomalies of urachus*

Cyst of urachus   Patent urachus

753.8   *Other specified anomalies of bladder and urethra*

Absence, congenital of: Congenital urethrorectal fistula
  bladder   Congenital prolapse of:
  urethra   bladder (mucosa)
Accessory: urethra
  bladder   Double:
  urethra   urethra
Congenital: urinary meatus
  diverticulum of bladder
  hernia of bladder

753.9   *Unspecified anomalies of urinary system*

Congenital:
  anomaly NOS   } of urinary system [any part, except urachus]
  deformity NOS

754   Certain congenital musculoskeletal deformities

754.0   *Of skull, face and jaw*

Asymmetry of face   Dolichocephaly
Compression facies   Plagiocephaly
Depressions in skull   Potter's facies
Deviation of nasal septum, congenital Squashed or bent nose, congenital

Excludes: dentofacial anomalies (524.–)
           syphilitic saddle nose (090.5)

754.1   *Of sternocleidomastoid muscle*

Congenital sternomastoid torticollis   Sternomastoid tumour
Contracture of sternocleidomastoid
   (muscle)

754.2   *Of spine*

Congenital postural:
  lordosis
  scoliosis

754.3   *Congenital dislocation of hip*

Congenital: Predislocation status of hip at birth
  dislocatable hip
  preluxation hip

754.4   *Congenital genu recurvatum and bowing of long bones of leg*

Congenital bowing of: Congenital dislocation of knee
  femur
  tibia and fibula

754.5 *Varus deformities of feet*

Metatarsus varus   Talipes equinovarus
Talipes calcaneovarus
Excludes: acquired (736.7)

754.6 *Valgus deformities of feet*

Congenital pes planus   Congenital valgus deformity of
Talipes calcaneovalgus   foot

Excludes: pes planus (acquired) (734)
                  valgus deformity of foot (acquired) (736.7)

754.7 *Other deformities of feet*

Asymmetric talipes   Congenital deformity of foot NOS
Clubfoot NOS   Talipes NOS

Excludes: acquired (736.7)

754.8 *Other specified*

Congenital: Clubhand (congenital)
    deformity of chest wall   Generalized flexion contractures of
    dislocation of elbow   lower limb joints, congenital
    funnel chest   Pectus excavatum
    pigeon chest   Spade-like hand (congenital)

755   Other congenital anomalies of limbs

Excludes: those deformities classified to 754.–

755.0 *Polydactyly*

Accessory fingers or toes   Supernumerary digits

755.1 *Syndactyly*

Fusion of fingers or toes   Webbed fingers or toes
Symphalangy

755.2 *Reduction deformities of upper limb*

Absence, congenital (complete or   Amelia   ⎫
    partial) of: Ectromelia ⎪
    arm   Hemimelia   ⎬ of upper limb
    finger   Phocomelia ⎭
    hand   Rudimentary arm
    radius   Shortening of arm, congenital

755.3 *Reduction deformities of lower limb*

Absence, congenital (complete or   Amelia   ⎫
    partial) of: Ectromelia ⎪
    femur   Hemimelia   ⎬ of lower limb
    foot   Phocomelia ⎭
    leg   Shortening of leg, congenital
    toe

755.4 *Reduction deformities, unspecified limb*

Absence, congenital (complete or partial) of limb NOS

Amelia
Ectromelia
Hemimelia
Phocomelia
} of unspecified limb

755.5 *Other anomalies of upper limb, including shoulder girdle*

Accessory carpal bones
Acrocephalosyndactyly
Cleidocranial dysostosis
Congenital deformity of:
  clavicle
  scapula

Lobster-claw hand
Macrodactylia (fingers)
Madelung's deformity
Radio-ulnar synostosis
Sprengel's deformity

755.6 *Other anomalies of lower limb, including pelvic girdle*

Astragalo-scaphoid synostosis
Congenital:
  absence of patella
  angulation of tibia
  anteversion of femur
  coxa valga
  coxa vara
  deformity (of):
    ankle (joint)
    knee (joint)
    sacroiliac (joint)

Congenital:
  fusion of sacroiliac joint
  genu valgum
  genu varum
  hallux varus
  hammer toe
Rudimentary patella

755.8 *Other specified anomalies of unspecified limb*

Arthrogryposis multiplex congenita

755.9 *Unspecified anomalies of unspecified limb*

Congenital:
  anomaly NOS
  deformity NOS
} of unspecified limb

Excludes: reduction deformity of unspecified limb (755.4)

756 Other congenital musculoskeletal anomalies

Excludes: those deformities classified to 754.–

756.0 *Anomalies of skull and face bones*

Absence of skull bone
Acrocephaly
Congenital deformity of forehead
Craniosynostosis
Crouzon's disease

Hypertelorism
Imperfect fusion of skull
Oxycephaly
Platybasia
Trigonocephaly

Excludes: dentofacial anomalies (524.–)
skull defects associated with anomalies of brain, such as:
anencephalus (740.0)
encephalocele (742.0)
hydrocephalus (742.3)
microcephalus (742.1)

756.1 *Anomalies of spine*

Congenital:
absence of vertebra
deformity, lumbosacral (joint)
(region)
fusion of spine
spondylolisthesis

Hemivertebra
Klippel-Feil syndrome
Spina bifida occulta
Supernumerary vertebra

756.2 *Cervical rib*

Supernumerary rib in cervical region

756.3 *Other anomalies of ribs and sternum*

Congenital:
absence of:
rib
sternum
fusion of ribs

Sternum bifidum

756.4 *Chondrodystrophy*

Achondroplasia
Chondrodystrophia (fetalis)

Dyschondroplasia
Ollier's disease

Excludes: lipochondrodystrophy (277.5)

756.5 *Osteodystrophies*

Albright(-McCune)-Sternberg
syndrome
Chondroectodermal dysplasia
Fragilitas ossium
Multiple epiphyseal dysplasia
Osteogenesis imperfecta

Osteopetrosis
Osteopoikilosis
Osteopsathyrosis
Polyostotic fibrous dysplasia

756.6 *Anomalies of diaphragm*

Absence of diaphragm
Congenital diaphragmatic hernia

Eventration of diaphragm

Excludes: congenital hiatus hernia (750.6)

756.7 *Anomalies of abdominal wall*

Exomphalos
Gastroschisis

Prune belly (syndrome)

Excludes: umbilical hernia (553.1)

756.8 *Other specified anomalies of muscle, tendon, fascia and connective tissue*

Absence of:
  muscle (pectoral)
  tendon
Accessory muscle

Amyotrophia congenita
Congenital shortening of tendon
Ehlers-Danlos syndrome

756.9 *Unspecified anomalies of musculoskeletal system*

Congenital:
  anomaly NOS } of musculoskeletal system, not elsewhere classified
  deformity NOS

757   Congenital anomalies of the integument
Includes: anomalies of skin, subcutaneous tissue, hair, nails and breast

757.0 *Hereditary oedema of legs*
Hereditary trophoedema

757.1 *Ichthyosis congenita*

757.2 *Dermatoglyphic anomalies*
Abnormal palmar creases

757.3 *Other specified anomalies of skin*

Accessory skin tags
Birthmarks
Congenital:
  ectodermal dysplasia
  poikiloderma
  scar

Epidermolysis bullosa
Harlequin foetus
Keratoderma (congenital)
Urticaria pigmentosa
Xeroderma pigmentosum

757.4 *Specified anomalies of hair*

Congenital:
  alopecia
  atrichosis
  beaded hair

Congenital:
  hypertrichosis
  monilethrix
Persistent lanugo

757.5 *Specified anomalies of nails*

Anonychia
Congenital:
  clubnail
  koilonychia

Congenital:
  leukonychia
  onychauxis
  pachyonychia

757.6 *Specified anomalies of breast*

Absent
Accessory   } breast or nipple
Supernumerary
Hypoplasia of breast
Excludes: absence of pectoral muscle (756.8)

757.8 *Other specified anomalies of the integument*

757.9 *Unspecified anomalies of the integument*

Congenital:
anomaly NOS ⎫
deformity NOS ⎭ of integument

758   Chromosomal anomalies

Includes: syndromes associated with anomalies in the number and form
of chromosomes

758.0 *Down's syndrome*

Trisomy: Translocation Down's syndrome
  21 or 22
  G

758.1 *Patau's syndrome*

Trisomy:
  13
  D$_1$

758.2 *Edwards's syndrome*

Trisomy:
  18
  E$_3$

758.3 *Autosomal deletion syndromes*

Antimongolism syndrome   Cri-du-chat syndrome

758.4 *Balanced autosomal translocation in normal individual*

758.5 *Other conditions due to autosomal anomalies*

758.6 *Gonadal dysgenesis*

Turner's syndrome   XO syndrome

Excludes: pure gonadal dysgenesis (752.7)

758.7 *Klinefelter's syndrome*

XYY syndrome

758.8 *Other conditions due to sex chromosome anomalies*

758.9 *Conditons due to anomaly of unspecified chromosome*

759   Other and unspecified congenital anomalies

759.0 *Anomalies of spleen*

759.1 *Anomalies of adrenal gland*

759.2 *Anomalies of other endocrine glands*

759.3 *Situs inversus*

Situs inversus or transversus:
  abdominalis
  thoracis

Transposition of viscera:
  abdominal
  thoracic

Excludes: dextrocardia (746.8) unless associated with complete transposition

759.4 *Conjoined twins*

Craniopagus
Dicephalus
Double monster

Pygopagus
Thoracopagus
Xiphopagus

759.5 *Tuberous sclerosis*

Bourneville's disease   Epiloia

759.6 *Other hamartoses, not elsewhere classified*

Syndrome:
  Peutz-Jeghers
  Sturge-Weber(-Dimitri)
  von Hippel-Lindau

Excludes: neurofibromatosis (237.7)

759.7 *Multiple congenital anomalies, so described*

Congenital: Monster NOS
  anomaly, multiple NOS
  deformity, multiple NOS

759.8 *Other specified anomalies*

Monster (single), specified type
Congenital malformation syndromes affecting multiple systems, not elsewhere classified

759.9 *Congenital anomaly, unspecified*

XV. CERTAIN CONDITIONS ORIGINATING IN THE PERINATAL PERIOD

Includes: conditions which have their origin in the perinatal period
even though death or morbidity occurs later

760   Fetus or newborn affected by maternal conditions which may be unrelated to present pregnancy

Includes: the listed maternal conditions only when specified as a cause
of mortality or morbidity of the fetus or newborn

Excludes: maternal endocrine and metabolic disorders influencing
fetus (775.–)

760.0   *Maternal hypertensive disorders*

Fetus or newborn affected by maternal conditions classifiable to 642.–

760.1   *Maternal renal and urinary tract diseases*

Fetus or newborn affected by maternal conditions classifiable to 580-599

760.2   *Maternal infections*

Fetus or newborn affected by maternal infectious disease classifiable to
001-136 and 487, but not itself manifesting that disease

Excludes: congenital infectious diseases (771.–)
maternal genital tract, and other localised, infections (760.8)

760.3   *Other chronic maternal circulatory and respiratory diseases*

Fetus or newborn affected by chronic maternal conditions classifiable to
390-459, 490-519, 745-748

760.4   *Maternal nutritional disorders*

Fetus or newborn affected by maternal disorders classifiable to 260-269
Maternal malnutrition NOS

760.5   *Maternal injury*

Fetus or newborn affected by maternal conditions classifiable to 800-996

760.6   *Surgical operation on mother*

Excludes: caesarean section for present delivery (763.4)
previous surgery to uterus or pelvic organs (763.8)

— 439 —

760.7   *Noxious influences transmitted via placenta or breast milk*

Excludes: anaesthetic and analgesic drugs administered during labour
                and delivery (763.5)

760.8   *Other*

760.9   *Unspecified*

761   Fetus or newborn affected by maternal complications of pregnancy

Includes: the listed maternal conditions only when specified as a cause
                of mortality or morbidity of the fetus or newborn

761.0   *Incompetent cervix*

761.1   *Premature rupture of membranes*

761.2   *Oligohydramnios*

Excludes: when due to premature rupture of membranes (761.1)

761.3   *Polyhydramnios*

Hydramnios

761.4   *Ectopic pregnancy*

Abdominal pregnancy

761.5   *Multiple pregnancy*

Triplet (pregnancy)   Twin (pregnancy)

761.6   *Maternal death*

761.7   *Malpresentation before labour*

Breech presentation ⎤
External version   ⎥
Transverse lie   ⎬ before labour
Unstable lie   ⎦

761.8   *Other*

Spontaneous abortion, fetus

761.9   *Unspecified*

**762   Fetus or newborn affected by complications of placenta, cord and
            membranes**

Includes: the listed maternal conditions only when specified as a cause
                of mortality or morbidity in the fetus or newborn

762.0   *Placenta praevia*

762.1 *Other forms of placental separation and haemorrhage*

Abruptio placentae
Accidental haemorrhage
Antepartum haemorrhage
Damage to placenta from amniocentesis, caesarean section or surgical
    induction
Maternal blood loss
Premature separation of placenta

762.2 *Other and unspecified morphological and functional abnormalities
    of placenta*

Placental:
    dysfunction
    infarction
    insufficiency

762.3 *Placental transfusion syndromes*

Placental and cord abnormality resulting in twin-to-twin or other trans-
    placental transfusion

Use code 772.0 or 776.4, in addition, if desired, to indicate resultant
    condition in the fetus or newborn

762.4 *Prolapsed cord*

762.5 *Other compression of umbilical cord*

Cord around neck   Knot in cord
Entanglement of cord

762.6 *Other and unspecified conditions of umbilical cord*

Short cord   Vasa praevia

Excludes: single umbilical artery (747.5)

762.7 *Chorioamnionitis*

Membranitis   Placentitis

762.8 *Other abnormalities of chorion and amnion*

762.9 *Unspecified abnormality of chorion and amnion*

763   **Fetus or newborn affected by other complications of labour and
       delivery**

Includes: the listed conditions only when specified as a cause of mortal-
               ity or morbidity in the fetus or newborn

763.0 *Breech delivery and extraction*

763.1   *Other malpresentation, malposition and disproportion during labour
        and delivery*

Fetus or newborn affected by conditions classifiable to 652, 653 and 660
Contracted pelvis
Persistent occipitoposterior
Transverse lie

763.2   *Forceps delivery*

763.3   *Delivery by vacuum extractor*

763.4   *Caesarean delivery*

763.5   *Maternal anaesthesia and analgesia*

Reactions and intoxications from maternal opiates and tranquillizers
        during labour and delivery

Excludes: drug-withdrawal syndrome in newborn (779.5)

763.6   *Precipitate delivery*

Rapid second stage

763.7   *Abnormal uterine contractions*

Fetus or newborn affected by conditions classifiable to 661.–, except 661.3
Hypertonic labour
Uterine inertia

763.8   *Other complications of labour and delivery*

Fetus or newborn affected by other conditions classifiable to 650-669 and
        by other procedures used in labour and delivery
Abnormality of maternal soft tissues
Destructive operation to facilitate delivery
Induction of labour

763.9   *Unspecified*

764   Slow fetal growth and fetal malnutrition

764.0   *"Light-for-dates" without mention of fetal malnutrition*

Infants underweight for gestational age
"Small-for-dates"

764.1   *"Light-for-dates" with signs of fetal malnutrition*

Infants "light-for-dates" as in .0, who in addition show signs of fetal
        malnutrition, such as dry, peeling skin and loss of subcutaneous
        tissue

764.2   *Fetal malnutrition without mention of "light-for-dates"*

Infants, not underweight for gestational age, showing signs of fetal mal-
        nutrition, such as dry, peeling skin and loss of subcutaneous tissue

764.9   *Fetal growth retardation, unspecified*

765   Disorders relating to short gestation and unspecified low birth-weight

Includes: the listed conditions, without further specification, as causes of mortality, morbidity or additional care, in fetus or newborn

Excludes: low birthweight due to slow fetal growth and fetal malnutrition (764.–)

765.0   *Extreme immaturity*

Note: Usually implies a birthweight of less than 1000 g. and/or a gestation of less than 28 completed weeks.

765.1   *Other preterm infants*

Prematurity or small size, not classifiable to 765.0 or as "light-for-dates" in 764.–
Prematurity NOS

766   Disorders relating to long gestation and high birthweight

Includes: the listed conditions, without further specification, as causes of mortality, morbidity or additional care, in fetus or newborn

766.0   *Exceptionally large baby*

Note: Usually implies a birthweight of 4500 g. or more.

766.1   *Other "heavy-for-dates" infants*

Other fetus or infant heavy-or large-for-dates regardless of period of gestation

766.2   *Post-term infant, not "heavy-for-dates"*

Fetus or infant with gestation period of 294 days or more [42 or more completed weeks], not heavy- or large-for-dates
Postmaturity NOS

767   Birth trauma

767.0   *Subdural and cerebral haemorrhage*

Subdural and cerebral haemorrhage, whether described as due to birth trauma or to intrapartum anoxia or hypoxia
Subdural haematoma (localized)
Tentorial tear
Use additional code, if desired, to identify cause

Excludes: intraventricular haemorrhage (772.1)
                 subarachnoid haemorrhage (772.2)

767.1   *Injuries to scalp*

Cephalhaematoma
Chignon (from vacuum extraction)
Massive epicranial subaponeurotic haemorrhage

767.2 *Fracture of clavicle*

767.3 *Other injuries to skeleton*

Fracture of:
  long bones
  skull

Excludes: fracture of spine (767.4)

767.4 *Injury to spine and spinal cord*

767.5 *Facial nerve injury*

Facial palsy

767.6 *Injury to brachial plexus*

Erb's palsy   Klumpke's palsy

767.7 *Other cranial and peripheral nerve injuries*

767.8 *Other*

Eye damage   Rupture of:
Haematoma of: liver
  liver (subcapsular)   spleen
  testes   Scalpel wound
  vulva   Traumatic glaucoma

767.9 *Unspecified*

768 **Intrauterine hypoxia and birth asphyxia**

768.0 *Fetal death from asphyxia or anoxia before onset of labour or at unspecified time*

768.1 *Fetal death from asphyxia or anoxia during labour*

768.2 *Fetal distress before onset of labour, in liveborn infant*

Liveborn infant showing evidence of intrauterine hypoxia before onset of labour
Abnormal fetal heart rate ⎤
Fetal or intrauterine: ⎥
  acidosis   ⎥
  anoxia   ⎥ first noted before onset of labour, liveborn
  asphyxia   ⎬ infant
  distress   ⎥
  hypoxia   ⎥
Meconium in liquor   ⎥
Passage of meconium   ⎦

768.3 *Fetal distress first noted during labour, in liveborn infant*

Liveborn infant showing evidence of intrauterine hypoxia during labour
or delivery

Abnormal fetal heart rate ⎫
Fetal or intrauterine: ⎪
  acidosis ⎪
  anoxia ⎪ first noted during labour or delivery, live-
  asphyxia ⎬ born infant
  distress ⎪
  hypoxia ⎪
Meconium in liquor ⎪
Passage of meconium ⎭

768.4 *Fetal distress, unspecified, in liveborn infant*

Liveborn infant showing evidence of intrauterine hypoxia before delivery,
but not stated whether before or after onset of labour

Abnormal fetal heart rate ⎫
Fetal or intrauterine: ⎪
  acidosis ⎪
  anoxia ⎪ not stated whether first noted before or after
  asphyxia ⎬ onset of labour, liveborn infant
  distress ⎪
  hypoxia ⎪
Meconium in liquor ⎪
Passage of meconium ⎭

768.5 *Severe birth asphyxia*

Pulse less than 100 per minute at birth and falling or steady, respiration
absent or gasping, colour poor, tone absent
1-minute Apgar score 0-3[1]
"White asphyxia"

768.6 *Mild or moderate birth asphyxia*

Normal respiration not established within one minute, but heart rate 100
or above, some muscle tone present, some response to stimulation
1-minute Apgar score 4-7[1]
"Blue asphyxia"

768.9 *Unspecified birth asphyxia in liveborn infant*

Anoxia ⎫
Asphyxia ⎬ NOS, in liveborn infant
Hypoxia ⎭

---

[1] The Apgar scoring system is described in: Apgar, V. Anesthesia and Analgesia...
Current Researches, **32**: 260 (1953)

769 Respiratory distress syndrome

Hyaline membrane (disease) (pulmonary)
Idiopathic respiratory distress syndrome of newborn [IRDS or RDS]

Excludes: transient tachypnoea of newborn (770.6)

770 Other respiratory conditions of fetus and newborn

770.0 *Congenital pneumonia*

Infective pneumonia acquired prenatally

770.1 *Massive aspiration syndrome*

Meconium aspiration syndrome
Pneumonitis:
  fetal aspiration
  meconium

770.2 *Interstitial emphysema and related conditions*

Pneumomediastinum ⎫
Pneumopericardium ⎬ originating in the perinatal period
Pneumothorax ⎭

770.3 *Pulmonary haemorrhage*

Haemorrhage: ⎫
  alveolar (lung) ⎪
  intraalveolar (lung) ⎬ originating in the perinatal period
  massive pulmonary ⎭

770.4 *Primary atelectasis*

Pulmonary immaturity NOS

770.5 *Other and unspecified atelectasis*

Atelectasis: ⎫
  NOS ⎪
  partial ⎬ originating in the perinatal period
Pulmonary collapse ⎭

770.6 *Transitory tachypnoea of newborn*

Tachypnoea commencing to resolve, usually, within 6 hours of birth

Excludes: respiratory distress syndrome (769)

770.7 *Chronic respiratory disease arising in the perinatal period*

Bronchopulmonary dysplasia   Wilson-Mikity syndrome

770.8   *Other respiratory problems after birth*

Apnoeic spells NOS ⎫
Cyanotic attacks NOS ⎪
Respiratory distress NOS ⎬ originating in the perinatal period
Respiratory failure NOS ⎭

770.9   *Unspecified*

771   Infections specific to the perinatal period

Includes: infections acquired before or during birth or via the umbilicus

Excludes: congenital pneumonia (770.0)
            congenital syphilis (090.–)
            ophthalmia neonatorum due to gonococcus (098.4)
            other infections acquired after birth (001-136, 480-486, etc.)
            maternal infectious disease as a cause of mortality or mor-
                bidity in fetus or newborn not itself manifesting the
                disease (760.2)

771.0   *Congenital rubella*

Congenital rubella pneumonitis

771.1   *Congenital cytomegalovirus infection*

771.2   *Other congenital infections*

Congenital: Congenital:
  herpes simplex   toxoplasmosis
  listeriosis   tuberculosis
  malaria

771.3   *Tetanus neonatorum*

771.4   *Omphalitis of newborn*

Excludes: tetanus omphalitis (771.3)

771.5   *Neonatal infective mastitis*

771.6   *Neonatal conjunctivitis and dacryocystitis*

Ophthalmia neonatorum NOS

Excludes: ophthalmia neonatorum due to gonococcus (098.4)

771.7   *Neonatal Candida infection*

Neonatal Monilia infection

771.8   *Other infection specific to the perinatal period*

Intraamniotic infection of fetus: Intrauterine sepsis of fetus
  NOS   Neonatal urinary tract infection
  Clostridial   Septicaemia [sepsis] of newborn
  Escherichia coli

772 Fetal and neonatal haemorrhage

Excludes: haematological disorders of fetus and newborn (776.–)

772.0 *Fetal blood loss*

Fetal blood loss from:
  cut end of co-twin's cord
  placenta
  ruptured cord
  vasa praevia

Fetal exsanguination
Fetal haemorrhage into:
  co-twin
  mother's circulation

772.1 *Intraventricular haemorrhage*

Intraventricular haemorrhage from any perinatal cause

772.2 *Subarachnoid haemorrhage*

Subarachnoid haemorrhage from any perinatal cause

772.3 *Umbilical haemorrhage after birth*

Slipped umbilical ligature

772.4 *Gastrointestinal haemorrhage*

Excludes: swallowed maternal blood (777.3)

772.5 *Adrenal haemorrhage*

772.6 *Cutaneous haemorrhage*

Bruising
Ecchymoses
Petechiae
Superficial haematomata
} in fetus or newborn

772.8 *Other*

Excludes: haemorrhagic disease of newborn (776.0)
          pulmonary haemorrhage (770.3)

772.9 *Unspecified*

773 Haemolytic disease of fetus or newborn, due to isoimmunization

773.0 *Haemolytic disease due to Rh isoimmunization*

Anaemia
Erythroblastosis (fetalis)
Haemolytic disease (fetus) (newborn)
Jaundice
Rh haemolytic disease
Rh isoimmunization
} due to Rh:
  antibodies
  isoimmunization
  maternal/fetal incompatibility

773.1 *Haemolytic disease due to ABO isoimmunization*

ABO haemolytic disease
ABO isoimmunization
Anaemia
Erythroblastosis (fetalis)
Haemolytic disease (fetus) (newborn)
Jaundice

due to ABO:
  antibodies
  isoimmunization
  maternal/fetal incompatibility

773.2 *Haemolytic disease due to other and unspecified isoimmunization*

Erythroblastosis (fetalis) NOS
Haemolytic disease (fetus) (newborn) NOS
Jaundice or anaemia due to other or unspecified blood-group incompatibility

773.3 *Hydrops fetalis due to isoimmunization*

773.4 *Kernicterus due to isoimmunization*

773.5 *Late anaemia due to isoimmunization*

774 Other perinatal jaundice

774.0* *Perinatal jaundice from hereditary haemolytic anaemias (282.–†)*

Jaundice due to excessive haemolysis from congenital spherocytosis, G-6-PD deficiency and other red-cell defects

774.1 *Perinatal jaundice from other excessive haemolysis*

Fetal or neonatal jaundice from:
  bruising
  drugs or toxins transmitted from mother
  infection
  polycythaemia
  swallowed maternal blood

Use additional code, if desired, to identify cause

Excludes: jaundice due to isoimmunization (773.0, 773.1, 773.2)

774.2 *Neonatal jaundice associated with preterm delivery*

Jaundice due to delayed conjugation associated with preterm delivery
Hyperbilirubinaemia of prematurity

774.3 *Neonatal jaundice due to delayed conjugation from other causes*

Jaundice due to delayed conjugation from causes such as breast-milk inhibitors, congenital hypothyroidism, and congenital absence or deficiency of enzyme systems for bilirubin conjugation
Neonatal jaundice associated with:
  Crigler-Najjar syndrome* (277.4†)
  Gilbert's syndrome* (277.4†)

774.4 *Perinatal jaundice due to hepatocellular damage*

Fetal or neonatal hepatitis   Inspissated bile syndrome

774.5 *Perinatal jaundice from other causes*

Fetal or neonatal jaundice associated with:
  congenital obstruction of bile duct* (751.6†)
  galactosaemia* (271.1†)
  mucoviscidosis* (277.0†)

774.6 *Unspecified fetal and neonatal jaundice*

Physiological jaundice NOS in newborn

774.7 *Kernicterus not due to isoimmunization*

Kernicterus NOS

Excludes: kernicterus due to isoimmunization (773.4)

775   Endocrine and metabolic disturbances specific to the fetus and newborn

Includes: transitory endocrine and metabolic disturbances caused by the infant's response to maternal endocrine and metabolic factors, its removal from them, or its adjustment to extrauterine existence

775.0 *Syndrome of "infant of a diabetic mother"*

Maternal diabetes mellitus affecting fetus or newborn (with hypoglycaemia)

775.1 *Neonatal diabetes mellitus*

775.2 *Neonatal myasthenia gravis*

775.3 *Neonatal thyrotoxicosis*

775.4 *Hypocalcaemia and hypomagnesaemia of newborn*

Cow's milk hypocalcaemia   Phosphate-loading hypocalcaemia
Neonatal hypoparathyroidism

775.5 *Other transitory neonatal electrolyte disturbances*

775.6 *Neonatal hypoglycaemia*

Excludes: infant of mother with diabetes mellitus (775.0)

775.7 *Late metabolic acidosis of newborn*

775.8 *Other transitory neonatal endocrine and metabolic disturbances*

Amino-acid metabolic disorders described as transitory

775.9 *Unspecified*

776 Haematological disorders of fetus and newborn

Includes: disorders specific to the fetus or newborn

776.0 *Haemorrhagic disease of newborn*

Vitamin K deficiency of newborn

776.1 *Transient neonatal thrombocytopenia*

Neonatal thrombocytopenia due to:
exchange transfusion
idiopathic maternal thrombocytopenia
isoimmunization

776.2 *Disseminated intravascular coagulation in newborn*

776.3 *Other transient neonatal disorders of coagulation*

776.4 *Polycythaemia neonatorum*

776.5 *Congenital anaemia*

Anaemia following fetal blood loss

Excludes: anaemia due to isoimmunization (773.–)
hereditary haemolytic anaemias (282.–)

776.6 *Anaemia of prematurity*

776.7 *Transient neonatal neutropenia*

Isoimmune neutropenia
Maternal transfer neutropenia

776.8 *Other specified transient haematological disorders*

776.9 *Unspecified*

777 Perinatal disorders of digestive system

Includes: disorders specific to the fetus and newborn
Excludes: intestinal obstruction classifiable to 560.–

777.0* *Meconium ileus (277.0†)*

Meconium obstruction in mucoviscidosis

777.1 *Other meconium obstruction*

Congenital faecaliths   Meconium plug syndrome

777.2 *Intestinal obstruction due to inspissated milk*

777.3 *Haematemesis and melaena due to swallowed maternal blood*

777.4 *Transitory ileus of newborn*

Excludes: Hirschsprung's disease (751.3)

777.5   *Necrotizing enterocolitis in fetus or newborn*

777.6   *Perinatal intestinal perforation*

Meconium peritonitis

777.8   *Other*

777.9   *Unspecified*

778   Conditions involving the integument and temperature regulation of fetus and newborn

778.0   *Hydrops fetalis not due to isoimmunization*

Idiopathic hydrops

Excludes: hydrops fetalis due to isoimmunization (773.3)

778.1   *Sclerema neonatorum*

778.2   *Cold injury syndrome of newborn*

778.3   *Other hypothermia of newborn*

778.4   *Other disturbances of temperature regulation of newborn*

Environmentally induced pyrexia and dehydration fever in newborn

778.5   *Other and unspecified oedema of newborn*

778.6   *Congenital hydrocele*

778.7   *Breast engorgement in newborn*

Noninfective mastitis of newborn

778.8   *Other*

Urticaria neonatorum

Excludes: impetigo neonatorum (684)
            pemphigus neonatorum (684)

778.9   *Unspecified*

779   Other and ill-defined conditions originating in the perinatal period

779.0   *Convulsions in newborn*

Fits ⎫
Seizures ⎬ in newborn

779.1   *Other and unspecified cerebral irritability in newborn*

779.2   *Cerebral depression, coma and other abnormal cerebral signs*

779.3 *Feeding problems in newborn*

Regurgitation of feeds ⎫
Slow feeding ⎬ in newborn
Vomiting ⎭

779.4 *Drug reactions and intoxications specific to newborn*

Grey syndrome from chloramphenicol administration in newborn

Excludes: reactions and intoxications from maternal opiates and tranquillizers (763.5)

779.5 *Drug withdrawal syndrome in newborn*

Drug withdrawal syndrome in infant of dependent mother

779.6 *Termination of pregnancy (fetus)*

779.8 *Other*

779.9 *Unspecified*

Congenital debility NOS

XVI. SYMPTOMS, SIGNS AND ILL-DEFINED CONDITIONS

This section includes symptoms, signs, abnormal results of laboratory or other investigative procedures, and ill-defined conditions regarding which no diagnosis classifiable elsewhere is recorded.

Signs and symptoms that point rather definitely to a given diagnosis are assigned to some category in the preceding part of the classification. In general, categories 780-796 include the more ill-defined conditions and symptoms that point with perhaps equal suspicion to two or more diseases or to two or more systems of the body, and without the necessary study of the case to make a final diagnosis. Practically all categories in this group could be designated as "not otherwise specified", or as "unknown etiology", or as "transient". The Alphabetical Index should be consulted to determine which symptoms and signs are to be allocated here and which to more specific sections of the classification; the residual subcategories numbered .9 are provided for other relevant symptoms which cannot be allocated elsewhere in the classification.

The conditions and signs or symptoms included in categories 780-796 consist of: *(a)* cases for which no more specific diagnosis can be made even after all facts bearing on the case have been investigated; *(b)* signs or symptoms existing at the time of initial encounter that proved to be transient and whose causes could not be determined; *(c)* provisional diagnoses in a patient who failed to return for further investigation or care; *(d)* cases referred elsewhere for investigation or treatment before the diagnosis was made; *(e)* cases in which a more precise diagnosis was not available for any other reason; *(f)* certain symptoms which represent important problems in medical care and which it might be desired to classify in addition to a known cause.

SYMPTOMS (780-789)

780   General symptoms

780.0   *Coma and stupor*

Drowsiness   Somnolence
Semicoma   Unconsciousness

Excludes: coma originating in the perinatal period (779.2)

780.1   *Hallucinations*

Excludes: visual hallucinations (368.1)
                 when part of a pattern of mental disorder

780.2 Syncope and collapse

Blackout   Vasovagal attack
Fainting

Excludes: carotid sinus syncope (337.0)
           neurocirculatory asthenia (306.2)
           orthostatic hypotension (458.0)
           shock NOS (785.5)

780.3 Convulsions

Convulsions: Fit NOS
  NOS
  febrile
  infantile

Excludes: convulsions in newborn (779.0)
           epileptic convulsions (345.–)

780.4 Dizziness and giddiness

Vertigo NOS

Excludes: Ménière's disease and other specified vertiginous syndromes
           (386.–)

780.5 Sleep disturbances

Insomnia   Inversion of sleep rhythm

Excludes: when of nonorganic origin (307.4)

780.6 Pyrexia of unknown origin

Chills with fever   Hyperpyrexia NOS
Fever NOS

Excludes: pyrexia of unknown origin during:
           labour (659.2)
           the puerperium (672)

780.7 Malaise and fatigue

Asthenia NOS   Postviral (asthenic) syndrome
Lethargy   Tiredness

Excludes: combat fatigue (308.–)
           fatigue during pregnancy (646.8)
           neurasthenia (300.5)
           senile asthenia (797)

780.8 Hyperhidrosis

Excessive sweating

780.9 *Other*

Amnesia (retrograde)
Generalized pain

Hypothermia, not associated with low environmental temperature

Excludes: hypothermia:
NOS (accidental) (991.6)
due to anaesthesia (995.8)
memory disturbance when part of a pattern of mental disorder

781   Symptoms involving nervous and musculoskeletal systems

Excludes: depression NOS (311)
disorders specifically relating to:
back (724.–)
hearing (388.–, 389.–)
joint (718.–, 719.–)
limb (729.–)
neck (723.–)
vision (368.–, 369.–)
pain in limb (729.5)

781.0 *Abnormal involuntary movements*

Abnormal head movements
Fasciculation

Spasms NOS
Tremor NOS

Excludes: chorea NOS (333.5)
infantile spasms (345.6)
spastic paralysis (342–344)
specified movement disorders classifiable to 333.– (333.–)
when of nonorganic origin (307.2, 307.3)

781.1 *Disturbances of sensation of smell and taste*

Anosmia

Parosmia

781.2 *Abnormality of gait*

Gait:
ataxic
paralytic

Gait:
spastic
staggering

Excludes: difficulty in walking (719.7)
locomotor ataxia (094.2)

781.3 *Lack of coordination*

Ataxia NOS

Muscular incoordination

Excludes: ataxic gait (781.2)
cerebellar ataxia (334.–)
vertigo NOS (780.4)

781.4 *Transient paralysis of limb*

Monoplegia, transient NOS

Excludes: paralysis (342–344)

781.5 *Clubbing of fingers*

781.6 *Meningismus*

781.7 *Tetany*

Carpopedal spasm

Excludes: hysterical (300.1)
psychogenic (306.0)

781.9 *Other*

Abnormal posture

782 Symptoms involving skin and other integumentary tissue

782.0 *Disturbance of skin sensation*

Anaesthesia of skin	Numbness
Burning or prickling sensation	Paraesthesia
Hyperaesthesia	Tingling
Hypoaesthesia	

782.1 *Rash and other nonspecific skin eruption*

782.2 *Localized superficial swelling, mass or lump*

Subcutaneous nodules

Excludes: localized adiposity (278.1)

782.3 *Oedema*

Localized oedema

Excludes: ascites (789.5)
fluid retention (276.6)
hydrops fetalis (773.3, 778.0)
hydrothorax (511.8)
nutritional oedema (262)
oedema of:
newborn NOS (778.5)
pregnancy (642.–, 646.1)

782.4 *Jaundice unspecified, not of newborn*

Cholaemia NOS   Icterus NOS

782.5 *Cyanosis*

Excludes: newborn (770.8)

782.6   *Pallor and flushing*

782.7   *Spontaneous ecchymoses*
Petechiae
Excludes: ecchymosis in fetus or newborn (772.6)
            purpura (287.–)

782.8   *Changes in skin texture*
Induration of skin   Thickening of skin

782.9   *Other*

783   Symptoms concerning nutrition, metabolism and development

783.0   *Anorexia*
Loss of appetite
Excludes: anorexia nervosa (307.1)
            loss of appetite of nonorganic origin (307.5)

783.1   *Abnormal weight gain*
Excludes: excessive weight gain in pregnancy (646.1)
            obesity (278.0)

783.2   *Abnormal loss of weight*

783.3   *Feeding difficulties and mismanagement*
Feeding problem (infant) (elderly)
Excludes: feeding problems in newborn (779.3)
            infantile feeding disturbance of nonorganic origin (307.5)

783.4   *Lack of expected normal physiological development*
Delayed milestone   Physical retardation
Failure to thrive   Short stature
Lack of growth
Excludes: delay in sexual development and puberty (259.0)
            specific delays in mental development (315.–)

783.5   *Polydipsia*
Excessive thirst

783.6   *Polyphagia*
Excessive eating   Hyperalimentation NOS
Excludes: disorders of eating of nonorganic origin (307.5)

783.9   *Other*
Excludes: abnormal basal metabolic rate (794.7)
            dehydratation (276.5)
            other disorders of fluid, electrolyte and acid-base balance
                (276.–)

784   Symptoms involving head and neck

Excludes: encephalopathy NOS (348.3)

784.0 *Headache*

Facial pain

Excludes: atypical face pain (350.2)
           migraine (346.–)
           tension headache (307.8)

784.1 *Throat pain*

Excludes: dysphagia (787.2)
           neck pain (723.1)
           sore throat (462, 472.1)

784.2 *Swelling, mass or lump in head and neck*

Space-occupying lesion, intracranial NOS

784.3 *Aphasia*

Excludes: developmental aphasia (315.3)

784.4 *Voice disturbance*

Aphonia   Hypernasality
Hoarseness   Hyponasality

784.5 *Other speech disturbance*

Dysarthria   Slurred speech
Dysphasia

Excludes: stammering and stuttering (307.0)
           when of nonorganic origin (307.0, 307.9)

784.6 *Other symbolic dysfunction*

Acalculia   Apraxia
Agnosia   Dyslexia
Agraphia

Excludes: developmental learning retardations (315.–)

784.7 *Epistaxis*

Haemorrhage from nose   Nosebleed

784.8 *Haemorrhage from throat*

Excludes: haemoptysis (786.3)

784.9 *Other*

Choking sensation   Mouth breathing
Halitosis   Sneezing

785   Symptoms involving cardiovascular system

Excludes: heart failure NOS (428.9)

785.0   *Tachycardia, unspecified*

Excludes: paroxysmal tachycardia (427.0-427.2)

785.1   *Palpitations*

Awareness of heart beat

Excludes: specified dysrhythmias (427.–)

785.2   *Functional and undiagnosed cardiac murmurs*

Heart murmur (benign) (innocent) NOS

785.3   *Other abnormal heart sounds*

Cardiac dullness, increased or   Precordial friction
    decreased
Friction fremitus, cardiac

785.4   *Gangrene*

Gangrene: Phagedaena
    NOS
    atherosclerotic* (440.2†)
    diabetic* (250.6†)
    spreading cutaneous

Excludes: gangrene of certain sites (see Alphabetical Index)
            gas gangrene (040.0)

785.5   *Shock without mention of trauma*

Failure of peripheral circulation   Shock:
Shock: endotoxic
    NOS   hypovolaemic
    cardiogenic   septic

Excludes: shock:
                anaesthetic (995.4)
                anaphylactic (995.0)
                    due to serum (999.4)
                electric (994.8)
                following abortion (639.5)
                lightning (994.0)
                obstetrical (669.1)
                postoperative (998.0)
                traumatic (958.4)

785.6   *Enlargement of lymph nodes*

Lymphadenopathy   "Swollen glands"

Excludes: lymphadenitis (289.–, 683)

785.9   *Other*

Bruit NOS

786   Symptoms involving respiratory system and other chest symptoms

786.0   *Dyspnoea and respiratory abnormalities*

Orthopnoea   Shortness of breath
Respiratory: Tachypnoea
  distress   Wheezing
  insufficiency

Excludes: hyperventilation, psychogenic (306.1)
            respiratory distress of newborn (770.8)
            respiratory distress syndrome (newborn) (769)
            respiratory failure (799.1)
                newborn (770.8)

786.1   *Stridor*

Excludes: congenital stridor (748.3)

786.2   *Cough*

Excludes: psychogenic cough (306.1)

786.3   *Haemoptysis*

Cough with haemorrhage   Pulmonary haemorrhage NOS
Excludes: pulmonary haemorrhage of newborn (770.3)

786.4   *Abnormal sputum*

Excessive sputum

786.5   *Chest pain*

Pain: Painful respiration
  anterior chest wall   Pleurodynia
  pleuritic
  precordial

Excludes: epidemic pleurodynia (074.1)
            pain in breast (611.7)

786.6   *Swelling, mass or lump in chest*

Excludes: lump in breast (611.7)

786.7   *Abnormal chest sounds*

Abnormal percussion, chest   Rales
Friction sounds, chest   Tympany, chest

Excludes: wheezing (786.0)

786.8   *Hiccough*
Excludes: psychogenic hiccough (306.1)

786.9   *Other*
Breath-holding spell

787   Symptoms involving digestive system
Excludes: pylorospasm (537.8)
                 congenital (750.5)

787.0   *Nausea and vomiting*
Excludes: haematemesis (531.– to 534.–, 578.0)
                 vomiting:
                    bilious, following gastrointestinal surgery (564.3)
                    cyclical (536.2)
                       psychogenic (306.4)
                    excessive, in pregnancy (643.–)
                    habit (536.2)
                    of newborn (779.3)
                    psychogenic NOS (307.5)

787.1   *Heartburn*
Excludes: dyspepsia (536.8)

787.2   *Dysphagia*
Difficulty in swallowing

787.3   *Flatulence, eructation and gas pain*
Bloating
Excludes: aerophagy (306.4)

787.4   *Visible peristalsis*

787.5   *Abnormal bowel sounds*

787.6   *Incontinence of faeces*
Encopresis NOS
Excludes: when of nonorganic origin (307.7)

787.7   *Abnormal faeces*
Excludes: melaena:
                 NOS (578.1)
                 newborn (772.4)

787.9   *Other*
Excludes: gastrointestinal haemorrhage (578.–)
                 intestinal obstruction (560.–)
                 specific functional digestive disorders (530.–, 536.–, 564.–)

788   Symptoms involving urinary system

Excludes: haematuria (599.7)
            small kidney of unknown cause (589.–)
            uraemia NOS (586.–)

788.0   *Renal colic*

788.1   *Dysuria*

788.2   *Retention of urine*

788.3   *Incontinence of urine*

Enuresis NOS

Excludes: when of nonorganic origin (307.6)
            stress incontinence (female) (625.6)

788.4   *Frequency of urination and polyuria*

Frequency of micturition   Nocturia

788.5   *Oliguria and anuria*

Excludes: when complicating:
            abortion (634-638 with fourth digit .3, 639.3)
            ectopic or molar pregnancy (639.3)
            pregnancy, childbirth or the puerperium (646.2)

788.6   *Other abnormality of urination*

Slowing of urinary stream   Splitting of urinary stream

788.7   *Urethral discharge*

788.8   *Extravasation of urine*

788.9   *Other*

Extrarenal uraemia

789   Other symptoms involving abdomen and pelvis

Excludes: symptoms referable to genital organs:
            female (625.–)
            male (302.7, 607.–, 608.–)

789.0   *Abdominal pain*

Abdominal tenderness   Epigastric pain
Colic:
  NOS
  infantile

Excludes: renal colic (788.0)

789.1   *Hepatomegaly*

789.2   *Splenomegaly*

789.3   *Abdominal or pelvic swelling, mass or lump*

789.4   *Abdominal rigidity*

789.5   *Ascites*

Fluid in peritoneal cavity

789.9   *Other*

Nonspecific abnormal findings (790-796)

790   Nonspecific findings on examination of blood

Excludes: abnormality of:
        coagulation (286.–)
        platelets (287.–)
        thrombocytes (287.–)
        white blood cells (288.–)

790.0   *Abnormality of red blood cells*

Abnormal red cell: Anisocytosis
  morphology NOS   Poikilocytosis
  volume NOS

Excludes: anaemias (280-285, 776.5, 776.6)
         polycythaemia (238.4, 289.0, 289.6, 776.4)

790.1   *Elevated sedimentation rate*

790.2   *Abnormal glucose tolerance test*

Diabetes: Prediabetes
  chemical
  latent

Excludes: when complicating pregnancy, childbirth or the puerperium
      (648.8)

790.3   *Excessive blood level of alcohol*

790.4   *Nonspecific elevation of levels of transaminase or lactic acid dehydrogenase [LDH]*

790.5   *Other nonspecific abnormal serum enzyme levels*

Abnormal serum level of: Abnormal serum level of:
  acid phosphatase   amylase
  alkaline phosphatase   lipase

Excludes: deficiency of circulating enzymes (277.6)

790.6   *Other abnormal blood chemistry*

Abnormal blood level of:
  cobalt
  copper
  iron
  lithium

Abnormal blood level of:
  magnesium
  mineral
  zinc

Excludes: abnormality of electrolyte or acid-base balance (276.–)
            hyperglycaemia NOS (250.9)
            hypoglycaemia NOS (251.2)
            specific findings indicating abnormality of:
              amino-acid transport and metabolism (270.–)
              carbohydrate transport and metabolism (271.–)
              lipid metabolism (272.–)
            uraemia (586)

790.7   *Bacteraemia, unspecified*

790.8   *Viraemia, unspecified*

790.9   *Other*

791   Nonspecific findings on examination of urine

Excludes: bacteriuria (599.0)
            haematuria NOS (599.7)
            specific findings indicating abnormality of:
              amino-acid transport and metabolism (270.–)
              carbohydrate transport and metabolism (271.–)

791.0   *Proteinuria*

Albuminuria   Bence-Jones proteinuria

Excludes: when arising during pregnancy or the puerperium (642.–,
            646.2)
            postural proteinuria (593.6)

791.1   *Chyluria*
Excludes: filarial (125.–)

791.2   *Haemoglobinuria*

791.3   *Myoglobinuria*

791.4   *Biliuria*

791.5   *Glycosuria*

791.6   *Acetonuria*

791.7   *Other cells and casts in urine*

791.9   *Other*

Crystalluria

792   Nonspecific abnormal findings in other body substances

Excludes: chromosomal studies (795.2)

792.0   *Cerebrospinal fluid*

792.1   *Stool contents*

Abnormal stool colour   Mucus in stool
Fat in stool   Pus in stool

792.2   *Semen*

Abnormal spermatozoa

Excludes: azoospermia (606)
            oligospermia (606)

792.3   *Amniotic fluid*

792.4   *Saliva*

Excludes: chromosomal studies (795.2)

792.9   *Other*

Peritoneal fluid   Synovial fluid
Pleural fluid   Vaginal fluids

793   Nonspecific abnormal findings on radiological and other examination of body structure

Includes: nonspecific abnormal findings of:
            thermography
            ultrasound examination [echogram]
            X-ray examination

Excludes: abnormal results of function studies (794.–)

793.0   *Skull and head*

793.1   *Lung field*

Coin lesion ⎫
            ⎬ lung
Shadow   ⎭

793.2   *Other intrathoracic organ*

Abnormal heart shadow   Mediastinal shift

793.3   *Biliary tract*

Nonvisualization of gallbladder

793.4   *Gastrointestinal tract*

793.5   *Genitourinary organs*

Filling defect:
  bladder
  kidney
  ureter

793.6   *Abdominal area, including retroperitoneum*

793.7   *Musculoskeletal system*

793.8   *Breast*

793.9   *Other*

794   Nonspecific abnormal results of function studies

794.0   *Brain and central nervous system*

Abnormal:
  echoencephalogram
  electroencephalogram [EEG]

794.1   *Peripheral nervous system and special senses*

Abnormal:
  electro-oculogram [EOG]
  electroretinogram [ERG]

Abnormal:
  response to nerve stimulation
  visually evoked potential [VEP]

794.2   *Pulmonary*

Reduced:
  ventilatory capacity
  vital capacity

794.3   *Cardiovascular*

Abnormal electrocardiogram
  [ECG] [EKG]

Abnormal phonocardiogram

794.4   *Kidney*

Abnormal renal function test

794.5   *Thyroid*

794.6   *Other endocrine function study*

794.7   *Basal metabolism*

Abnormal basal metabolic rate [BMR]

794.8   *Liver*

794.9 *Other*

Bladder   Spleen

795   Nonspecific abnormal histological and immunological findings
Excludes: nonspecific abnormalities of red blood cells (790.0)

795.0 *Nonspecific abnormal Papanicolaou smear of cervix*
Dyskaryotic cervical smear

795.1 *Nonspecific abnormal Papanicolaou smear of other origin*

795.2 *Nonspecific abnormal findings on chromosomal analysis*
Abnormal karyotype

795.3 *Nonspecific positive culture findings*
Positive culture findings in:
  nose
  sputum
  throat
  wound

795.4 *Other nonspecific abnormal histological findings*

795.5 *Nonspecific reaction to tuberculin test*
Abnormal result of Mantoux test

795.6 *False positive serological test for syphilis*
False positive Wasserman reaction

795.7 *Other nonspecific immunological findings*
Raised antibody titre   Raised level of immunoglobulins
Excludes: isoimmunization, in pregnancy (656.1, 656.2)
               affecting fetus or newborn (773)

796   Other nonspecific abnormal findings

796.0 *Nonspecific abnormal toxicological findings*

796.1 *Abnormal reflex*

796.2 *Elevated blood pressure reading without diagnosis of hypertension*
Note: This category is to be used to record an episode of elevated blood
       pressure in a patient in whom no formal diagnosis of hypertension
       has been made, or as an incidental finding.

796.3 *Nonspecific low blood pressure reading*

796.4 *Other abnormal clinical findings*

796.9 *Other*

ILL-DEFINED AND UNKNOWN CAUSES OF MORBIDITY AND
MORTALITY (797-799)

797   Senility without mention of psychosis

Old age

Excludes: senile psychoses (290.–)

798   Sudden death, cause unknown

798.0 *Sudden infant death syndrome*

Cot death   Sudden death of nonspecific cause
Crib death   in infancy

798.1 *Instantaneous death*

798.2 *Death occurring in less than 24 hours from onset of symptoms, not
otherwise explained*

Death known not to be violent or instantaneous, for which no cause
could be discovered
Died without sign of disease

798.9 *Unattended death*

Death in circumstances where the body of the deceased was found and no
cause could be discovered
Found dead

799   Other ill-defined and unknown causes of morbidity and mortality

799.0 *Asphyxia*

Excludes: asphyxia (due to):
carbon monoxide (986)
inhalation of food or foreign body (932-934)
newborn (768.–)
traumatic (994.7)

799.1 *Respiratory failure*

Cardiorespiratory failure   Respiratory arrest

Excludes: cardiac arrest (427.5)
failure of peripheral circulation (785.5)
respiratory failure, newborn (770.8)
respiratory insufficiency (786.0)

799.2 *Nervousness*

"Nerves"

799.3   *Debility, unspecified*

Excludes: asthenia 780.7
            nervous debility (300.5)
            neurasthenia (300.5)
            senile asthenia (797)

799.4   *Cachexia*

799.8   *Other ill-defined conditions*

799.9   *Other unknown and unspecified cause*

Undiagnosed disease, not specified as to site or system involved
Unknown cause of morbidity or mortality

XVII. INJURY AND POISONING

Note:

1. The principle of multiple coding of injuries should be followed wherever possible. Combination categories for multiple injuries are provided for use when there is insufficient detail as to the nature of the individual conditions, or for primary tabulation purposes when it is more convenient to record a single code; otherwise, the component injuries should be coded separately.

   Where multiple sites of injury are specified in the titles, the word "with" indicates involvement of both sites, and the word "and" indicates involvement of either or both sites. The word "finger" includes thumb.

2. Categories for "late effect" of injuries are to be found at 905-909.

FRACTURES (800-829)

Excludes: malunion (733.8)
            nonunion (733.8)
            pathological or spontaneous fracture (733.1)

The terms "condyle", "coronoid process", "ramus" and "symphysis" indicate the portion of the bone fractured, not the name of the bone involved

The descriptions "closed" and "open", used in the fourth-digit subdivisions, include the following terms:

closed:

comminuted		impacted	
depressed	with or without	linear	with or
elevated	delayed	march	without
fissured	healing	simple	delayed
greenstick		slipped epiphysis	healing
		spiral	

open:

compound	with or without	puncture	with or
infected	delayed	with foreign	without
missile	healing	body	delayed
			healing

A fracture not indicated as closed or open should be classified as closed

FRACTURE OF SKULL (800-804)

The following fourth-digit subdivisions are for use with categories 800-801, 803-804:

.0 Closed without mention of intracranial injury

.1 Closed with intracranial injury

.2 Open without mention of intracranial injury

.3 Open with intracranial injury

800 Fracture of vault of skull

[See above for fourth-digit subdivisions]

Frontal bone   Parietal bone

801 Fracture of base of skull

[See above for fourth-digit subdivisions]

Fossa: Sinus:
  anterior   ethmoid
  middle   frontal
  posterior   Sphenoid
Occiput   Temporal bone
Orbital roof

802 Fracture of face bones

802.0 *Nasal bones, closed*

802.1 *Nasal bones, open*

802.2 *Mandible, closed*

Inferior maxilla   Lower jaw (bone)

802.3 *Mandible, open*

802.4 *Malar and maxillary bones, closed*

Superior maxilla   Zygoma
Upper jaw (bone)

802.5 *Malar and maxillary bones, open*

802.6 *Orbital floor (blow-out), closed*

802.7 *Orbital floor (blow-out), open*

802.8 *Other facial bones, closed*

Alveolus   Palate
Orbit:
  NOS
  part other than roof or floor

Excludes: orbital:
          floor (802.6)
          roof (801.–)

802.9 *Other facial bones, open*

803 Other and unqualified skull fractures

[See page 474 for fourth-digit subdivisions]

Skull NOS   Skull multiple NOS

804 Multiple fractures involving skull or face with other bones

[See page 474 for fourth-digit subdivisions]

FRACTURE OF NECK AND TRUNK (805-809)

805 Fracture of vertebral column without mention of spinal cord lesion

Neural arch   Transverse process
Spine   Vertebra
Spinous process

805.0 *Cervical, closed*

805.1 *Cervical, open*

805.2 *Dorsal [thoracic], closed*

805.3 *Dorsal [thoracic], open*

805.4 *Lumbar, closed*

805.5 *Lumbar, open*

805.6 *Sacrum and coccyx, closed*

805.7 *Sacrum and coccyx, open*

805.8 *Unspecified, closed*

805.9 *Unspecified, open*

806   Fracture of vertebral column with spinal cord lesion

Any condition in 805.– with:

complete or incomplete transverse lesion (of cord)	paralysis
	paraplegia
haematomyelia	quadriplegia
injury to:	spinal concussion
cauda equina	
nerve	

806.0   *Cervical, closed*

806.1   *Cervical, open*

806.2   *Dorsal [thoracic], closed*

806.3   *Dorsal [thoracic], open*

806.4   *Lumbar, closed*

806.5   *Lumbar, open*

806.6   *Sacrum and coccyx, closed*

806.7   *Sacrum and coccyx, open*

806.8   *Unspecified, closed*

806.9   *Unspecified, open*

807   Fracture of rib(s), sternum, larynx and trachea

807.0   *Rib(s), closed*

807.1   *Rib(s), open*

807.2   *Sternum, closed*

807.3   *Sternum, open*

807.4   *Flail chest*

807.5   *Larynx and trachea, closed*

Hyoid bone	Trachea
Thyroid cartilage	

807.6   *Larynx and trachea, open*

808   Fracture of pelvis

808.0   *Acetabulum, closed*

808.1   *Acetabulum, open*

808.2   *Pubis, closed*

808.3   *Pubis, open*

808.4   *Other specified part, closed*

Ilium
Innominate bone

Ischium
Pelvic rim

808.5   *Other specified part, open*

808.8   *Unspecified, closed*

808.9   *Unspecified, open*

809   Ill-defined fractures of trunk

Bones of trunk with other bones except of skull and face
Multiple bones of trunk

Excludes: multiple fractures of:
          pelvic bones alone (808.–)
          ribs alone (807.–)
          ribs or sternum with limb bones (819.–, 828.–)
          skull or face with other bones (804.–)

809.0   *Fracture of trunk, closed*

809.1   *Fracture of trunk, open*

FRACTURE OF UPPER LIMB (810-819)

The following fourth-digit subdivisions are for use with those categories
   in 810-819 for which more detailed subdivision is not provided:

  .0   closed
  .1   open

810   Fracture of clavicle

[See above for fourth-digit subdivisions]

Clavicle:
  acromial end
  interligamentous

Clavicle shaft
Collar bone

811   Fracture of scapula

[See above for fourth-digit subdivisions]

Acromial process
Acromion (process)
Scapula (body) (neck)

Scapula, glenoid (cavity)
Shoulder blade

812 Fracture of humerus

812.0 *Upper end, closed*

Anatomical neck	Shoulder
Great tuberosity	Surgical neck
Proximal end	Upper epiphysis

812.1 *Upper end, open*

812.2 *Shaft or unspecified part, closed*

Humerus:	Upper arm NOS
NOS	
shaft	

812.3 *Shaft or unspecified part, open*

812.4 *Lower end, closed*

Articular process	External condyle
Distal end	Internal epicondyle
Elbow	Lower epiphysis

812.5 *Lower end, open*

813 Fracture of radius and ulna

813.0 *Upper end or unspecified part, closed*

Forearm NOS	Ulna:
Proximal end	coronoid process
Radius:	olecranon process
head	
neck	

813.1 *Upper end or unspecified part, open*

813.2 *Shaft, closed*

813.3 *Shaft, open*

813.4 *Lower end, closed*

Colles' fracture	Ulna:
Distal end	head
Dupuytren's fracture, radius	lower epiphysis
Radius, lower end	styloid process
Smith's fracture	

813.5 *Lower end, open .*

814   Fracture of carpal bone(s)

[See page 477 for fourth-digit subdivisions]

Cuneiform, wrist
Navicular, wrist
Os magnum
Scaphoid, wrist
Pisiform

Semilunar bone
Trapezium
Trapezoid bone
Unciform
Wrist

815   Fracture of metacarpal bone(s)

[See page 477 for fourth-digit subdivisions]

Bennett's fracture
Hand [except finger]

Metacarpus
Stave fractures

816   Fracture of one or more phalanges of hand

[See page 477 for fourth-digit subdivisions]

Finger(s)   Thumb

817   Multiple fractures of hand bones

[See page 477 for fourth-digit subdivisions]

Metacarpal bone(s) with phalanx or phalanges of same hand

818   Ill-defined fractures of upper limb

[See page 477 for fourth-digit subdivisions]

Arm NOS   Multiple bones of same upper limb

Excludes: multiple fractures of:
                    metacarpal bone(s) with phalanx or phalanges (817.–)
                    phalanges of hand alone (816.–)
                    radius with ulna (813.–)

819   Multiple fractures involving both upper limbs, and upper limb with rib(s) and sternum

[See page 477 for fourth-digit subdivisions]

Both arms [any bones]   Arm(s) with rib(s) or sternum

FRACTURE OF LOWER LIMB (820-829)

The following fourth-digit subdivisions are for use with those categories
in 820-829 for which more detailed subdivision is not provided:

.0 closed
.1 open

820   Fracture of neck of femur

820.0 *Transcervical fracture, closed*

Base of neck	Midcervical section
Cervicotrochanteric section	Subcapital
Epiphysis (separation) (upper)	Transepiphyseal
Head of femur	
Intracapsular section	

820.1 *Transcervical fracture, open*

820.2 *Pertrochanteric fracture, closed*

Intertrochanteric section	Trochanter:
Subtrochanteric section	NOS
	greater
	lesser

820.3 *Pertrochanteric fracture, open*

820.8 *Unspecified part, closed*

Hip NOS

820.9 *Unspecified part, open*

821   Fracture of other and unspecified parts of femur

821.0 *Shaft or unspecified part, closed*

Thigh	Upper leg

821.1 *Shaft or unspecified part, open*

821.2 *Lower end, closed*

Condyle	Epiphysis, lower
Distal end	

821.3 *Lower end, open*

822   Fracture of patella
[See above for fourth-digit subdivisions]
Knee cap

823   Fracture of tibia and fibula

Excludes: Dupuytren's fracture (824.–)
                  ankle (824.4, 824.5)
                  radius (813.4, 813.5)
                  Pott's fracture (824.4, 824.5)

823.0   *Upper end or unspecified part, closed*

Head	Tibia:
Lower leg NOS	condyles
Proximal end	tuberosity

823.1   *Upper end or unspecified part, open*

823.2   *Shaft, closed*

823.3   *Shaft, open*

824   Fracture of ankle

824.0   *Medial malleolus, closed*

Tibia involving:
  ankle
  malleolus

824.1   *Medial malleolus, open*

824.2   *Lateral malleolus, closed*

Fibula involving:
  ankle
  malleolus

824.3   *Lateral malleolus, open*

824.4   *Bimalleolar, closed*

Dupuytren's fracture, fibula   Pott's fracture

824.5   *Bimalleolar, open*

824.6   *Trimalleolar, closed*

Lateral and medial malleolus with anterior or posterior lip of tibia

824.7   *Trimalleolar, open*

824.8   *Unspecified, closed*

Ankle NOS

824.9   *Unspecified, open*

825   Fracture of one or more tarsal and metatarsal bones

825.0   *Fracture of calcaneus, closed*

Heel bone   Os calcis

825.1   *Fracture of calcaneus, open*

825.2   *Fracture of other tarsal and metatarsal bones, closed*

Astragalus   Navicular, foot
Cuboid   Scaphoid, foot
Cuneiform, foot   Talus
Foot [except toe]   Tarsal with metatarsal bone(s)
Instep   only

Excludes: calcaneus (825.0)

825.3   *Fracture of other tarsal and metatarsal bones, open*

826   Fracture of one or more phalanges of foot

[See page 480 for fourth-digit subdivisions]

Toe(s)

827   Other, multiple and ill-defined fractures of lower limb

[See page 480 for fourth-digit subdivisions]

Leg NOS   Multiple bones of same lower limb

Excludes: multiple fractures of:
                 ankle bones alone (824.–)
                 phalanges of foot alone (826.–)
                 tarsal with metatarsal bones (825.–)
                 tibia with fibula (823.–)

**828   Multiple fractures involving both lower limbs, lower with upper
          limb, and lower limb(s) with rib(s) and sternum**

[See page 480 for fourth-digit subdivisions]

Arm(s) and leg(s) [any bones]   Leg(s) with rib(s) or sternum
Both legs [any bones]

829   Fracture of unspecified bones

[See page 480 for fourth-digit subdivisions]

DISLOCATION (830-839)

Includes: displacement
               subluxation

Excludes: congenital dislocation (754-755)
pathological dislocation (718.2)
recurrent dislocation (718.3)

The descriptions "simple" and "compound", used in the fourth-digit subdivisions, include the following terms:

simple:
NOS   partial
closed   uncomplicated
complete

compound:
infected   with foreign body
open

The following fourth-digit subdivisions are for use with those categories
in 830-838 for which more detailed subdivision is not provided:

.0 simple dislocation
.1 compound dislocation

830 Dislocation of jaw
[See above for fourth-digit subdivisions]
Jaw (cartilage) (meniscus)   Maxilla (inferior)
Mandible   Temporomandibular (joint)

831 Dislocation of shoulder
[See above for fourth-digit subdivisions]
Acromioclavicular (joint)   Scapula
Excludes: sternoclavicular joint (839.6, 839.7)
          sternum (839.6, 839.7)

832 Dislocation of elbow
[See above for fourth-digit subdivisions]

833 Dislocation of wrist
[See above for fourth-digit subdivisions]
Carpal (bone)   Radiocarpal (joint)
Carpometacarpal (joint)   Radio-ulnar (joint), distal
Metacarpal (bone), proximal end Radius, distal end
Midcarpal (joint)   Ulna, distal end

834 Dislocation of finger
[See above for fourth-digit subdivisions]
Finger(s)   Metacarpophalangeal (joint)
Interphalangeal (joint), hand   Phalanx, of hand
Metacarpal (bone), distal end   Thumb

835 Dislocation of hip

[See page 483 for fourth-digit subdivisions]

836 Dislocation of knee

Excludes: dislocation of knee:
        old (718.2)
        pathological (718.2)
        recurrent (718.3)
        internal derangement of knee joint (717.–)
        old tear of cartilage or meniscus of knee (717.–)

836.0 *Tear of medial cartilage or meniscus of knee, current*

Bucket handle tear:
  NOS } current injury
  medial meniscus

836.1 *Tear of lateral cartilage or meniscus of knee, current*

836.2 *Other tear of cartilage or meniscus of knee, current*

Tear of:
  meniscus } not specified as medial or lateral
  cartilage (semilunar)

836.3 *Dislocation of patella, simple*

836.4 *Dislocation of patella, compound*

836.5 *Other dislocation of knee, simple*

Dislocation of knee NOS

836.6 *Other dislocation of knee, compound*

837 Dislocation of ankle

[See page 483 for fourth-digit subdivisions]

Astragalus	Scaphoid, foot
Fibula, distal end	Tibia, distal end
Navicular, foot	

838 Dislocation of foot

[See page 483 for fourth-digit subdivisions]

Interphalangeal (joint), foot	Phalanx, of foot
Metatarsal (bone)	Tarsal (bone) (joint)
Metatarsophalangeal (joint)	Tarsometatarsal (joint)
Midtarsal (joint)	Toe(s)

839   Other, multiple and ill-defined dislocations

839.0   *Cervical vertebra, simple*

Cervical spine   Neck

839.1   *Cervical vertebra, compound*

839.2   *Thoracic and lumbar vertebra, simple*

Dorsal [thoracic] vertebra

839.3   *Thoracic and lumbar vertebra, compound*

839.4   *Other vertebra, simple*

Coccyx   Sacrum
Sacroiliac (joint)   Spine NOS
                                              Vertebra NOS

839.5   *Other vertebra, compound*

839.6   *Other location, simple*

Pelvis   Sternum
Sternoclavicular joint

839.7   *Other location, compound*

839.8   *Multiple and ill-defined, simple*

Arm   Multiple locations, except fingers
Back   alone and toes alone
Hand   Other ill-defined locations
                                              Unspecified location

839.9   *Multiple and ill-defined, compound*

SPRAINS AND STRAINS OF JOINTS AND ADJACENT MUSCLES
(840-848)

Includes: avulsion
            haemarthrosis   of:
            laceration
            rupture   joint capsule
            sprain   ligament
            strain   muscle   } (attachment) (insertion)
            tear   tendon

Excludes: laceration of tendon in open wounds (880.2-884.2, 890.2-
            894.2)

840   Sprains and strains of shoulder and upper arm

840.0   *Acromioclavicular (joint) (ligament)*

840.1   *Coracoclavicular (ligament)*

840.2   *Coracohumeral (ligament)*

840.3   *Infraspinatus (muscle) (tendon)*

840.4   *Rotator cuff (capsule)*

840.5   *Subscapularis (muscle)*

840.6   *Supraspinatus (muscle) (tendon)*

840.8   *Other*

840.9   *Unspecified*

Shoulder NOS

841   Sprains and strains of elbow and forearm

841.0   *Radial collateral ligament*

841.1   *Ulnar collateral ligament*

841.2   *Radiohumeral (joint)*

841.3   *Ulnohumeral (joint)*

841.8   *Other*

841.9   *Unspecified*

Elbow NOS

842   Sprains and strains of wrist and hand

842.0   *Wrist*

Carpal (joint)   Radiocarpal (joint) (ligament)

842.1   *Hand*

Carpometacarpal (joint)   Metacarpophalangeal (joint)
Interphalangeal (joint)   Midcarpal (joint)

843   Sprains and strains of hip and thigh

843.0   *Iliofemoral (ligament)*

843.1   *Ischiocapsular (ligament)*

843.8   *Other*

843.9   *Unspecified*

Hip NOS   Thigh NOS

844   Sprains and strains of knee and leg

Excludes: current tear of cartilage or meniscus of knee (836.–)
                    old tear of cartilage or meniscus of knee (717.–)

844.0   *Lateral collateral ligament of knee*

844.1   *Medial collateral ligament of knee*

844.2   *Cruciate ligament of knee*

844.3   *Tibiofibular (joint) (ligament), superior*

844.8   *Other*

844.9   *Unspecified*
Knee NOS   Leg NOS

845   Sprains and strains of ankle and foot

845.0   *Ankle*
Achilles tendon   Internal collateral (ligament),
Calcaneofibular (ligament)   ankle
Deltoid (ligament), ankle   Tibiofibular (ligament), distal

845.1   *Foot*
Interphalangeal (joint), toe   Tarsometatarsal (joint) (ligament)
Metatarsophalangeal (joint)

846   Sprains and strains of sacroiliac region

846.0   *Lumbosacral (joint) (ligament)*

846.1   *Sacroiliac (ligament)*

846.2   *Sacrospinatus (ligament)*

846.3   *Sacrotuberous (ligament)*

846.8   *Other*

846.9   *Unspecified*

847   Sprains and strains of other and unspecified parts of back

Excludes: lumbosacral (846.0)

847.0   *Neck*
Anterior longitudinal (ligament), cervical
Atlanto-axial (joints)
Atlanto-occipital (joints)
Whiplash injury

847.1   *Thoracic*

847.2 *Lumbar*

847.3 *Sacrum*

Sacrococcygeal (ligament)

847.4 *Coccyx*

847.9 *Unspecified*

Back NOS

848   Other and ill-defined sprains and strains

848.0 *Septal cartilage of nose*

848.1 *Jaw*

Temporomandibular (joint) (ligament)

848.2 *Thyroid region*

Cricoarytenoid (joint) (ligament)   Thyroid cartilage
Cricothyroid (joint) (ligament)

848.3 *Ribs*

Chondrocostal (joint) ⎫
Costal cartilage   ⎬ without mention of injury to sternum
                              ⎭

848.4 *Sternum*

Chondrosternal (joint)   Xiphoid cartilage
Sternoclavicular (ligament)

848.5 *Pelvis*

Symphisis pubis
Excludes: in childbirth (665.6)

848.8 *Other specified sites*

848.9 *Unspecified site*

INTRACRANIAL INJURY, EXCLUDING THOSE WITH SKULL
FRACTURE (850-854)

Excludes: intracranial injury with skull fracture (800-801, 803-804
                with .1, .3)
            nerve injury (950.–, 951.–)
            open wound of head without intracranial injury (870-873)
            skull fracture alone (800-801, 803-804 with .0, .2)
The following fourth-digit subdivisions are for use with categories 851-
    854:
    .0 Without mention of open intracranial wound
    .1 With open intracranial wound

850 Concussion

Commotio cerebri

851 Cerebral laceration and contusion

[See page 488 for fourth-digit subdivisions]

Brain [any part]	Cerebellum
cortex	Cortex (cerebral)
membrane	

852 Subarachnoid, subdural and extradural haemorrhage, following injury

[See page 488 for fourth-digit subdivisions]

Middle meningeal haemorrhage ⎱
Subdural haematoma   ⎰ following injury

853 Other and unspecified intracranial haemorrhage following injury

[See page 488 for fourth-digit subdivisions]

Cerebral compression due to injury   Traumatic cerebral haemorrhage

854 Intracranial injury of other and unspecified nature

[See page 488 for fourth-digit subdivisions]

Brain injury NOS   Head injury NOS

INTERNAL INJURY OF CHEST, ABDOMEN AND PELVIS (860-869)

Includes: blast injuries ⎫
           bruise
           concussion injuries (except cerebral)
           crushing
           haematoma   ⎬ of internal organs
           laceration
           puncture
           tear
           traumatic rupture ⎭

Excludes: concussion NOS (850)
          foreign body entering through orifice (930-939)
          injury to blood vessels (901-902)

The description "with open wound", used in the fourth-digit subdivisions, includes those with mention of infection or foreign body

The following fourth-digit subdivisions are for use with categories 864-866, 868-869:

  .0   Without mention of open wound into cavity
  .1   With open wound into cavity

860 Traumatic pneumothorax and haemothorax

860.0 *Pneumothorax without mention of open wound into thorax*

860.1 *Pneumothorax with open wound into thorax*

860.2 *Haemothorax without mention of open wound into thorax*

860.3 *Haemothorax with open wound into thorax*

860.4 *Pneumohaemothorax without mention of open wound into thorax*

860.5 *Pneumohaemothorax with open wound into thorax*

861 Injury to heart and lung

861.0 *Heart, without mention of open wound into thorax*

861.1 *Heart, with open wound into thorax*

861.2 *Lung, without mention of open wound into thorax*

861.3 *Lung, with open wound into thorax*

862 Injury to other and unspecified intrathoracic organs

862.0 *Diaphragm, without mention of open wound into cavity*

862.1 *Diaphragm, with open wound into cavity*

862.2 *Other specified intrathoracic organ without mention of open wound into cavity*

Bronchus   Pleura
Oesophagus   Thymus gland

862.3 *Other specified intrathoracic organ, with open wound into cavity*

862.8 *Multiple and unspecified intrathoracic organs without mention of open wound into cavity*

Crushed chest   Multiple intrathoracic organs

862.9 *Multiple and unspecified intrathoracic organs, with open wound into cavity*

863 Injury to gastrointestinal tract

Excludes: anal sphincter laceration during delivery (664.2)
bile duct (868.–)
gallbladder (868.–)

863.0 *Stomach, without mention of open wound into cavity*

863.1 *Stomach, with open wound into cavity*

863.2 *Small intestine, without mention of open wound into cavity*

863.3 *Small intestine, with open wound into cavity*

863.4 *Colon or rectum, without mention of open wound into cavity*

863.5 *Colon or rectum, with open wound into cavity*

863.8 *Other and unspecified sites, without mention of open wound into cavity*

Gastrointestinal tract NOS   Pancreas
Intestine NOS

863.9 *Other and unspecified sites, with open wound into cavity*

864   Injury to liver
[See page 489 for fourth-digit subdivisions]

865   Injury to spleen
[See page 489 for fourth-digit subdivisions]

866   Injury to kidney
[See page 489 for fourth-digit subdivisions]

867   Injury to pelvic organs
Excludes: injury during delivery (664-665)

867.0 *Bladder and urethra, without mention of open wound into cavity*

867.1 *Bladder and urethra, with open wound into cavity*

867.2 *Ureter, without mention of open wound into cavity*

867.3 *Ureter, with open wound into cavity*

867.4 *Uterus, without mention of open wound into cavity*

867.5 *Uterus, with open wound into cavity*

867.6 *Other pelvic organ, without mention of open wound into cavity*

Fallopian tube   Seminal vesicle
Ovary   Vas deferens
Prostate

867.7 *Other pelvic organ, with open wound into cavity*

867.8 *Unspecified part, without mention of open wound into cavity*

867.9 *Unspecified part, with open wound into cavity*

868   Injury to other intraabdominal organs

[See page 489 for fourth-digit subdivisions]

Adrenal gland   Peritoneum
Bile duct   Multiple intraabdominal organs
Gallbladder

869   Internal injury to unspecified or ill-defined organs

[See page 489 for fourth-digit subdivisions]

Multiple extreme injury NOS   Severe crushing of unspecified site

OPEN WOUND (870-897)

Includes: animal bite
             avulsion
             cut
             laceration
             puncture wound
             traumatic amputation

Excludes: burn (940-949)
             crushing (925-929)
             puncture of internal organs (860-869)
             superficial injury (910-919)
             when incidental to:
                 dislocation (830-839)
                 fracture (800-829)
                 internal injury (860-869)
                 intracranial injury (851-854)

The description "complicated" used in the fourth-digit subdivisions includes those with mention of delayed healing, delayed treatment, foreign body or major infection

OPEN WOUND OF HEAD, NECK AND TRUNK (870-879)

The following fourth-digit subdivisions are for use with categories 875-877:

.0   Without mention of complication
.1   Complicated

870   Open wound of ocular adnexa

870.0   *Laceration of skin of eyelid and periocular area*

870.1   *Laceration of eyelid, full thickness, not involving lacrimal passages*

870.2   *Laceration of eyelid involving lacrimal passages*

870.3 *Penetrating wound of orbit without mention of foreign body*

870.4 *Penetrating wound of orbit with foreign body*
Excludes: retained (old) foreign body in orbit (376.6)

870.8 *Other open wounds of ocular adnexa*

870.9 *Unspecified open wound of ocular adnexa*

871 Open wound of eyeball
Excludes: 2nd cranial nerve [optic] injury (950.–)
3rd cranial nerve [oculomotor] injury (951.0)

871.0 *Ocular laceration without prolapse of intraocular tissue*

871.1 *Ocular laceration with prolapse or exposure of intraocular tissue*

871.2 *Rupture of eye with partial loss of intraocular tissue*

871.3 *Avulsion of eye*
Traumatic enucleation

871.4 *Unspecified laceration of eye*

871.5 *Penetration of eyeball with magnetic foreign body*
Excludes: retained (old) magnetic foreign body in globe (360.5)

871.6 *Penetration of eyeball with (nonmagnetic) foreign body*
Excludes: retained (old) (nonmagnetic) foreign body in globe (360.6)

871.7 *Unspecified ocular penetration*

871.9 *Unspecified open wound of eyeball*

872 Open wound of ear

872.0 *External ear, without mention of complication*
Auricle, ear   Pinna
Auditory canal

872.1 *External ear, complicated*

872.6 *Other specified parts, without mention of complication*
Ear drum

872.7 *Other specified parts, complicated*

872.8 *Part unspecified, without mention of complication*
Ear NOS

872.9 *Part unspecified, complicated*

873 Other open wound of head

Excludes: with mention of intracranial injury (851-854)

873.0 *Scalp, without mention of complication*

873.1 *Scalp, complicated*

873.2 *Nose, without mention of complication*
Nasal septum   Nasal sinus

873.3 *Nose, complicated*

873.4 *Face, without mention of complication*
Cheek   Forehead
Eyebrow   Jaw
Face: Lip
  NOS
  multiple sites

873.5 *Face, complicated*

873.6 *Internal structures of mouth, without mention of complication*
Gum   Palate
Mouth NOS   Tongue
                                                Tooth (broken)

873.7 *Internal structures of mouth, complicated*

873.8 *Other and unspecified open wound of head without mention of complication*
Head NOS

873.9 *Other and unspecified open wound of head, complicated*

874 Open wound of neck

874.0 *Larynx and trachea, without mention of complication*

874.1 *Larynx and trachea, complicated*

874.2 *Thyroid gland, without mention of complication*

874.3 *Thyroid gland, complicated*

874.4 *Pharynx, without mention of complication*
Cervical oesophagus

874.5 *Pharynx, complicated*

874.8 *Other and unspecified parts, without mention of complication*
Nape   Throat NOS
Supraclavicular region

874.9   *Other and unspecified parts, complicated*

875   Open wound of chest (wall)
[See page 492 for fourth-digit subdivisions]
Excludes: open wound into thoracic cavity (860-862)

876   Open wound of back
[See page 492 for fourth-digit subdivisions]
Loin   Lumbar region

877   Open wound of buttock
[See page 492 for fourth-digit subdivisions]
Sacroiliac region

878   Open wound of genital organs (external), including traumatic amputation
Excludes: internal genital organs (867.–)

878.0   *Penis, without mention of complication*

878.1   *Penis, complicated*

878.2   *Scrotum and testes, without mention of complication*

878.3   *Scrotum and testes, complicated*

878.4   *Vulva, without mention of complication*
Labium (majus) (minus)

878.5   *Vulva, complicated*

878.6   *Vagina, without mention of complication*

878.7   *Vagina, complicated*

878.8   *Other and unspecified parts, without mention of complication*

878.9   *Other and unspecified parts, complicated*

879   Open wound of other and unspecified sites, except limbs

879.0   *Breast, without mention of complication*

879.1   *Breast, complicated*

879.2   *Abdominal wall, anterior, without mention of complication*
Abdominal wall NOS   Pubic region
Epigastric region   Umbilical region
Hypogastric region

879.3   *Abdominal wall, anterior, complicated*

879.4   *Abdominal wall, lateral, without mention of complication*

Flank   Iliac (region)
Groin   Inguinal region
Hypochondrium

879.5   *Abdominal wall, lateral, complicated*

879.6   *Other and unspecified parts of trunk, without mention of complication*

Pelvic region   Trunk NOS
Perineum

879.7   *Other and unspecified parts of trunk, complicated*

879.8   *Open wound(s) (multiple) of unspecified site(s) without mention of complication*

Multiple open wounds NOS   Open wound NOS

879.9   *Open wound(s) (multiple) of unspecified site(s), complicated*

OPEN WOUND OF UPPER LIMB (880-887)

The following fourth-digit subdivisions are for use with categories 880-884:

   .0 Without mention of complication
   .1 Complicated
   .2 With tendon involvement

The subdivisions .0 and .1 are for use also with categories 885-886

880   Open wound of shoulder and upper arm
[See above for fourth-digit subdivisions]
Axilla   Scapular region

881   Open wound of elbow, forearm and wrist
[See above for fourth-digit subdivisions]

882   Open wound of hand except finger(s) alone
[See above for fourth-digit subdivisions]

883   Open wound of finger(s)
[See above for fourth-digit subdivisions]
Finger (nail)   Thumb (nail)

884   Multiple and unspecified open wound of upper limb
[See page 496 for fourth-digit subdivisions]
Arm NOS   Upper limb NOS
Multiple sites of one upper limb

885   Traumatic amputation of thumb (complete) (partial)
[See page 496 for fourth-digit subdivisions]
Thumb(s) (with finger(s) of either hand)

886   Traumatic amputation of other finger(s) (complete) (partial)
[See page 496 for fourth-digit subdivisions]
Finger(s) of one or both hands, without mention of thumb(s)

887   Traumatic amputation of arm and hand (complete) (partial)

887.0   *Unilateral, below elbow, without mention of complication*

887.1   *Unilateral, below elbow, complicated*

887.2   *Unilateral, at or above elbow, without mention of complication*

887.3   *Unilateral, at or above elbow, complicated*

887.4   *Unilateral, level not specified, without mention of complication*

887.5   *Unilateral, level not specified, complicated*

887.6   *Bilateral [any level], without mention of complication*

887.7   *Bilateral [any level], complicated*

OPEN WOUND OF LOWER LIMB (890-897)

The following fourth-digit subdivisions are for use with categories 890-894:
.0   Without mention of complication
.1   Complicated
.2   With tendon involvement
The subdivisions .0 and .1 are for use also with category 895.–

890   Open wound of hip and thigh
[See above for fourth-digit subdivisions]

891   Open wound of knee, leg [except thigh] and ankle
[See page 497 for fourth-digit subdivisions]
Leg NOS   Multiple sites of leg, except thigh

892   Open wound of foot except toe(s) alone
[See page 497 for fourth-digit subdivisions]
Heel

893   Open wound of toe(s)
[See page 497 for fourth-digit subdivisions]
Toe (nail)

894   Multiple and unspecified open wound of lower limb
[See page 497 for fourth-digit subdivisions]
Lower limb NOS   Multiple sites of one lower limb,
                                             except as in 891.–

895   Traumatic amputation of toe(s) (complete) (partial)
[See page 497 for fourth-digit subdivisions]
Toe(s) of one or both feet

896   Traumatic amputation of foot (complete) (partial)
896.0   *Unilateral, without mention of complication*
896.1   *Unilateral, complicated*
896.2   *Bilateral, without mention of complication*
Excludes: one foot and other leg (897.6, 897.7)
896.3   *Bilateral, complicated*

897   Traumatic amputation of leg(s) (complete) (partial)
897.0   *Unilateral, below knee, without mention of complication*
897.1   *Unilateral, below knee, complicated*
897.2   *Unilateral, at or above knee, without mention of complication*
897.3   *Unilateral, at or above knee, complicated*
897.4   *Unilateral, level not specified, without mention of complication*
897.5   *Unilateral, level not specified, complicated*

897.6 *Bilateral [any level], without mention of complication*

One foot and other leg

897.7 *Bilateral [any level], complicated*

INJURY TO BLOOD VESSELS (900-904)

Includes: arterial haematoma
avulsion
cut
laceration
rupture
traumatic aneurysm, or fistula
(arteriovenous)

of blood vessel, secondary to other injuries, e.g., fracture or open wound

Excludes: accidental puncture or laceration during medical procedure (998.2)
intracranial haemorrhage following injury (851-854)

900 Injury to blood vessels of head and neck

900.0 *Carotid artery*

Carotid artery (common) (external) (internal)

900.1 *Internal jugular vein*

900.8 *Other*

External jugular vein

Multiple blood vessels of head and neck

900.9 *Unspecified*

901 Injury to blood vessels of thorax

Excludes: traumatic haemothorax (860.2-860.5)

901.0 *Thoracic aorta*

901.1 *Innominate and subclavian arteries*

901.2 *Superior vena cava*

901.3 *Innominate and subclavian veins*

901.4 *Pulmonary blood vessel*

901.8 *Other*

Azygos vein
Intercostal artery or vein

Mammary artery or vein
Multiple blood vessels of thorax

901.9 *Unspecified*

902   Injury to blood vessels of abdomen and pelvis

902.0   *Abdominal aorta*

902.1   *Inferior vena cava*
Hepatic veins

902.2   *Coeliac and mesenteric arteries*

Gastric artery   Mesenteric artery
Hepatic artery   inferior
                                          superior
                                        Splenic artery

902.3   *Portal and splenic veins*
Mesenteric vein
  inferior
  superior

902.4   *Renal blood vessels*
Renal artery or vein

902.5   *Iliac blood vessels*

Hypogastric artery or vein   Uterine artery or vein
Iliac artery or vein

902.8   *Other*

Ovarian artery or vein   Multiple blood vessels of abdomen
                                          and pelvis

902.9   *Unspecified*

903   Injury to blood vessels of upper extremity

903.0   *Axillary blood vessels*

903.1   *Brachial blood vessels*

903.2   *Radial blood vessels*

903.3   *Ulnar blood vessels*

903.4   *Palmar artery*

903.5   *Digital blood vessels*

903.8   *Other*
Multiple blood vessels of upper extremity

903.9   *Unspecified*

904 Injury to blood vessels of lower extremity and unspecified sites

904.0 *Common femoral artery*

Femoral artery above profunda origin

904.1 *Superficial femoral artery*

904.2 *Femoral veins*

904.3 *Saphenous veins*

Saphenous vein
  greater
  lesser

904.4 *Popliteal blood vessels*

904.5 *Tibial blood vessels*

Tibial artery or vein
  anterior
  posterior

904.6 *Deep plantar blood vessels*

904.7 *Other blood vessels of lower extremity*

Multiple blood vessels of lower extremity

904.8 *Unspecified blood vessels of lower extremity*

904.9 *Unspecified site*

Injury to blood vessel NOS

LATE EFFECTS OF INJURIES, POISONINGS, TOXIC EFFECTS
AND OTHER EXTERNAL CAUSES (905-909)

Note: These categories are to be used to indicate conditions in 800-999 as the cause of late effects, which are themselves classified elsewhere. The "late effects" include those specified as such, or as sequelae, or those which are present one year or more after the acute injury [See III Late effects, page 723].

905 Late effects of musculoskeletal and connective tissue injuries

905.0 *Late effect of fracture of skull and face bones*

Late effect of injury classifiable to 800-804

905.1 *Late effect of fracture of spine and trunk without mention of spinal cord lesion*

Late effect of injury classifiable to 805, 807-809

905.2   *Late effect of fracture of upper extremities*
Late effect of injury classifiable to 810-819

905.3   *Late effect of fracture of neck of femur*
Late effect of injury classifiable to 820

905.4   *Late effect of fracture of lower extremities*
Late effect of injury classifiable to 821-827

905.5   *Late effect of fracture of multiple and unspecified bones*
Late effect of injury classifiable to 828-829

905.6   *Late effect of dislocation*
Late effect of injury classifiable to 830-839

905.7   *Late effect of sprain and strain without mention of tendon injury*
Late effect of injury classifiable to 840-848, except tendon injury

905.8   *Late effect of tendon injury*
Late effect of tendon injury due to:
   sprain and strain [injury classifiable to 840-848]
   open wound [injury classifiable to 880.2-884.2, 890.2-894.2]

905.9   *Late effect of traumatic amputation*
Late effect of injury classifiable to 885-887, 895-897
Excludes: late amputation stump complication (997.6)

906   Late effects of injuries to skin and subcutaneous tissues

906.0   *Late effect of open wound of head, neck and trunk*
Late effect of injury classifiable to 870-879

906.1   *Late effect of open wound of extremities without mention of tendon injury*
Late effect of injury classifiable to 880-884, 890-894 except .2

906.2   *Late effect of superficial injury*
Late effect of injury classifiable to 910-919

906.3   *Late effect of contusion*
Late effect of injury classifiable to 920-924

906.4   *Late effect of crushing*
Late effect of injury classifiable to 925-929

906.5   *Late effect of burn of eye, face, head and neck*
Late effect of injury classifiable to 940-941

906.6 *Late effect of burn of wrist and hand*
Late effect of injury classifiable to 944

906.7 *Late effect of burn of other extremities*
Late effect of injury classifiable to 943 or 945

906.8 *Late effect of burns of other specified sites*
Late effect of injury classifiable to 942, 946-947

906.9 *Late effect of burn of unspecified site*
Late effect of injury classifiable to 948-949

907 Late effects of injuries to the nervous system

907.0 *Late effect of intracranial injury without mention of skull fracture*
Late effect of injury classifiable to 850-854

907.1 *Late effect of injury to cranial nerve*
Late effect of injury classifiable to 950-951

907.2 *Late effect of spinal cord injury*
Late effect of injury classifiable to 806, 952

907.3 *Late effect of injury to nerve root(s), spinal plexus(es) and other nerves of trunk*
Late effect of injury classifiable to 953-954

907.4 *Late effect of injury to peripheral nerve of shoulder girdle and upper limb*
Late effect of injury classifiable to 955

907.5 *Late effect of injury to peripheral nerve of pelvic girdle and lower limb*
Late effect of injury classifiable to 956

907.9 *Late effect of injury to other and unspecified ner*
Late effect of injury classifiable to 957

908 Late effects of other and unspecified injuries

908.0 *Late effect of internal injury to chest*
Late effect of injury classifiable to 860-862

908.1 *Late effect of internal injury to intraabdominal organs*
Late effect of injury classifiable to 863-866, 868

908.2 *Late effect of internal injury to other internal organs*
Late effect of injury classifiable to 867 or 869

908.3 *Late effect of injury to blood vessel of head, neck and extremities*
Late effect of injury classifiable to 900, 903-904

908.4 *Late effect of injury to blood vessel of thorax, abdomen and pelvis*
Late effect of injury classifiable to 901-902

908.5 *Late effect of foreign body in orifice*
Late effect of injury classifiable to 930-939

908.6 *Late effect of certain complications of trauma*
Late effect of complications classifiable to 958

908.9 *Late effect of unspecified injury*
Late effect of injury classifiable to 959

909   Late effects of other and unspecified external causes

909.0 *Late effect of poisoning due to drug, medicament, or biological substance*
Late effect of condition classifiable to 960-979

909.1 *Late effect of toxic effects of nonmedical substances*
Late effect of condition classifiable to 980-989

909.2 *Late effect of radiation*
Late effect of condition classifiable to 990

909.3 *Late effect of complications of surgical and medical care*
Late effect of condition classifiable to 996-999

909.4 *Late effect of certain other external causes*
Late effect of condition classifiable to 991-994

909.9 *Late effect of other and unspecified external causes*
Late effect of condition classifiable to 995

SUPERFICIAL INJURY (910-919)

Excludes: burn (blisters) (940-949)
contusion (920-924)
foreign body:
    granuloma (728.8)
    inadvertently left in operation wound (998.4)
    residual, in soft tissue (729.6)
insect bite, venomous (989.5)
open wound with incidental foreign body (870-897)

The following fourth-digit subdivisions are for use with categories 910-917 and 919:

.0 Abrasion or friction burn without mention of infection
.1 Abrasion or friction burn, infected
.2 Blister without mention of infection
.3 Blister, infected
.4 Insect bite, nonvenomous, without mention of infection
.5 Insect bite, nonvenomous, infected
.6 Superficial foreign body (splinter) without major open wound and without mention of infection
.7 Superficial foreign body (splinter) without major open wound, infected
.8 Other and unspecified superficial injury without mention of infection
.9 Other and unspecified superficial injury, infected

910 Superficial injury of face, neck and scalp except eye

[See above for fourth-digit subdivisions]

Cheek	Lip
Ear	Nose
Gum	Throat

Excludes: eye and adnexa (918.–)

911 Superficial injury of trunk

[See above for fourth-digit subdivisions]

Abdominal wall	Interscapular region
Anus	Labium (majus) (minus)
Back	Penis
Breast	Perineum
Buttock	Scrotum
Chest wall	Testis
Flank	Vagina
Groin	Vulva

Excludes: scapular region (912.–)

912   Superficial injury of shoulder and upper arm
[See page 505 for fourth-digit subdivisions]
Axilla   Scapular region

913   Superficial injury of elbow, forearm and wrist
[See page 505 for fourth-digit subdivisions]

914   Superficial injury of hand(s) except finger(s) alone
[See page 505 for fourth-digit subdivisions]

915   Superficial injury of finger(s)
[See page 505 for fourth-digit subdivisions]
Finger (nail)   Thumb (nail)

916   Superficial injury of hip, thigh, leg and ankle
[See page 505 for fourth-digit subdivisions]

917   Superficial injury of foot and toe(s)
[See page 505 for fourth-digit subdivisions]
Heel   Toe (nail)

918   Superficial injury of eye and adnexa
Excludes: foreign body on external eye (930.–)
918.0   *Eyelids and periocular area*
918.1   *Cornea*
918.2   *Conjunctiva*
918.9   *Other and unspecified*
Eye(ball) NOS

919   Superficial injury of other, multiple and unspecified sites
[See page 505 for fourth-digit subdivisions]
Excludes: multiple sites classifiable to the same three-digit category
                (910-918)

CONTUSION WITH INTACT SKIN SURFACE (920-924)

Includes: bruice } without fracture or open wound
haematoma

Excludes: concussion (850)
haemarthrosis (840-848)
internal organs (860-869)
when incidental to:
crushing injury (925-929)
dislocation (830-839)
fracture (800-829)
internal injury (860-869)
intracranial injury (850-854)
nerve injury (950-957)
open wound (870-897)

920 Contusion of face, scalp, and neck except eye(s)

Cheek   Mandibular joint area
Ear (auricle)   Nose
Gum   Throat
Lip

921 Contusion of eye and adnexa

921.0 *Black eye, not otherwise specified*

921.1 *Contusion of eyelids and periocular area*

921.2 *Contusion of orbital tissues*

921.3 *Contusion of eyeball*

921.9 *Unspecified contusion of eye*

922 Contusion of trunk

922.0 *Breast*

922.1 *Chest wall*

922.2 *Abdominal wall*
Flank   Groin

922.3 *Back*
Buttock   Interscapular region
Excludes: scapular region (923.0)

922.4 *Genital organs*

Labium (majus) (minus)
Penis
Perineum

Scrotum
Testis
Vagina
Vulva

922.8 *Multiple sites of trunk*

922.9 *Unspecified part*

Trunk NOS

923 Contusion of upper limb

923.0 *Shoulder and upper arm*

Axilla

Scapular region

923.1 *Elbow and forearm*

923.2 *Wrist and hand(s), except finger(s) alone*

923.3 *Finger*

Finger (nail)

Thumb (nail)

923.8 *Multiple sites of upper limb*

923.9 *Unspecified part of upper limb*

Arm NOS

924 Contusion of lower limb and of other and unspecified sites

924.0 *Hip and thigh*

924.1 *Knee and lower leg*

924.2 *Ankle and foot, excluding toe(s)*

Heel

924.3 *Toe*

Toe (nail)

924.4 *Multiple sites of lower limb*

924.5 *Unspecified part of lower limb*

Leg NOS

924.8 *Multiple sites, not elsewhere classified*

924.9 *Unspecified site*

CRUSHING INJURY (925-929)

Excludes: concussion (850)
internal organs (860-869)
when incidental to:
internal injury (860-869)
intracranial injury (850-854)

925 Crushing injury of face, scalp and neck

Cheek	Pharynx
Ear	Throat
Larynx	

Excludes: head (800.3-803.3)
nose (802.0, 802.1)

926 Crushing injury of trunk

Excludes: crush injury of internal organs (860-869)

926.0 *External genitalia*

Labium (majus) (minus)	Testis
Penis	Vulva
Scrotum	

926.1 *Other specified sites*

Back	Buttock
Breast	

Excludes: crushing of chest (862.–)

926.8 *Multiple sites of trunk*

926.9 *Unspecified part*

Trunk NOS

927 Crushing injury of upper limb

927.0 *Shoulder and upper arm*

Axilla	Scapular region

927.1 *Elbow and forearm*

927.2 *Wrist and hand(s), except finger(s) alone*

927.3 *Finger*

927.8 *Multiple sites of upper limb*

927.9 *Unspecified part*

Arm NOS

928   Crushing injury of lower limb

928.0   *Hip and thigh*

928.1   *Knee and lower leg*

928.2   *Ankle and foot, excluding toe(s) alone*
Heel

928.3   *Toe*

928.8   *Multiple sites of lower limb*

928.9   *Unspecified part*
Leg NOS

929   Crushing injury of multiple and unspecified sites
Excludes: multiple extreme injury NOS (869.–)

929.0   *Multiple sites, not elsewhere classified*

929.9   *Unspecified site*
Excludes: severe crushing injury of unspecified site (869.–)

EFFECTS OF FOREIGN BODY ENTERING THROUGH ORIFICE
(930-939)

Excludes: foreign body:
                granuloma (728.8)
                inadvertently left in operation wound (998.4, 998.7)
                in open wound (800-839, 851-897)
                residual, in soft tissues (729.6)
                superficial without major open wound (910-919)

930   Foreign body on external eye
Excludes: foreign body in penetrating wound of:
                eyeball (871.5, 871.6)
                    retained (old) (360.5, 360.6)
                ocular adnexa (870.4)
                    retained (old) (376.6)

930.0   *Corneal foreign body*

930.1   *Foreign body in conjunctival sac*

930.2   *Foreign body in lacrimal punctum*

930.8   *Other and combined sites*

930.9 *Unspecified*
External eye NOS

931   Foreign body in ear
Auditory canal   Auricle

932   Foreign body in nose
Nasal sinus   Nostril

933   Foreign body in pharynx and larynx
933.0 *Pharynx*
Nasopharynx   Throat NOS
933.1 *Larynx*
Asphyxia due to foreign body   Choked on:
                                 food (regurgitated)
                                 phlegm

934   Foreign body in trachea, bronchus and lung
934.0 *Trachea*
934.1 *Main bronchus*
934.8 *Other specified part*
Bronchioles   Lung
934.9 *Respiratory tree, unspecified*
Inhalation of liquid or vomitus NOS

935   Foreign body in mouth, oesophagus and stomach
935.0 *Mouth*
935.1 *Oesophagus*
935.2 *Stomach*

936   Foreign body in intestine and colon

937   Foreign body in anus and rectum
Rectosigmoid (junction)

938   Foreign body in digestive system, unspecified
Alimentary tract NOS   Swallowed foreign body

939   Foreign body in genitourinary tract

939.0   *Bladder and urethra*

939.1   *Uterus, any part*

Excludes: intrauterine contraceptive device:
            complications from (996.3, 996.6)
            presence of (V45.5)

939.2   *Vulva and vagina*

939.3   *Penis*

939.9   *Unspecified*

BURNS (940-949)

Includes: burns from:
            electrical heating appliance
            electricity
            flame
            hot object
            lightning
            radiation
            chemical burns
              external
              internal
            scalds

Excludes: friction burns (910-919)
            sunburn (692.7)

The following fourth-digit subdivisions are for use with categories 941-946, 949:

.0   Unspecified degree
.1   Erythema [first degree]
.2   Blisters, epidermal loss [second degree]
.3   Full-thickness skin loss [third degree NOS]
.4   Deep necrosis of underlying tissues [deep third degree]

940   Burn confined to eye and adnexa

940.0   *Chemical burn of eyelids and periocular area*

940.1   *Other burns of eyelids and periocular area*

940.2   *Alkaline chemical burn of cornea and conjunctival sac*

940.3   *Acid chemical burn of cornea and conjunctival sac*

940.4   *Other burn of cornea and conjunctival sac*

940.5 *Burn with resulting rupture and destruction of eyeball*

940.9 *Unspecified burn of eye and adnexa*

941 Burn of face, head and neck

[See page 512 for fourth-digit subdivisions]

Ear [any part]
Eye with other parts of face, head
 and neck
Lip

Nose (septum)
Scalp [any part]
Temple (region)

Excludes: mouth (947.0)

942 Burn of trunk

[See page 512 for fourth-digit subdivisions]

Abdominal wall
Anus
Back [any part]
Breast
Buttock
Chest wall
Flank
Groin

Interscapular region
Labium (majus) (minus)
Penis
Perineum
Scrotum
Testis
Vulva

Excludes: scapular region (943.–)

943 Burn of upper limb, except wrist and hand

[See page 512 for fourth-digit subdivisions]

Arm [any part except wrist or hand]
Axilla

Scapular region
Shoulder

944 Burn of wrist(s) and hand(s)

[See page 512 for fourth-digit subdivisions]

Finger (nail)
Palm

Thumb (nail)

945 Burn of lower limb(s)

[See page 512 for fourth-digit subdivisions]

Foot [any part]
Leg [any part]

Thigh [any part]
Toe (nail)

946   Burns of multiple specified sites

[See page 512 for fourth-digit subdivisions]

Burns of sites classifiable to more than one category in 940-945

Excludes: multiple burns NOS (949.–)

947   Burn of internal organs

Includes: burns from ingested chemical agents

947.0   *Mouth and pharynx*

Gum   Tongue

947.1   *Larynx, trachea and lung*

947.2   *Oesophagus*

947.3   *Gastrointestinal tract*

Colon   Small intestine
Rectum   Stomach

947.4   *Vagina and uterus*

947.8   *Other*

947.9   *Unspecified*

948   Burns classified according to extent of body surface involved

Note: This category is to be used as the primary code only when the
       site of the burn is unspecified; it may be used as a supplementary
       code, if desired, with categories 940-947 when the site is specified.

948.0   *Less than 10% of body surface*

948.1   *10-19%*

948.2   *20-29%*

948.3   *30-39%*

948.4   *40-49%*

948.5   *50-59%*

948.6   *60-69%*

948.7   *70-79%*

948.8   *80-89%*

948.9   *90% or more*

949   Burn, unspecified

[See page 512 for fourth-digit subdivisions]

Burn NOS   Multiple burns NOS

Excludes: burn of unspecified site but with statement of the extent of
           body surface involved (948.–)

INJURY TO NERVES AND SPINAL CORD (950-957)

Includes: division of nerve
           lesion in continuity   } (with open wound)
           traumatic neuroma
           traumatic transient paralysis

Excludes: accidental puncture or laceration during medical procedure
           (998.2)

950   Injury to optic nerve and pathways

950.0 *Optic nerve injury*

Second cranial nerve

950.1 *Injury to optic chiasm*

950.2 *Injury to optic pathways*

950.3 *Injury to visual cortex*

950.9 *Unspecified*

Traumatic blindness NOS

951   Injury to other cranial nerve(s)

951.0 *Injury to oculomotor nerve*

Third cranial nerve

951.1 *Injury to trochlear nerve*

Fourth cranial nerve

951.2 *Injury to trigeminal nerve*

Fifth cranial nerve

951.3 *Injury to abducent nerve*

Sixth cranial nerve

951.4 *Injury to facial nerve*

Seventh cranial nerve

951.5 *Injury to acoustic nerve*

Auditory nerve   Traumatic deafness NOS
Eighth cranial nerve

951.6 *Injury to accessory nerve*

Eleventh cranial nerve

951.7 *Injury to hypoglossal nerve*

Twelfth cranial nerve

951.8 *Injury to other specified cranial nerves*

Glossopharyngeal [9th cranial] nerve Traumatic anosmia NOS
Olfactory [1st cranial] nerve   Vagus [10th cranial] nerve
Pneumogastric [10th cranial] nerve

951.9 *Injury to unspecified cranial nerve*

952 **Spinal cord lesion without evidence of spinal bone injury**

952.0 *Cervical*

952.1 *Dorsal [thoracic]*

952.2 *Lumbar*

952.3 *Sacral*

952.4 *Cauda equina*

952.8 *Multiple sites*

952.9 *Unspecified*

953 **Injury to nerve roots and spinal plexus**

953.0 *Cervical root*

953.1 *Dorsal root*

953.2 *Lumbar root*

953.3 *Sacral root*

953.4 *Brachial plexus*

953.5 *Lumbosacral plexus*

953.8 *Multiple sites*

953.9 *Unspecified*

954   Injury to other nerve(s) of trunk excluding shoulder and pelvic girdles

954.0   *Cervical sympathetic*

954.1   *Other sympathetic*

Coeliac ganglion or plexus   Splanchnic nerve(s)
Inferior mesenteric plexus   Stellate ganglion

954.8   *Other*

954.9   *Unspecified*

955   Injury to peripheral nerve(s) of shoulder girdle and upper limb

955.0   *Axillary nerve*

955.1   *Median nerve*

955.2   *Ulnar nerve*

955.3   *Radial nerve*

955.4   *Musculocutaneous nerve*

955.5   *Cutaneous sensory nerve, upper limb*

955.6   *Digital nerve*

955.7   *Other specified nerve(s)*

955.8   *Multiple nerves*

955.9   *Unspecified*

956   Injury to peripheral nerve(s) of pelvic girdle and lower limb

956.0   *Sciatic nerve*

956.1   *Femoral nerve*

956.2   *Posterior tibial nerve*

956.3   *Peroneal nerve*

956.4   *Cutaneous sensory nerve, lower limb*

956.5   *Other specified nerve(s)*

956.8   *Multiple nerves*

956.9   *Unspecified*

957   Injury to other and unspecified nerves

957.0   *Superficial nerves of head and neck*

957.1   *Other specified nerve(s)*

957.8   *Multiple nerves in several parts*

Multiple nerve injury NOS

957.9   *Unspecified site*

Nerve injury NOS

CERTAIN TRAUMATIC COMPLICATIONS AND UNSPECIFIED INJURIES
(958-959)

958   Certain early complications of trauma

Excludes: adult respiratory distress syndrome (518.5)
            shock lung (518.5)
            when occurring during or following medical procedures (996-
            999)

958.0   *Air embolism*

Pneumathaemia

Excludes: when complicating:
            abortion (634-638 with fourth digit .6, 639.6)
            ectopic or molar pregnancy (639.6)
            pregnancy, childbirth or the puerperium (673.0)

958.1   *Fat embolism*

Excludes: when complicating:
            abortion (634-638 with fourth digit .6, 639.6)
            ectopic or molar pregnancy (639.6)
            pregnancy, childbirth or the puerperium (673.8)

958.2   *Secondary and recurrent haemorrhage*

958.3   *Post-traumatic wound infection, not elsewhere classified*

958.4   *Traumatic shock*

Shock (immediate) (delayed) following injury

Excludes: shock:
            anaesthetic (995.4)
            anaphylactic (995.0)
              due to serum (999.4)
            electric (994.8)
            following abortion (639.5)
            lightning (994.0)
            nontraumatic NOS (785.5)
            obstetric (669.1)
            postoperative (998.0)

958.5 *Traumatic anuria*

Crush syndrome   Renal failure following crushing

958.6 *Volkmann's ischaemic contracture*

958.7 *Traumatic subcutaneous emphysema*

Excludes: subcutaneous emphysema resulting from a procedure (998.8)

958.8 *Other early complications of trauma*

959   Injury, other and unspecified

Includes: injury NOS

Excludes: injury NOS of:
   blood vessels (900-904)
   eye (921.–)
   head (854.–)
   internal organs (860-869)
   intracranial sites (850-854)
   nerves (950, 951, 953-957)
   spinal cord (952.–)

959.0 *Face and neck*

Cheek   Mouth
Ear   Nose
Eyebrow   Throat
Lip

959.1 *Trunk*

Abdominal wall   External genital organs
Back   Flank
Breast   Groin
Buttock   Interscapular region
Chest wall   Perineum

Excludes: scapular region (959.2)

959.2 *Shoulder and upper arm*

Axilla   Scapular region

959.3 *Elbow, forearm and wrist*

959.4 *Hand, except finger*

959.5 *Finger*

Finger (nail)   Thumb (nail)

959.6 *Hip and thigh*

Upper leg

959.7   *Knee, leg, ankle and foot*

959.8   *Other specified sites, including multiple*

Excludes: multiple sites classifiable to the same four-digit category (959.0-959.7)

959.9   *Unspecified site*

POISONING BY DRUGS, MEDICAMENTS AND BIOLOGICAL SUBSTANCES (960-979)

Includes: overdose of these substances
wrong substance given or taken in error

Excludes: adverse effects ["hypersensitivity", "reaction", etc.] of correct substance properly administered. Such cases are to be classified according to the nature of the adverse effect, such as:
allergic lymphadenitis (289.3)
aspirin gastritis (535.–)
blood disorders (280-289)
dermatitis:
   contact (692.–)
   due to ingestion (693.–)
nephropathy (583.8)
adverse effect NOS (995.2)
The drug giving rise to the adverse effect may be identified by use of categories E930-E949. If the E code is not being used, categories 960-979 may be used as *additional* codes to identify the drug. For this reason categories 960-979 are more detailed than would otherwise be necessary.
drug dependence (304.–)
drug reaction and poisoning affecting the newborn (760-779)
nondependent abuse of drugs (305.–)
pathological drug intoxication (292.2)

960   Poisoning by antibiotics

Excludes: antibiotics:
ear, nose and throat (976.6)
eye (976.5)
local (976.0)

960.0   *Penicillins*

960.1 *Antifungal antibiotics*

Excludes: preparations intended for topical use (976.–)

960.2 *Chloramphenicol group*

Chloramphenicol   Thiamphenicol

960.3 *Erythromycin and other macrolides*

960.4 *Tetracycline group*

960.5 *Cefalosporin group*

960.6 *Antimycobacterial antibiotics*

960.7 *Antineoplastic antibiotics*

960.8 *Other*

960.9 *Unspecified*

961   Poisoning by other anti-infectives

Excludes: anti-infectives:
           ear, nose and throat (976.6)
           eye (976.5)
           local (976.0)

961.0 *Sulfonamides*

961.1 *Arsenical anti-infectives*

961.2 *Heavy metal anti-infectives*

Excludes: mercurial diuretics (974.0)

961.3 *Quinoline and hydroxyquinoline derivatives*

Excludes: antimalarial drugs (961.4)

961.4 *Antimalarials and drugs acting on other blood protozoa*

Quinine

961.5 *Other antiprotozoal drugs*

961.6 *Anthelminthics*

961.7 *Antiviral drugs*

961.8 *Other antimycobacterial drugs*

961.9 *Other and unspecified anti-infectives*

962   Poisoning by hormones and synthetic substitutes

Excludes: oxytocic hormones (975.0)

962.0   *Adrenal cortical steroids*

962.1   *Androgens and anabolic congeners*

962.2   *Ovarian hormones and synthetic substitutes*

962.3   *Insulins and antidiabetic agents*

962.4   *Anterior pituitary hormones*

962.5   *Posterior pituitary hormones*

962.6   *Parathyroid and parathyroid derivatives*

962.7   *Thyroid and thyroid derivatives*

962.8   *Antithyroid agents*

962.9   *Other and unspecified hormones and synthetic substitutes*

963   Poisoning by primarily systemic agents

963.0   *Antiallergic and antiemetic drugs*

Chlorphenamine	Thonzylamine
Diphenhydramine	Tripelennamine
Diphenylpyraline	

Excludes: phenothiazine-based tranquillizers (969.1)

963.1   *Antineoplastic and immunosuppressive drugs*
Excludes: antineoplastic antibiotics (960.7)

963.2   *Acidifying agents*

963.3   *Alkalizing agents*

963.4   *Enzymes, not elsewhere classified*

963.5   *Vitamins, not elsewhere classified*
Excludes: nicotinic acid (972.2)
                  vitamin K (964.3)

963.8   *Other*

963.9   *Unspecified*

964   Poisoning by agents primarily affecting blood constituents

964.0   *Iron and its compounds*

964.1   *Liver preparations and other antianaemic agents*

964.2   *Anticoagulants*

| Coumarin | Warfarin sodium |
| Phenindione | |

964.3 *Vitamin K [Phytomenadione]*

964.4 *Fibrinolysis-affecting drugs*

964.5 *Anticoagulant antagonists and other coagulants*

964.6 *Gamma globulin*

964.7 *Natural blood and blood products*

964.8 *Other*

964.9 *Unspecified*

965   Poisoning by analgesics, antipyretics and antirheumatics
Excludes: drug dependence (304.–)
                 nondependent abuse (305.–)

965.0 *Opiates and related narcotics*
Codeine [methylmorphine]   Methadone
Heroin [diacetylmorphine]   Morphine
Pethidine [meperidine]   Opium (alkaloids)

965.1 *Salicylates*
Acetylsalicylic acid [aspirin]   Salicylic acid salts

965.4 *Aromatic analgesics, not elsewhere classified*
Acetanilide   Phenacetin [acetophenetidin]
Paracetamol [acetaminophen]

965.5 *Pyrazole derivatives*
Aminophenazone [amidopyrine]   Phenylbutazone

965.6 *Antirheumatics [antiphlogistics]*
Indometacin   Gold salts
Excludes: salicylates (965.1)
                 steroids (962.–)

965.7 *Other non-narcotic analgesics*
Pyrabital

965.8 *Other*
Pentazocine

965.9 *Unspecified*

966   Poisoning by anticonvulsants and anti-Parkinsonism drugs

966.0 *Oxazolidine derivatives*
Paramethadione   Trimethadione

966.1 *Hydantoin derivatives*

Phenytoin

966.2 *Succinimides*

Ethosuximide   Phensuximide

966.3 *Other and unspecified anticonvulsants*

Excludes: sulfonamides (961.0)

966.4 *Anti-Parkinsonism drugs*

Amantadine   Levodopa

967   Poisoning by sedatives and hypnotics

Excludes: drug dependence (304.–)
          nondependent abuse (305.–)

967.0 *Barbiturates*

Amobarbital [amylobarbitone]   Pentobarbital [pentobarbitone]
Barbital [barbitone]   Phenobarbital [phenobarbitone]
Butobarbital [butobarbitone]   Secobarbital [quinalbarbitone]

Excludes: thiobarbiturates (968.3)

967.1 *Chloral hydrate group*

967.2 *Paraldehyde*

967.3 *Bromine compounds*

Bromide   Carbromal (derivatives)
Carbamic esters

967.4 *Methaqualone compounds*

967.5 *Glutethimide group*

967.6 *Mixed sedatives, not elsewhere classified*

967.8 *Other*

967.9 *Unspecified*

Sleeping:
   draught
   drug   } NOS
   tablet

968   Poisoning by other central nervous system depressants

Excludes: drug dependence (304.–)
          nondependent abuse (305.–)

968.0 *Central nervous system muscle-tone depressants*

968.1 *Halothane*

968.2 *Other gaseous anaesthetics*

Ether
Halogenated hydrocarbon derivatives, except halothane
Nitrous oxide

968.3 *Intravenous anaesthetics*

Ketamine
Methohexital [methohexitone]

Thiobarbiturates, such as
   thiopental sodium

968.4 *Other and unspecified general anaesthetics*

968.5 *Surface and infiltration anaesthetics*

Cocaine
Lignocaine

Procaine
Tetracaine

968.6 *Peripheral nerve- and plexus-blocking anaesthetics*

968.7 *Spinal anaesthetics*

968.9 *Other and unspecified local anaesthetics*

969 Poisoning by psychotropic agents

Excludes: drug dependence (304.–)
          nondependent abuse (305.–)

969.0 *Antidepressants*

Amitriptyline
Imipramine

Monoamine oxidase inhibitors

969.1 *Phenothiazine-based tranquillizers*

Chlorpromazine
Fluphenazine

Prochlorperazine
Promazine

969.2 *Butyrophenone-based tranquillizers*

Haloperidol
Spiperone

Trifluperidol

969.3 *Other antipsychotics, neuroleptics and major tranquillizers*

969.4 *Benzodiazepine-based tranquillizers*

Chlordiazepoxide
Diazepam
Flurazepam

Lorazepam
Medazepam
Nitrazepam

969.5 *Other tranquillizers*

Hydroxyzine   Meprobamate

969.6 *Psychodysleptics [hallucinogens]*

Cannabis (derivatives)   Mescaline
Lysergide [LSD]   Psilocin
Marihuana (derivatives)   Psilocybine

969.7 *Psychostimulants*

Amphetamine   Caffeine

Excludes: central appetite depressants (977.0)

969.8 *Other psychotropic agents*

969.9 *Unspecified*

970   Poisoning by central nervous system stimulants

970.0 *Analeptics*

Lobeline   Nikethamide

970.1 *Opiate antagonists*

Levallorphan   Naloxone
Nalorphine

970.8 *Other*

970.9 *Unspecified*

971   Poisoning by drugs primarily affecting the autonomic nervous system

971.0 *Parasympathomimetics [cholinergics]*

Acetylcholine   Pilocarpine
Anticholinesterase:
  organophosphorus
  reversible

971.1 *Parasympatholytics [anticholinergics and antimuscarinics] and spasmolytics*

Atropine   Hyoscine [scopolamine]
Homatropine   Quaternary ammonium derivatives

Excludes: papaverine (972.5)

971.2 *Sympathomimetics [adrenergics]*

Epinephrine [adrenalin]   Levarterenol [noradrenalin]

971.3   *Sympatholytics [antiadrenergics]*

971.9   *Unspecified*

972   Poisoning by agents primarily affecting the cardiovascular system

972.0   *Cardiac rhythm regulators*

Practolol	Propranolol
Procainamide	Quinidine

972.1 • *Cardiotonic glycosides and drugs of similar action*

Digitalis glycosides

972.2   *Antilipaemic and antiarteriosclerotic drugs*

Clofibrate	Nicotinic acid derivatives

972.3   *Ganglion-blocking agents*

Pentamethonium bromide

972.4   *Coronary vasodilators*

972.5   *Other vasodilators*

Cyclandelate	Papaverine

972.6   *Other antihypertensive agents*

Guanethidine	Reserpine
Rauwolfia alkaloids	

972.7   *Antivaricose drugs, including sclerosing agents*

972.8   *Capillary-active drugs*

972.9   *Other and unspecified*

973   Poisoning by agents primarily affecting the gastrointestinal system

973.0   *Antacids and antigastric secretion drugs*

973.1   *Irritant cathartics*

973.2   *Emollient cathartics*

973.3   *Other cathartics, including intestinal atonia drugs*

973.4   *Digestants*

973.5   *Antidiarrhoeal drugs*

Excludes: anti-infectives (960-961)

973.6   *Emetics*

973.8   *Other*

973.9 *Unspecified*

974   Poisoning by water, mineral and uric acid metabolism drugs

974.0 *Mercurial diuretics*

974.1 *Purine derivative diuretics*

Excludes: aminophylline (975.7)

974.2 *Carbonic acid anhydrase inhibitors*

974.3 *Saluretics*

974.4 *Other diuretics*

974.5 *Electrolytic, caloric and water-balance agents*

974.6 *Other mineral salts, not elsewhere classified*

974.7 *Uric acid metabolism drugs*

Colchicine

975   Poisoning by agents primarily acting on the smooth and skeletal muscles and respiratory system

975.0 *Oxytocic agents*

975.1 *Smooth muscle relaxants*

Excludes: papaverine (972.5)

975.2 *Skeletal muscle relaxants*

975.3 *Other and unspecified drugs acting on muscles*

975.4 *Antitussives*

975.5 *Expectorants*

975.6 *Anti-common-cold drugs*

975.7 *Antiasthmatics*

975.8 *Other and unspecified respiratory drugs*

976   Poisoning by agents primarily affecting skin and mucous membrane, ophthalmological, otorhinolaryngological and dental drugs

976.0 *Local anti-infectives and anti-inflammatory drugs*

976.1 *Antipruritics*

976.2 *Local astringents and local detergents*

976.3 *Emollients, demulcents and protectants*

976.4   *Keratolytics, keratoplastics, other hair treatment drugs and preparations*

976.5   *Eye anti-infectives and other eye drugs*

Idoxuridine

976.6   *Anti-infectives and other drugs and preparations for ear, nose and throat*

976.7   *Dental drugs topically applied*

976.8   *Other*

Spermicides

976.9   *Unspecified*

977   Poisoning by other and unspecified drugs and medicaments

977.0   *Dietetics*

977.1   *Lipotropic drugs*

977.2   *Antidotes and chelating agents, not elsewhere classified*

977.3   *Alcohol deterrents*

977.4   *Pharmaceutical excipients*

977.8   *Other drugs and medicaments*

Diagnostic agents and kits
Contrast media used for diagnostic X-ray procedures

977.9   *Unspecified drug or medicament*

978   Poisoning by bacterial vaccines

978.0   *BCG*

978.1   *Typhoid and paratyphoid*

978.2   *Cholera*

978.3   *Plague*

978.4   *Tetanus*

978.5   *Diphtheria*

978.6   *Pertussis vaccine, including combinations with a pertussis component*

978.8   *Other and unspecified bacterial vaccines*

978.9   *Mixed bacterial vaccines, except combinations with a pertussis component*

979 Poisoning by other vaccines and biological substances

Excludes: gamma globulin (964.6)

979.0 *Smallpox vaccine*

979.1 *Rabies vaccine*

979.2 *Typhus vaccine*

979.3 *Yellow fever vaccine*

979.4 *Measles vaccine*

979.5 *Poliomyelitis vaccine*

979.6 *Other and unspecified viral and rickettsial vaccines*

979.7 *Mixed viral-rickettsial and bacterial vaccines, except combinations with a pertussis component*

979.9 *Other and unspecified vaccines and biological substances*

TOXIC EFFECTS OF SUBSTANCES CHIEFLY NONMEDICINAL AS
TO SOURCE (980-989)

Excludes: burns from ingested chemical agents (947.–)
respiratory conditions due to external agents (506-508)

980 Toxic effect of alcohol

980.0 *Ethyl alcohol*

Excludes: acute alcohol intoxication or "hangover" effects (305.0)
drunkenness (simple) 305.0
pathological (291.4)

980.1 *Methyl alcohol*

980.2 *Isopropyl alcohol*

980.3 *Fusel oil*

Alcohol:
  amyl
  butyl
  propyl

980.8 *Other*

980.9 *Unspecified*

981 Toxic effect of petroleum products

Benzine
Gasoline or petrol
Kerosine or paraffin oil
Paraffin wax

Petroleum:
ether
naphtha
spirit

982 Toxic effect of solvents other than petroleum-based

982.0 *Benzene and homologues*

982.1 *Carbon tetrachloride*

982.2 *Carbon disulfide*

982.3 *Other chlorinated hydrocarbon solvents*

Tetrachloroethylene   Trichloroethylene

Excludes: chlorinated hydrocarbon preparations other than solvents
(989.2)

982.4 *Nitroglycol*

982.8 *Other*

Acetone

983 Toxic effect of corrosive aromatics, acids and caustic alkalis

983.0 *Corrosive aromatics*

Carbolic acid or phenol   Cresol

983.1 *Acids*

Acid:
hydrochloric
nitric
sulphuric

983.2 *Caustic alkalis*

Potassium hydroxide   Sodium hydroxide

983.9 *Caustic, unspecified*

984 Toxic effect of lead and its compounds (including fumes)

Includes: from all sources except medicinal substances

984.0 *Inorganic lead compounds*

984.1 *Organic lead compounds*

984.8 *Other*

984.9 *Unspecified*

985   Toxic effect of other metals

Includes: from all sources except medicinal substances

985.0 *Mercury and its compounds*

Minamata disease

985.1 *Arsenic and its compounds*

985.2 *Manganese and its compounds*

985.3 *Beryllium and its compounds*

985.4 *Antimony and its compounds*

985.5 *Cadmium and its compounds*

985.6 *Chromium*

985.8 *Other*

985.9 *Unspecified*

986   Toxic effect of carbon monoxide

Includes: from all sources

987   Toxic effect of other gases, fumes or vapours

987.0 *Liquefied petroleum gases*

Butane   Propane

987.1 *Other hydrocarbon gas*

987.2 *Nitrogen oxides*

Nitrogen dioxide   Nitrous fumes

987.3 *Sulphur dioxide*

987.4 *Freon*

987.5 *Lacrimogenic gas*

Brombenzyl cyanide   Ethyliodoacetate
Chloroacetophenone

987.6 *Chlorine gas*

987.7 *Hydrocyanic acid gas*

987.8   *Other*

Polyester fumes

987.9   *Unspecified*

988   Toxic effect of noxious substances eaten as food

Excludes: allergic reaction to food, such as:
              gastroenteritis (558)
              rash (692.5, 693.1)
              food poisoning (bacterial) (005.–)
              toxic effects of food contaminants, such as:
              aflatoxin and other mycotoxin (989.7)
              mercury (985.0)

988.0   *Fish and shellfish*

988.1   *Mushrooms*

988.2   *Berries and other plants*

988.8   *Other*

988.9   *Unspecified*

989   Toxic effect of other substances, chiefly nonmedicinal as to source

989.0   *Hydrocyanic acid and cyanides*

Potassium cyanide   Sodium cyanide

Excludes: gas and fumes (987.7)

989.1   *Strychnine and salts*

989.2   *Chlorinated hydrocarbons*

Aldrin   DDT
Chlordane   Dieldrin

Excludes: chlorinated hydrocarbon solvents (982.–)

989.3   *Organophosphate and carbamate*

Carbaryl   Parathion
Dichlorvos

989.4   *Other pesticides, not elsewhere classified*

989.5   *Venom*

Tick paralysis

989.6   *Soaps and detergents*

989.7   *Aflatoxin and other mycotoxin [food contaminants]*

989.8 *Other*

989.9 *Unspecified*

OTHER AND UNSPECIFIED EFFECTS OF EXTERNAL CAUSES (990-995)

990   Effects of radiation, unspecified

Radiation sickness

Excludes: sunburn (692.7)
           specified adverse effects of radiation. Such cases are to be
           classified according to the nature of the adverse effect,
           such as:
              burns (940-949)
              dermatitis (692.7, 692.8)
              leukaemia (204-208)
              pneumonia (508.0)
           The type of radiation giving rise to the adverse effect may
           be identified by use of the E codes. If the E code is not
           being used, category 990 may be used as an *additional*
           code to identify radiation as the cause.

991   Effects of reduced temperature

991.0 *Frostbite of face*

991.1 *Frostbite of hand*

991.2 *Frostbite of foot*

991.3 *Frostbite of other and unspecified sites*

991.4 *Immersion foot*

Trench foot

991.5 *Chilblains*

991.6 *Hypothermia*

Hypothermia (accidental)

Excludes: hypothermia following anaesthesia (995.8)
           hypothermia not associated with low environmental tem-
           perature (780.9)

991.8 *Other*

991.9 *Unspecified*

Effects of freezing or excessive cold NOS

992 Effects of heat and light

Excludes: burns (940-949)
diseases of sweat glands due to heat (705.–)
malignant hyperpyrexia following anaesthesia (995.8)

992.0 *Heat stroke and sunstroke*

Heat apoplexy   Siriasis
Heat pyrexia   Thermoplegia
Ictus solaris

992.1 *Heat syncope*

Heat collapse

992.2 *Heat cramps*

992.3 *Heat exhaustion, anhydrotic*

Heat prostration due to water depletion

Excludes: when associated with salt depletion (992.4)

992.4 *Heat exhaustion due to salt depletion*

Heat prostration due to salt (and water) depletion

992.5 *Heat exhaustion, unspecified*

Heat prostration NOS

992.6 *Heat fatigue, transient*

992.7 *Heat oedema*

992.8 *Other heat effects*

992.9 *Unspecified*

993 Effects of air pressure

993.0 *Barotrauma, otitic*

Aero-otitis media   Effects of high altitude on ears

993.1 *Barotrauma, sinus*

Aerosinusitis   Effects of high altitude on sinuses

993.2 *Other and unspecified effects of high altitude*

Alpine sickness   Hypobaropathy
Andes disease   Mountain sickness
Anoxia due to high altitude

993.3 *Caisson disease*

Compressed-air disease   Divers' palsy or paralysis
Decompression sickness

993.4   *Effects of air pressure caused by explosion*

993.8   *Other*

993.9   *Unspecified*

994   Effects of other external causes

Excludes: certain adverse effects not elsewhere classified (995.–)

994.0   *Effects of lightning*

Shock from lightning	Struck by lightning NOS

Excludes: burns (940-949)

994.1   *Drowning and nonfatal submersion*

Bathing cramp	Immersion

994.2   *Effects of hunger*

Deprivation of food	Starvation

994.3   *Effects of thirst*

Deprivation of water

994.4   *Exhaustion due to exposure*

994.5   *Exhaustion due to excessive exertion*

Overexertion

994.6   *Motion sickness*

Air sickness	Travel sickness
Seasickness	

994.7   *Asphyxiation and strangulation*

Suffocation (by):	Suffocation (by):
bedclothes	plastic bag
cave-in	pressure
constriction	strangulation
mechanical	

Excludes: asphyxia from:
          carbon monoxide (986)
          inhalation of food or foreign body (932-934)
          other gases, fumes and vapours (987.–)

994.8   *Electrocution and nonfatal effects of electric current*

Shock from electric current

Excludes: electric burns (940-949)

994.9 *Other*

Effects of:
abnormal gravitational [G] forces or states
weightlessness

995   Certain adverse effects not elsewhere classified

Excludes: complications of surgical and medical care (996-999)

Note: This category is to be used for single-cause coding to identify
the effects not elsewhere classifiable of unknown, undetermined
or ill-defined causes. For multiple coding purposes this category
may be used as an additional code to identify the effects of conditions classified elsewhere.

995.0 *Anaphylactic shock*

Allergic shock
Anaphylactic reaction } NOS or due to adverse effect of correct medici-
Anaphylaxis   nal substance properly administered

Excludes: anaphylactic reaction to serum (999.4)

995.1 *Angioneurotic oedema*

Giant urticaria

Excludes: urticaria:
due to serum (999.5)
other specified (698.2, 708.–, 757.3)

995.2 *Unspecified adverse effect of drug, medicament and biological*

Adverse effect
Allergic reaction
Hypersensitivity } to correct medicinal substance properly administered
Idiosyncracy
Drug:
hypersensitivity NOS
reaction NOS

Excludes: pathological drug intoxication (292.2)

995.3 *Allergy, unspecified*

Allergic reaction NOS   Idiosyncracy NOS
Hypersensitivity NOS

Excludes: specified types of allergic reaction such as:
allergic diarrhoea (558)
dermatitis (691.–, 692.–, 693.–)
hay fever (477.–)
allergic reaction NOS to correct medicinal substance properly
administered (995.2)

995.4   *Shock due to anaesthesia*

Shock due to anaesthesia in which the correct substance was properly administered

Excludes: complications of anaesthesia in labour or delivery (668.–)
   overdose or wrong substance given (968-969)
   postoperative shock NOS (998.0)
   specified adverse effects of anaesthesia classified elsewhere, such as:
      anoxic brain damage (348.1)
      hepatitis (070.–), etc.
   unspecified adverse effect of anaesthesia (995.2)

995.5   *Child maltreatment syndrome*

Battered baby or child syndrome NOS
Emotional and/or nutritional maltreatment of child

995.8   *Other specified adverse effects not elsewhere classified*

Malignant hyperpyrexia or hypothermia due to anaesthesia

COMPLICATIONS OF SURGICAL AND MEDICAL CARE NOT ELSEWHERE CLASSIFIED (996-999)

Excludes: adverse effects of medicinal agents (001-799, 995.–)
   burns from local applications and irradiation (940-949)
   complications of:
      conditions for which the procedure was performed
      surgical procedures during abortion, labour and delivery (630-676)
   poisoning and toxic effects of drugs and chemicals (960-989)
   specified complications classified elsewhere:
      anaesthetic shock (995.4)
      blind-loop syndrome (579.2)
      colostomy malfunction (569.6)
      electrolyte imbalance (276.–)
      functional cardiac disturbances due to cardiac surgery (429.4)
      postgastric surgery syndromes (564.2)
      postlaminectomy syndrome (722.8)
      postmastectomy lymphoedema syndrome (457.0)
      postoperative psychosis (293.–)
      any other condition classified elsewhere in the Alphabetical Index when described as due to a procedure

Note: A supplementary classification (V code) is provided for classifying encounters with medical care for postoperative conditions in which *no* complications are present, such as:
      artificial opening status (V44.–)
      closure of external stoma (V55.–)
      fitting of prosthetic device (V52.–)

996   Complications peculiar to certain specified procedures

Includes: complications not elsewhere classified due to:

anastomosis (internal)
graft (bypass) (patch)
implant
internal device:
    catheter
    electronic
    fixation
    prosthetic
reimplant
transplant

    of natural source, such as:
        bone, blood vessel, etc.
    or artificial substitute, such as:
        Dacron, metal, Silastic,
        silicone, Teflon, etc.

Excludes: accidental puncture or laceration during procedure (998.2)
    complications of anastomosis, internal, of:
        gastrointestinal tract (997.4)
        urinary tract (997.5)
    other specified complications classified elsewhere, such as:
        haemolytic anaemia (283.1)
        functional cardiac disturbances (429.4)
        serum hepatitis (070.–)

996.0   *Mechanical complication of cardiac device, implant and graft*

Breakdown (mechanical)
Displacement
Leakage
Malposition
Obstruction, mechanical
Perforation
Protrusion

due to:
    cardiac pacemaker (electrode)
    coronary bypass graft
    heart valve prosthesis

996.1   *Mechanical complication of other vascular device, implant and graft*

Conditions listed in 996.0 due to:
  aortic (bifurcation) graft (replacement)
  arteriovenous:
    fistula
    shunt
        surgically created
  balloon (counterpulsation) device, intra-aortic
  carotid artery bypass graft
  dialysis catheter
  umbrella device, vena cava

996.2 *Mechanical complication of nervous system device, implant and graft*

Conditions listed in 996.0 due to:
 dorsal column stimulator
 electrodes implanted in brain [brain "pacemaker"]
 peripheral nerve graft
 ventricular (communicating) shunt

996.3 *Mechanical complication of genitourinary device, implant and graft*

Conditions listed in 996.0 due to:
 catheter:
  cystostomy
  urethral, indwelling
 intrauterine contraceptive device
 prosthetic reconstruction of vas deferens
 repair (graft) of ureter without mention of resection

Excludes: complications due to:
       external stoma of urinary tract (997.5)
       internal anastomosis of urinary tract (997.5)
       functioning intrauterine contraceptive device (V45.5)

996.4 *Mechanical complication of internal orthopaedic device, implant and graft*

Conditions listed in 996.0 due to:
 grafts of bone, cartilage, muscle or tendon
 internal (fixation) device such as nail, plate, rod, etc.

Excludes: complications of external orthopaedic device, such as:
       pressure ulcer due to cast (707.0)

996.5 *Mechanical complication of other specificied prosthetic device, implant and graft*

Conditions listed in 996.0 due to:
 prosthetic implant in:
  bile duct
  breast
  chin
  orbit of eye
 nonabsorbable surgical material NOS
 other graft, implant and internal device, not elsewhere classified

996.6 *Infection and inflammatory reaction due to internal prosthetic device, implant and graft*

Infection (causing obstruction) } due to (presence of) any device, implant
Inflammation } or graft listed in 996.0-996.5

996.7 *Other complications of internal prosthetic device, implant and graft*

Complication NOS ⎫
Embolism ⎪
Fibrosis ⎪ due to (presence of) any device, implant and graft
Haemorrhage ⎬ listed in 996.0-996.5
Pain ⎪
Stenosis ⎪
Thrombus ⎭

Excludes: transplant rejection (996.8)

996.8 *Complications of transplanted organ*

Transplant failure or rejection

996.9 *Complications of reattached extremity*

997 Complications affecting specified body systems, not elsewhere classified

Excludes: the listed conditions when specified as:
causing shock (998.0)
complications of:
anaesthesia:
adverse effect (001-799, 995.-)
in labour or delivery (668.-)
poisoning (968-969)
implanted device or graft (996.-)
obstetrical procedures (669.4)
reattached extremity (996.9)
transplanted organ (996.8)

997.0 *Central nervous system complications*

Anoxic brain damage } during or resulting from a procedure
Cerebral hypoxia }

997.1 *Cardiac complications*

Cardiac: ⎫
arrest ⎪
insufficiency ⎬ during or resulting from a procedure
Cardiorespiratory failure ⎪
Heart failure ⎭

Excludes: the listed conditions as long-term effects of cardiac surgery
or due to the presence of cardiac prosthetic device (429.4)

997.2   *Peripheral vascular complications*

Phlebitis
Thrombophlebitis } of any site during or resulting from a procedure

Excludes: the listed conditions due to:
          implant or catheter device (996.6)
          infusion, perfusion or transfusion (999.2)
      complications affecting internal blood vessels, such as:
          mesenteric artery (997.4)
          renal artery (997.5)

997.3   *Respiratory complications*

Mendelson's syndrome
Pneumonia (aspiration) } resulting from a procedure

Excludes: Mendelson's syndrome in labour and delivery (668.0)
      specified complications classified elsewhere, such as:
          adult respiratory distress syndrome (518.5)
          pulmonary oedema, postoperative (518.4)
          respiratory insufficiency, acute, postoperative (518.5)
          shock lung (518.5)
          tracheostomy malfunction (519.0)

997.4   *Gastrointestinal complications*

Complications of:
  external stoma of gastrointestinal tract, not elsewhere classified
  intestinal (internal) anastomosis and bypass, not elsewhere classified,
      except that involving urinary tract
Hepatic failure
Hepatorenal syndrome } specified as due to a procedure
Intestinal obstruction NOS

Excludes: specified gastrointestinal complications classified elsewhere,
      such as:
          colostomy or enterostomy malfunction (569.6)
          gastrojejunal ulcer (534.–)
          postcholecystectomy syndrome (576.0)
          postgastric surgery syndromes (564.2)

997.5   *Urinary complications*

Complications of:
  external stoma of urinary tract
  internal anastomosis and bypass of urinary tract, including that
      involving intestinal tract
Oliguria or anuria
Renal:
  failure (acute) } specified as due to a procedure
  insufficiency (acute)
Tubular necrosis (acute)

Excludes: specified complications classified elsewhere, such as:
postoperative stricture of:
ureter (539.3)
urethra (598.2)

997.6 *Late amputation stump complication*

997.9 *Complications affecting other specified body systems, not elsewhere classified*

Vitreous touch syndrome

Excludes: specified complications classified elsewhere, such as:
broad ligament laceration syndrome (620.6)
post-artificial-menopause syndrome (627.–)
postoperative stricture of vagina (623.2)

998 Other complications of procedures, not elsewhere classified

998.0 *Postoperative shock*

Collapse NOS ⎱ during or resulting from a
Shock (endotoxic) (hypovolaemic) (septic) ⎰ surgical procedure

Excludes: shock:
anaesthetic (995.4)
anaphylactic due to serum (999.4)
electric (994.8)
following abortion (639.5)
obstetric (669.1)
traumatic (958.4)

998.1 *Haemorrhage or haematoma complicating a procedure*

Haemorrhage of any site resulting from a procedure

Excludes: haemorrhage due to implanted device or graft (996.7)
when complicating caesarean section, or perineal, wound (674.3)

998.2 *Accidental puncture or laceration during a procedure*

Accidental perforation of: ⎱ by: catheter ⎱
blood vessel ⎟ endoscope ⎟ during a procedure
nerve ⎟ instrument ⎟
organ ⎰ probe ⎰

Excludes: puncture or laceration caused by implanted device intentionally left in operation wound (996.–)
specified complications classified elsewhere, such as:
broad ligament laceration syndrome (620.6)
trauma from instruments during delivery (664.–, 665.–)

998.3 *Disruption of operation wound*

Dehiscence } of operation wound
Rupture

Excludes: disruption of:
caesarean wound (674.1)
perineal wound, puerperal (674.2)

998.4 *Foreign body accidentally left during a procedure*

Adhesions } due to foreign body accidentally left in operation wound
Obstruction } or body cavity following a procedure
Perforation

Excludes: obstruction or perforation caused by implanted device intentionally left in body (996.–)

998.5 *Postoperative infection*

Abscess:
intra-abdominal
stitch
subphrenic } postoperative
wound
Septicaemia

Excludes: infection due to:
implanted device (996.6)
infusion, perfusion or transfusion (999.3)
postoperative obstetrical wound infection (674.3)

998.6 *Persistent postoperative fistula*

998.7 *Acute reaction to foreign substance accidentally left during a
procedure*

Peritonitis:
aseptic
chemical

998.8 *Other specified complications of procedures, not elsewhere classified*

Emphysema (subcutaneous) (surgical) resulting from a procedure

998.9 *Unspecified complication of procedure, not elsewhere classified*

Postoperative complication NOS

Excludes: complication NOS of obstetrical surgery or procedure (669.4)

999   Complications of medical care, not elsewhere classified

Includes: complications not elsewhere classified of:
dialysis (haemodialysis) (peritoneal) (renal)
extracorporeal circulation
hyperalimentation therapy
immunization
infusion
inhalation therapy
injection
inoculation
perfusion
transfusion
vaccination
ventilation therapy

Excludes: specified complications classified elsewhere, such as:
complications of implanted device (996.–)
contact dermatitis due to drugs (692.3)
dementia due to dialysis (293.–)
dialysis disequilibrium syndrome (276.–)
poisoning and toxic effects of drugs and chemicals (960-989)
postvaccinal encephalitis (323.5)
water and electrolyte imbalance (276.–)

999.0   *Generalized vaccinia*

999.1   *Air embolism*

Air embolism to any site following infusion, perfusion or transfusion

Excludes: embolism specified as:
complicating:
abortion (634-638 with fourth digit .6, 639.6)
ectopic or molar pregnancy (639.6)
pregnancy, childbirth or the puerperium (673.0)
due to implanted device (996.7)
traumatic (958.0)

999.2   *Other vascular complications*

Phlebitis
Thromboembolism } following infusion, perfusion or transfusion
Thrombophlebitis

Excludes: the listed conditions when specified as:
due to implanted device (996.7)
postoperative NOS (997.2)

999.3   *Other infection*

Infection ⎫
Sepsis   ⎬ following infusion, injection, transfusion or vaccination
Septicaemia ⎭

Excludes: the listed conditions when specified as:
                due to implanted device (996.6)
                postoperative NOS (998.5)

999.4   *Anaphylactic shock due to serum*

Excludes: shock:
                allergic NOS (995.0)
                anaphylactic:
                    NOS (995.0)
                    due to drugs and chemicals (995.0)

999.5   *Other serum reaction*

Intoxication by serum   Serum rash
Protein sickness   Serum sickness

Excludes: serum hepatitis (070.2, 070.3)

999.6   *ABO incompatibility reaction*

Incompatible blood transfusion
Reaction to blood group incompatibility in infusion or transfusion

999.7   *Rh incompatibility reaction*

Reactions due to Rh factor in infusion or transfusion

999.8   *Other transfusion reaction*

Septic shock due to transfusion   Transfusion reaction NOS

Excludes: postoperative shock (998.0)

**999.9   *Other and unspecified complications of medical care, not elsewhere
          classified***

Complications, not elsewhere classified, of:
  therapy:
    electroshock
    inhalation
    ultrasound
    ventilation
Unspecified misadventure of medical care

Excludes: unspecified complication of:
                phototherapy (990)
                radiation therapy (990)

SUPPLEMENTARY CLASSIFICATION OF
EXTERNAL CAUSES OF INJURY AND POISONING

This section is provided to permit the classification of environmental events, circumstances and conditions as the cause of injury, poisoning and other adverse effects. Where a code from this section is applicable, it is intended that it shall be used in addition to a code from one of the main chapters of the International Classification of Diseases, Injuries and Causes of Death, indicating the nature of the condition. Most often, the nature of the condition will be classifiable to Chapter XVII, Injuries, Poisoning and Violence, and for the classification of the underlying cause of death these will always require an "E" code in addition. Causes of death should preferably be tabulated according to both the Chapter XVII and the "E" codes, but if only one code is tabulated then the "E" code should be used in preference to the Chapter XVII code. Certain other conditions which may be stated to be due to external causes are classified in Chapters I to XVI of ICD, and for these the "E" code classification should be used as an additional code for multiple-condition analysis only.

Machinery accidents [other than connected with transport] are classifiable to category E919, in which the fourth digit allows a broad classification of the type of machinery involved. If a more detailed classification of type of machinery is required, it is suggested that the "Classification of Industrial Accidents according to Agency", prepared by the International Labour Office, be used in addition. This is reproduced on page 691 of this Manual for optional use.

Categories for "late effects" of accidents and other external causes are to be found at E929, E959, E969, E977, E989 and E999.

Definitions and examples related to transport accidents

(a) A **transport accident** (E800-E848) is any accident involving a device designed primarily for, or being used at the time primarily for, conveying persons or goods from one place to another.

Includes: accidents involving:
aircraft and spacecraft (E840-E848)
watercraft (E830-E838)
motor vehicle (E810-E825)
railway (E800-E807)
other road vehicles (E826-E829)

In classifying accidents which involve more than one kind of transport, the above order of precedence of transport accidents should be used.

Accidents involving agricultural and construction machines, such as tractors, cranes and bulldozers, are regarded as transport accidents only when these vehicles are under their own power on a highway [otherwise the vehicles are regarded as machinery]. Vehicles which can travel on land or water, such as hovercraft and other amphibious vehicles, are regarded as watercraft when on the water, as motor vehicles when on the highway, and as off-road motor vehicles when on land, but off the highway.

Excludes: accidents:
in sports which involve the use of transport but where the transport vehicle itself is not involved in the accident
involving vehicles which are part of industrial equipment used entirely on industrial premises
occurring during transportation but unrelated to the hazards associated with the means of transportation [e.g., injuries received in a fight on board ship; transport vehicle involved in a cataclysm such as an earthquake]
to persons engaged in the maintenance or repair of transport equipment or vehicle not in motion, unless injured by another vehicle in motion

(b) A **railway accident** is a transport accident involving a railway train or other railway vehicle operated on rails, whether in motion or not.

Excludes: accidents:
in repair shops
in roundhouse or on turntable
on railway premises but not involving a train or other railway vehicle

(c) A **railway train** or **railway vehicle** is any device with or without cars coupled to it, designed for traffic on a railway.

Includes: railway train, any power [steam] [electric] [diesel]
subterranean or elevated
monorail or two-rail
funicular

interurban:
electric car ⎫ (operated chiefly on its own right-of-way,
streetcar ⎭　　　not open to other traffic)
other vehicle designed to run on a railway track

Excludes: interurban electric cars [streetcars] specified to be operating on a right-of-way that forms part of the public street or highway [definition (n)]

(d) A **railway** or **railroad** is a right-of-way designed for traffic on rails, which is used by carriages or wagons transporting passengers or freight, and by other rolling stock, and which is not open to other public vehicular traffic.

(e) A **motor vehicle accident** is a transport accident involving a motor vehicle. It is defined as a motor vehicle traffic accident or as a motor vehicle nontraffic accident according to whether the accident occurs on a public highway or elsewhere.

Excludes: injury or damage due to cataclysm
injury or damage while a motor vehicle, not under its own power, is being loaded on, or unloaded from, another conveyance

(f) A **motor vehicle traffic accident** is any motor vehicle accident occurring on a public highway [i.e., originating, terminating or involving vehicle partially on the highway]. A motor vehicle accident is assumed to have occurred on the highway unless another place is specified, except in the case of accidents involving only off-road motor vehicles, which are classified as nontraffic accidents unless the contrary is stated.

(g) A **motor vehicle nontraffic accident** is any motor vehicle accident which occurs entirely in any place other than a public highway.

(h) A **public highway** [**trafficway**] or **street** is the entire width between property lines [or other boundary lines] of every way or place, of which any part is open to the use of the public for purposes of vehicular traffic as a matter of right or custom. A **roadway** is that part of the public highway designed, improved and ordinarily used, for vehicular travel.

Includes: approaches (public) to:
docks
public building
station

Excludes: driveway (private)   roads in:
parking lot   industrial premises
ramp   mine
roads in: private grounds
airfield   quarry
farm

(i) A **motor vehicle** is any mechanically or electrically powered device, not operated on rails, upon which any person or property may be transported or drawn upon a highway. Any object such as a trailer, coaster, sled, or wagon being towed by a motor vehicle is considered a part of the motor vehicle.

Includes: automobile [any type]
bus
construction machinery, farm and industrial machinery, steam roller, tractor, army tank, highway grader or similar vehicle on wheels or treads, while in transport under own power

fire engine (motorized)
motorcycle
motorized bicycle [moped] or scooter
trolley bus not operating on rails
truck
van

Excludes: devices used solely to move persons or materials within the confines of a building and its premises, such as:
building elevator
coal car in mine
electric baggage or mail truck used solely within a railroad station
electric truck used solely within an industrial plant
moving overhead crane

(j) A **motorcycle** is a two-wheeled motor vehicle having one or two riding saddles and sometimes having a third wheel for the support of a sidecar. The sidecar is considered part of the motorcycle.

Includes: motorized:
bicycle
scooter
tricycle

(k) An **off-road motor vehicle** is a motor vehicle of special design, to enable it to negotiate rough or soft terrain or snow. Examples of special design are high construction, special wheels and tyres, drive by tracks, or support on a cushion of air.

Includes: army tank
hovercraft, on land or swamp
snowmobile

(l) A **driver** of a motor vehicle is the occupant of the motor vehicle operating it or intending to operate it. A **motorcyclist** is the driver of a motor cycle. Other authorized occupants of a motor vehicle are **passengers.**

(m) An **other road vehicle** is any device, except a motor vehicle, in, on, or by which any person or property may be transported on a highway.

Includes: animal carrying a person or goods
animal-drawn vehicle
animal harnessed to conveyance
bicycle [pedal cycle]
street car
tricycle (pedal)

Excludes: pedestrian conveyance [definition (q)]

(n) A **streetcar** is a device designed and used primarily for transporting persons within a municipality, running on rails, usually subject to normal traffic control signals, and operated principally on a right-of-way that forms part of the traffic way. A trailer being towed by a streetcar is considered a part of the streetcar.

Includes: interurban electric or streetcar, when specified to be operating on a street or public highway
tram (car)
trolley (car)

(o) A **pedal cycle** is any road transport vehicle operated solely by pedals.

Includes: bicycle
pedal cycle
tricycle

Excludes: motorized bicycle [definition (i)]

(p) A **pedal cyclist** is any person riding on a pedal cycle or in a sidecar attached to such vehicle.

(q) A **pedestrian conveyance** is any human powered device by which a pedestrian may move other than by walking or by which a walking person may move another pedestrian.

Includes: baby carriage   roller skates
coaster wagon   scooter
ice skates   skateboard
perambulator   skis
pushcart   sled
pushchair   wheelchair

(r) A **pedestrian** is any person involved in an accident who was not at the time of the accident riding in or on a motor vehicle, railroad train, streetcar, animal-drawn or other vehicle, or on a bicycle or animal.

Includes: person:
changing tyre of vehicle
in or operating a pedestrian conveyance
making adjustment to motor of vehicle
on foot

(s) A **watercraft** is any device for transporting passengers or goods on the water.

(t) A **small boat** is any watercraft propelled by paddle, oars, or small motor, with a passenger capacity of less than ten.

Includes: boat NOS   row boat
            canoe   rowing shell
            coble   scull
            dinghy   skiff
            punt   small motorboat
            raft
Excludes: barge
            lifeboat (used after abandoning ship)
            raft (anchored) being used as a diving platform
            yacht

(u) An **aircraft** is any device for transporting passengers or goods in the air.
Includes: aeroplane [any type]   glider
            balloon   military aircraft
            bomber   parachute
            dirigible

(v) A **commercial transport aircraft** is any device for collective passenger or freight transportation by air, whether run on commercial lines for profit or by government authorities, with the exception of military craft.

RAILWAY ACCIDENTS (E800-E807)

For definitions of railway accident and related terms see definitions (a) to (d).
Excludes: accidents involving railway train and:
                aircraft (E840-E845)
                motor vehicle (E810-E825)
                watercraft (E830-E838)
The following fourth digits are for use with categories E800-E807 to identify the injured person.

    .0 *Railway employee*
        Any person who by virtue of his employment in connection with a railway, whether by the railway company or not, is at increased risk of involvement in a railway accident.
        Includes: catering staff on train   porter
                    driver   postal staff on train
                    railway fireman   shunter
                    guard   sleeping car attendant
    .1 *Passenger on railway*
        Any authorized person travelling on a train, except a railway employee.
        Excludes: intending passenger waiting at station (.8)
                    unauthorized rider on railway vehicle (.8)

.2 *Pedestrian*
See definition (n)
.3 *Pedal cyclist*
See definition (p)
.8 *Other specified person*
Includes: intending passenger waiting at station
unauthorized rider on railway vehicle
.9 *Unspecified person*

E800   Railway accident involving collision with rolling stock
Includes: collision between railway trains or railway vehicles, any kind
collision NOS on railway
derailment with antecedent collision with rolling stock or
NOS

E801   Railway accident involving collision with other object
Includes: collision of railway train   collision of railway train
with: with:
buffers   rock on railway
fallen tree on railway   street car
gates   other nonmotor vehicle
platform   other object
Excludes: collision with:
aircraft (E840-E842)
motor vehicle (E810.–, E820-E822)

E802   Railway accident involving derailment without antecedent collision

E803   Railway accident involving explosion, fire or burning
Excludes: explosion or fire, with mention of antecedent collision (E800.–,
E801.–)
explosion or fire, with antecedent derailment (E802.–)

E804   Fall in, on or from railway train
Includes: fall while alighting from or boarding railway train
Excludes: fall related to collision, derailment or explosion of railway
train (E800-E803)

E805   Hit by rolling stock
Includes: crushed   ⎤
injured   ⎟
killed   ⎬ by railway train or part of it
knocked down ⎟
run over   ⎦
Excludes: pedestrian hit by object set in motion by railway train
(E806.–)

E806   Other specified railway accident

Includes: hit by object falling in railway train
            injured by door or window on railway train
            nonmotor road vehicle or pedestrian hit by object set in
                motion by railway train
            railway train hit by falling:
                earth NOS
                rock
                tree
                other object

Excludes: railway accident due to cataclysm (E908-E909)

E807   Railway accident of unspecified nature

Includes: found dead $\Big\}$ on railway right-of-way NOS
            injured
            railway accident NOS

MOTOR VEHICLE TRAFFIC ACCIDENTS (E810-E819)

For definitions of motor vehicle traffic accident, and related terms see
definitions (e) to (k).

Excludes: accidents involving motor vehicle and aircraft (E840-E845)

The following fourth digits are for use with categories E810-E819 to
identify the injured person.

.0   *Driver of motor vehicle other than motorcycle*
     See definition (1)
.1   *Passenger in motor vehicle other than motorcycle*
     See definition (1)
.2   *Motorcyclist*
     See definition (1)
.3   *Passenger on motorcycle*
     See definition (1)
.4   *Occupant of streetcar*
.5   *Rider of animal; occupant of animal-drawn vehicle*
.6   *Pedal cyclist*
     See definition (p)
.7   *Pedestrian*
     See definition (r)
.8   *Other specified person*

     Includes: occupant of vehicle other than above
                 person in railway train involved in accident
                 unauthorized rider of motor vehicle

.9   *Unspecified person*

E810   Motor vehicle traffic accident involving collision with train

Excludes: motor vehicle collision with object set in motion by railway
               train (E815.–)
             railway train hit by object set in motion by motor vehicle
               (E818.–)

**E811   Motor vehicle traffic accident involving re-entrant collision with
           another motor vehicle**

Includes: collision between motor vehicle which accidentally leaves the
               roadway then re-enters the same roadway, or the oppo-
               site roadway on a divided highway, and another motor
               vehicle
Excludes: collision on the same roadway when none of the motor
               vehicles involved have left and re-entered the roadway
               (E812.–)

**E812   Other motor vehicle traffic accident involving collision with
           another motor vehicle**

Includes: collision with another motor vehicle parked, stopped, stalled,
               disabled, or abandoned on the highway
             motor vehicle collision NOS
Excludes: collision with object set in motion by another motor vehicle
               (E815.–)
             re-entrant collision with another motor vehicle (E811.–)

**E813   Motor vehicle traffic accident involving collision with other
           vehicle**

Includes: collision between motor vehicle, any kind, and:
               other road (nonmotor transport) vehicle such as:
                 animal carrying a person
                 animal-drawn vehicle
                 pedal cycle
                 street car
Excludes: collision with:
               object set in motion by nonmotor road vehicle (E815.–)
               pedestrian (E814.–)
             nonmotor road vehicle hit by object set in motion by motor
               vehicle (E818.–)

E814   Motor vehicle traffic accident involving collision with pedestrian

Includes: collision between motor vehicle, any kind, and pedestrian
             pedestrian dragged, hit, or run over by motor vehicle, any
               kind
Excludes: pedestrian hit by object set in motion by motor vehicle
               (E818.–)

E815   **Other motor vehicle traffic accident involving collision on the highway**

Includes: collision (due to loss of control) (on highway) between motor
                  vehicle, any kind, and:
              abutment (bridge) (overpass)
              animal (herded) (unattended)
              fallen stone, traffic sign, tree, utility pole
              guard rail or boundary fence
              inter-highway divider
              landslide (not moving)
              object set in motion by railway train or road vehicle
                  (motor) (nonmotor)
              object thrown in front of motor vehicle
              safety island
              temporary traffic sign or marker
              wall of cut made for road
              other object, fixed, movable or moving

Excludes: collision with:
              any object off the highway (resulting from loss of control)
                  (E816.–)
              any object which normally would have been off the high-
                  way and is not stated to have been on it (E816.–)
              motor vehicle parked, stopped, stalled, disabled, or
                  abandoned on highway (E812.–)
              moving landslide (E909)
              motor vehicle hit by object:
              set in motion by railway train or road vehicle (motor)
                  (nonmotor) (E818.–)
              thrown into or on vehicle (E818.–)

E816   **Motor vehicle traffic accident due to loss of control, without colli-
            sion on the highway**

Includes: motor vehicle:
              failing to make curve   and:
              going out of control (due to)   overturning
                burst tyre, blowout   colliding with object off
                driver falling asleep   the highway
                driver inattention   stopping abruptly off the
                excessive speed   highway
                failure of mechanical part

Excludes: collision on highway following loss of control (E810–E815)
              loss of control of motor vehicle following collision on the
                  highway (E810–E815)

E817   **Noncollision motor vehicle traffic accident while boarding or alighting**

Includes: fall down stairs of motor bus ⎫
            fall from car in street   ⎪ while boarding or
            injured by moving part of the vehicle ⎬   alighting
            trapped by door of motor bus   ⎭

E818   **Other noncollision motor vehicle traffic accident**

Includes: accidental poisoning from exhaust ⎫
              gas generated by   ⎪
            breakage of any part of   ⎪
            explosion of any part of   ⎪
            fall, jump or being accidentally ⎪
              pushed from   ⎬ motor vehicle while in
            fire starting in   ⎪   motion
            hit by object thrown into or on ⎪
            injured by being thrown against ⎪
              some part of, or object in ⎪
            injury from moving part of ⎪
            object falling in or on ⎪
            object thrown on ⎭
            collision of railway train or road vehicle, except motor vehicle, with object set in motion by motor vehicle
            motor vehicle hit by object set in motion by railway train or road vehicle (motor) (nonmotor)
            pedestrian, railway train or road vehicle (motor) (nonmotor) hit by object set in motion by motor vehicle

Excludes: collision between motor vehicle and:
            object set in motion by railway train or road vehicle (motor) (nonmotor) (E815.–)
            object thrown towards the motor vehicle (E815.–)
            person overcome by carbon monoxide generated by stationary motor vehicle off the roadway with motor running (E868.2)

E819   **Motor vehicle traffic accident of unspecified nature**

Includes: motor vehicle traffic accident NOS
            traffic accident NOS

Motor vehicle nontraffic accidents (E820-E825)

For definitions of motor vehicle nontraffic accident and related terms see definitions (a) to (k).

Includes: accidents involving motor vehicles being used in recreational or sporting activities off the highway
collision and noncollision motor vehicle accidents occurring entirely off the highway

Excludes: accidents involving motor vehicle and:
aircraft (E840-E845)
watercraft (E830-E838)
accidents, not on the public highway, involving agricultural and construction machinery but not involving another motor vehicle (E919.0, E919.2, E919.7)

The following fourth digits are for use with categories E820-E825 to identify the injured person.

.0 *Driver of motor vehicle other than motorcycle*
See definition (1)

.1 *Passenger in motor vehicle other than motorcycle*
See definition (1)

.2 *Motor cyclist*
See definition (1)

.3 *Passenger on motorcycle*
See definition (1)

.4 *Occupant of streetcar*

.5 *Rider of animal; occupant of animal-drawn vehicle*

.6 *Pedal cyclist*
See definition (o)

.7 *Pedestrian*
See definition (r)

.8 *Other specified person*
Includes: occupant of vehicle other than above
person on railway train involved in accident
unauthorized rider of motor vehicle

.9 *Unspecified person*

E820   Nontraffic accident involving motor-driven snow vehicle

Includes: breakage of part of ⎫
        fall from   ⎬ motor-driven snow vehicle (not on
        hit by   public highway)
        overturning of   ⎬
        run over or dragged by ⎭
        collision of motor-driven snow vehicle with:
           animal (being ridden) (-drawn vehicle)
           another off-road motor vehicle
           other motor vehicle, not on public highway
           railway train
           other object, fixed or movable
        injury caused by rough landing of motor-driven snow vehicle
           (after leaving ground on rough terrain)

Excludes: accident on the public highway, involving motor-driven snow
        vehicle (E810-E819)

E821   Nontraffic accident involving other off-road motor vehicle

Includes: breakage of part of ⎫
        fall from   ⎬
        hit by   off-road motor vehicle, except
        overturning of   ⎬ snow vehicle (not on public
        run over or dragged by   highway)
        thrown against some part ⎬
           of or object in   ⎭
        collision with:
           animal (being ridden)
           animal-drawn vehicle
           another off-road motor vehicle, except snow vehicle
           other motor vehicle, not on public highway
           other object, fixed or movable

Excludes: accident on public highway involving off-road motor vehicle
        (E810-E819)
        collision between motor-driven snow vehicle and other off-
        road motor vehicle (E820.–)
        hovercraft accident on water (E830-E838)

E822   Other motor vehicle nontraffic accident involving collision with moving object

Includes: collision, not on public highway, between motor vehicle,
        except off-road motor vehicle, and:
        animal
        nonmotor vehicle
        other motor vehicle except off-road motor vehicle
        pedestrian
        railway train
        other moving object

Excludes: collision with:
　　　　 motor-driven snow vehicle (E820.–)
　　　　 other off-road motor vehicle (E821.–)

E823　Other motor vehicle nontraffic accident involving collision with stationary object

Includes: collision, not on public highway, between motor vehicle, except off-road motor vehicle, and any object, fixed or movable, but not in motion

E824　Other motor vehicle nontraffic accident while boarding and alighting

Includes: fall
　　　　 injury from moving part of motor vehicle
　　　　 trapped by door of motor vehicle
} while boarding or alighting from motor vehicle, except off-road motor vehicle, not on public highway

E825　Other motor vehicle nontraffic accident of other and unspecified nature

Includes: accidental poisoning from carbon monoxide generated by
breakage of any part of
explosion of any part of
fall, jump or being accidentally pushed from
fire starting in
hit by object thrown into, towards or on
injured by being thrown against some part of, or object in
injury from moving part of
object falling in or on
} motor vehicle, except off-road motor vehicle, while in motion, not on public highway

motor vehicle nontraffic accident NOS

Excludes: fall from or in stationary motor vehicle (E884.9, E885)
　　　　 overcome by carbon monoxide or exhaust gas generated by stationary motor vehicle off the roadway with motor running (E868.2)
　　　　 struck by falling object from or in stationary motor vehicle (E916)

OTHER ROAD VEHICLE ACCIDENTS (E826-E829)

Other road vehicle accidents are transport accidents involving road vehicles other than motor vehicles.

For definitions of other road vehicle and related terms see definitions (m) to (o).

Includes: accidents involving other road vehicles being used in recreational or sporting activities

Excludes: collision of other road vehicle [any] with:
aircraft (E840-E845)
motor vehicle (E813.-, E820-E822)
railway train (E801.-)

The following fourth digits are for use with categories E826-E829 to identify the injured person.

.0 *Pedestrian*

See definition (r)

.1 *Pedal cyclist*

See definition (p)

.2 *Rider of animal*

.3 *Occupant of animal-drawn vehicle*

.4 *Occupant of streetcar*

.8 *Other specified person*

.9 *Unspecified person*

E826 Pedal cycle accident

Includes: breakage of any part of pedal cycle
collision between pedal cycle and:
animal (being ridden) (herded) (unattended)
another pedal cycle
nonmotor road vehicle, any
pedestrian
other object, fixed, movable or moving, not set in motion
by motor vehicle, railway train or aircraft
entanglement in wheel of pedal cycle
fall from pedal cycle
hit by object falling or thrown on the pedal cycle
pedal cycle accident NOS
pedal cycle overturned

E827 Animal-drawn vehicle accident

Includes: breakage of any part of vehicle
collision between animal-drawn vehicle and:
animal (being ridden) (herded) (unattended)
nonmotor road vehicle, except pedal cycle
pedestrian, pedestrian conveyance or pedestrian vehicle
other object, fixed, movable or moving, not set in motion
by motor vehicle, railway train or aircraft

fall from ⎫
knocked down by ⎪
overturning of ⎬ animal-drawn vehicle
run over by ⎪
thrown from ⎭

Excludes: collision of animal-drawn vehicle with pedal cycle (E826.–)

E828 Accident involving animal being ridden

Includes: collision between animal being ridden and:
another animal
nonmotor road vehicle except pedal cycle and animal-
drawn vehicle
pedestrian, pedestrian conveyance or pedestrian vehicle
other object, fixed, movable or moving, not set in motion
by motor vehicle, railway train or aircraft

fall from ⎫
knocked down by ⎪
thrown from ⎬ animal being ridden
trampled by ⎭
ridden animal stumbled and fell

Excludes: collision of animal being ridden with:
animal-drawn vehicle (E827.–)
pedal cycle (E826.–)

E829 Other road vehicle accidents

Includes: accident while boarding or ⎫
alighting from ⎪
blow from object in ⎪ streetcar
breakage of any part of ⎪ nonmotor road vehicle not
caught in door of ⎬ classifiable to E826 to
derailment of ⎪ E828
fall in, on, or from ⎪
fire in ⎭
collision between streetcar or nonmotor road vehicle, except
as in E826 to E828, and:
animal (not being ridden)

another nonmotor road vehicle not classifiable to E826 to
    E828
pedestrian
other object, fixed, movable or moving, not set in motion
    by motor vehicle, railway train or aircraft
nonmotor road vehicle accident NOS
street car accident NOS

Excludes: collision with:
    animal being ridden (E828.–)
    animal-drawn vehicle (E827.–)
    pedal cycle (E826.–)

WATER TRANSPORT ACCIDENTS (E830-E838)

For definitions of water transport accident and related terms see definitions (a), (s) and (t).

Includes: watercraft accidents in the course of recreational activities

Excludes: accidents involving both aircraft, including objects set in
    motion by aircraft, and watercraft (E840-E845)

The following fourth digits are for use with categories E830-E838 to
identify the injured person.

.0 *Occupant of small boat, unpowered*

.1 *Occupant of small boat, powered*

See definition (t)

Excludes: water skier (.3)

.2 *Occupant of other watercraft — crew*

Includes: persons:
    engaged in operation of watercraft
    providing passenger services [cabin attendants,
        ship's physician, catering personnel]
    working on ship during voyage in other capacity
        [musician in band, operators of shops and
        beauty parlours]

.3 *Occupant of other watercraft — other than crew*

Includes: passenger
    occupant of lifeboat, other than crew, after aban-
        doning ship

.4 *Water skier*

.5 *Swimmer*

.6   *Dockers, stevedores*
Includes: longshoreman employed on the dock in loading and
unloading ships

.8   *Other specified person*
Includes: immigration and customs officials on board ship
person:
accompanying passenger or member of crew
visiting boat
pilot (guiding ship into port)

.9   *Unspecified person*

E830   Accident to watercraft causing submersion
Includes: submersion and drowning due to:
boat overturning
boat submerging
falling or jumping from burning ship
falling or jumping from crushed watercraft
ship sinking
other accident to watercraft

E831   Accident to watercraft causing other injury
Includes: any injury except submersion and drowning as a result of an
accident to watercraft
burned while ship on fire
crushed between ships by collision
crushed by lifeboat after abandoning ship
fall due to collision or other accident to watercraft
hit by falling object due to accident to watercraft
injured in watercraft accident involving collision
struck by boat or part thereof after fall or jump from damaged
boat
Excludes: burns from localized fire or explosion on board ship (E837.–)

**E832   Other accidental submersion or drowning in water transport
accident**
Includes: submersion or drowning as a result of an accident other than
accident to the watercraft, such as:
fall:
from gangplank
from ship
overboard
thrown overboard by motion of ship
washed overboard
Excludes: submersion or drowning of swimmer or diver who voluntarily
jumps from boat not involved in an accident (E910.–)

E833   Fall on stairs or ladders in water transport

Excludes: fall due to accident to watercraft (E831.–)

E834   Other fall from one level to another in water transport

Excludes: fall due to accident to watercraft (E831.–)

E835   Other and unspecified fall in water transport

Excludes: fall due to accident to watercraft (E831.–)

E836   Machinery accident in water transport

Includes: injuries in water transport caused by:
deck
engine room
galley   } machinery
laundry
loading

E837   Explosion, fire or burning in watercraft

Includes: explosion of boiler on steamship
localized fire on ship

Excludes: burning ship (due to collision or explosion) resulting in:
submersion or drowning (E830.–)
other injury (E831.–)

E838   Other and unspecified water transport accident

Includes: accidental poisoning by gases or fumes on ship
atomic power plant malfunction in watercraft
crushed between ships without accident to watercraft
crushed by falling object on ship or while loading or unloading
excessive heat in:
boiler room
engine room
evaporator room
fire room
hit by boat while water skiing
struck by boat or part thereof (after fall from boat)
watercraft accident NOS

AIR AND SPACE TRANSPORT ACCIDENTS (E840–E845)

For definition of aircraft and related terms see definitions (u) and (v).
The following fourth digits are for use with categories E840–E845 to
identify the injured person.

.0 *Occupant of spacecraft*

.1 *Occupant of military aircraft, any*

Includes: crew
passenger (civilian)
(military)
troops

} in military aircraft [air force]
[army] [national guard]
[navy]

Excludes: occupants of aircraft operated under jurisdiction of
police departments (.5)
parachutist (.7)

.2 *Crew of commercial aircraft (powered) in surface to surface transport*

.3 *Other occupant of commercial aircraft (powered) in surface to surface transport*

Includes: flight personnel:
not part of crew
on familiarization flight
passenger on aircraft (powered) NOS

.4 *Occupant of commercial aircraft (powered) in surface to air transport*

Includes: occupant [crew] [passenger] of aircraft (powered)
engaged in activities such as:
aerial spraying (crops) (fire retardants)
air drops of emergency supplies
air drops of parachutists, except from military
craft
crop dusting
lowering of construction material [bridge or
telephone pole]
sky writing

.5 *Occupant of other powered aircraft*

Includes: occupant [crew] [passenger] of aircraft (powered)
engaged in activities such as:
aerobatic flying
aircraft racing
rescue operation
storm surveillance
traffic surveillance
occupant of private plane NOS

.6 *Occupant of unpowered aircraft, except parachutist*

Includes: occupant of aircraft listed in E842

.7 *Parachutist (military) (other)*

Includes: person making voluntary descent

Excludes: person making descent after accident to aircraft (.1-.6)

.8 *Ground crew, airline employee*

Includes: persons employed at airfields (civil) (military) or launching pads, not occupants of aircraft

.9 *Other person*

E840   Accident to powered aircraft at takeoff or landing

Includes: collision of aircraft with any object, fixed, movable or moving

crash

explosion on aircraft

fire on aircraft

forced landing

} while taking off or landing

E841   Accident to powered aircraft, other and unspecified

Includes: aircraft accident NOS

aircraft crash or wreck NOS

any accident to powered aircraft while in transit or when not specified whether in transit, taking off or landing

collision of aircraft with another aircraft, bird or any object, while in transit

explosion on aircraft while in transit

fire on aircraft while in transit

E842   Accident to unpowered aircraft

Includes: any accident, except collision with powered aircraft, to:

balloon

glider

hang glider

kite carrying a person

hit by object falling from unpowered aircraft

E843   Fall in, on or from aircraft

Includes: accident in boarding or alighting from aircraft, any kind

fall in, on or from aircraft [any kind], while in transit, taking off or landing, except when as a result of an accident to aircraft

E844   Other specified air transport accidents

Includes: hit by:
      aircraft
      object falling from aircraft
    injury by or from:
      machinery on aircraft
      rotating propeller   } without accident to aircraft
      voluntary parachute descent
    poisoning by carbon monoxide
      from aircraft while in
      transit
    sucked into jet
    any accident involving other transport vehicle (motor) (non-motor) due to being hit by object set in motion by aircraft (powered)

Excludes: air sickness (E903)
    effects of:
      high altitude (E902.–)
      pressure change (E902.–)
    injury in parachute descent due to accident to aircraft (E840-E842)

E845   Accident involving spacecraft

Includes: launching pad accident
Excludes: effects of weightlessness in spacecraft (E928.0)

VEHICLE ACCIDENTS NOT ELSEWHERE CLASSIFIABLE (E846-E848)

E846   Accidents involving powered vehicles used solely within the buildings and premises of an industrial or commercial establishment

Includes: accident to, on or involving:
    battery powered airport passenger vehicle
    battery powered trucks (baggage) (mail)
    coal car in mine
    logging car
    self propelled truck, industrial
    station baggage truck (powered)
    tram, truck or tub (powered) in mine or quarry
    breakage of any part of vehicle
    collision with:
      pedestrian
      other vehicle or object within premises
    explosion of
    fall from
    overturning of   } powered vehicle, industrial or commercial
    struck by

Excludes: accidental poisoning by exhaust gas from vehicle not elsewhere classifiable (E868.2)
injury by crane, lift (fork) or elevator (E919.2)

E847   Accidents involving cable cars not running on rails
Includes: accident to, on or involving:
cable car, not on rails
ski chair-lift
ski-lift with gondola
téléférique
breakage of cable
caught or dragged by ⎫
fall or jump from   ⎬ cable car, not on rails
object thrown from or in ⎭

E848   Accidents involving other vehicles not elsewhere classifiable
Includes: accident to, on or involving:
ice yacht
land yacht
nonmotor, nonroad vehicle NOS

Place of Occurence
The following fifth digit sub-classification may be used, if desired, with
categories E850-E869 and E880-E928, to denote the place where the
accident or poisoning occurred:

    .0   *Home*

Apartment	Private:
Boarding house	driveway to home
Farm house	garage
Home premises	garden to home
House (residential)	walk to home
Noninstitutional place of residence	Swimming pool in private house or garden
	Yard to home

Excludes: home under construction but not yet occupied (.3)
institutional place of residence (.7)

    .1   *Farm*

Farm:
   buildings
   land under cultivation
Excludes: farm house and home premises of farm (.0)

    .2   *Mine and quarry*

Gravel pit	Tunnel under construction
Sand pit	

.3 *Industrial place and premises*

Building under construction
Dockyard
Dry dock
Factory
  building
  premises
Garage — place of work

Industrial yard
Loading platform (factory) (store)
Plant, industrial
Railway yard
Shop — place of work
Warehouse
Workshop

.4 *Place for recreation and sport*

Amusement park
Baseball field
Basketball court
Beach resort
Cricket ground
Fives court
Football field
Golf course
Gymnasium
Hockey field
Holiday camp
Ice palace
Lake resort
Mountain resort
Playground, including
  school playground
Public park

Racecourse
Resort NOS
Riding school
Rifle range
Seashore resort
Skating rink
Sports ground
Sports palace
Stadium
Swimming pool, public
Tennis court
Vacation resort

Excludes: swimming pool in private house or garden (.0)

.5 *Street and highway*

.6 *Public building*

Building (including adjacent grounds) used by the general public or by a
  particular group of the public, such as:

airport
bank
cafe
casino
church
cinema
clubhouse
court house
dance hall
garage building (for car storage)
hotel
market (grocery or other commodity)
movie house
music hall

night club
office
office building
opera house
post office
public hall
radio broadcasting station
restaurant
school (private) (public) (state)
shop, commercial
station (bus) (railway)
store
theatre

Excludes: home garage (.0)
             industrial building or workplace (.3)

.7 *Residential institution*

Children's home	Old people's home
Dormitory	Orphanage
Hospital	Prison
Jail	Reform school

.8 *Other specified places*

Beach NOS	Parking place
Canal	Pond or pool (natural)
Caravan site NOS	Prairie
Derelict house	Public place NOS
Desert	Railway line
Dock	Reservoir
Forest	River
Harbour	Sea
Hill	Seashore NOS
Lake NOS	Stream
Mountain	Swamp
Parking lot	Woods

.9 *Unspecified place*

ACCIDENTAL POISONING BY DRUGS, MEDICAMENTS
AND BIOLOGICALS (E850-E858)

Includes: accidental overdose of drug, wrong drug given or taken in error, and drug taken inadvertently
accidents in the use of drugs and biologicals in medical and surgical procedure

Excludes: correct drug properly administered in therapeutic or prophylactic dosage, as the cause of any adverse effect (E930-E949)
administration with suicidal or homicidal intent, or intent to harm, or in circumstances classifiable to E980-E989 (E950.0 to E950.4, E962.0, E980.0 to E980.4)

See Alphabetical Index for more complete list of specific drugs to be classified under the fourth-digit subdivisions.

E850   Accidental poisoning by analgesics, antipyretics, antirheumatics

E850.0 *Opiates and related narcotics*

Codeine [methylmorphine]	Morphine
Heroin [diacetylmorphine]	Opium (alkaloids)
Methadone	Pethidine [meperidine]

E850.1   *Salicylates*

Acetylsalicylic acid [aspirin]   Salicylic acid salts
Amino derivatives of salicylic acid

E850.2   *Aromatic analgesics, not elsewhere classified*

Acetanilide   Phenacetin [acetophenetidin]
Paracetamol [acetaminophen]

E850.3   *Pyrazole derivatives*

Aminophenazone [amidopyrine]   Phenylbutazone

E850.4   *Antirheumatics [antiphlogistics]*

Indometacin   Gold salts

Excludes: salicylates (E850.1)
            steroids (E858.0)

E850.5   *Other non-narcotic analgesics*

Pyrabital

E850.8   *Other*

Pentazocine

E850.9   *Unspecified*

E851   Accidental poisoning by barbiturates

Amobarbital [amylobarbitone]   Phenobarbital [phenobarbitone]
Barbital [barbitone]   Secobarbital [quinalbarbitone]
Pentobarbital [pentobarbitone]

Excludes: thiobarbiturates (E855.1)

E852   Accidental poisoning by other sedatives and hypnotics

E852.0   *Chloral hydrate group*

E852.1   *Paraldehyde*

E852.2   *Bromine compounds*

Bromides   Carbromal (derivatives)
Carbamic esters

E852.3   *Methaqualone compounds*

E852.4   *Glutethimide group*

E852.5   *Mixed sedatives, not elsewhere classified*

E852.8   *Other*

E852.9   *Unspecified*

Sleeping:
  draught ⎤
  drug   ⎬ NOS
  tablet ⎦

E853   Accidental poisoning by tranquillizers

E853.0   *Phenothiazine-based tranquillizers*

Chlorpromazine   Promazine
Fluphenazine
Prochlorperazine

E853.1   *Butyrophenone-based tranquillizers*

Haloperidol   Trifluperidol
Spiperone .

E853.2   *Benzodiazepine based*

Chlordiazepoxide   Lorazepam
Diazepam   Medazepam
Flurazepam   Nitrazepam

E853.8   *Other*

E853.9   *Unspecified*

E854   Accidental poisoning by other psychotropic agents

E854.0   *Antidepressants*

Amitriptyline   Monoamine oxidase inhibitors
Imipramine

E854.1   *Psychodysleptics [hallucinogens]*

Cannabis (derivatives)   Psilocin
Lysergide [LSD]   Psilocybine
Marihuana (derivatives)
Mescaline

E854.2   *Psychostimulants*

Amphetamine   Caffeine

Excludes: central appetite depressants (E858.8)

E854.3   *Central nervous system stimulants*

Analeptics   Opiate antagonists

E855   Accidental poisoning by other drugs acting on central and auto-nomic nervous systems

E855.0 *Anticonvulsant and anti-Parkinsonism drugs*

Amantidine
Hydantoin derivatives
Levodopa

Oxazolidine derivatives
   [paramethadione]
   [trimethadione]
Succinimides

E855.1 *Other central nervous system depressants*

Ether
Gaseous anaesthetics
Halogenated hydrocarbon
   derivatives

Intravenous anaesthetics
Thiobarbiturates, such as
   thiopental sodium

E855.2 *Local anaesthetics*

Cocaine
Lidocaine [lignocaine]

Procaine
Tetracaine

E855.3 *Parasympathomimetics [cholinergics]*

Acetylcholine
Anticholinesterase:
   organophosphorus
   reversible

Pilocarpine

E855.4 *Parasympatholytics [anticholinergics and antimuscarinics] and*
        spasmolytics

Atropine
Homatropine

Hyoscine [scopolamine]
Quaternary ammonium derivatives

E855.5 *Sympathomimetics [adrenergics]*

Epinephrine [adrenalin]

Levarterenol [noradrenalin]

E855.6 *Sympatholytics [antiadrenergics]*

Phenoxybenzamine

Tolazoline hydrochloride

E855.8 *Other*

E855.9 *Unspecified*

E856   Accidental poisoning by antibiotics

E857   Accidental poisoning by anti-infectives

E858   Accidental poisoning by other drugs

E858.0 *Hormones and synthetic substitutes*

E858.1 *Primarily systemic agents*

E858.2 *Agents primarily affecting blood constituents*

E858.3 *Agents primarily affecting cardiovascular system*

E858.4 *Agents primarily affecting gastrointestinal system*

E858.5 *Water, mineral and uric acid metabolism drugs*

E858.6 *Agents primarily acting on the smooth and skeletal muscles and respiratory system*

E858.7 *Agents primarily affecting skin and mucous membrane, ophthalmological, otorhinolaryngological and dental drugs*

E858.8 *Other*

E858.9 *Unspecified*

ACCIDENTAL POISONING BY OTHER SOLID AND LIQUID
SUBSTANCES, GASES AND VAPOURS (E860-E869)

Note: Categories in this section are intended primarily to indicate the external cause of poisoning states classifiable to 980-989. They may also be used to indicate external causes of localized effects classifiable to 001-799.

E860 Accidental poisoning by alcohol, not elsewhere classified

E860.0 *Alcoholic beverages*

Alcohol in preparations intended for consumption

E860.1 *Other and unspecified ethyl alcohol and its products*

Denatured alcohol   Grain alcohol NOS
Ethanol NOS

E860.2 *Methyl alcohol*

Methanol
Methylated spirit
Wood alcohol

E860.3 *Isopropyl alcohol*

Dimethylcarbinol   Secondary propyl alcohol
Isopropanol
Rubbing alcohol substitute

E860.4 *Fusel oil*

Fusel oil:
  amyl
  butyl
  propyl

E860.8   *Other*

E860.9   *Unspecified*

E861   Accidental poisoning by cleansing and polishing agents, disinfectants, paints and varnishes

E861.0   *Synthetic detergents and shampoos*

E861.1   *Soap products*

E861.2   *Polishes*

E861.3   *Other cleansing and polishing agents*
Scouring powders

E861.4   *Disinfectants*
Household and other disinfectants not ordinarily used on the person
Excludes: carbolic acid or phenol (E864.1)

E861.5   *Lead paints*

E861.6   *Other paints and varnishes*
Laquers   Paints, other than lead
Oil colours   White washes

E861.9   *Unspecified*

E862   Accidental poisoning by petroleum products, other solvents and their vapours, not elsewhere classified

E862.0   *Petroleum solvents*
Petroleum:
  ether
  benzine
  naphtha

E862.1   *Petroleum fuels and cleaners*
Antiknock additives to petroleum   Gas oils
    fuels   Gasoline or petrol
Benzine   Kerosene or paraffin
Excludes: kerosene insecticides (E863.4)

E862.2   *Lubricating oils*

E862.3   *Petroleum solids*
Paraffin wax

E862.4   *Other solvents*
Benzene   Solvent naphtha

E862.9   *Unspecified*

E863 **Accidental poisoning by agricultural and horticultural chemical and pharmaceutical preparations other than plant foods and fertilizers**

Excludes: plant foods and fertilizers (E866.5)

E863.0 *Insecticides of organochlorine compounds*

Benzene hexachlorine
Chlordane
DDT

Dieldrin
Endrine
Toxaphene

E863.1 *Insecticides of organophosphorus compounds*

Demeton
Diazinon
Dichlorous
Malathion
Methyl parathion

Parathion
Phenylsulphthion
Phorate
Phosdrin

E863.2 *Carbamates*

Aldicarb
Carbaryl

Propoxur

E863.3 *Mixtures of insecticides*

E863.4 *Other and unspecified insecticides*

E863.5 *Herbicides*

Chlorates
Diquat
Mixtures of plant foods and
    fertilizers with herbicides

Paraquat
2,4 - D
2,4,5 - T

E863.6 *Fungicides*

Organic mercurials (used in seed dressing)
Pentachlorphenols

E863.7 *Rodenticides*

Fluoracetates
Squill and derivatives
Thallium

Warfarin
Zinc phosphide

E863.8 *Fumigants*

Cyanides
Methyl bromide

Phosphine

E863.9   *Other and unspecified*

E864   Accidental poisoning by corrosives and caustics, not elsewhere classified

Excludes: when component of disinfectant (E861.4)

E864.0   *Corrosive aromatics*

E864.1   *Acids*

Carbolic acid or phenol

E864.2   *Caustic alkalis*

E864.3   *Other*

E864.4   *Unspecified*

E865   Accidental poisoning from foodstuffs and poisonous plants

Includes: any meat, fish or shellfish
food additives and contaminants
plants, berries and fungi eaten as, or in mistake for, food, or
by a child

Excludes: food poisoning (bacterial) (005.–)
poisoning and toxic reactions to venomous plants (E905.6, E905.7)

E865.0   *Meat*

E865.1   *Shellfish*

E865.2   *Other fish*

E865.3   *Berries and seeds*

E865.4   *Other plants*

E865.5   *Mushrooms and other fungi*

E865.8   *Other food*

E865.9   *Unspecified*

E866   Accidental poisoning by other and unspecified solid and liquid substances

Excludes: these substances as a component of:
food contaminants (E865.–)
medicines (E850-E858)
paints (E861.5, E861.6)
pesticides (E863.–)
petroleum fuels (E862.1)

E866.0   *Lead and its compounds and fumes*

E866.1   *Mercury and its compounds and fumes*

E866.2   *Antimony and its compounds and fumes*

E866.3   *Arsenic and its compounds and fumes*

E866.4   *Other metals and their compounds and fumes*

Beryllium and its compounds	Iron compounds
Brass fumes	Manganese and its compounds
Cadmium and its compounds	Nickel compounds
Copper salts	Thallium compounds

E866.5   *Plant foods and fertilizers*

Excludes: mixtures with herbicides (E863.5)

E866.6   *Glues and adhesives*

E866.7   *Cosmetics*

E866.8   *Other*

E866.9   *Unspecified*

E867   Accidental poisoning by gas distributed by pipeline

Includes: carbon monoxide from incomplete combustion of piped gas
coal gas NOS
liquefied petroleum gas distributed through pipes (pure or
mixed with air)
piped gas (natural) (manufactured)

E868   Accidental poisoning by other utility gas and other carbon monoxide

E868.0   *Liquefied petroleum gas distributed in mobile containers*

Butane	Propane

Liquefied hydrocarbon gas NOS
Carbon monoxide from incomplete combustion of above gases

E868.1   *Other and unspecified utility gas*

Acetylene	Water gas

Gas NOS used for lighting,
heating or cooking
Carbon monoxide from incomplete combustion of above gases

E868.2 *Motor vehicle exhaust gas*

Exhaust gas from:
  farm tractor, not in transit
  gas engine
  motor pump
  motor vehicle, not in transit
  any type of combustion engine not in watercraft

Excludes: poisoning by carbon monoxide from:
           aircraft while in transit (E844)
           motor vehicle while in transit (E818)
           watercraft whether or not in transit (E838)

E868.3 *Carbon monoxide from incomplete combustion of other domestic fuels*

Carbon monoxide from incomplete combustion of:
  coal
  coke
  kerosene or paraffin } in domestic stove or fireplace
  wood

Excludes: carbon monoxide from smoke and fumes due to conflagration (E890-E893)

E868.8 *Carbon monoxide from other sources*

Carbon monoxide from:
  blast furnace gas
  incomplete combustion of fuels in industrial use
  kiln vapour

E868.9 *Unspecified carbon monoxide*

E869 Accidental poisoning by other gases and vapours

Excludes: effects of gases used as anaesthetics (E855.1, E938.2)
           fumes from heavy metals (E866.0-E866.4)
           smoke and fumes due to conflagration or explosion (E890-E899)

E869.0 *Nitrogen oxides*

E869.1 *Sulphur dioxide*

E869.2 *Freon*

E869.3 *Lacrimogenic gas [tear gas]*

Brombenzyl cyanide   Ethyliodoacetate
Chloroacetophenone

E869.8 *Other specified gases and vapours*

Chlorine   Hydrocyanic acid gas

E869.9 *Unspecified gases and vapours*

MISADVENTURES TO PATIENTS DURING SURGICAL AND MEDICAL CARE (E870-E876)

Excludes: accidental overdose of drug and wrong drug given in error (E850-E858)
surgical and medical procedures as the cause of abnormal reaction by the patient, without mention of misadventure at the time of procedure (E878-E879)

E870 Accidental cut, puncture, perforation or haemorrhage during medical care

E870.0 *Surgical operation*

E870.1 *Infusion or transfusion*

E870.2 *Kidney dialysis or other perfusion*

E870.3 *Injection or vaccination*

E870.4 *Endoscopic examination*

E870.5 *Aspiration of fluid or tissue, puncture and catheterization [any, except heart catheterization]*

Abdominal paracentesis   Lumbar puncture
Aspirating needle biopsy   Thoracentesis
Blood sampling

E870.6 *Heart catheterization*

E870.7 *Administration of enema*

E870.8 *Other*

E870.9 *Unspecified*

E871 Foreign object left in body during procedure

E871.0 *Surgical operation*

E871.1 *Infusion or transfusion*

E871.2 *Kidney dialysis or other perfusion*

E871.3 *Injection or vaccination*

E871.4 *Endoscopic examination*

E871.5   *Aspiration of fluid or tissue, puncture and catheterization [any, except heart catheterization]*

Abdominal paracentesis˙   Lumbar puncture
Aspirating needle biopsy   Thoracentesis
Blood sampling

E871.6   *Heart catheterization*

E871.7   *Removal of catheter or packing*

E871.8   *Other*

E871.9   *Unspecified*

E872   Failure of sterile precautions during procedure

E872.0   *Surgical operation*

E872.1   *Infusion or transfusion*

E872.2   *Kidney dialysis and other perfusion*

E872.3   *Injection or vaccination*

E872.4   *Endoscopic examination*

E872.5   *Aspiration of fluid or tissue, puncture and catheterization [any, except heart catheterization]*

Abdominal paracentesis   Lumbar puncture
Aspirating needle biopsy   Thoracentesis
Blood sampling

E872.6   *Heart catheterization*

E872.8   *Other*

E872.9   *Unspecified*

E873   Failure in dosage

Excludes: accidental overdose of drug, medicament or biological substance (E850-E858)

E873.0   *Excessive amount of blood or other fluid during transfusion or infusion*

E873.1   *Incorrect dilution of fluid during infusion*

E873.2   *Overdose of radiation in therapy*

E873.3   *Inadvertent exposure of patient to radiation during medical care*

E873.4   *Failure in dosage in electroshock or insulin-shock therapy*

E873.5 *Inappropriate [too hot or too cold] temperature in local application and packing*

E873.6 *Nonadministration of necessary drug or medicament*

E873.8 *Other*

E873.9 *Unspecified*

E874 Mechanical failure of instrument or apparatus during procedure

E874.0 *Surgical operation*

E874.1 *Infusion and transfusion*

Air in system

E874.2 *Kidney dialysis and other perfusion*

E874.3 *Endoscopic examination*

E874.4 *Aspiration of fluid or tissue, puncture and catheterization [any, except heart catheterization]*

Abdominal paracentesis
Aspirating needle biopsy
Blood sampling

Lumbar puncture
Thoracentesis

E874.5 *Heart catheterization*

E874.8 *Other*

E874.9 *Unspecified*

E875 Contaminated or infected blood, other fluid, drug or biological substance

Presence of:
  bacterial pyrogens
  endotoxin-producing bacteria
  serum hepatitis-producing agent

E875.0 *Contaminated substance transfused or infused*

E875.1 *Contaminated substance injected or used for vaccination*

E875.2 *Contaminated drug or biological substance administered by other means*

E875.8 *Other*

E875.9 *Unspecified*

E876   **Other and unspecified misadventures during medical care**

E876.0 *Mismatched blood in transfusion*

E876.1 *Wrong fluid in infusion*

E876.2 *Failure in suture and ligature during surgical operation*

E876.3 *Endotracheal tube wrongly placed during anaesthetic procedure*

E876.4 *Failure to introduce or to remove other tube or instrument*

Excludes: foreign object left in body during procedure (E871.–)

E876.5 *Performance of inappropriate operation*

E876.8 *Other specified misadventures*

E876.9 *Unspecified misadventure*

SURGICAL AND MEDICAL PROCEDURES AS THE CAUSE OF ABNORMAL
REACTION OF PATIENT OR LATER COMPLICATION, WITHOUT MENTION
OF MISADVENTURE AT THE TIME OF PROCEDURE (E878-E879)

Includes: procedures as the cause of abnormal reaction such as:
            displacement or malfunction of prosthetic device
            hepatorenal failure, postoperative
            malfunction of external stoma
            postoperative intestinal obstruction
            rejection of transplanted organ

Excludes: anaesthetic management properly carried out as the cause of
            adverse effect (E937-E938)
            infusion and transfusion, without mention of misadventure
            in the technique of procedure (E930-E949)

E878   **Surgical operation and other surgical procedures as the cause of
abnormal reaction of patient, or of later complication, without
mention of misadventure at the time of operation**

E878.0 *Surgical operation with transplant of whole organ*

Transplantation of: Transplantation of:
  heart   .   liver
  kidney

E878.1 *Surgical operation with implant of artificial internal device*

Cardiac pacemaker   Heart valve prosthesis
Electrodes implanted in brain   Internal orthopaedic device

E878.2 *Surgical operation with anastomosis, bypass or graft, with natural or artificial tissues used as implant*

Anastomosis:
  arteriovenous
  gastrojejunal

Graft of blood vessel, tendon, or skin

Excludes: external stoma (E878.3)

E878.3 *Surgical operation with formation of external stoma*

Colostomy
Cystostomy
Duodenostomy

Gastrostomy
Ureterostomy

E878.4 *Other restorative surgery*

E878.5 *Amputation of limb(s)*

E878.6 *Removal of other organ (partial) (total)*

E878.8 *Other*

E878.9 *Unspecified*

E879 Other procedures, without mention of misadventure at the time of procedure, as the cause of abnormal reaction of patient, or of later complication

E879.0 *Cardiac catheterization*

E879.1 *Kidney dialysis*

E879.2 *Radiological procedure and radiotherapy*

Excludes: radio-opaque dyes for diagnostic X-ray procedures (E947.8)

E879.3 *Shock therapy*

Electroshock therapy

Insulin-shock therapy

E879.4 *Aspiration of fluid*

Lumbar puncture

Thoracentesis

E879.5 *Insertion of gastric or duodenal sound*

E879.6 *Urinary catheterization*

E879.7 *Blood sampling*

E879.8 *Other*

Blood transfusion

E879.9 *Unspecified*

ACCIDENTAL FALLS (E880–E888)

Excludes: falls (in or from):
                burning building (E890.8, E891.8)
                into fire (E890–E899)
                into water (with submersion or drowning) (E910.–)
                machinery (in operation) (E919.–)
                on edged, pointed, sharp object (E920.–)
                transport vehicle (E800–E845)
                vehicle not elsewhere classifiable (E846–E848)

E880   Fall on or from stairs or steps

E880.0   *Escalator*

E880.9   *Other stairs or steps*

E881   Fall on or from ladders or scaffolding

E881.0   *Fall from ladder*

E881.1   *Fall from scaffolding*

E882   Fall from or out of building or other structure

Fall from: Fall from:
    balcony   turret
    bridge   viaduct
    building   wall
    flagpole   window
    tower   Fall through roof

Excludes: collapse of a building or structure (E916)
                fall or jump from burning building (E890.8, E891.8)

E883   Fall into hole or other opening in surface

Fall into: Fall into:
    cavity   quarry
    dock   shaft
    hole   swimming pool
    pit   tank
                                      well

Excludes: fall into water NOS (E910.9)
                resulting in drowning or submersion without mention of
                    injury (E910.–)

E883.0　*Accident from diving or jumping into water [swimming pool]*

Strike or hit:
　against bottom when jumping or diving into shallow water
　wall or board of swimming pool
　water surface

Excludes:　diving with insufficient air supply (E913.2)
　　　　　　effects of air pressure from diving (E902.2)

E883.1　*Accidental fall into well*

E883.2　*Accidental fall into storm drain or manhole*

E883.9　*Fall into other hole or other opening in surface*

E884　Other fall from one level to another

E884.0　*Fall from playground equipment*

Excludes:　recreational machinery (E919.–)

E884.1　*Fall from cliff*

E884.2　*Fall from chair or bed*

E884.9　*Other fall from one level to another*

Fall from:　　　　　　　　　Fall from:
　embankment　　　　　　　　stationary vehicle
　haystack　　　　　　　　　tree

E885　Fall on same level from slipping, tripping or stumbling

E886　Fall on same level from collision, pushing or shoving, by or with other person

Excludes:　crushed or pushed by a crowd or human stampede (E917.1)

E886.0　*In sports*

Tackles in sports

Excludes:　kicked, stepped on, struck by object, in sports (E917.0)

E886.9　*Other and unspecified*

Fall from collision of pedestrian (conveyance) with another pedestrian (conveyance)

E887　Fracture, cause unspecified

E888   Other and unspecified fall

Accidental fall NOS
Fall on same level NOS
Fall from bumping against object

ACCIDENTS CAUSED BY FIRE AND FLAMES (E890-E899)

Includes: asphyxia or poisoning due to conflagration or ignition
             burning by fire
             secondary fires resulting from explosion

Excludes: arson (E968.0)
             fire in or on:
                 machinery (in operation) (E919.–)
                 transport vehicle other than stationary vehicle (E800-E845)
                 vehicle not elsewhere classifiable (E846-E848)

E890   Conflagration in private dwelling

Includes: conflagration in:
                 apartment   house
                 boarding house   lodging house
                 camping place   private garage
                 caravan   rooming house
                 farmhouse   tenement
             conflagration originating from
                 sources classifiable to E893-E898 in the above buildings

E890.0   *Explosion caused by conflagration*

E890.1   *Fumes from combustion of polyvinylchloride [PVC] and similar
          material in conflagration*

E890.2   *Other smoke and fumes from conflagration*

Carbon monoxide ⎫
Fumes NOS   ⎬ from conflagration in private building
Smoke NOS   ⎭

E890.3   *Burning caused by conflagration*

E890.8   *Other accident resulting from conflagration*

Collapse of   ⎫
Fall from   ⎪
Hit by object falling from ⎬ burning private building
Jump from   ⎭

E890.9   *Unspecified*

E891   Conflagration in other and unspecified building or structure

Conflagration in:
  barn
  church
  convalescent and other
    residential home
  dormitory of educational
    institution
  factory

Conflagration in:
  farm outbuildings
  hospital
  hotel
  school
  store
  theatre

Conflagration originating from
  sources classifiable to E893-
  E898 in the above buildings

E891.0 *Explosion caused by conflagration*

E891.1 *Fumes from combustion of polyvinylchloride [PVC] and similar*
  material in conflagration

E891.2 *Other smoke and fumes from conflagration*

Carbon monoxide ⎫
Fumes NOS   ⎬ from conflagration in building or structure
Smoke NOS   ⎭

E891.3 *Burning caused by conflagration*

E891.8 *Other accident resulting from conflagration*

Collapse of   ⎫
Fall from   ⎪
Hit by object falling from   ⎬ burning building or structure
Jump from   ⎭

E891.9 *Unspecified*

E892   Conflagration not in building or structure

Fire (uncontrolled) (in) (of):
  forest
  grass
  hay
  lumber
  mine
  prairie
  transport vehicle [any] except while in transit
  tunnel

E893   Accident caused by ignition of clothing

Excludes: ignition of clothing:
             from highly inflammable material (E894)
             with conflagration (E890-E892)

E893.0　*From controlled fire in private dwelling*

Ignition of clothing from:
　normal fire (charcoal) (coal) (electric)
　　(gas) (wood) in:
　　brazier
　　fireplace
　　furnace
　　stove
}　in private dwelling (as listed in E890)

E893.1　*From controlled fire in other building or structure*

Ignition of clothing from:
　normal fire (charcoal) (coal) (electric)
　　(gas) (wood) in:
　　brazier
　　fireplace
　　furnace
　　stove
}　in other building or structure (as listed in E891)

E893.2　*From controlled fire not in building or structure*

Ignition of clothing from:
　bonfire (controlled)
　brazier fire (controlled), not in building or structure
　trash fire (controlled)

Excludes:　conflagration not in building (E892)
　　　　　　trash fire out of control (E892)

E893.8　*From other sources*

Ignition of clothing from:

blowlamp	cigar
blowtorch	lighter
burning bedspread	matches
candle	pipe
cigarette	welding torch

E893.9　*Unspecified*

Includes:　ignition of clothing (from controlled fire NOS) (in building NOS) NOS

E894　**Ignition of highly inflammable material**

Ignition of:
　benzine
　gasoline
　fat
　kerosene
　paraffin
　petrol
}　(with ignition of clothing)

Excludes: ignition of highly inflammable material with:
conflagration (E890-E892)
explosion (E923.–)

E895   Accident caused by controlled fire in private dwelling
Burning by (flame of) normal fire (charcoal) (coal) (electric) (gas) (wood)
in:
brazier
fireplace
furnace   } in private dwelling (as listed in E890)
stove
Excludes: burning by hot objects not producing fire or flames (E924.–)
ignition of clothing from these sources (E893.0)
poisoning by carbon monoxide from incomplete combustion
of fuel (E867-E868)
with conflagration (E890)

**E896   Accident caused by controlled fire in other and unspecified building
or structure**
Burning by (flame of) normal fire (charcoal) (coal) (electric) (gas) (wood)
in:
brazier
fireplace   in other building or structure
furnace   (as listed in E891)
stove
Excludes: burning by hot objects not producing fire or flames (E924.–)
ignition of clothing from these sources (E893.1)
poisoning by carbon monoxide from incomplete combustion
of fuel (E867-E868)
with conflagration (E891)

E897   Accident caused by controlled fire not in building or structure
Burns from flame of:
  bonfire (controlled)
  brazier fire (controlled), not in building or structure
  trash fire (controlled)
Excludes: ignition of clothing from these sources (E893.2)
trash fire out of control (E892)
with conflagration (E892)

E898   Accident caused by other specified fire and flames
Excludes: conflagration (E890-E892)
ignition of:
  clothing (E893.8)   } originating from
  highly inflammable material (E894) }   these sources

E898.0 *Burning bedclothes*

Bed set on fire NOS

E898.1 *Other*

Burning by:
  blowlamp
  blowtorch
  candle
  cigarette
  cigar
  fire in room NOS

Burning by:
  lamp
  lighter
  matches
  pipe
  welding torch

E899 Accident caused by unspecified fire

Burning NOS

ACCIDENTS DUE TO NATURAL AND ENVIRONMENTAL
FACTORS (E900-E909)

E900 Excessive heat

E900.0 *Due to weather conditions*

Excessive heat as the external cause of:
  ictus solaris
  siriasis
  sunstroke

E900.1 *Of manmade origin*

Heat (in):
  boiler room
  drying room
  factory

Heat (in):
  furnace room
  generated in transport vehicle
  kitchen

E900.9 *Of unspecified origin*

E901 Excessive cold

E901.0 *Due to weather conditions*

Excessive cold as the cause of:
  chilblains NOS
  immersion foot

E901.1 *Of manmade origin*

Contact with $\Big\{$ dry ice
Inhalation of $\Big|$ liquid air
  liquid hydrogen
  liquid nitrogen

Prolonged exposure in:
  deep freeze unit
  refrigerator

E901.8   *Other*

E901.9   *Of unspecified origin*

E902   High and low air pressure and changes in air pressure

E902.0   *Residence or prolonged visit at high altitude*

Residence or prolonged visit at high altitude as the cause of:
  Acosta syndrome
  Alpine sickness
  altitude sickness
  Andes disease
  anoxia, hypoxia
  barotitis, barodontalgia,
      baro-sinusitis,
      barotrauma otitic
  hypobarism, hypobaropathy
  mountain sickness
  range disease

E902.1   *In aircraft*

Sudden change in air pressure in aircraft during ascent or descent as the
    cause of:
  aeroneurosis
  aviators' disease

E902.2   *Due to diving*

High air pressure from rapid descent ⎤ as the cause of:
    in water   ⎢   caisson disease
Reduction in atmospheric pressure while ⎢   divers' disease
    surfacing from deep water diving ⎦   divers' palsy or paralysis

E902.8   *Due to other specified causes*

Reduction in atmospheric pressure while surfacing from underground

E902.9   *Unspecified*

E903   Travel and motion

E904   Hunger, thirst, exposure, neglect

Excludes: any condition resulting from homicidal intent (E968.–)
            hunger, thirst and exposure resulting from accidents con-
                nected with transport (E800-E848)

E904.0   *Abandonment or neglect of infants and helpless persons*

Exposure to weather conditions ⎱ resulting from abandonment or
Hunger or thirst   ⎰   neglect
Desertion of newborn
Inattention at or after birth
Lack of care (helpless person) (infant)

Excludes: criminal neglect (E968.5)

E904.1   *Lack of food*

Lack of food as the cause of:
   inanition
   insufficient nourishment
   starvation

Excludes: hunger resulting from abandonment or neglect (E904.0)

E904.2   *Lack of water*

Lack of water as the cause of:
   dehydration
   inanition

Excludes: dehydration due to acute fluid loss (276.5)

E904.3   *Exposure (to weather conditions) not elsewhere classifiable*

Exposure NOS   Struck by hailstones
Humidity

Excludes: struck by lightning (E907)

E904.9   *Privation, unqualified*

Destitution

**E905   Venomous animals and plants as the cause of poisoning and toxic
           reactions**

Includes: chemical released by animal
            insects
            release of venom through fangs, hairs, spines, tentacles and
               other venom apparatus

Excludes: eating of poisonous animals or plants (E865.–)

E905.0   *Venomous snakes and lizards*

Cobra   Rattlesnake
Fer de lance   Sea snake
Gila monster   Snake (venomous)
Krait   Viper

Excludes: bites of snakes and lizards known to be nonvenomous
               (E906.2)

E905.1 *Venomous spiders*

Black widow spider   Tarantula (venomous)

E905.2 *Scorpion*

E905.3 *Hornets, wasps and bees*

Yellow jacket

E905.4 *Centipede and venomous millipede (tropical)*

E905.5 *Other venomous arthropods*

Sting of:
  ant
  caterpillar

E905.6 *Venomous marine animals and plants*

Puncture by sea urchin spine   Sting of:
Sting of: sea anemone
  coral   sea cucumber
  jelly fish   other marine animal or plant
  nematocysts

Excludes: bites and other injuries caused by nonvenomous marine
              animal (E906.–)
            bite of sea snake (venomous) (E905.0)

E905.7 *Poisoning and toxic reactions caused by other plants*

Injection of poisons or toxins into or through skin by plant thorns, spines
  or other mechanisms

Excludes: puncture wound NOS by plant thorns or spines (E920.8)

E905.8 *Other specified*

E905.9 *Unspecified*

Sting NOS   Venomous bite NOS

E906   **Other injury caused by animals**

Excludes: poisoning and toxic reactions caused by venomous animals
              and insects (E905.–)
            tripping, falling over an animal (E885)

E906.0 *Dog bite*

E906.1 *Rat bite*

E906.2 *Bite of nonvenomous snakes and lizards*

E906.3 *Bite of other animal except arthropod*

Cats   Rodents, except rats
Moray eel   Shark

E906.4 *Bite of nonvenomous arthropod*

Insect bite NOS

E906.8 *Other specified injury caused by animal*

Butted by animal
Fallen on by horse or other animal, not being ridden
Gored by animal
Implantation of quills of porcupine
Pecked by bird
Run over by animal, not being ridden
Stepped on by animal, not being ridden

Excludes: injury by animal being ridden (E828.–)

E906.9 *Unspecified*

E907 Lightning

Excludes: injury from:
fall of tree or other object caused by lightning (E916)
fire caused by lightning (E890-E892)

E908 Cataclysmic storms, and floods resulting from storms

Blizzard
Cloudburst
Cyclone
Flood
arising from remote storm
of cataclysmic nature arising from melting snow
resulting directly from storm
Hurricane
Tornado
Torrential rain
Transport vehicle washed off road by storm

Excludes: collapse of dam or manmade structure causing flood (E909)
transport accident occurring after storm (E800-E848)

E909 Cataclysmic earth surface movements and eruptions

Avalanche
Collapse of dam or manmade structure causing flood
Earthquake
Landslide
Mud slide of cataclysmic nature
Tidal wave
Volcanic eruption

Excludes: "tidal wave" caused by storm action (E908)
transport accident involving collision with avalanche or landslide not in motion (E800-E848)

ACCIDENTS CAUSED BY SUBMERSION, SUFFOCATION
AND FOREIGN BODIES (E910-E915)

E910   Accidental drowning and submersion

Includes: immersion
             swimmers' cramp

Excludes: diving accident (NOS) (resulting in injury except drowning)
                 (E883.0)
             diving with insufficient air supply (E913.2)
             drowning and submersion due to:
                 cataclysm (E908, E909)
                 machinery accident (E919.–)
                 transport accident (E800-E845)
             effect of high and low air pressure (E902.2)
             injury from striking against objects while in running water
                 (E917.2)

E910.0   *While water skiing*

Fall from water skis with submersion or drowning

Excludes: accident to water skier involving a watercraft and resulting
                 in submersion or other injury (E830.4, E831.4)

E910.1   *While engaged in other sport or recreational activity with diving
         equipment*

Scuba diving NOS   Underwater spear fishing NOS
Skin diving NOS

E910.2   *While engaged in other sport or recreational activity without
         diving equipment*

Fishing ⎤
Hunting ⎦ except from boat or with diving equipment
Ice skating
Playing in water
Swimming NOS
Surfboarding
Voluntarily jumping from boat, not involved in accident, for swim NOS
Wading in water

Excludes: jumping into water to rescue another person (E910.3)

E910.3   *While swimming or diving for purposes other than recreation or
         sport*

Marine salvage   ⎤
Pearl diving   ⎪
Placement of fishing nets   ⎬ (with diving equipment)
Rescue (attempt) of another person ⎪
Underwater construction or repairs ⎦

E910.4　*In bathtub*

E910.8　*Other*

Drowning (in):
　NOS
　quenching tank
　swimming pool

E910.9　*Unspecified*

Accidental fall into water NOS

E911　Inhalation and ingestion of food causing obstruction of respiratory tract or suffocation

Asphyxia by ⎫
Choked on　⎬ food [including bone, seed in food, regurgitated food]
Suffocation by ⎭
Aspiration and inhalation of food [any] (into respiratory tract) NOS
Compression of trachea　　　⎫
Interruption of respiration ⎬ by food lodged in oesophagus
Obstruction of respiration ⎭
Obstruction of pharynx by food (bolus)

Excludes:　injury, except asphyxia and obstruction of respiratory passage,
　　　　　　caused by food (E915)
　　　　　obstruction of oesophagus by food without mention of
　　　　　　asphyxia or obstruction of respiratory passage (E915)

E912　Inhalation and ingestion of other object causing obstruction of respiratory tract or suffocation

Asphyxia by ⎫ any object, except food, entering by nose or mouth
Choked on　⎬ mucus
Suffocation by ⎭ phlegm
Aspiration and inhalation of foreign body except food (into respiratory
　　tract) NOS
Foreign object [bean] [marble] in nose
Obstruction of pharynx by foreign body
Compression　　　　　　　　⎫
Interruption of respiration ⎬ by foreign body in oesophagus
Obstruction of respiration ⎭

Excludes:　injury, except asphyxia and obstruction of respiratory passage,
　　　　　　caused by foreign body (E915)
　　　　　obstruction of oesophagus by foreign body without mention
　　　　　　of asphyxia or obstruction of respiratory passage (E915)

E913   Accidental mechanical suffocation
Excludes: mechanical suffocation from or by:
        accidental inhalation or ingestion of:
           food (E911)
             foreign object (E912)
        cataclysm (E908-E909)
        explosion (E921.–, E923.–)
        machinery accident (E919.–)

E913.0   *In bed or cradle*
Excludes: suffocation by plastic bag (E913.1)

E913.1   *By plastic bag*

E913.2   *Due to lack of air (in closed place)*
Accidentally closed up in refrigerator or other airtight enclosed space
Excludes: suffocation by plastic bag (E913.1)

E913.3   *By falling earth or other substance*
Cave-in NOS
Excludes: cave-in caused by cataclysmic earth surface movements and
           eruptions (E909)
        struck by cave-in without asphyxiation or suffocation (E916)

E913.8   *Other specified means*
Accidental hanging, except in bed or cradle

E913.9   *Unspecified*
Asphyxia, mechanical NOS
Strangulation NOS
Suffocation NOS

E914   Foreign body accidentally entering eye and adnexa
Excludes: corrosive liquid

E915   Foreign body accidentally entering other orifice
Excludes: aspiration and inhalation of foreign body, any, (into respi-
        ratory tract) NOS (E911-E912)

OTHER ACCIDENTS (E916-E928)

E916   Struck accidentally by falling object

Collapse of building except on fire	Falling:
Falling:	stone
rock	tree
snowslide NOS	Object falling from:
	machine, not in operation
	stationary vehicle

Excludes: collapse of building on fire (E890-E891)
          falling object in:
              cataclysm (E908-E909)
              machinery accidents (E919.–)
              transport accidents (E800-E845)
              vehicle accidents not elsewhere classifiable (E846-E848)
          object set in motion by:
              explosion (E921.–, E923.–)
              firearm (E922.–)
          projected object (E917.–)

E917 Striking against or struck accidentally by objects or persons

Includes: bumping into or against ⎫
          colliding with   ⎬ object (moving) (projected)
          kicking against   ⎪   (stationary)
          stepping on   ⎪ person
          struck by   ⎭ pedestrian conveyance

Excludes: fall from:
              bumping into or against object (E888)
              collision with another person, except when caused by a
                  crowd (E886.–)
              stumbling over object (E885)
          injury caused by:
              assault (E960.–, E967.–)
              cutting or piercing instrument (E920.–)
              explosion (E921.–, E923.–)
              firearm (E922.–)
              machinery (E919.–)
              transport vehicle (E800-E845)
              vehicle not elsewhere classifiable (E846-E848)

E917.0 *In sports*

Kicked or stepped on during game (football) (rugby)
Knocked down while boxing
Struck by hit or thrown ball
Struck by hockey stick or puck

E917.1 *Caused by a crowd, by collective fear or panic*

Crushed   ⎫
Pushed   ⎬ by crowd or human stampede
Stepped on ⎭

E917.2 *In running water*

Excludes: drowning or submersion (E910.–)
          in sports (E917.0)

E917.9 *Other*

E918   Caught accidentally in or between objects

Caught, crushed, jammed, or pinched:

between:
  moving objects
  stationary and moving
    objects
in object
} such as {
  escalator
  folding object
  hand tools, appliances or imple-
    ments, not causing cut or
    puncture
  sliding door and door frame
  under packing crate due to los-
    ing grip
  washing machine wringer

Excludes: injury caused by:
        cutting or piercing instrument (E920.–)
        machinery (E919.–)
        transport vehicle (E800-E845)
        vehicle not elsewhere classifiable (E846-E848)
       struck accidentally by:
        falling object (E916)
        object (moving) (projected) (E917.–)

E919   Accidents caused by machinery

Includes: burned by
       caught in (moving parts) of
       collapse of
       crushed by
       cut or pierced by
       drowning or submersion
           caused by
       explosion of, on, in
       fall from or into moving part of
       fire starting in or on
       mechanical suffocation caused by
       object falling from, on, set in
           motion by
       overturning of
       pinned under
       run over by
       struck by
       thrown from
       } machinery (accident)
       caught between machinery and other object
       collision of machinery with:
           object (fixed) (movable) (moving) not set in motion by
               transport vehicle
           pedestrian
       machinery accident NOS

Excludes: accidents involving machinery, not in operation (E884.9, E916-E918)

injury caused by:

     electric current in connection with machinery (E925.–)

     escalator (E880.0, E918)

     explosion of pressure vessel in connection with machinery (E921.–)

     moving sidewalk (E885)

     powered hand tools, appliances and implements (E916-E918, E920, E921, E923-E926)

     transport vehicle accidents involving machinery (E800-E848)

poisoning by carbon monoxide generated by machine (E868.8)

E919.0   *Agricultural machines*

Animal powered agricultural machine	Harvester
Combine	Hay mower or rake
Derrick, hay	Reaper
Farm machinery NOS	Thresher
Farm tractor	

Excludes: when in transport under own power on the highway (E810-E819)

     when being towed by another vehicle on the highway (E810-E819, E827, E829)

     when involved in accident classifiable to E820-E829 (E820-E829)

E919.1   *Mining and earth-drilling machinery*

Bore or drill (land) (seabed)	Shaft lift
Shaft hoist	Under-cutter

Excludes: coal car, tram, truck and tub in mine (E846.–)

E919.2   *Lifting machines and appliances*

Chain hoist
Crane
Derrick
Elevator (building) (grain)   } except in agricultural or mining operations
Forklift truck
Lift
Pulley block
Winch

Excludes: when in transport under own power on the highway (E810-E819)

     when being towed by another vehicle on the highway (E810-E819, E827, E829)

     when involved in accident classifiable to E820-E829 (E820-E829)

E919.3 *Metalworking machines*

Abrasive wheel
Forging machine
Lathe
Mechanical shears

Metal:
  drilling machine
  milling machine
  power press
  rolling-mill
  sawing machine

E919.4 *Woodworking and forming machines*

Band saw
Bench saw
Circular saw
Moulding machine

Overhead plane
Powered saw, except hand
Radial saw
Sander

E919.5 *Prime movers, except electrical motors*

Gas turbine
Internal combustion engine

Steam engine
Water driven turbine

Excludes: when in transport under own power on the highway (E810-E819)
  when being towed by other vehicle on the highway (E810-E819, E827, E829)

E919.6 *Transmission machinery*

Transmission:
  belt
  cable
  chain
  gear

Transmission:
  pinion
  pulley
  shaft

E919.7 *Earth moving, scraping and other excavating machines*

Bulldozer
Road scraper

Steam shovel

Excludes: when in transport under own power on the highway (E810-E819)
  when being towed by other vehicle on the highway (E810-E819, E827, E829)

E919.8 *Other*

Machines for manufacture of:
  clothing
  foodstuffs and beverages
  paper

Printing machine
Spinning, weaving and textile machines

E919.9 *Unspecified*

E920   Accidents caused by cutting and piercing instruments or objects

Includes: fall on ⎤   object:
          accidental injury by ⎫   edged
                             ⎭   pointed
                                 sharp

E920.0   *Powered lawn mower*

E920.1   *Other powered hand tools*

Any powered hand tool [compressed air] [electric] [explosive cartridge]
   [hydraulic power] such as:
   drill   rivet gun
   hand saw   staple gun
   hedge clipper

Excludes: band saw (E919.4)
           bench saw (E919.4)

E920.2   *Powered household appliances and implements*

Blender   Electric:
Electric: knife
   beater or mixer   sewing machine
   can opener   Garbage disposal appliance
   fan

E920.3   *Knives, swords and daggers*

E920.4   *Other hand tools and implements*

Axe   Paper cutter
Can opener NOS   Pitchfork
Chisel   Rake
Fork   Scissors
Hand saw   Screwdriver
Hoe   Sewing machine, not powered
Ice pick   Shovel
Needle

E920.8   *Other*

Arrow   Lathe turnings
Broken glass   Nail
Dart   Plant thorn
Edge of stiff paper   Splinter
                                 Tin can lid

Excludes: animal spines or quills (E906.8)
           flying glass due to explosion (E921-E923)

E920.9   *Unspecified*

E921   Accident caused by explosion of pressure vessel

Includes: accidental explosion of pressure vessels, whether or not part of machinery

Excludes: explosion of pressure vessel on transport vehicle (E800-E845)

E921.0   *Boilers*

E921.1   *Gas cylinders*

Air tank   Pressure gas tank

E921.8   *Other*

Aerosol can   Pressure cooker
Automobile tyre

E921.9   *Unspecified*

E922   Accident caused by firearm missile

E922.0   *Hand gun*

Pistol   Revolver

Excludes: Verey pistol (E922.8)

E922.1   *Shotgun (automatic)*

E922.2   *Hunting rifle*

Excludes: air rifle [BB gun] (E917.9)

E922.3   *Military firearms*

Army rifle   Machine gun

E922.8   *Other*

Verey pistol [flare]

E922.9   *Unspecified*

Gunshot wound NOS   Shot NOS

E923   Accident caused by explosive material

Includes: flash burns and other injuries resulting from explosion of explosive material
             ignition of highly explosive material with explosion

Excludes: explosion:
             in or on machinery (E919.–)
             on any transport vehicle except stationary motor vehicle (E800-E848)
             secondary fires resulting from explosion (E890-E899)
             with conflagration (E892, E890-E892)

E923.0 *Fireworks*

E923.1 *Blasting materials*

Blasting cap
Detonator

Dynamite
Explosive [any] used in blasting
   operations

E923.2 *Explosive gases*

Acetylene
Butane
Coal gas
Explosion NOS in mine
Fire damp

Gasoline fumes
Methane
Propane

E923.8 *Other*

Bomb
Explosive missile
Grenade
Mine
Shell
Torpedo

Explosion in:
   grain store
   munitions:
      dump
      factory

E923.9 *Unspecified*

Includes: explosion NOS

E924 Accident caused by hot substance or object, caustic or corrosive material and steam

Excludes: burning NOS (E899.–)
   chemical burn resulting from swallowing a corrosive sub-
      stance (E860-E864)
   fire caused by these substances and objects (E890-E894)
   radiation burns (E926.–)
   therapeutic misadventures (E870-E876)

E924.0 *Hot liquids and vapours, including steam*

Burning or scalding by:
   boiling water
   hot or boiling liquids not primarily caustic or corrosive
   liquid metal
   steam
   other hot vapour

E924.1 *Caustic and corrosive substances*

Burning by:
   acid [any kind]
   ammonia
   caustic oven cleaner or other substance
   corrosive substance
   lye
   vitriol

E924.8 *Other*

Burning by:
  heat from electric heating appliance
  hot object NOS
  steam pipe

E924.9 *Unspecified*

E925   Accident caused by electric current

Includes: electric current from: burning
              exposed wire   cardiac fibrillation
              faulty appliance or   as the convulsions
                electric machine   } cause { electric shock
              high voltage cable   of: electrocution
              live rail   puncture wound
              open electric socket   respiratory paralysis

Excludes: burn by heat from electrical appliance (E924.8)
            lightning (E907)

E925.0 *Domestic wiring and appliances*

E925.1 *Electric power generating plants, distribution stations, transmission lines*

Broken power line

E925.2 *Industrial wiring, appliances and electrical machinery*

Conductors   Electrical equipment and machines
Control apparatus   Transformers

E925.8 *Other*

Wiring and appliances in or on: Wiring and appliances in or on:
  farm [not farmhouse]   residential institutions
  outdoors   schools
  public building

E925.9 *Unspecified*

Burns or other injury from electric current NOS
Electric shock NOS
Electrocution NOS

E926   Exposure to radiation

Excludes: abnormal reaction to a complication of treatment, without
              mention of misadventure (E879.2)
            atomic power plant malfunction in water transport (E838.–)
            misadventure to patient in surgical and medical procedures
              (E873.2-E873.3)
            use of radiation in war operations (E996, E997)

E926.0 *Radiofrequency radiation*

Overexposure to: } from:
  microwave radiation   high-powered radio and television
  radar radiation   transmitters
  radiofrequency   industrial radiofrequency induction heaters
    radiation [any]   radar installations

E926.1 *Infrared heaters and lamps*

                    blistering
Exposure to infrared radiation from burning
  heaters and lamps as the cause of: charring
                    inflammatory changes

Excludes: physical contact with heater or lamp (E924.8)

E926.2 *Visible and ultraviolet light sources*

Arclamps   Oxygas welding torch
Black light sources   Sun rays
Electrical welding arc

Excludes: excessive heat from these sources (E900.–)

E926.3 *X-rays and other electromagnetic ionizing radiation*

Gamma rays   X-rays (hard) (soft)

E926.4 *Lasers*

E926.5 *Radioactive isotopes*

Radiobiologicals   Radiopharmaceuticals

E926.8 *Other specified*

Artificially accelerated beams of ionized particles, generated by:
  betatrons
  synchrotrons

E926.9 *Unspecified*

Radiation NOS

E927   Overexertion and strenuous movements

Excessive physical exercise   Strenuous movements in:
Overexertion (from)   recreational activities
  lifting   other activities
  pulling
  pushing

E928   Other and unspecified environmental and accidental causes

E928.0 *Prolonged stay in weightless environment*

Weightlessness in spacecraft (simulator)

E928.1 *Exposure to noise*

Noise (pollution)   Supersonic waves
Sound waves

E928.2 *Vibration*

E928.8 *Other*

E928.9 *Unspecified accidents*

Accident NOS
Blow NOS   ⎫
Casualty (not due to war)   ⎪
Decapitation   ⎪
Injury [any part of body,   ⎬ stated as accidentally inflicted but not
     or unspecified]   ⎪   otherwise specified
Killed   ⎪
Knocked down   ⎪
Mangled   ⎪
Wound   ⎭

Excludes: fracture, cause unspecified (E887)
           injuries undetermined whether accidentally or purposely
           inflicted (E980-E989)

LATE EFFECTS OF ACCIDENTAL INJURY (E929)

Note: This category is to be used to indicate accidental injury as the
        cause of death or disability from late effects, which are them-
        selves classifiable elsewhere. The "late effects" include condi-
        tions reported as such, or occurring as sequelae one year or more
        after accidental injury. [See III Late effects, page 723].

E929   Late effects of accidental injury

Excludes: late effects of:
           surgical and medical procedures (E870-E879)
           therapeutic use of drugs and medicaments (E930-E949)

E929.0 *Late effects of motor vehicle accident*

Late effects of accidents classifiable to E810-E825

E929.1 *Late effects of other transport accident*

Late effects of accidents classifiable to E800-E807, E826-E838, E840-E848

E929.2 *Late effects of accidental poisoning*

Late effects of accidents classifiable to E850-E858, E860-E869

E929.3   *Late effects of accidental fall*
Late effects of accidents classifiable to E880-E888

E929.4   *Late effects of accident caused by fire*
Late effects of accidents classifiable to E890-E899

E929.5   *Late effects of accident due to natural and environmental factors*
Late effects of accidents classifiable to E900-E909

E929.8   *Late effects of other accidents*
Late effects of accidents classifiable to E910-E928.8

E929.9   *Late effects of unspecified accident*
Late effects of accidents classifiable to E928.9

DRUGS, MEDICAMENTS AND BIOLOGICAL SUBSTANCES CAUSING
ADVERSE EFFECTS IN THERAPEUTIC USE (E930-E949)

Includes: correct drug properly administered in therapeutic or prophy-
             lactic dosage, as the cause of any adverse effect
Excludes: accidental overdose of drug and wrong drug given or taken
             in error (E850-E858)
             accidents in the technique of administration of drug or bio-
             logical substance, such as accidental puncture during
             injection, or contamination of drug (E870-E876)
             administration with suicidal or homicidal intent or intent to
             harm, or in circumstances classifiable to E980-E989
             (E950.0 to E950.4, E962.0, E980.0 to E980.4)
See Alphabetical Index for more complete list of specific drugs to be
classified under the fourth-digit subdivisions.

E930   Antibiotics
Excludes: if used as eye, ear, nose and throat [ENT], and local anti-
             infectives (E946.-)

E930.0   *Penicillins*
Natural   Semisynthetic, such as
Synthetic   ampicillin
                                   cloxacillin
                                   nafcillin
                                   oxacillin

E930.1   *Antifungal antibiotics*
Amphotericin B   Nystatin
Griseofulvin
Hachimycin [trichomycin]

E930.2   *Chloramphenicol group*

Chloramphenicol   Thiamphenicol

E930.3   *Erythromycin and other macrolides*

Oleandomycin   Spiramycin

E930.4   *Tetracycline group*

Doxycycline   Oxytetracycline
Minocycline

E930.5   *Cefalosporin group*

Cefalexin   Cefaloridine
Cefaloglycin   Cefalotin

E930.6   *Antimycobacterial antibiotics*

Cycloserine   Rifampicin
Kanamycin   Streptomycin

E930.7   *Antineoplastic antibiotics*

Actinomycins, such as   Bleomycin
   cactinomycin   Daunorubicin
   dactinomycin   Mitomycin

Excludes: other antineoplastic drugs (E933.1)

E930.8   *Other specified antibiotics*

E930.9   *Unspecified*

E931   Other anti-infectives

Excludes: ENT, and local anti-infectives (E946.–)

E931.0   *Sulfonamides*

Sulfadiazine   Sulfamethoxazole
Sulfadimethoxine   Sulfamethoxypyridazine
Sulfafurazole

E931.1   *Arsenical anti-infectives*

E931.2   *Heavy metal anti-infectives*

Compounds of: Compounds of:
   antimony   lead
   bismuth   mercury

Excludes: mercurial diuretics (E944.0)

E931.3   *Quinoline and hydroxyquinoline derivatives*

Chiniofon   Diiodohydroxyquinoline

Excludes: antimalarial drugs (E931.4)

E931.4 *Antimalarials and drugs acting on other blood protozoa*

Chloroquine phosphate
Cycloguanil
Primaquine

Proguanil [chloroguanide]
Pyrimethamine
Quinine (sulphate)

E931.5 *Other antiprotozoal drugs*

Emetine

E931.6 *Anthelminthics*

Hexylresorcinol
Male fern oleoresin

Piperazine
Tiabendazole

E931.7 *Antiviral drugs*

Metisazone

Excludes: amantadine (E936.4)
         cytarabine (E933.1)
         idoxuridine (E946.5)

E931.8 *Other antimycobacterial drugs*

Isoniazid
Ethionamide
Ethambutol

Para-aminosalicylic acid
   derivatives
Sulfones

E931.9 *Other and unspecified anti-infectives*

Nitrofuran derivatives

Flucytosine

E932   Hormones and synthetic substitutes

E932.0 *Adrenal cortical steroids*

Cortisone derivatives
Desoxycortone derivatives

Fluorinated corticosteroids

E932.1 *Androgens and anabolic congeners*

Metandienone
Nandrolone phenylpropionate
Norethandrolone

Oxymetholone
Testosterone and preparations

E932.2 *Ovarian hormones and synthetic substitutes*

Contraceptives, oral
Oestrogens

Progestogens
Oestrogens and progestogens,
   combined

E932.3 *Insulins and antidiabetic agents*

Acetohexamide
Biguanide derivatives, oral
Chlorpropamide
Glucagon

Insulin
Phenformin
Sulfonylurea derivatives, oral
Tolbutamide

Excludes: adverse effect of insulin administered for shock therapy
      (E879.3)

E932.4   *Anterior pituitary hormones*

Corticotrophin   Somatotrophin
Gonadotrophin

E932.5   *Posterior pituitary hormones*

Vasopressin

Excludes: oxytocic agents (E945.0)

E932.6   *Parathyroid and parathyroid derivatives*

E932.7   *Thyroid and thyroid derivatives*

Dextrothyroxine   Thyroglobulin
Liothyronine   Levothyroxine sodium

E932.8   *Antithyroid agents*

Iodides   Thiourea
Thiouracil

E932.9   *Other and unspecified hormones and synthetic substitutes*

E933   Primarily systemic agents

E933.0   *Antiallergic and antiemetic drugs*

Antihistamines   Diphenylpyraline
Chlorphenamine   Thonzylamine
Diphenhydramine   Tripelennamine

Excludes: phenothiazine-based tranquillizers (E939.1)

E933.1   *Antineoplastic and immunosuppressive drugs*

Azathioprine   Cytarabine
Busulfan   Fluorouracil
Chlorambucil   Mercaptopurine
Chlormethine hydrochloride   Thiotepa
Cyclophosphamide

Excludes: antineoplastic antibiotics (E930.7)

E933.2   *Acidifying agents*

E933.3   *Alkalizing agents*

E933.4   *Enzymes not elsewhere classified*

Penicillinase

E933.5   *Vitamins, not elsewhere classified*

Excludes: nicotinic acid (E942.5)
            vitamin K (E934.3)

E933.8   *Other systemic agents, not elsewhere classified*

Heavy metal antagonists

E933.9   *Unspecified*

E934   **Agents primarily affecting blood constituents**

E934.0   *Iron and its compounds*

Ferric salts
Ferrous sulphate and other ferrous salts

E934.1   *Liver preparations and other antianemic agents*

Folic acid

E934.2   *Anticoagulants*

Coumarin
Heparin
Phenindione

Prothrombin synthesis inhibitor
Warfarin sodium

E934.3   *Vitamin K [phytomenadione]*

E934.4   *Fibrinolysis-affecting drugs*

Aminocaproic acid
Streptokinase

Streptodornase
Urokinase

E934.5   *Anticoagulant antagonists and other coagulants*

Hexadimethrine bromide

Protamine sulfate

E934.6   *Gamma globulin*

E934.7   *Natural blood and blood products*

Blood plasma
Human fibrinogen

Packed red cells
Whole blood

E934.8   *Other*

Macromolecular blood substitutes

E934.9   *Unspecified*

E935   **Analgesics, antipyretics and antirheumatics**

E935.0   *Opiates and related narcotics*

Codeine [methylmorphine]
Heroin [diacetylmorphine]
Methadone

Morphine
Opium (alkaloids)
Pethidine [meperidine]

E935.1   *Salicylates*

Acetylsalicylic acid [aspirin]
Amino derivatives of salicylic acid

Salicylic acid salts

E935.2 *Aromatic analgesics, not elsewhere classified*

Acetanilide
Paracetamol [acetaminophen]
Phenacetin [acetophenetedin]

E935.3 *Pyrazole derivatives*

Aminophenazone [amidopyrine]
Phenylbutazone

E935.4 *Antirheumatics [antiphlogistics]*

Gold salts
Indometacin

Excludes: salicylates (E935.1)
steroids (E932.0)

E935.5 *Other non-narcotic analgesics*

Pyrabital

E935.8 *Other*

Pentazocine

E935.9 *Unspecified*

E936 **Anticonvulsants and anti-Parkinsonism drugs**

E936.0 *Oxazolidine derivatives*

Paramethadione
Trimethadione

E936.1 *Hydantoin derivatives*

Phenytoin

E936.2 *Succinimides*

Ethosuximide
Phensuximide

E936.3 *Other and unspecified anticonvulsants*

Beclamide
Primidone

E936.4 *Anti-Parkinsonism drugs*

Amantadine
Levodopa
Profenamine [ethopropazine]

E937 **Sedatives and hypnotics**

E937.0 *Barbiturates*

Amobarbital [amylobarbitone]
Barbital [barbitone]
Butobarbital [butobarbitone]
Pentobarbital [pentobarbitone]
Phenobarbital [phenobarbitone]
Secobarbital [quinalbarbitone]

Excludes: thiobarbiturates (E938.3)

E937.1 *Chloral hydrate group*

E937.2   *Paraldehyde*

E937.3   *Bromine compounds*

Bromide   Carbromal (derivatives)
Carbamic esters

E937.4   *Methaqualone compounds*

E937.5   *Glutethimide group*

E937.6   *Mixed sedatives, not elsewhere classified*

E937.8   *Other*

Methyprylon

E937.9   *Unspecified*

Sleeping:
  draught
  drug   } NOS
  tablet

E938   Other central nervous system depressants

E938.0   *Central nervous system muscle-tone depressants*

Chlorphenesin (carbamate)   Methocarbamol
Mephenesin

E938.1   *Halothane*

E938.2   *Other gaseous anaesthetics*

Ether
Halogenated hydrocarbon derivatives, except halothane
Nitrous oxide

E938.3   *Intravenous anaesthetics*

Ketamine   Thiobarbiturates, such as
Methohexital [methohexitone]   thiopental sodium

E938.4   *Other and unspecified general anaesthetics*

E938.5   *Surface and infiltration anaesthetics*

Cocaine   Procaine
Lidocaine [lignocaine]   Tetracaine

E938.6   *Peripheral nerve- and plexus-blocking anaesthetics*

E938.7   *Spinal anaesthetics*

E938.9   *Other and unspecified local anaesthetics*

E939   Psychotropic agents

E939.0 *Antidepressants*

Amitriptyline
Imipramine

Monoamine oxidase inhibitors

E939.1 *Phenothiazine-based tranquillizers*

Chlorpromazine
Fluphenazine
Phenothiazine

Prochlorperazine
Promazine

E939.2 *Butyrophenone-based tranquillizers*

Haloperidol
Spiperone

Trifluperidol

E939.3 *Other antipsychotics, neuroleptics and major tranquillizers*

E939.4 *Benzodiazepine-based tranquillizers*

Chlordiazepoxide
Diazepam
Flurazepam

Lorazepam
Medazepam
Nitrazepam

E939.5 *Other tranquillizers*

Hydroxyzine

Meprobamate

E939.6 *Psychodysleptics [hallucinogens]*

Cannabis (derivatives)
Lysergide [LSD]
Marihuana (derivatives)

Mescaline
Psilocin
Psilocybine

E939.7 *Psychostimulants*

Amphetamine

Caffeine

Excludes: central appetite depressants (E947.8)

E939.8 *Other psychotropic agents*

E939.9 *Unspecified*

E940   Central nervous system stimulants

E940.0 *Analeptics*

Lobeline

Nikethamide

E940.1 *Opiate antagonists*

Levallorphan
Nalorphine

Naloxone

E940.8 *Other*

E940.9 *Unspecified*

E941 Drugs primarily affecting the autonomic nervous system

E941.0 *Parasympathomimetics [cholinergics]*

Acetylcholine
Anticholinesterase:
  organophosphorus
  reversible

Pilocarpine

E941.1 *Parasympatholytics [anticholinergics and antimuscarinics] and spasmolytics*

Atropine
Homatropine

Hyoscine [scopolamine]
Quaternary ammonium derivatives

Excludes: papaverine (E942.5)

E941.2 *Sympathomimetics [adrenergics]*

Epinephrine [adrenalin]

Levarterenol [noradrenalin]

E941.3 *Sympatholytics [antiadrenergics]*

Phenoxybenzamine

Tolazoline hydrochloride

E941.9 *Unspecified*

E942 Agents primarily affecting the cardiovascular system

E942.0 *Cardiac rhythm regulators*

Practolol
Procainamide

Propranolol
Quinidine

E942.1 *Cardiotonic glycosides and drugs of similar action*

Digitalis glycosides
Digoxin

Strophantins

E942.2 *Antilipaemic and antiarteriosclerotic drugs*

Clofibrate
Colestyramine

Nicotinic acid derivatives
Sitosterols

Excludes: dextrothyroxine (E932.7)

E942.3 *Ganglion-blocking agents*

Pentamethonium bromide

E942.4 *Coronary vasodilators*

Dipyridamole
Nitrates [nitroglycerin]

Nitrites
Prenylamine

E942.5 *Other vasodilators*

Cyclandelate
Diazoxide
Hydralazine

Nicotinic acid
Papaverine

E942.6   *Other antihypertensive agents*

Clonidine
Guanethidine

Rauwolfia alkaloids
Reserpine

E942.7   *Antivaricose drugs, including sclerosing agents*

Monoethanolamine

Zinc salts

E942.8   *Capillary-active drugs*

Adrenochrome derivatives
Bioflavonoids

Metaraminol

E942.9   *Other and unspecified*

E943   Agents primarily affecting gastrointestinal system

E943.0   *Antacids and anti-gastric-secretion drugs*

Aluminium hydroxide

Magnesium trisilicate

E943.1   *Irritant cathartics*

Bisacodyl
Castor oil

Phenolphthalein

E943.2   *Emollient cathartics*

Sodium dioctyl sulfosuccinate

E943.3   *Other cathartics, including intestinal atonia drugs*

Magnesium sulphate

E943.4   *Digestants*

Pancreatin
Papain

Pepsin

E943.5   *Antidiarrhoeal drugs*

Bismuth subcarbonate
Kaolin

Pectin

Excludes: anti-infectives (E930-E931)

E943.6   *Emetics*

E943.8   *Other*

E943.9   *Unspecified*

E944   Water, mineral and uric acid metabolism drugs

E944.0   *Mercurial diuretics*

Chlormerodrin
Mercaptomerin

Mercurophylline
Mersalyl

E944.1 *Purine derivative diuretics*

Theobromine   Theophylline

Excludes: aminophylline [theophylline ethylenediamine] (E945.7)

E944.2 *Carbonic acid anhydrase inhibitors*

Acetazolamide

E944.3 *Saluretics*

Chlorothiazide group

E944.4 *Other diuretics*

Etacrynic acid   Furosemide

E944.5 *Electrolytic, caloric and water-balance agents*

E944.6 *Other mineral salts, not elsewhere classified*

E944.7 *Uric acid metabolism drugs*

Cinchopen and congeners   Phenoquin
Colchicine   Probenecid

E945   Agents primarily acting on the smooth and skeletal muscles and respiratory system

E945.0 *Oxytocic agents*

Ergot alkaloids

E945.1 *Smooth muscle relaxants*

Adiphenine   Orciprenaline [metaproterenol]

Excludes: papaverine (E942.5)

E945.2 *Skeletal muscle relaxants*

Alcuronium chloride   Suxamethonium chloride

E945.3 *Other and unspecified drugs acting on muscles*

E945.4 *Antitussives*

Dextromethorphan   Pipazetate hydrochloride

E945.5 *Expectorants*

Acetylcysteine   Ipecacuanha
Cocillana   Terpin hydrate
Glyceryl guaiacolate

E945.6 *Anti-common-cold drugs*

E945.7 *Antiasthmatics*

Aminophylline [theophylline ethylenediamine]

E945.8 *Other and unspecified respiratory drugs*

E946 **Agents primarily affecting skin and mucous membrane, ophthalmological, otorhinolaryngological and dental drugs**

E946.0 *Local anti-infectives and anti-inflammatory drugs*

E946.1 *Antipruritics*

E946.2 *Local astringents and local detergents*

E946.3 *Emollients, demulcents and protectants*

E946.4 *Keratolytics, keratoplastics, other hair treatment drugs and preparations*

E946.5 *Eye anti-infectives and other eye drugs*

Idoxuridine

E946.6 *Anti-infective and other drugs and preparations for ear, nose and throat*

E946.7 *Dental drugs topically applied*

E946.8 *Other*

Spermicides

E946.9 *Unspecified*

E947 **Other and unspecified drugs and medicaments**

E947.0 *Dietetics*

E947.1 *Lipotropic drugs*

E947.2 *Antidotes and chelating agents, not elsewhere classified*

E947.3 *Alcohol deterrents*

E947.4 *Pharmaceutical excipients*

E947.8 *Other drugs and medicaments*

Contrast media used for diagnostic X-ray procedures
Diagnostic agents and kits

E947.9 *Unspecified drug or medicament*

E948 **Bacterial vaccines**

E948.0 *BCG vaccine*

E948.1 *Typhoid and paratyphoid·*

E948.2 *Cholera*

E948.3 *Plague*

E948.4 .Tetanus

E948.5 Diphtheria

E948.6 Pertussis vaccine, including combinations with a pertussis component

E948.8 Other and unspecified bacterial vaccines

E948.9 Mixed bacterial vaccines, except combinations with a pertussis component

E949   Other vaccines and biological substances

Excludes: gamma globulin (E934.6)

E949.0 Smallpox vaccine

E949.1 Rabies vaccine

E949.2 Typhus vaccine

E949.3 Yellow fever vaccine

E949.4 Measles vaccine

E949.5 Poliomyelitis vaccine

E949.6 Other and unspecified viral and rickettsial vaccines

E949.7 Mixed viral-rickettsial and bacterial vaccines, except combinations with a pertussis component

E949.9 Other and unspecified vaccines and biological substances

SUICIDE AND SELFINFLICTED INJURY (E950-E959)

Includes: injuries in suicide and attempted suicide
           selfinflicted injuries specified as intentional

E950   Suicide and selfinflicted poisoning by solid or liquid substances

E950.0 Analgesics, antipyretics and antirheumatics

E950.1 Barbiturates

E950.2 Other sedatives and hypnotics

E950.3 Tranquillizers and other psychotropic agents

E950.4 Other specified drugs and medicaments

E950.5 Unspecified drug or medicament

E950.6 Agricultural and horticultural chemical and pharmaceutical preparations other than plant foods and fertilizers

E950.7   *Corrosive and caustic substances*

Suicide and selfinflicted poisoning by substances classifiable to E864.–

E950.8   *Arsenic and its compounds*

E950.9   *Other and unspecified solid and liquid substances*

E951   Suicide and selfinflicted poisoning by gases in domestic use

E951.0   *Gas distributed by pipeline*

E951.1   *Liquefied petroleum gas distributed in mobile containers*

E951.8   *Other utility gas*

E952   Suicide and selfinflicted poisoning by other gases and vapours

E952.0   *Motor vehicle exhaust gas*

E952.1   *Other carbon monoxide*

E952.8   *Other specified gases and vapours*

E952.9   *Unspecified gases and vapours*

E953   Suicide and selfinflicted injury by hanging, strangulation and suffocation

E953.0   *Hanging*

E953.1   *Suffocation by plastic bag*

E953.8   *Other specified means*

E953.9   *Unspecified means*

E954   Suicide and selfinflicted injury by submersion [drowning]

E955   Suicide and selfinflicted injury by firearms and explosives

E955.0   *Hand gun*

E955.1   *Shot gun*

E955.2   *Hunting rifle*

E955.3   *Military firearms*

E955.4   *Other and unspecified firearm*

Gunshot NOS   Shot NOS

E955.5   *Explosives*

E955.9   *Unspecified*

E956   **Suicide and selfinflicted injury by cutting and piercing instruments**

E957   **Suicide and selfinflicted injuries by jumping from high place**

E957.0   *Residential premises*

E957.1   *Other manmade structures*

E957.2   *Natural sites*

E957.9   *Unspecified*

E958   **Suicide and selfinflicted injury by other and unspecified means**

E958.0   *Jumping or lying before moving object*

E958.1   *Burns, fire*

E958.2   *Scald*

E958.3   *Extremes of cold*

E958.4   *Electrocution*

E958.5   *Crashing of motor vehicle*

E958.6   *Crashing of aircraft*

E958.7   *Caustic substances, except poisoning*

E958.8   *Other specified means*

E958.9   *Unspecified means*

E959   **Late effects of selfinflicted injury**

Note: This category is to be used to indicate circumstances classifiable
to E950-E958 as the cause of death or disability from late effects,
which are themselves classified elsewhere. The "late effects"
include conditions reported as such, or occurring as sequelae one
year or more after attempted suicide or selfinflicted injury.
[See III Late effects, page 723].

HOMICIDE AND INJURY PURPOSELY INFLICTED BY OTHER PERSONS
(E960-E969)

Includes: injuries inflicted by another person with intent to injure or
kill, by any means

Excludes: injuries due to:
legal intervention (E970-E978)
operations of war (E990-E999)

E960　　**Fight, brawl, rape**

E960.0　*Unarmed fight or brawl*

Brawl or fight with hands, fists, feet　　Injured or killed in fight NOS

Excludes:　homicidal:
　　　　　　　injury by weapons (E965, E966, E969)
　　　　　　　strangulation (E963)
　　　　　　　submersion (E964)

E960.1　*Rape*

E961　　**Assault by corrosive or caustic substance, except poisoning**

Injury or death purposely caused by corrosive or caustic substance such as:
　acid [any]
　corrosive substance
　vitriol

Excludes:　burns from hot liquid (E968)
　　　　　　　chemical burns from swallowing a corrosive substance (E962)

E962　　**Assault by poisoning**

E962.0　*Drugs and medicaments*

Homicidal poisoning by any drug or medicament

E962.1　*Other solid and liquid substances*

E962.2　*Other gases and vapours*

E962.9　*Unspecified poisoning*

E963　　**Assault by hanging and strangulation**

Homicidal (attempt):
　garrotting or ligature
　hanging
　strangulation
　suffocation

E964　　**Assault by submersion [drowning]**

E965　　**Assault by firearms and explosives**

E965.0　*Handgun*

Pistol　　　　　　　　　　　　　　Revolver

E965.1　*Shotgun*

E965.2 *Hunting rifle*

E965.3 *Military firearms*

E965.4 *Other and unspecified firearm*

E965.5 *Antipersonnel bomb*

E965.6 *Petrol bomb*

E965.7 *Letter bomb*

E965.8 *Other specified explosive*

Bomb NOS (placed in)   Dynamite
  car
  house

E965.9 *Unspecified explosive*

E966   Assault by cutting and piercing instrument

Assassination (attempt), homicide (attempt) by any instrument classifiable under E920

Homicidal:
  cut
  puncture
  stab } any part of body
Stabbed

E967   Child battering and other maltreatment

E967.0 *By parent*

E967.1 *By other specified person*

E967.9 *By unspecified person*

E968   Assault by other and unspecified means

E968.0 *Fire*

Arson   Homicidal burns NOS

Excludes: burns from hot liquid (E968.3)

E968.1 *Pushing from high place*

E968.2 *Striking by blunt or thrown object*

E968.3 *Hot liquid*

Homicidal burns by scalding

E968.4 *Criminal neglect*

Abandonment of child or infant with intent to injure or kill

E968.8 *Other specified means*

Bite of human being

E968.9 *Unspecified means*

Assassination (attempt) NOS
Homicidal (attempt):
  injury NOS
  wound NOS

Manslaughter (nonaccidental)
Murder (attempt) NOS
Violence, nonaccidental

E969   Late effects of injury purposely inflicted by other person

Note: This category is to be used to indicate circumstances classifiable to E960-E968 as the cause of death or disability from late effects, which are themselves classified elsewhere. The "late effects" include conditions reported as such, or occurring as sequelae one year or more after injury purposely inflicted by another person. [See III Late effects, page 723].

LEGAL INTERVENTION (E970-E978)

Includes: injuries inflicted by the police or other law-enforcing agents, including military on duty, in the course of arresting or attempting to arrest lawbreakers, suppressing disturbances, maintaining order, and other legal action
  legal execution

Excludes: injuries caused by civil insurrections (E990-E999)

E970   Injury due to legal intervention by firearms

Gun shot wound
Injury by:
  machine gun
  revolver

Injury by:
  rifle pellet or rubber bullet
  shot NOS

E971   Injury due to legal intervention by explosives

Injury by:
  dynamite
  explosive shell
  grenade
  mortar bomb

E972   Injury due to legal intervention by gas

Asphyxiation by gas
Injury by tear gas

Poisoning by gas

E973 Injury due to legal intervention by blunt object

Hit, struck by:
 baton
 blunt object
 stave

E974 Injury due to legal intervention by cutting and piercing instruments

Cut	Injured by bayonet
Incised wound	Stab wound

E975 Injury due to legal intervention by other specified means

Blow	Man-handling

E976 Injury due to legal intervention by unspecified means

E977 Late effects of injuries due to legal intervention

Note: This category is to be used to indicate circumstances classifiable to E970-E976 as the cause of death or disability from late effects, which are themselves classified elsewhere. The "late effects" include conditions reported as such, or occurring as sequelae one year or more after injury due to legal intervention. [See III Late effects, page 723].

E978 Legal execution

All executions performed at the behest of the judiciary or ruling authority [whether permanent or temporary], such as:

asphyxiation by gas	hanging
beheading, decapitation	poisoning
(by guillotine)	shooting
capital punishment	other specified means
electrocution	

INJURY UNDETERMINED WHETHER ACCIDENTALLY OR PURPOSELY INFLICTED (E980-E989)

Note: Categories E980-E989 are for use when it is stated that an investigation by a medical or legal authority has not determined whether the injuries are accidental, suicidal or homicidal. They include selfinflicted injuries, but not poisoning, when not specified whether accidental or with intent to harm.

E980 Poisoning by solid or liquid substances, undetermined whether accidentally or purposely inflicted

E980.0 *Analgesics, antipyretics and antirheumatics*

E980.1 *Barbiturates*

E980.2 *Other sedatives and hypnotics*

E980.3 *Tranquillizers and other psychotropic agents*

E980.4 *Other specified drugs and medicaments*

E980.5 *Unspecified drug or medicament*

E980.6 *Corrosive and caustic substances*

Poisoning, undetermined whether accidental or purposeful, by substances classifiable to E864.–

E980.7 *Agricultural and horticultural chemical and pharmaceutical preparations other than plant foods and fertilizers*

E980.8 *Arsenic and its compounds*

E980.9 *Other and unspecified solid and liquid substances*

E981 Poisoning by gases in domestic use, undetermined whether accidentally or purposely inflicted

E981.0 *Gas distributed by pipeline*

E981.1 *Liquefied petroleum gas distributed in mobile containers*

E981.8 *Other utility gas*

E982 Poisoning by other gases, undetermined whether accidentally or purposely inflicted

E982.0 *Motor vehicle exhaust gas*

E982.1 *Other carbon monoxide*

E982.8 *Other specified gases and vapours*

E982.9 *Unspecified gases and vapours*

E983 Hanging, strangulation or suffocation, undetermined whether accidentally or purposely inflicted

E983.0 *Hanging*

E983.1 *Suffocation by plastic bag*

E983.8 *Other specified means*

E983.9 *Unspecified means*

E984   **Submersion [drowning], undetermined whether accidentally or purposely inflicted**

E985   **Injury by firearms and explosives, undetermined whether accidentally or purposely inflicted**

E985.0   *Hand gun*

E985.1   *Shot gun*

E985.2   *Hunting rifle*

E985.3   *Military firearms*

E985.4   *Other and unspecified firearm*

E985.5   *Explosives*

E986   **Injury by cutting and piercing instruments, undetermined whether accidentally or purposely inflicted**

E987   **Falling from high place, undetermined whether accidentally or purposely inflicted**

E987.0   *Residential premises*

E987.1   *Other man-made structures*

E987.2   *Natural sites*

E987.9   *Unspecified*

E988   **Injury by other and unspecified means, undetermined whether accidentally or purposely inflicted**

E988.0   *Jumping or lying before moving object*

E988.1   *Burns, fire*

E988.2   *Scald*

E988.3   *Extremes of cold*

E988.4   *Electrocution*

E988.5   *Crashing of motor vehicle*

E988.6   *Crashing of aircraft*

E988.7   *Caustic substances, except poisoning*

E988.8   *Other specified means*

E988.9   *Unspecified means*

E989　**Late effects of injury, undetermined whether accidentally or purposely inflicted**

Note:　This category is to be used to indicate circumstances classifiable to E980-E988 as the cause of death or disability from late effects, which are themselves classified elsewhere. The "late effects" include conditions reported as such, or occurring as sequelae one year or more after injury undetermined whether accidentally or purposely inflicted.　[See III Late effects, page 723].

INJURY RESULTING FROM OPERATIONS OF WAR (E990-E999)

Includes:　injuries to military personnel and civilians caused by war and civil insurrections and occurring during the time of war and insurrection

injuries due to operations of war, occurring after cessation of hostilities

Excludes:　accidents during training of military personnel, manufacture of war material and transport, unless attributable to enemy action

E990　**Injury due to war operations by fires and conflagrations**

Includes:　asphyxia ⎫ originating from fire caused directly by a fire-
　　　　　 burns 　⎬　producing device or indirectly by any
　　　　　 other injury ⎭ conventional weapon

E990.0　*From petrol bomb*

E990.9　*From other and unspecified sources*

E991　**Injury due to war operations by bullets and fragments**

E991.0　*Rubber bullets (rifle)*

E991.1　*Pellets (rifle)*

E991.2　*Other bullets*

Bullet [any except rubber bullets, and pellets]
　carbine
　machine gun
　pistol
　rifle
　shotgun

E991.3　*Antipersonnel bomb (fragments)*

E991.9   *Other and unspecified fragments*

Fragments from:

artillery shell	land mine
bombs, except antipersonnel	rockets
grenade	shell
guided missile	shrapnel

E992   Injury due to war operations by explosion of marine weapons

Depth charge	Sea-based artillery shell
Marine mines	Torpedo
Mine NOS, at sea or in harbour	Underwater blast

E993   Injury due to war operations by other explosion

Accidental explosion of	Explosion of:
munitions being used in war	artillery shell
Accidental explosion of	breech block
own weapons	cannon block
Air blast NOS	mortar bomb
Blast NOS	Injury by weapon burst
Explosion NOS	

E994   Injury due to war operations by destruction of aircraft

Aeroplane:	Crushed by falling aeroplane
burned	
exploded	
shot down	

E995   Injury due to war operations by other and unspecified forms of conventional warfare

Battle wounds	Drowned in war operations
Bayonet injury	

E996   Injury due to war operations by nuclear weapons

Blast effects	Heat
Fireball effects	Exposure to ionizing radiation
Other direct and secondary effects of	from nuclear weapon
nuclear weapons	

E997   Injury due to war operations by other forms of unconventional warfare

E997.0   *Lasers*

E997.1   *Biological warfare*

E997.2   *Gases, fumes and chemicals*

E997.8   *Other*

E997.9   *Unspecified*

E998   Injury due to war operations but occurring after cessation of hostilities

Injuries due to operations of war but occurring after cessation of hostilities by any means classifiable under E990-E997

Injuries by explosion of bombs or mines placed in the course of operations of war, if the explosion occurred after cessation of hostilities

E999   Late effects of injury due to war operations

Note: This category is to be used to indicate circumstances classifiable to E990-E998 as the cause of death or disability from late effects, which are themselves classified elsewhere. The "late effects" include conditions reported as such, or occurring as sequelae one year or more after injury resulting from operations of war. [See III Late effects page 723].

SUPPLEMENTARY CLASSIFICATION OF FACTORS INFLUENCING HEALTH STATUS AND CONTACT WITH HEALTH SERVICES

This classification is provided to deal with occasions when circumstances other than a disease or injury classifiable to categories 000-999, the main part of ICD, or to the E code, are recorded as "diagnoses" or "problems". This can arise in two main ways:

a) When a person who is not currently sick encounters the health services for some specific purpose, such as to act as a donor of an organ or tissue, to receive prophylactic vaccination or to discuss a problem which is in itself not a disease or injury. This will be a fairly rare occurrence amongst hospital inpatients but will be relatively more common amongst hospital outpatients and patients of family practitioners, health clinics, etc. In these circumstances, it is permissible for the V code to be used in providing single cause tabulations.

b) When some circumstance or problem is present which influences the person's health status but is not in itself a current illness or injury. Such factors may be elicited during population surveys, when the person may or may not be currently sick, or be recorded as an additional factor to be borne in mind when the person is receiving care for some illness or injury. In the latter circumstances the V code should be used only as a supplementary code and should not be the one selected for use in primary, single cause tabulations. Examples of these circumstances are a personal history of certain diseases, or a person with an artificial heart valve in situ.

PERSONS WITH POTENTIAL HEALTH HAZARDS RELATED TO COMMUNICABLE DISEASES (V01-V07)

Excludes: family history of infectious and parasitic diseases (V18.8)
personal history of infectious and parasitic diseases (V12.0)

V01   Contact with or exposure to communicable diseases

V01.0   *Cholera*
Conditions in 001.–

V01.1   *Tuberculosis*
Conditions in 010.– to 018.–

V01.2   *Poliomyelitis*
Conditions in 045.–

V01.3   *Smallpox*
Conditions in 050.–

V01.4   *Rubella*

Conditions in 056.–

V01.5   *Rabies*

Conditions in 071

V01.6   *Venereal diseases*

Conditions in 090.– to 099.–

V01.7   *Other viral diseases*

Conditions in 045.– to 078.–, except as above

V01.8   *Other communicable diseases*

Conditions in 001 to 136, except as above

V01.9   *Unspecified*

V02   Carrier or suspected carrier of infectious diseases

V02.0   *Cholera*

V02.1   *Typhoid*

V02.2   *Amoebiasis*

V02.3   *Other gastrointestinal pathogens*

V02.4   *Diphtheria*

V02.5   *Other specified bacterial diseases*

Bacterial disease due to:
  meningococci
  staphylococci
  streptococci

V02.6   *Viral hepatitis*

Hepatitis Australia-antigen [HAA] [SH] carrier

V02.7   *Gonorrhoea*

V02.8   *Other venereal diseases*

V02.9   *Other specified infectious organism*

V03   Need for prophylactic vaccination and inoculation against bacterial diseases

Excludes: vaccination not carried out because of contraindication (V64.0)
            vaccines against combinations of diseases (V06.–)

V03.0　*Cholera alone*

V03.1　*Typhoid-paratyphoid alone [TAB]*

V03.2　*Tuberculosis [BCG]*

V03.3　*Plague*

V03.4　*Tularaemia*

V03.5　*Diphtheria alone*

V03.6　*Pertussis alone*

V03.7　*Tetanus toxoid alone*

V03.8　*Other specified vaccinations against single bacterial diseases*

V03.9　*Unspecified*

V04　Need for prophylactic vaccination and inoculation against certain viral diseases

Excludes:　vaccines against combinations of diseases (V06.–)

V04.0　*Poliomyelitis*

V04.1　*Smallpox*

V04.2　*Measles alone*

V04.3　*Rubella alone*

V04.4　*Yellow fever*

V04.5　*Rabies*

V04.6　*Mumps alone*

V04.7　*Common cold*

V04.8　*Influenza*

V05　Need for other prophylactic vaccination and inoculation against single diseases

Excludes:　vaccines against combinations of diseases (V06.–)

V05.0　*Arthropod-borne viral encephalitis*

V05.1　*Other arthropod-borne viral diseases*

V05.2　*Leishmaniasis*

V05.8　*Other specified disease*

V05.9　*Unspecified*

V06   Need for prophylactic vaccination and inoculation against combinations of diseases

V06.0   *Cholera with typhoid-paratyphoid [cholera + TAB]*

V06.1   *Diphtheria-tetanus-pertussis, combined [DTP]*

V06.2   *Diphtheria-tetanus-pertussis with typhoid-paratyphoid [DTP + TAB]*

V06.3   *Diphtheria-tetanus-pertussis with poliomyelitis [DTP + polio]*

V06.4   *Measles-mumps-rubella [MMR]*

V06.8   *Other combinations*

V06.9   *Unspecified combined vaccine*

V07   Need for isolation and other prophylactic measures

V07.0   *Isolation*

Admission to protect the individual from his surroundings or for isolation of individual after contact with infectious diseases

V07.1   *Desensitization to allergens*

V07.2   *Prophylactic immunotherapy*

Administration of immune sera [gamma globulin]

V07.3   *Other prophylactic chemotherapy*

Administration for prophylactic purposes of:
   antibiotics
   other chemotherapeutic agents
Chemoprophylaxis

Excludes: maintenance chemotherapy following disease (V58.1)

V07.8   *Other specified prophylactic measure*

V07.9   *Unspecified*

PERSONS WITH POTENTIAL HEALTH HAZARDS RELATED TO
PERSONAL AND FAMILY HISTORY (V10-V19)

Excludes: aftercare and follow-up (V50-V58)
              when the possibility that the fetus might be affected is the
              reason for observation or action during pregnancy (655.–)

V10   Personal history of malignant neoplasm
Includes: the conditions "in remission"

V10.0   *Gastrointestinal tract*
History of condition classifiable to 140-159

V10.1   *Trachea, bronchus and lung*
History of condition classifiable to 162

V10.2   *Other respiratory and intrathoracic organs*
History of condition classifiable to 160, 161, 163-165

V10.3   *Breast*
History of condition classifiable to 174 and 175

V10.4   *Genital organs*
History of condition classifiable to 179-187

V10.5   *Urinary organs*
History of condition classifiable to 188 and 189

V10.6   *Leukaemia*
Condition classifiable to 204-208, in remission

V10.7   *Other lymphatic and haematopoietic neoplasms*
Condition classifiable to 200-203 and 209, in remission

V10.8   *Other*
Skin

V10.9   *Unspecified*

V11   Personal history of mental disorder

V12   Personal history of certain other diseases

V12.0   *Infectious and parasitic diseases*

V12.1   *Nutritional deficiency*

V12.2   *Endocrine, metabolic and immunity disorders*
Excludes: history of allergy (V14.–, V15.0)

V12.3   *Diseases of blood and blood-forming organs*

V12.4   *Disorders of nervous system and sense organs*

V12.5   *Diseases of circulatory system*
Excludes: old myocardial infarction (412)
             post-myocardial infarction syndrome (411)

V12.6   *Diseases of respiratory system*

V12.7   *Diseases of digestive system*

V13   Personal history of other diseases

V13.0   *Disorders of urinary system*

V13.1   *Trophoblastic disease*

Excludes: supervision during a current pregnancy (V23.1)

V13.2   *Other genital system and obstetric disorders*

Excludes: supervision during a current pregnancy of a woman with poor obstetric history (V23.–)

V13.3   *Diseases of skin and subcutaneous tissue*

V13.4   *Arthritis*

V13.5   *Other musculoskeletal disorders*

V13.6   *Congenital malformations*

V13.7   *Perinatal problems*

V13.8   *Other*

V13.9   *Unspecified*

V14   Personal history of allergy to medicinal agents

V14.0   *Penicillin*

V14.1   *Other antibiotic agent*

V14.2   *Sulfonamides*

V14.3   *Other anti-infective agent*

V14.4   *Anaesthetic agent*

V14.5   *Narcotic agent*

V14.6   *Analgesic agent*

V14.7   *Serum or vaccine*

V14.8   *Other*

V14.9   *Unspecified*

V15   Other personal history presenting hazards to health

V15.0   *Allergy, other than to medicinal agents*

V15.1   *Surgery to heart and great vessels*

Excludes: replacement by transplant or other means (V42.–, V43.–)

V15.2   *Surgery to other major organs*

Excludes: replacement by transplant or other means (V42.–, V43.–)

V15.3   *Irradiation*

Previous exposure to therapeutic or other ionising radiation

V15.4   *Psychological trauma*

Excludes: history of condition classifiable to 290-316 (V11)

V15.5   *Injury*

V15.6   *Poisoning*

V15.7   *Contraception*

Excludes: current contraceptive management (V25.–)
              presence of intrauterine contraceptive device as incidental
              finding (V45.5)

V15.8   *Other*

V15.9   *Unspecified*

V16   Family history of malignant neoplasm

V16.0   *Gastrointestinal tract*

Family history of condition classifiable to 140-159

V16.1   *Trachea, bronchus and lung*

Family history of condition classifiable to 162

V16.2   *Other respiratory and intrathoracic organs*

Family history of condition classifiable to 160, 161, 163 to 165

V16.3   *Breast*

Family history of condition classifiable to 174

V16.4   *Genital organs*

Family history of condition classifiable to 179-187

V16.5   *Urinary organs*

Family history of condition classifiable to 189

V16.6   *Leukaemia*

Family history of condition classifiable to 204-208

V16.7   *Other lymphatic and haematopoietic neoplasms*

Family history of condition classifiable to 200-203

V16.8   *Other*
Family history of other condition classifiable to 140-199
V16.9   *Unspecified*

V17   Family history of certain chronic disabling diseases
V17.0   *Psychiatric condition*
V17.1   *Stroke (cerebrovascular)*
V17.2   *Other neurological diseases*
Epilepsy   Huntington's chorea
V17.3   *Ischaemic heart disease*
V17.4   *Other cardiovascular diseases*
V17.5   *Asthma*
V17.6   *Other chronic respiratory conditions*
V17.7   *Arthritis*
V17.8   *Other musculoskeletal diseases*

V18   Family history of certain other specific conditions
V18.0   *Diabetes mellitus*
V18.1   *Other endocrine and metabolic diseases*
V18.2   *Anaemia*
V18.3   *Other blood disorders*
V18.4   *Mental retardation*
V18.5   *Digestive disorders*
V18.6   *Kidney diseases*
V18.7   *Other genitourinary diseases*
V18.8   *Infectious diseases*

V19   Family history of other conditions
V19.0   *Blindness or visual loss*
V19.1   *Other eye disorders*
V19.2   *Deafness or hearing loss*
V19.3   *Other ear disorders*

V19.4   *Skin conditions*

V19.5   *Congenital anomalies*

V19.6   *Allergic disorders*

V19.7   *Consanguinity*

V19.8   *Other*

PERSONS ENCOUNTERING HEALTH SERVICES IN CIRCUMSTANCES
RELATED TO REPRODUCTION AND DEVELOPMENT (V20-V28)

V20   Health supervision of infant or child

V20.0   *Foundling*

V20.1   *Other healthy infant receiving care*

V20.2   *Routine child health check*
Development testing of infant or child
Excludes: special screening for developmental handicaps (V79.3)

V21   Constitutional states in development

V21.0   *Period of rapid growth in childhood*

V21.1   *Puberty*

V21.2   *Other adolescence*

V21.8   *Other*

V21.9   *Unspecified*

V22   Normal pregnancy
Excludes: pregnancy   examination   or   test,   pregnancy   unconfirmed
(V72.4)

V22.0   *Supervision of normal first pregnancy*

V22.1   *Supervision of other normal pregnancy*

V22.2   *Pregnant state, incidental*
Pregnant state NOS

V23   Supervision of high-risk pregnancy

V23.0   *Pregnancy with history of infertility*

V23.1   *Pregnancy with history of trophoblastic disease*
Pregnancy with history of:
  hydatidiform mole
  vesicular mole

V23.2 *Pregnancy with history of abortion*

Pregnancy with history of conditions in 634.– to 638.–
Excludes: habitual aborter:
        care during pregnancy (646.3)
        without current pregnancy (629.9)

V23.3 *Grand multiparity*

Excludes: care in relation to labour and delivery (659.4)
        without current pregnancy (V61.5)

V23.4 *Pregnancy with other poor obstetric history*

Pregnancy with history of other conditions in 630 to 676.–

V23.5 *Pregnancy with other poor reproductive history*

Pregnancy with history of stillbirth or neonatal death

V23.8 *Other high-risk pregnancy*

V23.9 *Unspecified high-risk pregnancy*

V24 Postpartum care and examination

V24.0 *Immediately after delivery*

Care and observation in uncomplicated cases

V24.1 *Lactating mother*

V24.2 *Routine postpartum follow-up*

V25 Contraceptive management

V25.0 *General counselling and advice*

Family planning advice NOS   Prescription of contraceptives

V25.1 *Insertion of intrauterine contraceptive device*

V25.2 *Sterilization*

Admission for interruption of fallopian tubes or vas deferens

V25.3 *Menstrual extraction*

Interception of pregnancy   Menstrual regulation

V25.4 *Surveillance of previously prescribed contraceptive methods*

Checking, reinsertion or removal of (intrauterine) contraceptive device
Repeat prescription for contraceptive pill or other contraceptive method
Routine examination in connection with contraceptive maintenance

Excludes: presence of intrauterine contraceptive device as an incidental
        finding (V45.5)

V25.8   *Other*

V25.9   *Unspecified*

V26   Procreative management

V26.0   *Tuboplasty or vasoplasty after previous sterilization*

V26.1   *Artificial insemination*

V26.2   *Investigation and testing*

Fallopian insufflation   Sperm counts

V26.3   *Genetic counselling*

V26.4   *General counselling and advice*

V26.8   *Other*

V26.9   *Unspecified*

V27   Outcome of delivery

Note: This category is intended for the coding of the outcome of delivery
        on the mother's record.

V27.0   *Single live birth*

V27.1   *Single stillbirth*

V27.2   *Twins, both live born*

V27.3   *Twins, one live born and one stillborn*

V27.4   *Twins, both stillborn*

V27.5   *Other multiple birth, all live born*

V27.6   *Other multiple birth, some live born*

V27.7   *Other multiple birth, all stillborn*

V27.9   *Unspecified*

Multiple birth ⎫
Single birth   ⎬ outcome to infant unspecified

V28   Antenatal screening

Excludes: routine prenatal care (V22.–, V23.–)

V28.0   *Screening for chromosomal anomalies by amniocentesis*

V28.1   *Screening for raised alphafetoprotein levels in amniotic fluid*

V28.2   *Other screening based on amniocentesis*

V28.3 *Screening for malformations using ultrasonics*

V28.4 *Screening for fetal growth retardation using ultrasonics*

V28.5 *Screening for isoimmunization*

V28.8 *Other*

V28.9 *Unspecified*

HEALTHY LIVEBORN INFANTS ACCORDING TO TYPE OF BIRTH (V30-V39)

Note: These categories are intended for the coding of liveborn infants who are not sick but who are nevertheless consuming health care [e.g., cot occupancy].

The following fourth-digit subdivisions are for use with categories V30-V39:

.0 Born in hospital
.1 Born before admission to hospital
.2 Born outside hospital and not hospitalized

V30 Singleton

V31 Twin, mate live born

V32 Twin, mate stillborn

V33 Twin, unspecified

V34 Other multiple, mates all live born

V35 Other multiple, mates all stillborn

V36 Other multiple, mates live- and stillborn

V37 Other multiple, unspecified

V39 Unspecified

PERSONS WITH A CONDITION INFLUENCING THEIR HEALTH STATUS
(V40-V49)

Note: These categories are intended for use when the listed conditions are recorded as "diagnoses" or "problems".

V40   Mental and behavioural problems

V40.0   *Problems with learning*

V40.1   *Problems with communication [including speech]*

V40.2   *Other mental problems*

V40.3   *Other behavioural problems*

V40.9 · *Unspecified mental or behavioural problems*

V41   Problems with special senses and other special functions

V41.0   *Problems with sight*

V41.1   *Other eye problems*

V41.2   *Problems with hearing*

V41.3   *Other ear problems*

V41.4   *Problems with voice production*

V41.5   *Problems with smell and taste*

V41.6   *Problems with swallowing and mastication*

V41.7   *Problems with sexual function*

Excludes: marital problems (V61.1)
            psychosexual disorders (302.–)

V41.8   *Other problems with special functions*

V41.9   *Unspecified*

V42   Organ or tissue replaced by transplant

Includes: homologous or heterologous (animal) (human) transplant
            organ status

V42.0   *Kidney*

V42.1   *Heart*

V42.2   *Heart valve*

V42.3   *Skin*

V42.4   *Bone*

V42.5   *Cornea*

V42.6   *Lung*

V42.7   *Liver*

V42.8   *Other specified organ or tissue*

Intestine   Pancreas

V42.9   *Unspecified*

V43   Organ or tissue replaced by other means

Includes: replacement of organ by:
               artificial device
               mechanical device
               prosthesis

Excludes: cardiac pacemaker (V45.0)
               renal dialysis status (V45.1)

V43.0   *Eye globe*

V43.1   *Lens*

Pseudophakia

V43.2   *Heart*

V43.3   *Heart valve*

V43.4   *Blood vessel*

V43.5   *Bladder*

V43.6   *Joint*

Finger joint replacement   Hip joint replacement (partial)
                                                   (total)

V43.7   *Limb*

V43.8   *Other*

Larynx

V44   Artificial opening status

Excludes: artificial openings requiring attention or management (V55.–)

V44.0   *Tracheostomy*

V44.1   *Gastrostomy*

V44.2   *Ileostomy*

V44.3   *Colostomy*

V44.4   *Other artificial opening of gastrointestinal tract*

V44.5   *Cystostomy*

V44.6 *Other artificial opening of urinary tract*
Nephrostomy   Urethrostomy
Ureterostomy

V44.7 *Artificial vagina*

V44.8 *Other*

V44.9 *Unspecified*

V45 Other postsurgical states
Excludes: follow-up or aftercare management (V51-V58)
          malfunction or other complication—code to condition

V45.0 *Cardiac pacemaker in situ*
Excludes: admission for adjustment or other care (V52.3)
          malfunction (996.0)

V45.1 *Renal dialysis status*
Patient requiring intermittent renal dialysis
Presence of arterial-venous shunt (for dialysis)
Excludes: admission for dialysis session (V56.0)

V45.2 *Presence of cerebrospinal fluid drainage device*
Cerebral ventricle (communicating) shunt, valve or device in situ
Excludes: malfunction (996.2)

V45.3 *Intestinal bypass or anastomosis status*

V45.4 *Arthrodesis status*

V45.5 *Presence of intrauterine contraceptive device*
Excludes: checking, re-insertion or removal of device (V25.4)
          complications from device (996.3)
          insertion of device (V25.1)

V45.6 *States following surgery of eye and adnexa*
Excludes: artificial:
          eye globe (V43.0)
          lens (V43.1)

V45.8 *Other*
Excludes: artificial heart valve (V43.3)
          vascular prosthesis (V43.4)

V46 Other dependence on machines

V46.0 *Aspirator*

V46.1 *Respirator*

V46.8 *Other enabling machines*

V46.9 *Unspecified*

V47 Other problems with internal organs

V47.0 *Deficiences of internal organs*

V47.1 *Mechanical and motor problems with internal organs*

V47.2 *Other cardiorespiratory problems*

V47.3 *Other digestive problems*

V47.4 *Other urinary problems*

V47.5 *Other genital problems*

V47.9 *Unspecified*

V48 Problems with head, neck and trunk

V48.0 *Deficiences of head*

V48.1 *Deficiences of neck and trunk*

V48.2 *Mechanical and motor problems with head*

V48.3 *Mechanical and motor problems with neck and trunk*

V48.4 *Sensory problem with head*

V48.5 *Sensory problem with neck and trunk*

V48.6 *Disfigurements of head*

V48.7 *Disfigurements of neck and trunk*

V48.8 *Other problems with head, neck and trunk*

V48.9 *Unspecified*

V49 Problems with limbs and other problems

V49.0 *Deficiencies of limbs*

V49.1 *Mechanical problems with limbs*

V49.2 *Motor problems with limbs*

V49.3 *Sensory problems with limbs*

V49.4 *Disfigurements of limbs*

V49.5 *Other problems with limbs*

V49.8 *Other specified problems influencing health status*

V49.9 *Unspecified*

PERSONS ENCOUNTERING HEALTH SERVICES FOR SPECIFIC
PROCEDURES AND AFTERCARE (V50-V59)

Note: Categories V51-V58 are intended for use to indicate a reason for
care in patients who have already been treated for some disease or
injury not now present, but who are receiving follow-up medical
surveillance or care to consolidate the treatment, to deal with
residual states, to ensure that the condition has not recurred or
to prevent recurrence. The codes should be used alternatively
or additionally to the code indicating the original disease or
injury (001-999), which will be the one to be tabulated for
underlying cause purposes.

V50   Elective surgery for purposes other than remedying health states

V50.0 *Hair transplant*

V50.1 *Other plastic surgery for unacceptable cosmetic appearance*
Excludes: plastic surgery following healed injury or operation (V51)

V50.2 *Routine or ritual circumcision*
Circumcision in the absence of significant medical indication

V50.3 *Ear piercing*

V50.8 *Other*

V50.9 *Unspecified*

V51   Aftercare involving the use of plastic surgery
Plastic surgery following healed injury or operation
Repair of scarred tissue
Excludes: cosmetic plastic surgery (V50.1)
plastic surgery as treatment for current injury—code to
condition

V52   Fitting and adjustment of prosthetic device

V52.0 *Artificial arm (complete) (partial)*

V52.1 *Artificial leg (complete) (partial)*

V52.2 *Artificial eye*

V52.3 *Dental prosthetic device*

V52.4 *Breast prosthesis*
Excludes: breast implant (V50.1)

V52.8 *Other specified prosthetic device*

V52.9 *Unspecified*

V53 Fitting and adjustment of other device

V53.0 *Devices related to nervous system and special senses*

Auditory ⎫
Visual ⎭ substitution device

V53.1 *Spectacles and contact lenses*

V53.2 *Hearing aid*

V53.3 *Cardiac pacemaker*

V53.4 *Orthodontic devices*

V53.5 *Ileostomy or other intestinal appliance*

V53.6 *Urinary devices*

V53.7 *Orthopaedic devices*

Orthopaedic:
  brace
  cast

Orthopaedic:
  corset
  shoes

V53.8 *Wheelchair*

V53.9 *Other and unspecified*

V54 Other orthopaedic aftercare

V54.0 *Aftercare involving removal of fracture plate or other internal fixation device*

Removal of:
  pins
  plates

Removal of:
  rods
  screws

Excludes: malfunction of internal orthopaedic device (996.4)
other complication of nonmechanical nature (996.6, 996.7)
removal of external fixation device (V54.8)

V54.8 *Other orthopaedic aftercare*

Change, checking or removal of:
  Kirschner wire
  plaster cast
  splint, external
  other external fixation or traction device

V54.9 *Unspecified*

V55   Attention to artificial openings

Includes: closure
                   passage of sounds or bougies
                   reforming
                   removal of catheter
                   toilet or cleansing

Excludes: complications of external stoma (519.0, 569.6, 997.4, 997.5)
                   status only, without need for care (V44.–)

V55.0   *Tracheostomy*

V55.1   *Gastrostomy*

V55.2   *Ileostomy*

V55.3   *Colostomy*

V55.4   *Other artificial opening of digestive tract*

V55.5   *Cystostomy*

V55.6   *Other artificial opening of urinary tract*
Nephrostomy   Urethrostomy

V55.7   *Artificial vagina*

V55.8   *Other specified*

V55.9   *Unspecified*

V56   Aftercare involving intermittent dialysis

Includes: dialysis preparation and treatment

V56.0   *Extracorporeal dialysis*
Dialysis (renal) NOS
Excludes: dialysis status (V45.1)

V56.8   *Other dialysis*
Peritoneal dialysis

V57   Care involving use of rehabilitation procedures

V57.0   *Breathing exercises*

V57.1   *Other physical therapy*
Therapeutic and remedial exercises, except breathing

V57.2   *Occupational therapy and vocational rehabilitation*

V57.3   *Speech therapy*

V57.4 *Orthoptic training*

V57.8 *Other*

V57.9 *Unspecified*

V58 Other and unspecified aftercare

V58.0 *Radiotherapy session*

Admission solely for radiotherapy, the main part of the treatment (for malignant disease) already having been completed

V58.1 *Maintenance chemotherapy*

Excludes: prophylactic chemotherapy against disease which has never been present (V03.– to V07.–)

V58.2 *Blood transfusion, without reported diagnosis*

V58.3 *Attention to surgical dressings and sutures*

Change of dressings   Removal of sutures

V58.4 *Other aftercare following surgery*

Excludes: attention to artificial openings (V55.–)
orthopaedic aftercare (V54.–)

V58.5 *Orthodontics*

V58.8 *Other*

V58.9 *Unspecified*

V59 Donors

Excludes: examination of potential donor (V70.8)

V59.0 *Blood*

V59.1 *Skin*

V59.2 *Bone*

V59.3 *Bone marrow*

V59.4 *Kidney*

V59.5 *Cornea*

V59.8 *Other specified organ or tissue*

V59.9 *Unspecified*

PERSONS ENCOUNTERING HEALTH SERVICES IN OTHER
CIRCUMSTANCES (V60-V68)

V60 Housing, household and economic circumstances

V60.0 *Lack of housing*

Hobos
Social migrants
Tramps

Transients
Vagabonds

V60.1 *Inadequate housing*

Lack of heating
Restriction of space

Technical defects in home prevent-
ing adequate care

V60.2 *Inadequate material resources*

Economic problem

Poverty NOS

V60.3 *Person living alone*

V60.4 *No other household member able to render care*

Person requiring care (has) (is):
  family member too handicapped, ill or otherwise unsuited to render
    care
  partner temporarily away from home
  temporarily away from usual place of abode

Excludes: holiday relief care (V60.5)

V60.5 *Holiday relief care*

Provision of health care facilities to a person normally cared for at home,
  to enable relatives to take a vacation

V60.6 *Person living in residential institution*

Boarding school resident

V60.8 *Other*

V60.9 *Unspecified*

V61 Other family circumstances

Includes: when these circumstances or fear of them, affecting the person
  directly involved or others, are mentioned as the reason,
  justified or not, for seeking or receiving medical advice
  or care

V61.0 *Family disruption*

Divorce

Estrangement

V61.1   *Marital problems*

Marital conflict

Excludes: problems related to:
         psychosexual disorders (302.–)
         sexual function (V41.7)

V61.2   *Parent-child problems*

Child:
  abuse
  battering
  neglect

Concern about behaviour of child
Parent-child conflict
Problem concerning adopted or foster child

Excludes: effect of maltreatment on the child (995.5)

V61.3   *Problems with aged parents or in-laws*

V61.4   *Health problems within family*

Alcoholism in family

Care of
Presence of } sick or handicapped person in family or household

V61.5   *Multiparity*

V61.6   *Illegitimacy or illegitimate pregnancy*

V61.7   *Other unwanted pregnancy*

V61.8   *Other*

V61.9   *Unspecified*

V62   Other psychosocial circumstances

Includes: when these circumstances or fear of them, affecting the person
        directly involved or others, are mentioned as the reason,
        justified or not, for seeking or receiving medical advice
        or care

Excludes: previous psychological trauma (V15.4)

V62.0   *Unemployment*

Excludes: when main problem is inadequate material resources (V60.2)

V62.1   *Adverse effects of work environment*

V62.2   *Other occupational circumstances or maladjustment*

Career choice problem   Dissatisfaction with employment

V62.3   *Educational circumstances*

Dissatisfaction with school   Educational handicap
  environment

V62.4 *Social maladjustment*

Cultural deprivation
Political, religious or sex
   discrimination

Social:
   isolation
   persecution

V62.5 *Legal circumstances*

Imprisonment
Litigation

Prosecution

V62.6 *Refusal of treatment for reasons of religion or conscience*

V62.8 *Other psychological or physical strain, not elsewhere classified*

V62.9 *Unspecified*

V63   Unavailability of other medical facilities for care

V63.0 *Residence remote from hospital or other health care facility*

V63.1 *Medical services in home not available*

Excludes: no other household member able to render care (V60.4)

V63.2 *Person awaiting admission to adequate facility elsewhere*

V63.8 *Other*

Person on waiting list undergoing social agency investigation

V63.9 *Unspecified*

V64   Persons encountering health services for specific procedures, not carried out

V64.0 *Vaccination not carried out because of contraindication*

V64.1 *Surgical or other procedure not carried out because of contra-indication*

V64.2 *Surgical or other procedure not carried out because of patient's decision*

V64.3 *Procedure not carried out for other reasons*

V65   Other persons seeking consultation without complaint or sickness

V65.0 *Healthy person accompanying sick person*

Boarder

V65.1 *Person consulting on behalf of another person*

Advice or treatment for nonattending third party

Excludes: anxiety (normal) about sick person in family (V61.4)

V65.2   *Person feigning illness*
Malingerer   Peregrinating patient

V65.3   *Dietary surveillance and counselling*
Dietary surveillance and counselling   Dietary surveillance and counsell-
    (in):   ing (in):
  NOS   gastritis
  colitis   hypercholesterolaemia
  diabetes mellitus   hypoglycaemia
  food allergies or intolerance   obesity

V65.4   *Other counselling, not elsewhere classified*
Health: Explanation of:
  advice   investigation findings
  education   medication
  instruction
Excludes: counselling (for):
              contraception (V25.0)
              genetic (V26.3)
              procreative management (V26.4)

V65.5   *Person with feared complaint in whom no diagnosis was made*
Feared condition not demonstrated   "Worried well"
Problem was normal state

V65.8   *Other*
Excludes: specified symptoms

V65.9   *Unspecified*

V66   Convalescence

V66.0   *Following surgery*

V66.1   *Following radiotherapy*

V66.2   *Following chemotherapy*

V66.3   *Following psychotherapy and other treatment for mental disorder*

V66.4   *Following treatment of fracture*

V66.5   *Following other treatment*

V66.6   *Following combined treatment*

V66.9   *Unspecified*

V67   Follow-up examination
Includes: surveillance only following treatment
Excludes: surveillance of contraception (V25.4)

V67.0   *Following surgery*

V67.1   *Following radiotherapy*

V67.2   *Following chemotherapy*

V67.3   *Following psychotherapy and other treatment for mental disorder*

V67.4   *Following treatment of fracture*

V67.5   *Following other treatment*

V67.6   *Following combined treatment*

V67.9   *Unspecified*

V68   Encounters for administrative purposes

V68.0   *Issue of medical certificates*

Issue of medical certificate of:
  cause of death
  fitness
  incapacity

Excludes: encounter for general medical examination (V70.–)

V68.1   *Issue of repeat prescriptions*

Issue of repeat prescription for:
  appliance
  glasses
  medicaments

Excludes: repeat prescription for contraceptives (V25.4)

V68.2   *Request for expert evidence*

V68.8   *Other*

V68.9   *Unspecified*

PERSONS WITHOUT REPORTED DIAGNOSIS ENCOUNTERED
DURING EXAMINATION AND INVESTIGATION
OF INDIVIDUALS AND POPULATIONS (V70-V82)

Note: Nonspecific abnormal findings disclosed at the time of these examinations are classifiable to categories 790-795.

V70   General medical examination

V70.0   *Routine general medical examination at a health care facility*

Health checkup

V70.1 *General psychiatric examination, requested by the authority*

V70.2 *General psychiatric examination, other and unspecified*

V70.3 *Other medical examination for administrative purposes*

General medical examination for:
  admission to old age home
  adoption
  camp
  driving licence
  immigration and naturalization

General medical examination for:
  insurance certification
  marriage
  prison
  school admission
  sports competition

Excludes: attendance for issue of medical certificates (V68.0)
  pre-employment screening (V70.5)

V70.4 *Examination for medicolegal reasons*

Blood-alcohol tests   Blood-drug tests

Excludes: examination and observation following:
  accidents (V71.3, V71.4)
  assault (V71.6)
  rape (V71.5)

V70.5 *Health examination of defined subpopulations*

Armed forces personnel   Prostitutes
Inhabitants of institutions   Refugees
Occupational health examinations   School children
Pre-employment screening   Students
Preschool children

V70.6 *Health examination in population surveys*

Excludes: special screening (V73.– to V82.–)

V70.7 *Examination for normal comparison or control in clinical research*

V70.8 *Other*

V70.9 *Unspecified*

V71   Observation and evaluation for suspected conditions

Includes: cases which present some symptoms or evidence of an abnormal condition which required study, but which, after examination and observation show no need for further treatment or medical care

V71.0 *Mental*

Dyssocial behaviour ⎫
Gang activity   ⎬ without manifest psychiatric behaviour

V71.1 *Observation for suspected malignant neoplasm*

V71.2   *Observation for suspected tuberculosis*

V71.3   *Observation following accident at work*

V71.4   *Observation following other accident*

Examination of individual involved in motor vehicle traffic accident

V71.5   *Observation following alleged rape or seduction*

Examination of victim or culprit

V71.6   *Observation following other inflicted injury*

Examination of victim or culprit

V71.7   *Observation for suspected cardiovascular disease*

V71.8   *Observation for other specified suspected condition*

V71.9   *Unspecified*

V72   Special investigations and examinations

Includes: routine examination of specific system

Excludes: general screening examination of defined population groups
(V70.5, V70.6, V70.7)
screening examination for specific disorders (V73.– to V82.–)

V72.0   *Examination of eyes and vision*

V72.1   *Examination of ears and hearing*

V72.2   *Dental examination*

V72.3   *Gynaecological examination*

Pelvic examination (annual) (periodic)

Excludes: routine examination in contraceptive management (V25.4)

V72.4   *Pregnancy examination or test, pregnancy unconfirmed*

Possible pregnancy, not (yet) confirmed

Excludes: pregnancy examination with immediate confirmation (V22.0,
V22.1)

V72.5   *Radiological examination, not elsewhere classified*

Routine chest X-ray

Excludes: examination for suspected tuberculosis (V71.2)

V72.6   *Laboratory examination*

Excludes: that for suspected disorder (V71.–)

V72.7   *Diagnostic skin and sensitization tests*
Allergy tests   Skin tests for hypersensitivity
Excludes: diagnostic skin tests for bacterial diseases (V74.–)

V72.8   *Other specified examination*

V72.9   *Unspecified*

V73   **Special screening examination for viral diseases**

V73.0   *Poliomyelitis*

V73.1   *Smallpox*

V73.2   *Measles*

V73.3   *Rubella*

V73.4   *Yellow fever*

V73.5   *Other arthropod-borne viral diseases*
Dengue fever   Viral encephalitis:
Haemorrhagic fever   mosquito-borne
                                tick-borne

V73.6   *Trachoma*

V73.8   *Other*

V73.9   *Unspecified*

V74   **Special screening examination for bacterial and spirochaetal diseases**
Includes: diagnostic skin tests for these diseases

V74.0   *Cholera*

V74.1   *Pulmonary tuberculosis*

V74.2   *Leprosy*

V74.3   *Diphtheria*

V74.4   *Bacterial conjunctivitis*

V74.5   *Venereal disease*

V74.6   *Yaws*

V74.8   *Other*
Brucellosis   Tetanus
Leptospirosis   Whooping cough
Plague

V74.9   *Unspecified*

V75   Special screening examination for other infectious diseases

V75.0   *Rickettsial diseases*

V75.1   *Malaria*

V75.2   *Leishmaniasis*

V75.3   *Trypanosomiasis*

Chagas's disease   Sleeping sickness

V75.4   *Mycotic infections*

V75.5   *Schistosomiasis*

V75.6   *Filariasis*

V75.7   *Intestinal helminthiasis*

V75.8   *Other specified parasitic infections*

V75.9   *Unspecified infectious disease*

V76   Special screening for malignant neoplasms

V76.0   *Respiratory organs*

V76.1   *Breast*

V76.2   *Cervix*

Routine cervical Papanicolaou smear

Excludes: when part of a general gynaecological examination (V72.3)

V76.3   *Bladder*

V76.4   *Other sites*

V76.8   *Other neoplasm*

V76.9   *Unspecified*

V77   Special screening for endocrine, nutritional, metabolic and immunity disorders

V77.0   *Thyroid disorders*

V77.1   *Diabetes mellitus*

V77.2   *Malnutrition*

V77.3   *Phenylketonuria*

V77.4   *Galactosaemia*

V77.5   *Gout*

V77.6 *Cystic fibrosis*

V77.7 *Other inborn errors of metabolism*

V77.8 *Obesity*

V77.9 *Other and unspecified*

V78   Special screening for disorders of blood and blood-forming organs

V78.0 *Iron deficiency anaemia*

V78.1 *Other and unspecified deficiency anaemia*

V78.2 *Sickle-cell disease or trait*

V78.3 *Other haemoglobinopathies*

V78.8 *Other*

V78.9 *Unspecified*

V79   Special screening for mental disorders and developmental handicaps

V79.0 *Depression*

V79.1 *Alcoholism*

V79.2 *Mental retardation*

V79.3 *Developmental handicaps in early childhood*

V79.8 *Other*

V79.9 *Unspecified*

V80   Special screening for neurological, eye and ear diseases

V80.0 *Neurological conditions*

V80.1 *Glaucoma*

V80.2 *Other eye conditions*

Screening for:
  cataract
  congenital anomaly of eye
  senile macular lesions

Excludes: general vision examination (V72.0)

V80.3 *Ear diseases*

Excludes: general hearing examination (V72.1)

V81   Special screening for cardiovascular, respiratory and genitourinary diseases

V81.0   *Ischaemic heart disease*

V81.1   *Hypertension*

V81.2   *Other and unspecified cardiovascular conditions*

V81.3   *Chronic bronchitis and emphysema*

V81.4   *Other and unspecified respiratory conditions*

Excludes: screening for:
            lung neoplasm (V76.0)
            pulmonary tuberculosis (V74.1)

V81.5   *Nephropathy*

Screening for asymptomatic bacteriuria

V81.6   *Other and unspecified genitourinary conditions*

V82   Special screening for other conditions

V82.0   *Skin conditions*

V82.1   *Rheumatoid arthritis*

V82.2   *Other rheumatic disorders*

V82.3   *Congenital dislocation of hip*

V82.4   *Postnatal screening for chromosomal anomalies*

V82.5   *Chemical poisoning and other contamination*

Screening for:
  heavy metal poisoning
  ingestion of radioactive
    substance

Screening for:
  poisoning from contaminated
    water supply
  radiation exposure

V82.6   *Multiphasic screening*

V82.8   *Other*

V82.9   *Unspecified*

MORPHOLOGY OF NEOPLASMS

As explained in the Introduction, the World Health Organization has published an adaptation of the International Classification of Diseases for oncology (ICD-O). It contains a coded nomenclature for the morphology of neoplasms, which is reproduced here for those who wish to use it in conjunction with Chapter II of the International Classification of Diseases.

The morphology code numbers consist of five digits; the first four identify the histological type of the neoplasm and the fifth indicates its behaviour. The one-digit behaviour code is as follows:

/0 Benign

/1 Uncertain whether benign or malignant
    Borderline malignancy

/2 Carcinoma in situ
    Intraepithelial
    Noninfiltrating
    Noninvasive

/3 Malignant, primary site

/6 Malignant, metastatic site
    Secondary site

/9 Malignant, uncertain whether primary or metastatic site

In the nomenclature below, the morphology code numbers include the behaviour code appropriate to the histological type of neoplasm, but this behaviour code should be changed if other reported information makes this necessary. For example, "chordoma (M9370/3)" is assumed to be malignant; the term "benign chordoma" should be coded M9370/0. Similarly, "superficial spreading adenocarcinoma (M8143/3)" described as "noninvasive" should be coded M8143/2 and "melanoma (M8720/3)" described as "secondary" should be coded M8720/6.

The following table shows the correspondence between the morphology code and the different sections of Chapter II:

Morphology Code Histology/Behaviour		ICD Chapter II	
Any	0	210-229	Benign neoplasms
M8000-M8002	1	239	Neoplasms of unspecified nature
M8010+	1	235-238	Neoplasms of uncertain behaviour
Any	2	230-234	Carcinoma in situ
Any	3	140-195	Malignant neoplasms, stated or
		200-208	presumed to be primary
Any	6	196-198	Malignant neoplasms, stated or
			presumed to be secondary

The ICD-O behaviour digit /9 is inapplicable in an ICD context, since all malignant neoplasms are presumed to be primary (/3) or secondary (/6) according to other information on the medical record.

Only the first-listed term of the full ICD-O morphology nomenclature appears against each code number in the list below. The ICD Alphabetical Index (Volume 2), however, includes all the ICD-O synonyms as well as a number of other morphological names still likely to be encountered on medical records but omitted from ICD-O as outdated or otherwise undesirable.

A coding difficulty sometimes arises where a morphological diagnosis contains two qualifying adjectives that have different code numbers. An example is "transitional cell epidermoid carcinoma". "Transitional cell carcinoma NOS" is M8120/3 and "epidermoid carcinoma NOS" is M8070/3. In such circumstances, the higher number (M8120/3 in this example) should be used, as it is usually more specific. For other information about the coding of morphology see pages 724, 725.

CODED NOMENCLATURE FOR MORPHOLOGY OF NEOPLASMS

M800   **Neoplasms NOS**

M8000/0	*Neoplasm, benign*
M8000/1	*Neoplasm, uncertain whether benign or malignant*
M8000/3	*Neoplasm, malignant*
M8000/6	*Neoplasm, metastatic*
M8000/9	*Neoplasm, malignant, uncertain whether primary or metastatic*
M8001/0	*Tumour cells, benign*
M8001/1	*Tumour cells, uncertain whether benign or malignant*
M8001/3	*Tumour cells, malignant*
M8002/3	*Malignant tumour, small cell type*
M8003/3	*Malignant tumour, giant cell type*
M8004/3	*Malignant tumour, fusiform cell type*

M801-M804 **Epithelial neoplasms NOS**

M8010/0	*Epithelial tumour, benign*
M8010/2	*Carcinoma in situ NOS*
M8010/3	*Carcinoma NOS*
M8010/6	*Carcinoma, metastatic NOS*
M8010/9	*Carcinomatosis*
M8011/0	*Epithelioma, benign*
M8011/3	*Epithelioma, malignant*

M8012/3	*Large cell carcinoma NOS*
M8020/3	*Carcinoma, undifferentiated type NOS*
M8021/3	*Carcinoma, anaplastic type NOS*
M8022/3	*Pleomorphic carcinoma*
M8030/3	*Giant cell and spindle cell carcinoma*
M8031/3	*Giant cell carcinoma*
M8032/3	*Spindle cell carcinoma*
M8033/3	*Pseudosarcomatous carcinoma*
M8034/3	*Polygonal cell carcinoma*
M8035/3	*Spheroidal cell carcinoma*
M8040/1	*Tumourlet*
M8041/3	*Small cell carcinoma NOS*
M8042/3	*Oat cell carcinoma*
M8043/3	*Small cell carcinoma, fusiform cell type*

M805-M808 Papillary and squamous cell neoplasms

M8050/0	*Papilloma NOS (except Papilloma of urinary bladder M8120/1)*
M8050/2	*Papillary carcinoma in situ*
M8050/3	*Papillary carcinoma NOS*
M8051/0	*Verrucous papilloma*
M8051/3	*Verrucous carcinoma NOS*
M8052/0	*Squamous cell papilloma*
M8052/3	*Papillary squamous cell carcinoma*
M8053/0	*Inverted papilloma*
M8060/0	*Papillomatosis NOS*
M8070/2	*Squamous cell carcinoma in situ NOS*
M8070/3	*Squamous cell carcinoma NOS*
M8070/6	*Squamous cell carcinoma, metastatic NOS*
M8071/3	*Squamous cell carcinoma, keratinizing type NOS*
M8072/3	*Squamous cell carcinoma, large cell, non-keratinizing type*
M8073/3	*Squamous cell carcinoma, small cell, non-keratinizing type*
M8074/3	*Squamous cell carcinoma, spindle cell type*
M8075/3	*Adenoid squamous cell carcinoma*
M8076/2	*Squamous cell carcinoma in situ with questionable stromal invasion*
M8076/3	*Squamous cell carcinoma, microinvasive*
M8080/2	*Queyrat's erythroplasia*
M8081/2	*Bowen's disease*
M8082/3	*Lymphoepithelial carcinoma*

M809-M811 Basal cell neoplasms

M8090/1   *Basal cell tumour*
M8090/3   *Basal cell carcinoma NOS*
M8091/3   *Multicentric basal cell carcinoma*
M8092/3   *Basal cell carcinoma, morphoea type*
M8093/3   *Basal cell carcinoma, fibroepithelial type*
M8094/3   *Basosquamous carcinoma*
M8095/3   *Metatypical carcinoma*
M8096/0   *Intraepidermal epithelioma of Jadassohn*
M8100/0   *Trichoepithelioma*
M8101/0   *Trichofolliculoma*
M8102/0   *Tricholemmoma*
M8110/0   *Pilomatrixoma*

M812-M813 Transitional cell papillomas and carcinomas

M8120/0   *Transitional cell papilloma NOS*
M8120/1   *Urothelial papilloma*
M8120/2   *Transitional cell carcinoma in situ*
M8120/3   *Transitional cell carcinoma NOS*
M8121/0   *Schneiderian papilloma*
M8121/1   *Transitional cell papilloma, inverted type*
M8121/3   *Schneiderian carcinoma*
M8122/3   *Transitional cell carcinoma, spindle cell type*
M8123/3   *Basaloid carcinoma*
M8124/3   *Cloacogenic carcinoma*
M8130/3   *Papillary transitional cell carcinoma*

M814-M838 Adenomas and adenocarcinomas

M8140/0   *Adenoma NOS*
M8140/1   *Bronchial adenoma NOS*
M8140/2   *Adenocarcinoma in situ*
M8140/3   *Adenocarcinoma NOS*
M8140/6   *Adenocarcinoma, metastatic NOS*
M8141/3   *Scirrhous adenocarcinoma*
M8142/3   *Linitis plastica*
M8143/3   *Superficial spreading adenocarcinoma*
M8144/3   *Adenocarcinoma, intestinal type*
M8145/3   *Carcinoma, diffuse type*
M8146/0   *Monomorphic adenoma*

M8147/0	*Basal cell adenoma*
M8150/0	*Islet cell adenoma*
M8150/3	*Islet cell carcinoma*
M8151/0	*Insulinoma NOS*
M8151/3	*Insulinoma, malignant*
M8152/0	*Glucagonoma NOS*
M8152/3	*Glucagonoma, malignant*
M8153/1	*Gastrinoma NOS*
M8153/3	*Gastrinoma, malignant*
M8154/3	*Mixed islet cell and exocrine adenocarcinoma*
M8160/0	*Bile duct adenoma*
M8160/3	*Cholangiocarcinoma*
M8161/0	*Bile duct cystadenoma*
M8161/3	*Bile duct cystadenocarcinoma*
M8170/0	*Liver cell adenoma*
M8170/3	*Hepatocellular carcinoma NOS*
M8180/0	*Hepatocholangioma, benign*
M8180/3	*Combined hepatocellular carcinoma and cholangiocarcinoma*
M8190/0	*Trabecular adenoma*
M8190/3	*Trabecular adenocarcinoma*
M8191/0	*Embryonal adenoma*
M8200/0	*Eccrine dermal cylindroma*
M8200/3	*Adenoid cystic carcinoma*
M8201/3	*Cribriform carcinoma*
M8210/0	*Adenomatous polyp NOS*
M8210/3	*Adenocarcinoma in adenomatous polyp*
M8211/0	*Tubular adenoma NOS*
M8211/3	*Tubular adenocarcinoma*
M8220/0	*Adenomatous polyposis coli*
M8220/3	*Adenocarcinoma in adenomatous polyposis coli*
M8221/0	*Multiple adenomatous polyps*
M8230/3	*Solid carcinoma NOS*
M8231/3	*Carcinoma simplex*
M8240/1	*Carcinoid tumour NOS*
M8240/3	*Carcinoid tumour, malignant*
M8241/1	*Carcinoid tumour, argentaffin NOS*
M8241/3	*Carcinoid tumour, argentaffin, malignant*
M8242/1	*Carcinoid tumour, nonargentaffin NOS*
M8242/3	*Carcinoid tumour, nonargentaffin, malignant*
M8243/3	*Mucocarcinoid tumour, malignant*

M8244/3	*Composite carcinoid*
M8250/1	*Pulmonary adenomatosis*
M8250/3	*Bronchiolo-alveolar adenocarcinoma*
M8251/0	*Alveolar adenoma*
M8251/3	*Alveolar adenocarcinoma*
M8260/0	*Papillary adenoma NOS*
M8260/3	*Papillary adenocarcinoma NOS*
M8261/1	*Villous adenoma NOS*
M8261/3	*Adenocarcinoma in villous adenoma*
M8262/3	*Villous adenocarcinoma*
M8263/0	*Tubulovillous adenoma*
M8270/0	*Chromophobe adenoma*
M8270/3	*Chromophobe carcinoma*
M8280/0	*Acidophil adenoma*
M8280/3	*Acidophil carcinoma*
M8281/0	*Mixed acidophil-basophil adenoma*
M8281/3	*Mixed acidophil-basophil carcinoma*
M8290/0	*Oxyphilic adenoma*
M8290/3	*Oxyphilic adenocarcinoma*
M8300/0	*Basophil adenoma*
M8300/3	*Basophil carcinoma*
M8310/0	*Clear cell adenoma*
M8310/3	*Clear cell adenocarcinoma NOS*
M8311/1	*Hypernephroid tumour*
M8312/3	*Renal cell carcinoma*
M8313/0	*Clear cell adenofibroma*
M8320/3	*Granular cell carcinoma*
M8321/0	*Chief cell adenoma*
M8322/0	*Water-clear cell adenoma*
M8322/3	*Water-clear cell adenocarcinoma*
M8323/0	*Mixed cell adenoma*
M8323/3	*Mixed cell adenocarcinoma*
M8324/0	*Lipoadenoma*
M8330/0	*Follicular adenoma*
M8330/3	*Follicular adenocarcinoma NOS*
M8331/3	*Follicular adenocarcinoma, well differentiated type*
M8332/3	*Follicular adenocarcinoma, trabecular type*
M8333/0	*Microfollicular adenoma*
M8334/0	*Macrofollicular adenoma*
M8340/3	*Papillary and follicular adenocarcinoma*

M8350/3	*Nonencapsulated sclerosing carcinoma*
M8360/1	*Multiple endocrine adenomas*
M8361/1	*Juxtaglomerular tumour*
M8370/0	*Adrenal cortical adenoma NOS*
M8370/3	*Adrenal cortical carcinoma*
M8371/0	*Adrenal cortical adenoma, compact cell type*
M8372/0	*Adrenal cortical adenoma, heavily pigmented variant*
M8373/0	*Adrenal cortical adenoma, clear cell type*
M8374/0	*Adrenal cortical adenoma, glomerulosa cell type*
M8375/0	*Adrenal cortical adenoma, mixed cell type*
M8380/0	*Endometrioid adenoma NOS*
M8380/1	*Endometrioid adenoma, borderline malignancy*
M8380/3	*Endometrioid carcinoma*
M8381/0	*Endometrioid adenofibroma NOS*
M8381/1	*Endometrioid adenofibroma, borderline malignancy*
M8381/3	*Endometrioid adenofibroma, malignant*

M839-M842 Adnexal and skin appendage neoplasms

M8390/0	*Skin appendage adenoma*
M8390/3	*Skin appendage carcinoma*
M8400/0	*Sweat gland adenoma*
M8400/1	*Sweat gland tumour NOS*
M8400/3	*Sweat gland adenocarcinoma*
M8401/0	*Apocrine adenoma*
M8401/3	*Apocrine adenocarcinoma*
M8402/0	*Eccrine acrospiroma*
M8403/0	*Eccrine spiradenoma*
M8404/0	*Hidrocystoma*
M8405/0	*Papillary hydradenoma*
M8406/0	*Papillary syringadenoma*
M8407/0	*Syringoma NOS*
M8410/0	*Sebaceous adenoma*
M8410/3	*Sebaceous adenocarcinoma*
M8420/0	*Ceruminous adenoma*
M8420/3	*Ceruminous adenocarcinoma*

M843 Mucoepidermoid neoplasms

| M8430/0 | *Mucoepidermoid tumour* |
| M8430/3 | *Mucoepidermoid carcinoma* |

M844-M849 Cystic, mucinous and serous neoplasms

M8440/0	*Cystadenoma NOS*
M8440/3	*Cystadenocarcinoma NOS*
M8441/0	*Serous cystadenoma NOS*
M8441/1	*Serous cystadenoma, borderline malignancy*
M8441/3	*Serous cystadenocarcinoma NOS*
M8450/0	*Papillary cystadenoma NOS*
M8450/1	*Papillary cystadenoma, borderline malignancy*
M8450/3	*Papillary cystadenocarcinoma NOS*
M8460/0	*Papillary serous cystadenoma NOS*
M8460/1	*Papillary serous cystadenoma, borderline malignancy*
M8460/3	*Papillary serous cystadenocarcinoma*
M8461/0	*Serous surface papilloma NOS*
M8461/1	*Serous surface papilloma, borderline malignancy*
M8461/3	*Serous surface papillary carcinoma*
M8470/0	*Mucinous cystadenoma NOS*
M8470/1	*Mucinous cystadenoma, borderline malignancy*
M8470/3	*Mucinous cystadenocarcinoma NOS*
M8471/0	*Papillary mucinous cystadenoma NOS*
M8471/1	*Papillary mucinous cystadenoma, borderline malignancy*
M8471/3	*Papillary mucinous cystadenocarcinoma*
M8480/0	*Mucinous adenoma*
M8480/3	*Mucinous adenocarcinoma*
M8480/6	*Pseudomyxoma peritonei*
M8481/3	*Mucin-producing adenocarcinoma*
M8490/3	*Signet ring cell carcinoma*
M8490/6	*Metastatic signet ring cell carcinoma*

M850-M854 Ductal, lobular and medullary neoplasms

M8500/2	*Intraductal carcinoma, noninfiltrating NOS*
M8500/3	*Infiltrating duct carcinoma*
M8501/2	*Comedocarcinoma, noninfiltrating*
M8501/3	*Comedocarcinoma NOS*
M8502/3	*Juvenile carcinoma of the breast*
M8503/0	*Intraductal papilloma*
M8503/2	*Noninfiltrating intraductal papillary adenocarcinoma*
M8504/0	*Intracystic papillary adenoma*
M8504/2	*Noninfiltrating intracystic carcinoma*
M8505/0	*Intraductal papillomatosis NOS*

M8506/0	*Subareolar duct papillomatosis*
M8510/3	*Medullary carcinoma NOS*
M8511/3	*Medullary carcinoma with amyloid stroma*
M8512/3	*Medullary carcinoma with lymphoid stroma*
M8520/2	*Lobular carcinoma in situ*
M8520/3	*Lobular carcinoma NOS*
M8521/3	*Infiltrating ductular carcinoma*
M8530/3	*Inflammatory carcinoma*
M8540/3	*Paget's disease, mammary*
M8541/3	*Paget's disease and infiltrating duct carcinoma of breast*
M8542/3	*Paget's disease, extramammary (except Paget's disease of bone)*

M855   **Acinar cell neoplasms**

M8550/0	*Acinar cell adenoma*
M8550/1	*Acinar cell tumour*
M8550/3	*Acinar cell carcinoma*

M856-M858   **Complex epithelial neoplasms**

M8560/3	*Adenosquamous carcinoma*
M8561/0	*Adenolymphoma*
M8570/3	*Adenocarcinoma with squamous metaplasia*
M8571/3	*Adenocarcinoma with cartilaginous and osseous metaplasia*
M8572/3	*Adenocarcinoma with spindle cell metaplasia*
M8573/3	*Adenocarcinoma with apocrine metaplasia*
M8580/0	*Thymoma, benign*
M8580/3	*Thymoma, malignant*

M859-M867   **Specialized gonadal neoplasms**

M8590/1	*Sex cord-stromal tumour*
M8600/0	*Thecoma NOS*
M8600/3	*Theca cell carcinoma*
M8610/0	*Luteoma NOS*
M8620/1	*Granulosa cell tumour NOS*
M8620/3	*Granulosa cell tumour, malignant*
M8621/1	*Granulosa cell-theca cell tumour*
M8630/0	*Androblastoma, benign*
M8630/1	*Androblastoma NOS*
M8630/3	*Androblastoma, malignant*

M8631/0	Sertoli-Leydig cell tumour
M8632/1	Gynandroblastoma
M8640/0	Tubular androblastoma NOS
M8640/3	Sertoli cell carcinoma
M8641/0	Tubular androblastoma with lipid storage
M8650/0	Leydig cell tumour, benign
M8650/1	Leydig cell tumour NOS
M8650/3	Leydig cell tumour, malignant
M8660/0	Hilar cell tumour
M8670/0	Lipid cell tumour of ovary
M8671/0	Adrenal rest tumour

M868-M871 Paragangliomas and glomus tumours

M8680/1	Paraganglioma NOS
M8680/3	Paraganglioma, malignant
M8681/1	Sympathetic paraganglioma
M8682/1	Parasympathetic paraganglioma
M8690/1	Glomus jugulare tumour
M8691/1	Aortic body tumour
M8692/1	Carotid body tumour
M8693/1	Extra-adrenal paraganglioma NOS
M8693/3	Extra-adrenal paraganglioma, malignant
M8700/0	Phaeochromocytoma NOS
M8700/3	Phaeochromocytoma, malignant
M8710/3	Glomangiosarcoma
M8711/0	Glomus tumour
M8712/0	Glomangioma

M872-M879 Naevi and melanomas

M8720/0	Pigmented naevus NOS
M8720/3	Malignant melanoma NOS
M8721/3	Nodular melanoma
M8722/0	Balloon cell naevus
M8722/3	Balloon cell melanoma
M8723/0	Halo naevus
M8724/0	Fibrous papule of the nose
M8725/0	Neuronaevus
M8726/0	Magnocellular naevus
M8730/0	Nonpigmented naevus

M8730/3	*Amelanotic melanoma*
M8740/0	*Junctional naevus*
M8740/3	*Malignant melanoma in junctional naevus*
M8741/2	*Precancerous melanosis NOS*
M8741/3	*Malignant melanoma in precancerous melanosis*
M8742/2	*Hutchinson's melanotic freckle*
M8742/3	*Malignant melanoma in Hutchinson's melanotic freckle*
M8743/3	*Superficial spreading melanoma*
M8750/0	*Intradermal naevus*
M8760/0	*Compound naevus*
M8761/1	*Giant pigmented naevus*
M8761/3	*Malignant melanoma in giant pigmented naevus*
M8770/0	*Epithelioid and spindle cell naevus*
M8771/3	*Epithelioid cell melanoma*
M8772/3	*Spindle cell melanoma NOS*
M8773/3	*Spindle cell melanoma, type A*
M8774/3	*Spindle cell melanoma, type B*
M8775/3	*Mixed epithelioid and spindle cell melanoma*
M8780/0	*Blue naevus NOS*
M8780/3	*Blue naevus, malignant*
M8790/0	*Cellular blue naevus*

M880	**Soft tissue tumours and sarcomas NOS**
M8800/0	*Soft tissue tumour, benign*
M8800/3	*Sarcoma NOS*
M8800/9	*Sarcomatosis NOS*
M8801/3	*Spindle cell sarcoma*
M8802/3	*Giant cell sarcoma (except of bone M9250/3)*
M8803/3	*Small cell sarcoma*
M8804/3	*Epithelioid cell sarcoma*

M881-M883	**Fibromatous neoplasms**
M8810/0	*Fibroma NOS*
M8810/3	*Fibrosarcoma NOS*
M8811/0	*Fibromyxoma*
M8811/3	*Fibromyxosarcoma*
M8812/0	*Periosteal fibroma*
M8812/3	*Periosteal fibrosarcoma*
M8813/0	*Fascial fibroma*

M8813/3	*Fascial fibrosarcoma*
M8814/3	*Infantile fibrosarcoma*
M8820/0	*Elastofibroma*
M8821/1	*Aggressive fibromatosis*
M8822/1	*Abdominal fibromatosis*
M8823/1	*Desmoplastic fibroma*
M8830/0	*Fibrous histiocytoma NOS*
M8830/1	*Atypical fibrous histiocytoma*
M8830/3	*Fibrous histiocytoma, malignant*
M8831/0	*Fibroxanthoma NOS*
M8831/1	*Atypical fibroxanthoma*
M8831/3	*Fibroxanthoma, malignant*
M8832/0	*Dermatofibroma NOS*
M8832/1	*Dermatofibroma protuberans*
M8832/3	*Dermatofibrosarcoma NOS*

M884 **Myxomatous neoplasms**

M8840/0	*Myxoma NOS*
M8840/3	*Myxosarcoma*

M885-M888 Lipomatous neoplasms

M8850/0	*Lipoma NOS*
M8850/3	*Liposarcoma NOS*
M8851/0	*Fibrolipoma*
M8851/3	*Liposarcoma, well differentiated type*
M8852/0	*Fibromyxolipoma*
M8852/3	*Myxoid liposarcoma*
M8853/3	*Round cell liposarcoma*
M8854/3	*Pleomorphic liposarcoma*
M8855/3	*Mixed type liposarcoma*
M8856/0	*Intramuscular lipoma*
M8857/0	*Spindle cell lipoma*
M8860/0	*Angiomyolipoma*
M8860/3	*Angiomyoliposarcoma*
M8861/0	*Angiolipoma NOS*
M8861/1	*Angiolipoma, infiltrating*
M8870/0	*Myelolipoma*
M8880/0	*Hibernoma*
M8881/0	*Lipoblastomatosis*

M889-M892 Myomatous neoplasms

M8890/0	*Leiomyoma NOS*
M8890/1	*Intravascular leiomyomatosis*
M8890/3	*Leiomyosarcoma NOS*
M8891/1	*Epithelioid leiomyoma*
M8891/3	*Epithelioid leiomyosarcoma*
M8892/1	*Cellular leiomyoma*
M8893/0	*Bizarre leiomyoma*
M8894/0	*Angiomyoma*
M8894/3	*Angiomyosarcoma*
M8895/0	*Myoma*
M8895/3	*Myosarcoma*
M8900/0	*Rhabdomyoma NOS*
M8900/3	*Rhabdomyosarcoma NOS*
M8901/3	*Pleomorphic rhabdomyosarcoma*
M8902/3	*Mixed type rhabdomyosarcoma*
M8903/0	*Fetal rhabdomyoma*
M8904/0	*Adult rhabdomyoma*
M8910/3	*Embryonal rhabdomyosarcoma*
M8920/3	*Alveolar rhabdomyosarcoma*

M893-M899 Complex mixed and stromal neoplasms

M8930/3	*Endometrial stromal sarcoma*
M8931/1	*Endolymphatic stromal myosis*
M8932/0	*Adenomyoma*
M8940/0	*Pleomorphic adenoma*
M8940/3	*Mixed tumour, malignant NOS*
M8950/3	*Mullerian mixed tumour*
M8951/3	*Mesodermal mixed tumour*
M8960/1	*Mesoblastic nephroma*
M8960/3	*Nephroblastoma NOS*
M8961/3	*Epithelial nephroblastoma*
M8962/3	*Mesenchymal nephroblastoma*
M8970/3	*Hepatoblastoma*
M8980/3	*Carcinosarcoma NOS*
M8981/3	*Carcinosarcoma, embryonal type*
M8982/0	*Myoepithelioma*
M8990/0	*Mesenchymoma, benign*

M8990/1   *Mesenchymoma NOS*
M8990/3   *Mesenchymoma, malignant*
M8991/3   *Embryonal sarcoma*

M900-M903 Fibroepithelial neoplasms

M9000/0   *Brenner tumour NOS*
M9000/1   *Brenner tumour, borderline malignancy*
M9000/3   *Brenner tumour, malignant*
M9010/0   *Fibroadenoma NOS*
M9011/0   *Intracanalicular fibroadenoma NOS*
M9012/0   *Pericanalicular fibroadenoma*
M9013/0   *Adenofibroma NOS*
M9014/0   *Serous adenofibroma*
M9015/0   *Mucinous adenofibroma*
M9020/0   *Cellular intracanalicular fibroadenoma*
M9020/1   *Cystosarcoma phyllodes NOS*
M9020/3   *Cystosarcoma phyllodes, malignant*
M9030/0   *Juvenile fibroadenoma*

M904   **Synovial neoplasms**

M9040/0   *Synovioma, benign*
M9040/3   *Synovial sarcoma NOS*
M9041/3   *Synovial sarcoma, spindle cell type*
M9042/3   *Synovial sarcoma, epithelioid cell type*
M9043/3   *Synovial sarcoma, biphasic type*
M9044/3   *Clear cell sarcoma of tendons and aponeuroses*

M905   **Mesothelial neoplasms**

M9050/0   *Mesothelioma, benign*
M9050/3   *Mesothelioma, malignant*
M9051/0   *Fibrous mesothelioma, benign*
M9051/3   *Fibrous mesothelioma, malignant*
M9052/0   *Epithelioid mesothelioma, benign*
M9052/3   *Epithelioid mesothelioma, malignant*
M9053/0   *Mesothelioma, biphasic type, benign*
M9053/3   *Mesothelioma, biphasic type, malignant*
M9054/0   *Adenomatoid tumour NOS*

M906-M909 Germ cell neoplasms

M9060/3	*Dysgerminoma*
M9061/3	*Seminoma NOS*
M9062/3	*Seminoma, anaplastic type*
M9063/3	*Spermatocytic seminoma*
M9064/3	*Germinoma*
M9070/3	*Embryonal carcinoma NOS*
M9071/3	*Endodermal sinus tumour*
M9072/3	*Polyembryoma*
M9073/1	*Gonadoblastoma*
M9080/0	*Teratoma, benign*
M9080/1	*Teratoma NOS*
M9080/3	*Teratoma, malignant NOS*
M9081/3	*Teratocarcinoma*
M9082/3	*Malignant teratoma, undifferentiated type*
M9083/3	*Malignant teratoma, intermediate type*
M9084/0	*Dermoid cyst*
M9084/3	*Dermoid cyst with malignant transformation*
M9090/0	*Struma ovarii NOS*
M9090/3	*Struma ovarii, malignant*
M9091/1	*Strumal carcinoid*

M910 Trophoblastic neoplasms

M9100/0	*Hydatidiform mole NOS*
M9100/1	*Invasive hydatidiform mole*
M9100/3	*Choriocarcinoma*
M9101/3	*Choriocarcinoma combined with teratoma*
M9102/3	*Malignant teratoma, trophoblastic*

M911 Mesonephromas

M9110/0	*Mesonephroma, benign*
M9110/1	*Mesonephric tumour*
M9110/3	*Mesonephroma, malignant*
M9111/1	*Endosalpingioma*

M912-M916 Blood vessel tumours

M9120/0	*Haemangioma NOS*
M9120/3	*Haemangiosarcoma*
M9121/0	*Cavernous haemangioma*

M9122/0	*Venous haemangioma*
M9123/0	*Racemose haemangioma*
M9124/3	*Kupffer cell sarcoma*
M9130/0	*Haemangioendothelioma, benign*
M9130/1	*Haemangioendothelioma NOS*
M9130/3	*Haemangioendothelioma, malignant*
M9131/0	*Capillary haemangioma*
M9132/0	*Intramuscular haemangioma*
M9140/3	*Kaposi's sarcoma*
M9141/0	*Angiokeratoma*
M9142/0	*Verrucous keratotic haemangioma*
M9150/0	*Haemangiopericytoma, benign*
M9150/1	*Haemangiopericytoma NOS*
M9150/3	*Haemangiopericytoma, malignant*
M9160/0	*Angiofibroma NOS*
M9161/1	*Haemangioblastoma*

M917　　**Lymphatic vessel tumours**

M9170/0	*Lymphangioma NOS*
M9170/3	*Lymphangiosarcoma*
M9171/0	*Capillary lymphangioma*
M9172/0	*Cavernous lymphangioma*
M9173/0	*Cystic lymphangioma*
M9174/0	*Lymphangiomyoma*
M9174/1	*Lymphangiomyomatosis*
M9175/0	*Haemolymphangioma*

M918-M920 Osteomas and osteosarcomas

M9180/0	*Osteoma NOS*
M9180/3	*Osteosarcoma NOS*
M9181/3	*Chondroblastic osteosarcoma*
M9182/3	*Fibroblastic osteosarcoma*
M9183/3	*Telangiectatic osteosarcoma*
M9184/3	*Osteosarcoma in Paget's disease of bone*
M9190/3	*Juxtacortical osteosarcoma*
M9191/0	*Osteoid osteoma NOS*
M9200/0	*Osteoblastoma*

M921-M924 Chondromatous neoplasms

M9210/0	*Osteochondroma*
M9210/1	*Osteochondromatosis NOS*
M9220/0	*Chondroma NOS*
M9220/1	*Chondromatosis NOS*
M9220/3	*Chondrosarcoma NOS*
M9221/0	*Juxtacortical chondroma*
M9221/3	*Juxtacortical chondrosarcoma*
M9230/0	*Chondroblastoma NOS*
M9230/3	*Chondroblastoma, malignant*
M9240/3	*Mesenchymal chondrosarcoma*
M9241/0	*Chondromyxoid fibroma*

M925 Giant cell tumours

M9250/1	*Giant cell tumour of bone NOS*
M9250/3	*Giant cell tumour of bone, malignant*
M9251/1	*Giant cell tumour of soft parts NOS*
M9251/3	*Malignant giant cell tumour of soft parts*

M926 Miscellaneous bone tumours

M9260/3	*Ewing's sarcoma*
M9261/3	*Adamantinoma of long bones*
M9262/0	*Ossifying fibroma*

M927-M934 Odontogenic tumours

M9270/0	*Odontogenic tumour, benign*
M9270/1	*Odontogenic tumour NOS*
M9270/3	*Odontogenic tumour, malignant*
M9271/0	*Dentinoma*
M9272/0	*Cementoma NOS*
M9273/0	*Cementoblastoma, benign*
M9274/0	*Cementifying fibroma*
M9275/0	*Gigantiform cementoma*
M9280/0	*Odontoma NOS*
M9281/0	*Compound odontoma*
M9282/0	*Complex odontoma*
M9290/0	*Ameloblastic fibro-odontoma*
M9290/3	*Ameloblastic odontosarcoma*
M9300/0	*Adenomatoid odontogenic tumour*

M9301/0	*Calcifying odontogenic cyst*
M9310/0	*Ameloblastoma NOS*
M9310/3	*Ameloblastoma, malignant*
M9311/0	*Odontoameloblastoma*
M9312/0	*Squamous odontogenic tumour*
M9320/0	*Odontogenic myxoma*
M9321/0	*Odontogenic fibroma NOS*
M9330/0	*Ameloblastic fibroma*
M9330/3	*Ameloblastic fibrosarcoma*
M9340/0	*Calcifying epithelial odontogenic tumour*

M935-M937 Miscellaneous tumours

M9350/1	*Craniopharyngioma*
M9360/1	*Pinealoma*
M9361/1	*Pineocytoma*
M9362/3	*Pineoblastoma*
M9363/0	*Melanotic neuroectodermal tumour*
M9370/3	*Chordoma*

M938-M948 Gliomas

M9380/3	*Glioma, malignant*
M9381/3	*Gliomatosis cerebri*
M9382/3	*Mixed glioma*
M9383/1	*Subependymal glioma*
M9384/1	*Subependymal giant cell astrocytoma*
M9390/0	*Choroid plexus papilloma NOS*
M9390/3	*Choroid plexus papilloma, malignant*
M9391/3	*Ependymoma NOS*
M9392/3	*Ependymoma, anaplastic type*
M9393/1	*Papillary ependymoma*
M9394/1	*Myxopapillary ependymoma*
M9400/3	*Astrocytoma NOS*
M9401/3	*Astrocytoma, anaplastic type*
M9410/3	*Protoplasmic astrocytoma*
M9411/3	*Gemistocytic astrocytoma*
M9420/3	*Fibrillary astrocytoma*
M9421/3	*Pilocytic astrocytoma*
M9422/3	*Spongioblastoma NOS*
M9423/3	*Spongioblastoma polare*

M9430/3	*Astroblastoma*
M9440/3	*Glioblastoma NOS*
M9441/3	*Giant cell glioblastoma*
M9442/3	*Glioblastoma with sarcomatous component*
M9443/3	*Primitive polar spongioblastoma*
M9450/3	*Oligodendroglioma NOS*
M9451/3	*Oligodendroglioma, anaplastic type*
M9460/3	*Oligodendroblastoma*
M9470/3	*Medulloblastoma NOS*
M9471/3	*Desmoplastic medulloblastoma*
M9472/3	*Medullomyoblastoma*
M9480/3	*Cerebellar sarcoma NOS*
M9481/3	*Monstrocellular sarcoma*

M949-M952 Neuroepitheliomatous neoplasms

M9490/0	*Ganglioneuroma*
M9490/3	*Ganglioneuroblastoma*
M9491/0	*Ganglioneuromatosis*
M9500/3	*Neuroblastoma NOS*
M9501/3	*Medulloepithelioma NOS*
M9502/3	*Teratoid medulloepithelioma*
M9503/3	*Neuroepithelioma NOS*
M9504/3	*Spongioneuroblastoma*
M9505/1	*Ganglioglioma*
M9506/0	*Neurocytoma*
M9507/0	*Pacinian tumour*
M9510/3	*Retinoblastoma NOS*
M9511/3	*Retinoblastoma, differentiated type*
M9512/3	*Retinoblastoma, undifferentiated type*
M9520/3	*Olfactory neurogenic tumour*
M9521/3	*Aesthesioneurocytoma*
M9522/3	*Aesthesioneuroblastoma*
M9523/3	*Aesthesioneuroepithelioma*

M953 Meningiomas

M9530/0	*Meningioma NOS*
M9530/1	*Meningiomatosis NOS*
M9530/3	*Meningioma, malignant*
M9531/0	*Meningotheliomatous meningioma*

M9532/0	Fibrous meningioma
M9533/0	Psammomatous meningioma
M9534/0	Angiomatous meningioma
M9535/0	Haemangioblastic meningioma
M9536/0	Haemangiopericytic meningioma
M9537/0	Transitional meningioma
M9538/1	Papillary meningioma
M9539/3	Meningeal sarcomatosis

M954-M957 Nerve sheath tumour

M9540/0	Neurofibroma NOS
M9540/1	Neurofibromatosis NOS
M9540/3	Neurofibrosarcoma
M9541/0	Melanotic neurofibroma
M9550/0	Plexiform neurofibroma
M9560/0	Neurilemmoma NOS
M9560/1	Neurinomatosis
M9560/3	Neurilemmoma, malignant
M9570/0	Neuroma NOS

M958　　　　　Granular cell tumours and alveolar soft part sarcoma

M9580/0	Granular cell tumour NOS
M9580/3	Granular cell tumour, malignant
M9581/3	Alveolar soft part sarcoma

M959-M963 Lymphomas, NOS or diffuse

M9590/0	Lymphomatous tumour, benign
M9590/3	Malignant lymphoma NOS
M9591/3	Malignant lymphoma, non Hodgkin's type
M9600/3	Malignant lymphoma, undifferentiated cell type NOS
M9601/3	Malignant lymphoma, stem cell type
M9602/3	Malignant lymphoma, convoluted cell type NOS
M9610/3	Lymphosarcoma NOS
M9611/3	Malignant lymphoma, lymphoplasmacytoid type
M9612/3	Malignant lymphoma, immunoblastic type
M9613/3	Malignant lymphoma, mixed lymphocytic-histiocytic NOS
M9614/3	Malignant lymphoma, centroblastic-centrocytic, diffuse
M9615/3	Malignant lymphoma, follicular centre cell NOS
M9620/3	Malignant lymphoma, lymphocytic, well differentiated NOS

M9621/3	*Malignant lymphoma, lymphocytic, intermediate differentiation NOS*
M9622/3	*Malignant lymphoma, centrocytic*
M9623/3	*Malignant lymphoma, follicular centre cell, cleaved NOS*
M9630/3	*Malignant lymphoma, lymphocytic, poorly differentiated NOS*
M9631/3	*Prolymphocytic lymphosarcoma*
M9632/3	*Malignant lymphoma, centroblastic type NOS*
M9633/3	*Malignant lymphoma, follicular centre cell, non-cleaved NOS*

M964 Reticulosarcomas

M9640/3	*Reticulosarcoma NOS*
M9641/3	*Reticulosarcoma, pleomorphic cell type*
M9642/3	*Reticulosarcoma, nodular*

M965-M966 Hodgkin's disease

M9650/3	*Hodgkin's disease NOS*
M9651/3	*Hodgkin's disease, lymphocytic predominance*
M9652/3	*Hodgkin's disease, mixed cellularity*
M9653/3	*Hodgkin's disease, lymphocytic depletion NOS*
M9654/3	*Hodgkin's disease, lymphocytic depletion, diffuse fibrosis*
M9655/3	*Hodgkin's disease, lymphocytic depletion, reticular type*
M9656/3	*Hodgkin's disease, nodular sclerosis NOS*
M9657/3	*Hodgkin's disease, nodular sclerosis, cellular phase*
M9660/3	*Hodgkin's paragranuloma*
M9661/3	*Hodgkin's granuloma*
M9662/3	*Hodgkin's sarcoma*

M969 Lymphomas, nodular or follicular

M9690/3	*Malignant lymphoma, nodular NOS*
M9691/3	*Malignant lymphoma, mixed lymphocytic-histiocytic, nodular*
M9692/3	*Malignant lymphoma, centroblastic-centrocytic, follicular*
M9693/3	*Malignant lymphoma, lymphocytic, well differentiated, nodular*
M9694/3	*Malignant lymphoma, lymphocytic, intermediate differentiation, nodular*
M9695/3	*Malignant lymphoma, follicular centre cell, cleaved, follicular*
M9696/3	*Malignant lymphoma, lymphocytic, poorly differentiated, nodular*
M9697/3	*Malignant lymphoma, centroblastic type, follicular*
M9698/3	*Malignant lymphoma, follicular centre cell, non-cleaved, follicular*

M970   **Mycosis fungoides**

M9700/3   *Mycosis fungoides*
M9701/3   *Sézary's disease*

M971-M972 Miscellaneous reticuloendothelial neoplasms

M9710/3   *Microglioma*
M9720/3   *Malignant histiocytosis*
M9721/3   *Histiocytic medullary reticulosis*
M9722/3   *Letterer-Siwe's disease*

M973   **Plasma cell tumours**

M9730/3   *Plasma cell myeloma*
M9731/0   *Plasma cell tumour, benign*
M9731/1   *Plasmacytoma NOS*
M9731/3   *Plasma cell tumour, malignant*

M974   **Mast cell tumours**

M9740/1   *Mastocytoma NOS*
M9740/3   *Mast cell sarcoma*
M9741/3   *Malignant mastocytosis*

M975   **Burkitt's tumour**

M9750/3   *Burkitt's tumour*

M980-M994 Leukaemias

M980   **Leukaemias NOS**

M9800/3   *Leukaemia NOS*
M9801/3   *Acute leukaemia NOS*
M9802/3   *Subacute leukaemia NOS*
M9803/3   *Chronic leukaemia NOS*
M9804/3   *Aleukaemic leukaemia NOS*

M981   **Compound leukaemias**

M9810/3   *Compound leukaemia*

M982	**Lymphoid leukaemias**
M9820/3	*Lymphoid leukaemia NOS*
M9821/3	*Acute lymphoid leukaemia*
M9822/3	*Subacute lymphoid leukaemia*
M9823/3	*Chronic lymphoid leukaemia*
M9824/3	*Aleukaemic lymphoid leukaemia*
M9825/3	*Prolymphocytic leukaemia*
M983	**Plasma cell leukaemias**
M9830/3	*Plasma cell leukaemia*
M984	**Erythroleukaemias**
M9840/3	*Erythroleukaemia*
M9841/3	*Acute erythraemia*
M9842/3	*Chronic erythraemia*
M985	**Lymphosarcoma cell leukaemias**
M9850/3	*Lymphosarcoma cell leukaemia*
M986	**Myeloid leukaemias**
M9860/3	*Myeloid leukaemia NOS*
M9861/3	*Acute myeloid leukaemia*
M9862/3	*Subacute myeloid leukaemia*
M9863/3	*Chronic myeloid leukaemia*
M9864/3	*Aleukaemic myeloid leukaemia*
M9865/3	*Neutrophilic leukaemia*
M9866/3	*Acute promyelocytic leukaemia*
M987	**Basophilic leukaemias**
M9870/3	*Basophilic leukaemia*
M988	**Eosinophilic leukaemias**
M9880/3	*Eosinophilic leukaemia*
M989	**Monocytic leukaemias**
M9890/3	*Monocytic leukaemia NOS*
M9891/3	*Acute monocytic leukaemia*
M9892/3	*Subacute monocytic leukaemia*
M9893/3	*Chronic monocytic leukaemia*
M9894/3	*Aleukaemic monocytic leukaemia*

M990-M994 Miscellaneous leukaemias

M9900/3	*Mast cell leukaemia*
M9910/3	*Megakaryocytic leukaemia*
M9920/3	*Megakaryocytic myelosis*
M9930/3	*Myeloid sarcoma*
M9940/3	*Hairy cell leukaemia*

M995-M997 Miscellaneous myeloproliferative and lymphoproliferative disorders

M9950/1	*Polycythaemia vera*
M9951/1	*Acute panmyelosis*
M9960/1	*Chronic myeloproliferative disease*
M9961/1	*Myelosclerosis with myeloid metaplasia*
M9962/1	*Idiopathic thrombocythaemia*
M9970/1	*Chronic lymphoproliferative disease*

CLASSIFICATION OF INDUSTRIAL ACCIDENTS ACCORDING TO AGENCY

Annex B to the Resolution concerning Statistics of Employment Injuries adopted by the Tenth International Conference of Labour Statisticians on 12 October 1962

1 MACHINES

11 Prime-Movers, except Electrical Motors

111 *Steam engines*
112 *Internal combustion engines*
119 *Others*

12 Transmission Machinery

121 *Transmission shafts*
122 *Transmission belts, cables, pulleys, pinions, chains, gears*
129 *Others*

13 Metalworking Machines

131 *Power presses*
132 *Lathes*
133 *Milling machines*
134 *Abrasive wheels*
135 *Mechanical shears*
136 *Forging machines*
137 *Rolling-mills*
139 *Others*

14 Wood and Assimilated Machines

141 *Circular saws*
142 *Other saws*
143 *Moulding machines*
144 *Overhand planes*
149 *Others*

15 Agricultural Machines

151 *Reapers (including combine reapers)*
152 *Threshers*
159 *Others*

16 Mining Machinery

    161   *Under-cutters*
    169   *Others*

19 Other Machines Not Elsewhere Classified

    191   *Earth-moving machines, excavating and scraping machines, except means of transport*
    192   *Spinning, weaving and other textile machines*
    193   *Machines for the manufacture of foodstuffs and beverages*
    194   *Machines for the manufacture of paper*
    195   *Printing machines*
    199   *Others*

2 MEANS OF TRANSPORT AND LIFTING EQUIPMENT

21 Lifting Machines and Appliances

    211   *Cranes*
    212   *Lifts and elevators*
    213   *Winches*
    214   *Pulley blocks*
    219   *Others*

22 Means of Rail Transport

    221   *Inter-urban railways*
    222   *Rail transport in mines, tunnels, quarries, industrial establishments, docks, etc.*
    229   *Others*

23 Other Wheeled Means of Transport, Excluding Rail Transport

    231   *Tractors*
    232   *Lorries*
    233   *Trucks*
    234   *Motor vehicles, not elsewhere classified*
    235   *Animal-drawn vehicles*
    236   *Hand-drawn vehicles*
    239   *Others*

24 Means of Air Transport

25 Means of Water Transport

    251   *Motorised means of water transport*
    252   *Non-motorised means of water transport*

26 Other Means of Transport

261 *Cable-cars*
262 *Mechanical conveyors, except cable-cars*
269 *Others*

3 OTHER EQUIPMENT

31 Pressure Vessels

311 *Boilers*
312 *Pressurised containers*
313 *Pressurised piping and accessories*
314 *Gas cylinders*
315 *Caissons, diving equipment*
319 *Others*

32 Furnaces, Ovens, Kilns

321 *Blast furnaces*
322 *Refining furnaces*
323 *Other furnaces*
324 *Kilns*
325 *Ovens*

33 Refrigerating Plants

34 Electrical Installations, Including Electric Motors, but Excluding Electric Hand Tools

341 *Rotating machines*
342 *Conductors*
343 *Transformers*
344 *Control apparatus*
349 *Others*

35 Electric Hand Tools

36 Tools, Implements and Appliances, except Electric Hand Tools

361 *Power-driven hand tools, except electric hand tools*
362 *Hand tools, not power-driven*
369 *Others*

37 Ladders, Mobile Ramps

38 Scaffolding

39 Other Equipment, Not Elsewhere Classified

4   MATERIALS, SUBSTANCES AND RADIATIONS

41   Explosives

42   Dusts, Gases, Liquids and Chemicals, Excluding Explosives

    421   *Dusts*
    422   *Gases, vapours, fumes*
    423   *Liquids, not elsewhere classified*
    424   *Chemicals, not elsewhere classified*
    429   *Others*

43   Flying Fragments

44   Radiations

    441   *Ionising radiations*
    449   *Others*

49   Other Materials and Substances Not Elsewhere Classified

5   WORKING ENVIRONMENT

51   Outdoor

    511   *Weather*
    512   *Traffic and working surfaces*
    513   *Water*
    519   *Others*

52   Indoor

    521   *Floors*
    522   *Confined quarters*
    523   *Stairs*
    524   *Other traffic and working surfaces*
    525   *Floor openings and wall openings*
    526   *Environmental factors (lighting, ventilation, temperature, noise, etc.)*
    529   *Others*

53   Underground

    531   *Roofs and faces of mine roads and tunnels, etc.*
    532   *Floors of mine roads and tunnels, etc.*
    533   *Working-faces of mines, tunnels, etc.*
    534   *Mine shafts*

535 *Fire*
536 *Water*
539 *Others*

6 OTHER AGENCIES, NOT ELSEWHERE CLASSIFIED

61 Animals

611 *Live animals*
612 *Animals products*

69 Other Agencies, Not Elsewhere Classified

7 AGENCIES NOT CLASSIFIED FOR LACK OF SUFFICIENT DATA

MEDICAL CERTIFICATION
AND RULES FOR CLASSIFICATION

MEDICAL CERTIFICATION
AND RULES FOR CLASSIFICATION

Reference should be made to the Introduction for information about the use in morbidity and mortality statistics of the dual classification of certain diagnostic entities (the "dagger and asterisk" system, page XXVI) and of the supplementary classification of external causes (the " E Code ", page XXIX).

MORTALITY

The Twentieth World Health Assembly defined the causes of death to be entered on the medical certificate of cause of death as " all those diseases, morbid conditions or injuries which either resulted in or contributed to death and the circumstances of the accident or violence which produced any such injuries " (see page 763). The purpose of the definition was to ensure that all the relevant information is recorded and that the certifier does not select some conditions for entry and reject others. It will be noted that the definition does not include symptoms and modes of dying, such as heart failure, asthenia, etc.

The problem of classifying causes of death for vital statistics is relatively simple when only one cause of death is involved. However, in many cases, two or more morbid conditions contribute to the death. In such cases, it has been the traditional practice in vital statistics to select one of the causes for tabulation. This cause has been variously described in the past as " the cause of death ", "primary cause of death", " principal cause of death ", " fundamental cause of death ", etc. In order to make uniform the terminology and procedure of selecting the cause of death for primary tabulations, it was agreed by the Sixth Decennial. International Revision Conference that the cause to be tabulated should be designated the *underlying cause of death*.

The Ninth International Revision Conference, while endorsing the principle of a single underlying cause for tabulation of mortality in general, considered that it was less useful in perinatal mortality, where two separate individuals (mother and baby) were involved and where causes or circumstances not necessarily attributable to either mother or child could contribute to the event of perinatal death. An alternative was therefore proposed for perinatal mortality; see page 731.

GENERAL MORTALITY

Definition of underlying cause of death

From the standpoint of prevention of deaths, it is important to cut the chain of events or institute the cure at some point. The most effective public health objective is to prevent the precipitating cause from operating. For this purpose, the underlying cause has been defined as " (a) the disease or injury which initiated the train of morbid events leading directly to death, or (b) the circumstances of the accident or violence which produced the fatal injury " (see page 763).

In order to secure uniform application of the above principle, it is implicit that the medical certification form recommended by the World Health Assembly should be used. The use of such a form places the responsibility for indicating the train of events on the physician or surgeon signing the medical certificate of death. It is assumed, and rightly so, that the certifying medical practitioner is in a better position than any other individual to decide which of the morbid conditions led directly to death and to state the antecedent conditions, if any, which gave rise to this cause.

International form of medical certificate of cause of death

The medical certificate of death shown below is designed to elicit the information which will facilitate the selection of the underlying cause of death when two or more causes are jointly recorded.

The form of medical certificate may be considered as consisting of two parts (I and II), which are designated for convenience as:

I (a) Direct cause,
      (due to)

  (b) Intervening antecedent cause,
      (due to)

  (c) Underlying antecedent cause;

II Other significant conditions contributing to the death but not related to the disease or condition causing it.

In Part I is reported the cause leading directly to death (stated on line (a)) and also the antecedent conditions (lines (b) and (c)) which gave rise to the cause reported in line (a), the underlying cause being stated last in the sequence of events. However, no entry is necessary in lines (b) and (c) if the disease or condition directly leading to death, stated in line (a), describes completely the train of events.

In Part II is entered any other significant condition which unfavourably influenced the course of the morbid process, and thus contributed to the fatal outcome, but which was not related to the disease or condition directly causing death.

The words " due to (or as a consequence of) " which appear on the form of medical certificate include not only actiological or pathological sequences, but also sequences where there is no such direct causation but where an antecedent condition is believed to have prepared the way for the direct cause by damage to tissues or impairment of function even after a long interval.

INTERNATIONAL FORM OF MEDICAL CERTIFICATE OF CAUSE OF DEATH

	CAUSE OF DEATH	Approximate interval between onset and death
I		
Disease or condition direct- ly leading to death *	(a) . . . . due to (or as a consequence of)	. . . .
Antecedent causes Morbid conditions, if any, giving rise to the above cause, stating the underlying con- dition last	(b) . . . . due to (or as a consequence of) (c)	. . . .
II		
Other significant conditions contributing to the death, but not related to the disease or condition causing it	. . . .	. . . .

* This does not mean the mode of dying, e.g., heart failure, asthenia, etc. It means the disease, injury, or complication which caused death.

Rules for selection of cause of death for primary mortality tabulation

When only one cause of death is recorded, this cause is selected for tabulation. When more than one cause of death is recorded, selection should be made in accordance with the rules which follow. The rules are based on the concept of the *underlying cause*, i.e. the disease or injury which initiated the sequence of events which led to death. Where the selected cause is an injury, either the circumstances which gave rise to the injury, or the nature of the injury, or preferably both should be coded.

Selection of the cause to be coded comprises two stages; selection of the underlying cause, and subsequent modification of the underlying cause. These two stages are described below.

Selection of the underlying cause

The rules for selecting the underlying cause are as follows. Either the General rule or Rule 1 or Rule 2 will apply to all certificates. Rule 3 may apply in addition to one of these.

General rule. Select the condition entered alone on the lowest used line of Part I unless it is highly improbable that this condition could have given rise to all the conditions entered above it.

Rule 1. If there is a reported sequence terminating in the condition first entered on the certificate, select the underlying cause of this sequence.

If there is more than one such sequence, select the underlying cause of the first-mentioned sequence.

Rule 2. If there is no reported sequence terminating in the condition first entered on the certificate, select this first mentioned condition.

Rule 3. If the condition selected by the *General rule* or *Rules 1 or 2* can be considered a direct sequel of another reported condition, whether in Part I or Part II, select this primary condition. If there are two or more such primary conditions, select the first mentioned of these.

In a properly completed certificate, the underlying cause will have been entered alone on the lowest used line of Part I and the conditions, if any, which arose as a consequence of this underlying cause will have been entered above it, one condition to a line, in ascending causal order of sequence.

Example 1:   I(*a*)   Uraemia
            (*b*)   Retention of urine
            (*c*)   Hypertrophy of prostate

Example 2:   I(*a*)   Bronchopneumonia
            (*b*)   Chronic bronchitis

         II   Chronic myocarditis

In a properly completed certificate, therefore, the *General rule* will apply. However, the fact that the certificate as a whole has not been completed in an entirely satisfactory manner does not preclude the application of the *General rule*. Provided that it is not highly improbable that the condition entered alone on the lowest used line of Part I could have given rise to all the conditions above it, the *General rule* should be applied, even though the conditions entered above it have not been entered in a correct causal order of sequence.

Example 3:   I(*a*)   Gangrene of intestine and
            (*b*)   peritonitis
            (*c*)   Volvulus of caecum

Example 4:   I(*a*)   Coronary thrombosis
            (*b*)   Cerebral haemorrhage
            (*c*)   Arteriosclerosis

The *General rule* should be discarded only when the certifier has entered more than one condition on the lowest used line of Part I or has entered there a single condition and it is highly improbable that this condition could have given rise to all the conditions entered above it. Guidance on the interpretation of " highly improbable " is given at the end of the rules, but it should be borne in mind that the medical certifier's statement indicates his opinion about the conditions leading to death and about their relationship one to another, and this opinion should not be lightly disregarded.

Where the *General rule* cannot be applied, clarification of the certificate should be sought from the certifier whenever this is possible, since the remaining selection rules are somewhat arbitrary and may not always lead to a satisfactory selection of the underlying cause. Where further clarification cannot be obtained, however, *Rule 1* or *Rule 2* must be applied.

In these rules, the term " reported sequence " means two or more conditions entered on successive lines of Part I, each condition being an acceptable cause of the one entered on the line above it. *Rule 1* is applicable only if such a reported sequence, terminating in the condition first entered on the certificate, is found. If such a sequence is not found, *Rule 2* applies and the first entered condition is selected.

The condition selected by the above rules may, however, be an obvious sequel of another condition which was not reported in a correct causal relationship with it, e.g. in Part II or on the same line in Part I. If so, then *Rule 3* also applies and the primary condition is selected. It applies, however, only when there is no doubt about the causal relationship between the two conditions; it is not sufficient that a causal relationship between them would have been accepted if the certifier had reported it.

Modification of the underlying cause

The underlying cause, as selected by the above rules, will not necessarily be the most useful and informative condition for tabulations of mortality data. For example, if senility or some generalized disease such as hypertension or arteriosclerosis has been selected, more useful information will be conveyed if the condition to be tabulated is some reported manifestation of the ageing or disease process. In other cases it may be necessary to modify the assignment to conform with provisions of the International Classification of Diseases for a single code for two or more causes jointly reported or for preference for a particular cause when reported with certain other conditions.

The modification rules (*Rules 4-12*), therefore, are intended to improve the usefulness and precision of mortality tabulations and should be applied after selection of the underlying cause by means of the selection rules. The processes of selection and modification have been separated for the sake of clarity, though they are closely interwoven; it will be seen, for example, that some of the modification rules require a renewed application of the selection rules. This should present no difficulty to experienced coders but for beginning coders the importance of going through the mental processes of selection, modification and, if necessary, re-selection, should be emphasized.

Examples of the selection rules

General rule. Select the condition on the lowest used line of Part I unless it is highly improbable that this condition could have given rise to all the conditions entered above it.

Example 5: I(*a*)   Abscess of lung
        (*b*)   Lobar pneumonia

Select lobar pneumonia.

Example 6: I(*a*)   Hepatic failure
        (*b*)   Bile duct obstruction
        (*c*)   Carcinoma of pancreas

Select carcinoma of pancreas.

Example 7: I(*a*)   Secondaries in lung with lung abscess
        (*b*)   Cancer of brain

Select cancer of brain.

Example 8: I(*a*)   Pulmonary oedema

     II   Secondary anaemia and chronic lymphatic leukaemia

Select pulmonary oedema. But *rule 3* also applies; see example 21.

Rule 1. If there is a reported sequence terminating in the condition first entered on the certificate, select the underlying cause of this sequence. If there is more than one such sequence, select the underlying cause of the first mentioned sequence.

Example 9: I(*a*)   Coronary embolism
        (*b*)   Arteriosclerotic heart disease
        (*c*)   Influenza

Select arteriosclerotic heart disease. The reported sequence terminating in the condition first entered on the certificate is coronary embolism due to arteriosclerotic heart disease. But *rule 7* also applies; see example 44.

Example 10: I(*a*)   Bronchopneumonia
         (*b*)   Cerebral thrombosis and hypertensive heart disease

Select cerebral thrombosis. There are two reported sequences terminating in the condition first entered on the certificate; bronchopneumonia due to cerebral thrombosis, and bronchopneumonia due to hypertensive heart disease. The underlying cause of the first mentioned sequence is selected.

Example 11: I(*a*)   Oesophageal varices and congestive heart failure
         (*b*)   Cirrhosis of liver and chronic rheumatic heart disease

Select cirrhosis of liver. The reported sequence terminating in the condition first entered on the certificate is oesophageal varices due to cirrhosis of liver.

Example 12: I(*a*)   Pericarditis
         (*b*)   Uraemia and pneumonia

Select uraemia. There are two reported sequences terminating in the condition first entered on the certificate; pericarditis due to uraemia, and pericarditis due to pneumonia. The underlying cause of the first mentioned sequence is selected. But *rule 8* also applies; see example 52.

Example 13: I(*a*)   Cerebral haemorrhage and hypostatic pneumonia
         (*b*)   Hypertension and diabetes
         (*c*)   Arteriosclerosis

Select arteriosclerosis. There are two reported sequences terminating in the condition first entered on the certificate; cerebral haemorrhage due to hypertension due to arteriosclerosis, and cerebral haemorrhage due to diabetes. The underlying cause of the first mentioned sequence is selected. But *rule 7* also applies; see example 46.

Example 14: I(*a*) Cerebral haemorrhage
         (*b*) Hypertension
         (*c*) Chronic pyelonephritis and prostatic obstruction

Select chronic pyelonephritis. This is the condition which is the underlying cause of the reported sequence terminating in the condition first entered on the certificate; the other condition on line (*c*) is not reported in sequence. But *rule 3* also applies; see example 22.

Rule 2. If there is no reported sequence terminating in the condition first entered on the certificate, select this first mentioned condition.

Example 15: I(*a*) Pernicious anaemia and gangrene of
         (*b*)   foot
         (*c*) Arteriosclerosis

Select pernicious anaemia. There is a reported sequence, gangrene of foot due to arteriosclerosis, but it does not terminate in the condition first entered on the certificate.

Example 16: I(*a*) Rheumatic and arteriosclerotic heart
         (*b*)   disease

Select rheumatic heart disease. There is no reported sequence.

Example 17: I(*a*) Senility and hypostatic pneumonia
         (*b*) Rheumatoid arthritis

Select senility. There is a reported sequence, hypostatic pneumonia due to rheumatoid arthritis, but it does not terminate in the condition first entered on the certificate. But *rule 4* also applies; see example 28.

Example 18: I(*a*) Fibrocystic disease of the pancreas
         (*b*) Bronchitis and bronchiectasis

Select fibrocystic disease of the pancreas. There is no reported sequence.

Example 19: I(*a*) Bursitis and ulcerative colitis

Select bursitis. There is no reported sequence. But *rule 6* also applies; see example 39.

Example 20: I(*a*) Acute nephritis, scarlet fever

Select acute nephritis. There is no reported sequence. But *rule 3* also applies; see example 23.

Rule 3. If the condition selected by the *General rule* or *Rules 1 or 2* can be considered a direct sequel of another reported condition, whether in Part I or Part II, select this primary condition. If there are two or more such primary conditions, select the first mentioned of these.

Certain conditions that are common post-operative complications (pneumonia (any type), haemorrhage, thrombophlebitis, embolism, thrombosis, infarction) can be considered as direct sequels to an operation unless it is stated to have occurred 4 or more weeks before death.

Example 21: I(a) Pulmonary oedema
          II   Secondary anaemia and chronic lymphatic leukaemia

Select chronic lymphatic leukaemia. Pulmonary oedema, selected by the *General rule* (see example 8), can be considered a direct sequel of either of the conditions in Part II, but secondary anaemia is itself a direct sequel of lymphatic leukaemia.

Example 22: I(a) Cerebral haemorrhage
        (b) Hypertension
        (c) Chronic pyelonephritis and prostatic obstruction

Select prostatic obstruction. Chronic pyelonephritis, selected by *rule 1* (see example 14), can be considered a direct sequel of prostatic obstruction.

Example 23: I(a) Acute nephritis, scarlet fever

Select scarlet fever. Acute nephritis, selected by *rule 2* (see example 20), can be considered a direct sequel of scarlet fever.

Example 24: I(a) Nephrectomy
          II   Embryoma of kidney

Select embryoma of kidney. There is no doubt that the nephrectomy was performed for the embryoma of kidney.

Example 25: I(a) Carcinomatosis
          II   Carcinoma of ovary, resected

Select carcinoma of ovary. There is little doubt that a causal relationship existed between these conditions. The certifier presumably entered the primary neoplasm in Part II because it was no longer present, but it is nevertheless the underlying cause.

Example 26: I(a) Hypostatic pneumonia, cerebral
        (b)   haemorrhage and cancer of
        (c)   breast

Select cerebral haemorrhage. Hypostatic pneumonia, selected by *rule 2*, can be considered a direct sequel of either of the other conditions reported; the one first mentioned is selected.

Example 27: I(a) Myocardial infarction (immediate)
          II   Left pneumonectomy of carcinoma of lung 3 weeks ago

Select carcinoma of lung.

Examples of the modification rules

Rule 4. Senility. Where the selected underlying cause is classifiable to 797 (Senility) and a condition classifiable elsewhere than to 780-799 is reported on the certificate, re-select the underlying cause as if the senility had not been reported, except to take account of the senility if it modifies the coding.

Example 28: I(a) Senility and hypostatic pneumonia
        (b) Rheumatoid arthritis

Code to rheumatoid arthritis (714.0). The senility, selected by *rule 2* (see example 17), is ignored and the *General rule* applied.

Example 29: I(*a*) Cerebral arteriosclerosis
        (*b*) Senility
      II Gastro-enteritis

Code to cerebral arteriosclerosis (437.0). The senility is ignored and the *General rule* applied.

Example 30: I(*a*) Myocardial degeneration and
        (*b*) emphysema
        (*c*) Senility

Code to myocardial degeneration (429.1). The senility is ignored and *rule 2* applied.

Example 31: I(*a*) Psychosis
        (*b*) Senility

Code to senile psychosis (290.2). The senility modifies the psychosis.

Rule 5. Ill-defined conditions. Where the selected underlying cause is classifiable to 780-796, 798-799 (the ill-defined conditions) and a condition classifiable elsewhere than to 780-799 is reported on the certificate, re-select the underlying cause as if the ill-defined condition had not been reported, except to take account of the ill-defined condition if it modifies the coding.

Example 32: I(*a*) Bacteraemia and haematemesis

Code to haematemesis (578.0). Bacteraemia (790.7), selected by rule *2*, is ignored.

Example 33: I(*a*) Terminal pneumonia
        (*b*) Spreading gangrene and cerebrovascular
        (*c*) accident

Code to cerebrovascular accident (436). Gangrene (785.4), selected by *rule 1*, is ignored and the *General rule* applied.

Example 34: I(*a*) Electrolyte imbalance
        (*b*) Vomiting and dehydration

Code to dehydration (276.5). Vomiting (787.0), selected by *rule 1*, is ignored and the *General rule* applied.

Example 35: I(*a*) Anaemia
        (*b*) Splenomegaly

Code to splenomegalic anaemia (285.8). Splenomegaly modifies the coding.

Rule 6. Trivial conditions. Where the selected underlying cause is a trivial condition unlikely to cause death, proceed as follows:

(a) if the death was the result of an adverse reaction to treatment of the trivial condition, select the adverse reaction.

Example 36: I(*a*) Cardiac arrest
        (*b*) Administration of nitrous oxide for dental extraction

Code to cardiac arrest (427.5) and adverse effect of gaseous anaesthetics (E938.2).

Example 37: I(*a*) Acute renal failure
        (*b*) Aspirin taken for recurrent headaches

Code to acute renal failure (584.9) and adverse effect of aspirin (E935.1).

Example 38: I(*a*) Postoperative haemorrhage
   (*b*) Tonsillectomy
   (*c*) Hypertrophy of tonsils

Code to postoperative haemorrhage (998.1) and removal of organ as cause of complication (E878.6).

(b)   if the trivial condition is not reported as the cause of a more serious complication, and a more serious unrelated condition is reported on the certificate, re-select the underlying cause as if the trivial condition had not been reported.

Example 39: I(*a*) Bursitis and ulcerative colitis

Code to ulcerative colitis (566).   Bursitis, selected by *rule 2* (see example 19), is ignored.

Example 40: I(*a*) Dental caries

   II Tetanus

Code to tetanus (037).   Dental caries, selected by the *General rule*, is ignored since this condition was not reported as the cause of a more serious complication.

Example 41: I(*a*) Dermatitis, perforating duodenal
   (*b*) ulcer, and hypertensive
   (*c*) heart disease

Code to perforating duodenal ulcer (532.5).   Dermatitis selected by *rule 2*, is ignored since it was not reported as the cause of a more serious complication. *Rule 2* is applied to the remaining conditions.

Rule 7.   Linkage.   Where the selected underlying cause is linked by a provision in the classification in the Notes for use in primary mortality coding on pages 713-721 with one or more of the other conditions on the certificate, code the combination.

Where the linkage provision is only for the combination of one condition specified as due to another, code the combination only when the correct causal relationship is stated or can be inferred from application of the selection rules.

Where a conflict in linkages occurs, link with the condition that would have been selected if the underlying cause initially selected had not been reported.   Apply any further linkage that is applicable.

Example 42: I(*a*) Intestinal obstruction
   (*b*) Femoral hernia

Code to femoral hernia with obstruction (552.0).

Example 43: I(*a*) Parkinsonism
   (*b*) Arteriosclerosis

Code to paralysis agitans (332.0).   The conditions are stated in the correct causal relationship for the " due to " linkage.

Example 44: I(a)   Coronary embolism
     (b)   Arteriosclerotic heart disease
     (c)   Influenza

Code to coronary embolism (410). Arteriosclerotic heart disease, selected by *rule 1* (see example 9), links with coronary embolism.

Example 45: I(a)   Cardiac dilatation and renal sclerosis
     (b)   Hypertension

Code to hypertensive heart and renal disease (404.9). All three conditions combine.

Example 46: I(a)   Cerebral haemorrhage and hypostatic pneumonia
     (b)   Hypertension and diabetes
     (c)   Arteriosclerosis

Code to cerebral haemorrhage (431). Arteriosclerosis, selected by *rule 1* (see example 13), links with hypertension, which itself links with cerebral haemorrhage.

Example 47: I(a)   Aortic aneurysm and generalized arteriosclerosis

Code to aortic aneurysm (nonsyphilitic) (441.6). The correct causal relationship for the " due to " linkage can be inferred from the use of *rule 3* to select arteriosclerosis as the underlying cause.

Example 48: I(a)   Cerebral haemorrhage
     (b)   Arteriosclerosis and hypertensive heart
     (c)   disease

Code to hypertensive heart disease (402.9). Link arteriosclerosis, selected by *rule 1*, with hypertensive heart disease since hypertensive heart disease would have been selected by the *General rule* if arteriosclerosis had not been reported.

Example 49: I(a)   Cerebral haemorrhage and hypertensive
     (b)   heart disease
     (c)   Arteriosclerosis

Code to cerebral haemorrhage (431). Link with cerebral haemorrhage since this condition would have been selected by *rule 2* if arteriosclerosis had not been reported.

Example 50: I(a)   Secondary polycythaemia
     (b)   Pulmonary emphysema
     (c)   Bronchitis

Code to obstructive chronic bronchitis (491.2). Bronchitis, selected by the *General rule*, links with emphysema.

Example 51: I(a)   Spastic quadriplegia and mental retardation 2 yrs.
     (b)   Intrauterine anoxia
     (c)   Premature separation of placenta

Code to quadriplegic infantile cerebral palsy (343.2). Provision has been made for classifying residual cerebral paralysis that occurs as a result of perinatal causes classifiable to 760–779 to cerebral palsy.

Example 52: I(a)   Coronary embolism
     (b)   Myocarditis and nephritis
     (c)   Hypertension

Code to coronary embolism (410). Link with myocarditis since this condition would have been selected by *rule 1* if hypertension had not been reported; there is a further linkage between myocarditis and coronary embolism.

Rule 8. Specificity. Where the selected underlying cause describes a condition in general terms and a term which provides more precise information about the site or nature of this condition is reported on the certificate, prefer the more informative term. This rule will often apply when the general term can be regarded as an adjective qualifying the more precise term.

Example 53: I(*a*)   Cerebral thrombosis
        (*b*)   Cerebrovascular accident

    Code to cerebral thrombosis (434.0).

Example 54: I(*a*)   Rheumatic heart disease, mitral stenosis
    Code to rheumatic mitral stenosis (394.0).

Example 55: I(*a*)   Meningitis
        (*b*)   Tuberculosis

    Code to tuberculous meningitis (013.0).   The conditions are stated in the correct causal relationship.

Example 56: I(*a*)   Toxaemia of pregnancy
        II   Eclamptic convulsions

    Code to eclampsia of pregnancy (642.6).

Example 57: I(*a*)   Aneurysm of aorta
        (*b*)   Syphilis

    Code to aneurysm of aorta, specified as syphilitic (093.0).   The conditions are stated in the correct causal relationship.

Example 58: I(*a*)   Internal injuries from automobile accident
        II   Ruptured spleen
        Accident: Automobile struck highway divider

    Code to rupture of spleen (865.0) and other motor vehicle traffic accident involving collision (E815.9).

Example 59: I(*a*)   Pericarditis
        (*b*)   Uraemia and pneumonia

    Code to uraemic pericarditis (585).   Uraemia, selected by *rule 1* (see example 12), may be used as an adjectival modifier since the conditions are stated in the correct causal relationship.

Rule 9. Early and late stages of disease. Where the selected underlying cause is an early stage of a disease and a more advanced stage of the same disease is reported on the certificate, code to the more advanced stage. This rule does not apply to a " chronic " form reported as due to an " acute " form unless the Classification gives special instructions to that effect.

Example 60: I(*a*)   Tertiary syphilis
        (*b*)   Primary syphilis

    Code to tertiary syphilis (097.0).

Example 61: I(*a*) Eclampsia during pregnancy
        (*b*) Pre-eclamptic toxaemia

Code to eclampsia of pregnancy (642.6).

Example 62: I(*a*) Chronic myocarditis
        (*b*) Acute myocarditis

Code to acute myocarditis (422.9).

Example 63: I(*a*) Chronic nephritis
        (*b*) Acute nephritis

Code to chronic nephritis, unspecified (582.9).   (See Notes, page 719.)

Rule 10.   Late effects.   Where the selected underlying cause is an early form of a condition for which the Classification provides a separate late effects category and there is evidence that death occurred from residual effects of this condition rather than in its active phase, code to the appropriate late effects category.

The following late effects categories, including those in the Supplementary E code, have been provided: 137, 138, 139, 268.1, 326, 438, 905-909, E929, E959, E969, E977, E989, and E999.   (See III Late effects, page 723.)

Example 64: I(*a*) Pulmonary fibrosis
        (*b*) Old pulmonary tuberculosis

Code to late effects of respiratory tuberculosis (137.0).

Example 65: I(*a*) Heart failure
        (*b*) Curvature of spine
        (*c*) Rickets in childhood

Code to late effects of rickets (268.1).

Example 66: I(*a*) Hydrocephalus
        (*b*) Cerebral abscess

Code to late effects of intracranial abscess (326).

Example 67: I(*a*) Hypostatic pneumonia
        (*b*) Hemiplegia
        (*c*) Cerebrovascular accident 10 years

Code to late effects of cerebrovascular disease (438).

Example 68: I(*a*) Chronic nephritis
        (*b*) Scarlet fever

Code to late effects of other infectious and parasitic diseases (139.8).   The description of the nephritis as " chronic " implies that the scarlet fever is no longer in its active phase.

Example 69: I(*a*) Paralysis
        (*b*) Fractured spine
        (*c*) Automobile accident, 18 months ago

Code to late effects of fracture of vertebral column with spinal cord lesion (907.2) and late effects of automobile accident (E929.0).

Rule 11.   Old pneumonia, influenza and maternal conditions. Where the selected underlying cause is pneumonia or influenza (480-487) and there is evidence that the date of onset was 1 year or more prior to death or a resultant chronic condition is reported, reselect the underlying cause as if the pneumonia or influenza had not been reported. Where the selected underlying cause is a maternal cause (630-678) and there is evidence that death occurred more than 42 days after termination of pregnancy or a resultant chronic condition is reported, reselect the underlying cause as if the maternal cause had not been reported. Take into account the pneumonia, influenza or maternal condition if it modifies the coding.

Example 70: I(*a*)   Cerebral haemorrhage
             (*b*)   Hypertension
             (*c*)   Childbirth 5 months ago

Code to cerebral haemorrhage (431). Since the childbirth occurred more than 42 days prior to death, hypertension is reselected and linked with cerebral haemorrhage.

Example 71: I(*a*)   Pneumonia 1 year

Code to other unknown and unspecified cause (799.9). The only cause reported is ignored.

Rule 12.   Errors and accidents in medical care. Where the selected underlying cause was subject to medical care and the reported sequence in Part I indicates explicitly that the death was the result of an error or accident occurring during medical care (conditions classifiable to categories E850-E858, E870-E876), regard the sequence of events leading to death as starting at the point at which the error or accident occurred. This does not apply to attempts at resuscitation.

Example 72: I(*a*)   Cerebral infarction
             (*b*)   Anoxia
             (*c*)   Wrong positioning of endotracheal tube during induction of
                     anaesthesia in operation for carcinoma of uterus

Code to anoxic brain damage resulting from a procedure (997.0) and endotracheal tube wrongly placed during anaesthetic procedure (E876.3).

Example 73: I(*a*)   Hypernatraemia
             (*b*)   Saline emetic and gastric lavage
             (*c*)   Double dose of morphine (treatment for pain control in carcinoma-
                     tosis)

Code to overdose of morphine (965.0 and E850.0).

Example 74: I(*a*)   Cardiac tamponade
             (*b*)   Perforation of auricle during cardiac catheterization
             (*c*)   Interventricular septal defect

Code to accidental puncture or laceration during heart catheterization (998.2, E870.6).

Example 75: I(*a*)   Cardiac arrest
             (*b*)   Overdose of potassium during rehydration
             (*c*)   Operation for hypernephroma

Code to overdose of potassium (974.5, E858.5).

Notes for use in underlying cause mortality coding

When a condition in one of the categories shown in the following list is reported as a cause of death, the provisions of the relevant note should be applied. Notes dealing with the linkage of conditions appear at the categories from which the combination is excluded.

012 *Other respiratory tuberculosis, except tuberculous pleurisy in 012.0*
013-017 *Tuberculosis of other organs*

Excludes with conditions in 011 (Pulmonary tuberculosis) **(011)** unless reported as the underlying cause of and with a specified duration exceeding that of the condition in 011.

035 *Erysipelas*
037 *Tetanus*
038 *Septicaemia*

Code to these diseases when they follow vaccination or a slight injury (any condition in N910-N919, prick, splinter, minor cut, puncture (except of trunk), bruise or contusion of superficial tissues or external parts, burn of first degree); when they follow a more serious injury, code to the injury.

036.2 *Meningococcaemia*

Excludes with conditions in:
　　036.0 Meningococcal meningitis **(036.0)**
　　036.1 Meningococcal encephalitis **(036.1)**
　　036.3 Waterhouse-Friderichsen syndrome, meningococcal **(036.3)**.

196 *Secondary and unspecified malignant neoplasm of lymph nodes*
197 *Secondary malignant neoplasm of respiratory and digestive systems*
198 *Other secondary malignant neoplasms*

Not to be used for underlying cause mortality coding. See page 727.

244.0 *Postsurgical hypothyroidism*

Not to be used for underlying cause mortality coding. If the reason for the surgery is not known and this information cannot be obtained, code to **246.9**. See Operations, page 724.

251.3 *Postsurgical hypoinsulinaemia*

Not to be used for underlying cause mortality coding. If the reason for the surgery is not known and this information cannot be obtained, code to **577.9**. See Operations, page 724.

292 *Drug psychosis*

Excludes with mention of drug dependence **(304)**.

293-294 *Transient and other organic psychotic conditions*
299.1 *Disintegrative psychosis*

Not to be used if the underlying physical condition is known.

303   *Alcohol dependence syndrome*

Excludes with:

alcoholic psychosis in 291.0-291.3, 291.5-291.9 **(291.0-291.3, 291.5-291.9)**
physical complication such as:
cirrhosis of liver **(571.2)**
epilepsy **(345.–)**
gastritis **(535.3)**.

304   *Drug dependence*

Includes drug dependence with mention of acute narcotism, drug abuse (acute), overdose of, intoxication by, or poisoning by dependence-producing drugs, accidental or undetermined whether accidental or purposeful.

305.1   *Nondependent abuse of tobacco*

Excludes when reported as the underlying cause of physical conditions such as:

bronchitis **(490-491)**
emphysema **(492)**
ischaemic heart disease **(410-414)**.

310   *Specific nonpsychotic mental disorders following organic brain damage*
317-319   *Mental retardation*

Not to be used if the underlying physical condition is known.

331.0   *Alzheimer's disease*
331.1   *Pick's disease*

Excludes with mention of dementia **(290.1)**.

331.2   *Senile degeneration of brain*

Excludes with mention of dementia **(290.0)**.

342   *Hemiplegia*

Not to be used if the cause of the hemiplegia is known.

344   *Other paralytic syndromes*

Not to be used if the cause of the paralysis is known.

345   *Epilepsy*

Includes accidents resulting from epilepsy.

Excludes epilepsy due to trauma (code to the appropriate categories in Chapter XVII and in the Supplementary E code; if the nature and cause of injury is not known, code to **854.0** and **E928.9**).

369   *Blindness and low vision*
389   *Deafness*

Not to be used if the antecedent condition is known.

383.3   *Complications following mastoidectomy*

Not to be used for underlying cause mortality coding. If the reason for the surgery is not known and this information cannot be obtained, code to **385.9**. See Operations, page 724.

394.9   *Diseases of mitral valve, other and unspecified*

Excludes the listed conditions when of unspecified cause with conditions in 424.0 **(424.0)**.

397   *Diseases of other endocardial structures*

Excludes with conditions in:

    394   (Diseases of mitral valve) **(394)**
    395   (Diseases of aortic valve) **(395)**
    396   (Diseases of mitral and aortic valves) **(396)**.

397.1   *Rheumatic diseases of pulmonary valve*

Excludes with conditions in:

    397.0   (Diseases of tricuspid valve) **(397.0)**.

401   *Essential hypertension*

Excludes with conditions in:

    402   (Hypertensive heart disease) **(402)**
    403   (Hypertensive renal disease) **(403)**
    404   (Hypertensive heart and renal disease) **(404)**
    410-414   (Ischaemic heart disease) **(410-414)**
    430-438   (Cerebrovascular disease) **(430-438)**
    580-583   (Nephritis and nephrotic syndrome, except nephropathy (chronic) and chronic renal disease) **(580-583)**
    585   (Chronic renal failure)   ⎫
    586   (Renal failure unspecified)   ⎬ **(403)**
    587   (Renal sclerosis, unspecified) ⎭

and when reported as the underlying cause of:

    362.1   (Retinopathy) **(362.1)**
    394.0   (Mitral stenosis not specified as rheumatic) **(424.0)**
    394.2   (Mitral stenosis with insufficiency not specified as rheumatic) **(424.0)**
    394.9   (Other and unspecified diseases of mitral valve not specified as rheumatic) **(424.0)**
    396   (Diseases of mitral and aortic valve not specified as rheumatic) **(424.0)**
    397.0   (Disease of tricuspid valve not specified as rheumatic) **(424.2)**

424   (Other diseases of endocardium) **(424)**
428   (Heart failure) **(402)**
429.0 (Myocarditis, unspecified) **(402)**
429.1 (Myocardial degeneration) **(402)**
429.2 (Cardiovascular disease, unspecified) **(402)**
429.3 (Cardiomegaly) **(402)**
429.8 (Other ill-defined descriptions of heart disease) **(402)**
429.9 (Unspecified descriptions of heart disease) **(402)**

and of the terms nephropathy (chronic) and renal disease (chronic) in 582, 583 and 593.9 **(403)**.

402   *Hypertensive heart disease*

Excludes with conditions in:

403   (Hypertensive renal disease) **(404)**
404   (Hypertensive heart and renal disease) **(404)**
410-414   (Ischaemic heart disease) **(410-414)**
585   (Chronic renal failure)
586   (Renal failure, unspecified)   } **(404)**.
587   (Renal sclerosis, unspecified)

403   *Hypertensive renal disease*

Excludes with conditions in:

402   (Hypertensive heart disease) **(404)**
404   (Hypertensive heart and renal disease) **(404)**
410-414   (Ischaemic heart disease) **(410-414)**

and when reported as the underlying cause of:
428   (Heart failure) **(404)**
429.0 (Myocarditis, unspecified) **(404)**
429.1 (Myocardial degeneration) **(404)**
429.2 (Cardiovascular disease, unspecified) **(404)**
429.3 (Cardiomegaly) **(404)**
429.8 (Other ill-defined descriptions of heart disease) **(404)**
429.9 (Unspecified descriptions of heart disease) **(404)**.

404   *Hypertensive heart and renal disease*

Excludes with conditions in:

410-414   (Ischaemic heart disease) **(410-414)**.

405   *Secondary hypertension*

Not to be used for underlying cause mortality coding.

411   *Other acute and subacute forms of ischaemic heart disease*
412   *Old myocardial infarction*
413   *Angina pectoris*
414   *Other forms of chronic ischaemic heart disease*

Excludes with conditions in 410 (Acute myocardial infarction) **(410)**.

416.9   *Pulmonary heart disease, unspecified*

Excludes with conditions in 737.3 (Kyphoscoliosis and scoliosis) **(416.1)**.

Not to be used if an underlying pulmonary condition is known.

428   *Heart failure*
429.9   *Unspecified descriptions of heart disease*

Excludes with conditions in 737.3 (Kyphoscoliosis and scoliosis) **(416.1)**.

424   *Other diseases of endocardium*

When more than one valve is mentioned, priority in classification is in the order listed, i.e., mitral, aortic, tricuspid, pulmonary.

426   *Conduction disorders*
427   *Cardiac dysrhythmias*
428   *Heart failure*
429   *Ill-defined descriptions and complications of heart disease, except conditions in 429.4*

Excludes with conditions in 410-414 (Ischaemic heart disease) **(410-414)**.

428.9   *Heart failure, unspecified*
429.9   *Unspecified descriptions of heart disease*

Excludes with conditions in 518.4 (Acute œdema of lung, unspecified) **(428.1)**.

429.4   *Functional disturbances following cardiac surgery*

Not to be used for underlying cause mortality coding. If the reason for the surgery is not known and this information cannot be obtained, code to **429.9**. See Operations, page 724.

437.0   *Cerebral atherosclerosis*

Excludes with conditions in:

    430-434   (Cerebral haemorrhage and infarction **(430-434)**
    436   (Acute but ill-defined cerebrovascular disease) **(436)**

and when reported as the underlying cause of conditions in:
    294.9   (Dementia, unspecified) **(290.4)**
    332.0   (Paralysis agitans) **(332.0)**.

440   *Atherosclerosis*

Excludes with conditions in:

    401-404   (Hypertensive disease) **(401-404)**
    410-414   (Ischaemic heart disease) **(410-414)**
    429.0   (Myocarditis, unspecified) **(429.0)**
    429.1   (Myocardial degeneration) **(429.1)**
    429.2   (Cardiovascular disease, unspecified) **(429.2)**
    430-438   (Cerebrovascular disease) **(430-438)**

and when reported as the underlying cause of:

394.0 (Mitral stenosis not specified as rheumatic) **(424.0)**

394.2 (Mitral stenosis with insufficiency not specified as rheumatic) **(424.0)**

394.9 (Other and unspecified diseases of mitral valve not specified as rheumatic) **(424.0)**

396 (Diseases of mitral and aortic valves not specified as rheumatic) **(424.0)**

397.0 (Diseases of tricuspid valve not specified as rheumatic) **(424.2)**

424 (Other diseases of endocardium) **(424)**

441-447 (Other diseases of arteries and arterioles) **(441-447)**

557 (Vascular insufficiency of intestine) **(557)**

587 (Renal sclerosis, unspecified) **(403)**

and of the terms Bright's disease (chronic), nephritis (chronic) (interstitial), nephropathy (chronic) and renal disease (chronic) only in 582, 583, 593.9 **(403)**.

440.9 *Atherosclerosis, generalized and unspecified*

Excludes with gangrene in 785.4 **(440.2)**

and when reported as the underlying cause of conditions in:

294.9 (Dementia, unspecified) **(290.4)**

332.0 (Paralysis agitans) **(332.0)**.

457.0 *Postmastectomy lymphoedema syndrome*

Not to be used for underlying cause mortality coding. If the reason for the surgery is not known and this information cannot be obtained, code to **611.9**. See Operations, page 724.

460 *Acute nasopharyngitis (common cold)*
465 *Acute upper respiratory infections of multiple and unspecified sites*

Excludes when reported as the underlying cause of serious conditions such as meningitis **(322.9)**, intracranial abscess **(324.0)**, otitis media **(381, 382)**, mastoiditis and related conditions **(383)**, pneumonia and influenza **(480-483, 485-487)**, bronchitis and bronchiolitis **(466, 490, 491)**, acute nephritis **(580.0-580.9)**.

466.0 *Acute bronchitis*

Excludes with conditions in 491 (Chronic bronchitis) **(491)**.

490 *Bronchitis not specified as acute or chronic*

Excludes with conditions in:

492 (Emphysema) **(491.2)**

496 (Chronic airways obstruction, not elsewhere classified) **(491.2)**.

491.9   *Chronic bronchitis, unspecified*

Excludes with conditions in 492 (Emphysema) **(491.2)**.

Excludes when selected as the underlying cause (see note at 493 below) if asthma is also mentioned **(491.2)**.

492   *Emphysema*

Excludes with conditions in:

  . 490   (Bronchitis not specified as acute or chronic) **(491.2)**
   491   (Chronic bronchitis) **(491.2)**.

493   *Asthma*

When asthma and bronchitis (acute) (chronic) are separately reported on the same certificate of cause of death, the underlying cause should be selected by applying the *General rule* or *Rules 1, 2* or *3* in the normal way. Neither term should be treated as an adjectival modifier of the other.

500   *Coalworkers' pneumoconiosis*
501   *Asbestosis*
502   *Pneumoconiosis due to other silica or silicates*
505   *Pneumoconiosis, unspecified*

Excludes with conditions in 011 (Pulmonary tuberculosis) **(011)**.

518.4   *Acute oedema of lung, unspecified*   .

Excludes with conditions in:

   428.9   (Heart failure, unspecified) **(428.1)**
   429.9   (Unspecified descriptions of heart disease) **(428.1)**.

564.2   *Postgastric surgery syndrome*
564.3   *Vomiting following gastrointestinal surgery*
569.6   *Colostomy or enterostostomy malfunction*
576.0   *Postcholecystectomy syndrome*
579.2   *Blind loop syndrome*
579.3   *Other and unspecified postsurgical nonabsorption*

Not to be used for underlying cause mortality coding. If the reason for the surgery is not known and this information cannot be obtained, code to **537.9, 537.9, 569.9, 575.9, 569.9** and **569.9** respectively. See Operations, page 724.

580   *Acute glomerulonephritis*

Exclude when reported as the underlying cause of conditions in 582 (Chronic glomerulonephritis) **(582)**.

585   *Chronic renal failure*
586   *Renal failure, unspecified*

587   *Renal sclerosis, unspecified*

Excludes with conditions in:

    401   (Essential hypertension) **(403)**
    402   (Hypertensive heart disease) **(404)**
    403   (Hypertensive renal disease) **(403)**.

606   *Infertility, male*
628   *Infertility, female*

Not to be used if the causative condition is known.

639   *Complications following abortion and ectopic and molar pregnancies*

Not to be used for underlying cause mortality coding.

652   *Malposition and malpresentation of fetus*

Excludes with conditions in 653 (Disproportion) **(653)**.

653.4   *Fetopelvic disproportion*

Excludes with conditions in 653.0-653.3 (Pelvic abnormality) **(653.0-653.3)**.

660.0   *Obstruction caused by malposition of fetus at onset of labour*

Excludes with conditions in 660.1 (Obstruction by bony pelvis) **(660.1)**.

737.3   *Kyphoscoliosis and scoliosis*

Excludes with conditions in:

    416.9   (Pulmonary heart disease, unspecified) **(416.1)**
    428   (Heart failure) **(416.1)**
    429.9   (Unspecified descriptions of heart disease) **(416.1)**.

760-779   *Certain conditions originating in the perinatal period*

Excludes residual cerebral paralysis at ages 4 weeks or over **(333.7, 343)**.

765   *Disorders relating to short gestation and unspecified low birthweight*
766   *Disorders relating to long gestation and high birthweight*

Not to be used if any other cause of perinatal mortality is reported.

800-999   *Injury and Poisoning*

Not to be used for underlying cause mortality coding except as an additional code to the relevant category in E800-E999.

800-803   *Fracture of skull*

When more than one site is mentioned, priority in classification is in the order base, vault, other.

958   *Certain early complications of trauma*

Not to be used if the nature of the antecedent injury is known.

960-999 *Poisoning by drugs, medicaments and biological substances*

Excludes poisoning, accidental or undetermined whether accidental or purposeful, by dependence-producing drugs if drug dependence is mentioned **(304)**.

E850-E858 *Accidental poisoning by drugs, medicaments and biologicals*
E980 *Poisoning by solid or liquid substances, undetermined whether accidentally or purposely inflicted*

Excludes poisoning by dependence-producing drugs if drug dependence is mentioned **(304)**.

Notes for interpretation of entries of causes of death

The foregoing rules will usually determine the underlying cause of death for primary mortality tabulation. Each country will need to amplify the rules, depending on the consistency and completeness of medical certification. The following paragraphs will be of assistance in formulating such additional instructions.

I. Guides for the determination of the probability of sequences

A. *Assumption of intervening cause*

The assumption of an intervening cause in Part I is permissible for the purpose of accepting a sequence as reported, but it must not be used to modify the coding.

Example 1: 1(*a*)   Cerebral haemorrhage
            (*b*)   Chronic nephritis

Code to chronic nephritis (582.9). It is necessary to assume hypertension as a condition intervening between cerebral haemorrhage and the underlying cause, chronic nephritis.

Example 2: 1(*a*)   Mental retardation
            (*b*)   Premature separation of placenta

Code to premature separation of placenta (762.1). It is necessary to assume birth trauma, anoxia or hypoxia as a condition intervening between mental retardation and the underlying cause, premature separation of placenta.

B. *Interpretation of "highly improbable"*

As a guide to the acceptability of sequences in the application of the selection rules, the following relationships should be regarded as "highly improbable":

(*a*) an infectious or parasitic disease (001-139) other than colitis, enteritis, gastroenteritis and diarrhoea (009.1, 009.3), diseases due to other mycobacteria (031), erysipelas (035), tetanus (037), septicaemia or pyaemia (038), gas gangrene (040.0), Vincent's angina (101) and mycoses (110-119) reported as "due to" any disease outside the group;

(*b*) a malignant neoplasm reported as " due to " any other disease;

(*c*) a congenital anomaly (740-759) reported as " due to " any other disease of the individual, including immaturity;

(*d*) diabetes (250) reported as " due to " any other disease except haemochromatosis (275.0), disease of pancreas (577) and pancreatic neoplasms;

(*e*) haemophilia (286.0-286.2) or influenza (487) reported as " due to " any other disease;

(*f*) rheumatic fever (390-392) or rheumatic heart disease (393-398) reported as " due to " any disease other than streptococcal sore throat (034.0), scarlet fever (034.1), streptococcal septicaemia (038.0), and acute tonsillitis (463);

(*g*) a non-inflammatory disease of the central nervous system (330-349, 430-438) reported as " due to " a disease of the digestive system (520-579) or, except for cerebral embolism (434.1), as " due to " endocarditis (394-397, 421, 424);

(*h*) chronic ischaemic heart disease (412-414) reported as " due to " any neoplasm;

(*i*) any condition described as atherosclerotic [arteriosclerotic] reported as " due to " neoplasm;

(*j*) any hypertensive condition reported as " due to " any neoplasm except carcinoid tumors or endocrine or renal neoplasms;

(*k*) a condition of stated date of onset " X " reported as " due to " a condition of stated date of onset " Y ", when " X " predates " Y ".

The above list does not cover all " highly improbable " sequences, but in other cases the general rule should be followed unless there are strong indications to the contrary.

The following should be accepted as possible sequences in Part I of the certificate:

Acute or terminal circulatory diseases when reported as due to malignant neoplasm, diabetes or asthma. The following conditions are regarded as acute or terminal circulatory diseases:

410 Acute myocardial infarction
411 Other acute and subacute forms of ischaemic heart disease
415 Acute pulmonary heart disease
420 Acute pericarditis
421 Acute and subacute endocarditis
422 Acute myocarditis
426 Conduction disorders
427 Cardiac dysrhythmias
428 Heart failure
429.8 Other ill-defined descriptions of heart disease
430-438 Cerebrovascular disease except 437.0-437.5, 437.9, 438

II. *Effect of duration on classification*

In evaluating the reported sequence of the direct and antecedent causes, consideration should be given to any statements of the interval between the onset of the disease or condition and time of death. This would apply in the interpretation of " highly improbable " relationships, item I(k), and in rule 11.

Conditions classified as congenital anomalies in the International Classification of Diseases (Nos. 740-759), even when not specified as congenital on the medical certificate, should be coded as such if the interval between onset and death and the age of the decedent indicate that the condition existed from birth.

The Classification provides specific categories to be used to indicate certain diseases and injuries as the cause of late effects. In many cases these late effects include conditions present one year or more after the onset of the disease or injury. (See also Late Effects below.)

III. *Late effects*

Certain categories in the Classification (Nos. 137, 138, 139, 268.1, 326, 438, 905-909) are to be used for underlying cause mortality coding to indicate that death resulted from late (residual) effects of a given disease or injury rather than during the active phase. (Categories E929, E959, E969, E977, E989, E999 in the Supplementary E code are to be used to indicate certain external causes as the cause of late effects.) Rule 10 applies in such circumstances. Guidance in interpreting late effects is given under each of the late effects categories in the tabular list of inclusions and in the E code. Further clarification of categories 137 and of the subcategories 139 is given below.

137   Late effects of tuberculosis

The " late effects " include conditions specified as such or as sequelae of past tuberculous disease and residuals of tuberculosis specified as arrested, cured, healed, inactive, old, or quiescent unless there is evidence of active tuberculosis.

139.0   Late effects of viral encephalitis

The " late effects " include conditions specified as such, or as sequelae, and those which were present one year or more after onset of the causal condition.

139.1   Late effects of trachoma

The " late effects " include residuals of trachoma specified as healed or inactive and certain specified sequelae such as blindness, cicatricial entropion and conjunctival scars unless there is evidence of active infection.

139.8   Late effects of other infectious and parasitic diseases

The " late effects " include conditions specified as such or as sequelae and residuals of these diseases described as arrested, cured, healed, inactive, old or quiescent unless there is evidence of active disease. " Late effects " also include chronic conditions reported as due to, or residual conditions present one year or more after onset of, condition classifiable to categories 001-003, 020-022, 027.0, 032-037, 047, 048, 049.0, 049.1, 050, 052-056, 060, 066.2, 071-073, 080-083, 130.

IV. *Sex limitations*

Certain categories in the Classification are limited to one sex (Nos. 175, 185-187, 222, 233.4-233.6, 236.4-236.6, 257, 600-608 for males only and Nos. 174, 179-184, 218-221, 233.1-233.3, 236.0-236.3, 256, 614-676 for females only). If, after verification, the sex and cause of death on the certificate are not consistent, the death should be coded to " Other unknown and unspecified causes (799.9) ".

V. *Operations*

If an operation appears on the certificate as the cause of death without mention of the condition for which it was performed, or of the findings at operation, and the index provides no assignment for it, it is to be assumed that the condition for which the operation is usually performed was present, and assignment will be made in accordance with the above rules for selection of the cause of death. However, if the name of the operation leaves in doubt what specific morbid condition was present, additional information is to be sought. Failing this, code to the residual category for the organ or site indicated by the name of the operation (e.g., code " gastrectomy " to 537.9); if the operation does not indicate an organ or site (e.g., " laparotomy "), code to " Other unknown and unspecified causes (799.9) ", unless there is mention of a postoperative complication or a therapeutic misadventure.

VI. *Malignant neoplasms*

A. *Morphological types*

The morphological types classified on pages 668 to 690 appear in the Alphabetical Index with their M codes and with an indication as to the coding by site. This may take the form of a reference to the "Neoplasm" listing in the index when the morphological type could occur in a variety of organs, e.g.

Adenoacanthoma (M8570/3) — see Neoplasm, malignant

or to a particular part of that listing when the morphological type arises in a particular type of tissue, e.g.

Sarcoma (M8800/3) — see Neoplasm, connective tissue, malignant

It may give the code for the site assumed to be most likely when no site is specified, e.g.

Astrocytoma (M9400/3)
    specified sites — see Neoplasm, malignant
    unspecified site 191.9

or it may give a code to be used whatever site is reported when the vast majority of neoplasms of the morphological type occur in a particular site, e.g.

Hepatocarcinoma (M8170/3) 155.0

Coders should, therefore, look up the morphological type in the Alphabetical Index before coding by site.

A morphological term ending in " osis ", unless it is specifically indexed, should be coded in the same way as the tumour name to which " osis " has been added. Thus, neuroblastomatosis should be coded in the same way as neuroblastoma but haemangiomatosis, which is specifically indexed, is not coded in the same way as haemangioma.

It has not been possible to index all combinations of the order of prefixes in compound morphological terms. For example, the coder will not find the term " Chondrofibrosarcoma " in the index, but he will find " Fibrochondrosarcoma (M9220/3) — see Neoplasm, cartilage, malignant ", which has the same prefixes in a different order, and he should code the former term in the same way as the latter.

B. *Multiple sites*

If malignant neoplasms of more than one site are entered on the certificate, the site indicated as primary should be selected, regardless of the position of the conditions on the certificate. This indication may be:

(a) the specification of one site as primary;

Example: I(a)   Carcinoma of bladder
                (b)   Primary in kidney

Code to carcinoma of kidney (189.0).

(b) the specification of other sites as " secondary", " metastases " or " spread ";

Example: I(a)   Carcinoma of breast with secondaries in brain

Code to carcinoma of breast (174.9).

Example: I(a)   Cancer of lung with spread to kidney, adrenal and brain

Code to cancer of lung (162.9).

(c) an acceptable order of entry pointing to one site as primary;

Example: I(a)   Cancer of liver
                (b)   Cancer of stomach

Code to cancer of stomach (151.9). The order of entry indicates that this was the primary site.

Malignant neoplasm of lymph nodes not specified as primary should be assumed to be secondary.

Example: I(*a*)   Cancer in supraclavicular lymph node
       (*b*)
       (*c*)

      II   Gastric carcinoma

Code to cancer of stomach (151.9).

If there is no indication as to which was the primary site or if it appears that there were two or more primary malignant neoplasms (for example, if sites are entered on the same line or in different Parts of the certificate), prefer a defined site to an ill-defined site in category 195. Otherwise, prefer the first mentioned.

Example: I(*a*)   Carcinoma, breast and caecum

Code to carcinoma of breast (174.9).

Example: I(*a*)   Carcinoma of adrenal gland
       (*b*)
       (*c*)

      II   Carcinoma of caecum

Code to carcinoma of adrenal gland (194.0).

Example: I(*a*)   Cancer of abdomen and stomach

Code to cancer of stomach (151.9).

C.   *Imprecise or doubtful descriptions of site*

Neoplasms of sites prefixed by " peri ", " para ", " pre ", " supra ", " infra ", etc. or described as in the " area " or " region " of a site, unless these terms are specifically indexed, should be coded as follows: for morphological types classifiable to one of the categories 170, 171, 172, 173, 191 or 192, code to the appropriate subdivision of that category; otherwise, code to the appropriate subdivision of 195 (Other and ill-defined sites).

Example: Fibrosarcoma in the region of the wrist

Code to 171.2 (fibrosarcoma of upper limb)

Example: Peribiliary carcinoma

Code to 195.2 (carcinoma of abdomen)

Neoplasms described as of one site *or* another should be coded to the rubric that embraces both sites or, if no appropriate rubric exists, to " unspecified site ".

Example: Osteosarcoma of lumbar vertebrae or sacrum

Code to 170.9 (osteosarcoma, unspecified site)

Example: Carcinoma of small intestine or colon

Code to 159.0 (carcinoma of intestine NOS)

Example: Cancer of pancreas or lung

Code to 199.1 (cancer of unspecified site)

D. Neoplasm of unspecified site

When there is no specification of the site of a neoplasm, code to " unspecified site " for the morphological type involved, even though the neoplasm is associated with some other condition (e.g. obstruction, haemorrhage, perforation) of a specified site.

Example: I(a)   Perforation of stomach
             (b)   Carcinoma

Code to 199.1

Example: I(a)   Ureteric obstruction
             (b)   Sarcoma

Code to 171.9

Example: I(a)   Haemorrhage of bladder
             (b)   Transitional cell carcinoma

Code to 199.1

E. " Primary site unknown "

When the statement " primary site unknown " appears on a certificate, code to the category for " unspecified site " for the morphological type involved (e.g. adenocarcinoma 199.1, fibrosarcoma 171.9, osteosarcoma 170.9); any other sites of malignant neoplasm reported elsewhere on the certificate should be assumed to be secondary.

F. Secondary sites

Categories 196, 197 and 198 are not to be used for underlying-cause mortality coding. Secondary neoplasm of specified sites, or of unspecified site, without mention of a primary site, should be coded to the category for " unspecified site " for the morphological type involved (e.g. carcinoma 199.1, sarcoma 171.9, melanoma 172.9).

Categories 196, 197 and 198 are for use in multiple-condition coding and in morbidity coding and for these purposes include all secondary neoplasms of specified site regardless of the morphological types of neoplasm (e.g. secondary melanoma of lung 197.0, secondary squamous cell carcinoma, cervical lymph node 196.0).

G. Leukaemia

Acute exacerbation of or blastic crisis in chronic leukaemia should be coded to the chronic form.

Example: I(a)   Acute and chronic lymphatic leukaemia

Code to 204.1 (chronic lymphatic leukaemia)

Acute leukaemia of any type should be coded to the acute form regardless of the interval between onset and death.

When a condition classifiable to categories 200-202 is reported as terminating in leukaemia, code to 200-202.

H. *Implication of malignancy*

Mention on a certificate that a neoplasm has given rise to metastases or secondaries means that the neoplasm is malignant and it should be so coded even though the name of the neoplasm without mention of metastases would be classified to some other section of Chapter II.

Example: I(*a*)   Metastatic involvement of lymph nodes
             (*b*)   Carcinoma-in-situ of cervix, resected 2 years ago

Code to malignant neoplasm of cervix uteri (180.9)

Example: I(*a*)   Secondaries in lymph nodes and lung
             (*b*)   Brenner tumour

Code to malignant neoplasm of ovary (183.0)

J. *"Metastatic" cancer*

The adjective " metastatic " is used ambiguously, sometimes to mean secondary deposits from a primary elsewhere and sometimes to mean a metastasizing primary.   No arbitrary rule can satisfactorily solve this problem since usage varies in different languages and different countries, but the following rule is proposed as an expedient when there is doubt as to the meaning intended:

(a)   Cancer described as " metastatic from " a site should be interpreted as primary of that site, and cancer described as " metastatic to " a site should be interpreted as secondary of that site.

Example: I(*a*)   Carcinoma in lymph nodes and lungs
             (*b*)   Metastatic from nasopharynx

Code to primary malignant neoplasm of nasopharynx (147.9)

Example: I(*a*)   Metastatic cancer from liver to lung

Code to primary malignant neoplasm of liver (155.0)

(b)   If two or more sites are reported and all are qualified as " metastatic ", code as for " primary site unknown " in E above.

Example: I(*a*)   Metastatic carcinoma of lung
             (*b*)   Metastatic carcinoma of breast
      Code to 199.1

Example: I(*a*)   Metastatic melanoma of lung and liver
      Code to 172.9

(c)   If only one site is reported and this is qualified as " metastatic ", proceed as follows:

   (1)   code to the category for " unspecified site " for the morphological type concerned unless this code is 199

Example: I(*a*)   Metastatic renal cell carcinoma of lung

Code to 189.0

Example: I(*a*)   Metastatic osteosarcoma of brain

Code to 170.9

    (2)   otherwise, code as for primary malignant neoplasm of the reported site except for the following sites, which should be coded to 199:

        bone
        brain, spinal cord, meninges
        liver
        lymph nodes
        pleura
        peritoneum, retroperitoneum, mediastinum, heart, diaphragm
        sites classifiable to 195

Example: I(*a*)   Metastatic lung cancer

Code to 162.9

Example: I(*a*)   Metastatic cancer of brain

Code to 199.1

Example: I(*a*)   Metastatic cancer of hip

Code to 199.1

(d) If no site is reported, but the morphological type is qualified as " metastatic " code as for " primary site unknown " in E above.

(e) If two or more sites are reported and some are qualified as " metastatic " while others are not, " metastatic " cancer of the sites listed under (c)(2) above should be interpreted as secondary. If sites other than these are qualified as " metastatic ", attempt to resolve the problem of selecting the underlying cause by taking into account the order of entry on the certificate and any statements of the duration of the conditions reported.

Example: I(*a*)   Abdominal carcinomatosis
         (*b*)   Bronchial carcinomatosis
         (*c*)   Metastatic mammary cancer

Code to 174.9

VII.   *Rheumatic fever with heart involvement*

If there is no statement that the rheumatic process was active at the time of death, assume activity if the heart condition (other than terminal conditions and bacterial endocarditis) which is specified as rheumatic or stated to be due to rheumatic fever is described as acute or subacute; in the absence of such description, the terms " carditis ", " endocarditis ", " heart disease ", " myocarditis ", and " pancarditis " can be regarded as acute if the interval between onset and death is less than one year or, if no interval is stated, if the age at death is under 15, and the term " pericarditis " can be regarded as acute at any age.

VIII. *Congenital anomalies*

The following conditions may be regarded as congenital when causing death at the ages stated provided there is no indication that they were acquired after birth.

Under 1 year: aneurysm, aortic stenosis, atresia, atrophy of brain, cyst of brain, deformity, displacement of organ, ectopia, hypoplasia of organ, malformation, pulmonary stenosis, valvular heart disease.

Under 4 weeks: endocarditis, heart disease NOS, hydrocephalus NOS, myocarditis.

IX. *Nature of injury*

Where more than one kind of injury in 800-959 is mentioned and there is no clear indication as to which caused death, the injury to be coded should be selected in accordance with the following order of preference, provided that there is no contrary instruction in the classification:

fracture of skull (800, 801, 803, 804) and broken neck (805.0, 805.1, 806.0, 806.1)
internal injury of chest, abdomen, pelvis (860-869)
fracture of face bones, spine, trunk (802, 805.2-805.9, 806.2-809)
other head injury (850-854), open wounds of neck and chest (874, 875), traumatic amputation of limbs (887, 897) and spinal cord lesion without evidence of spinal bone injury (952)
fracture of limbs (810-829)
burn (940-949)
others in 800-959

X. *Poisoning by drugs, medicaments and biological substances*

When combinations of medicinal agents classified differently are involved, proceed as follows. If one component of the combination is specified as the cause of death, code to that component. If one component is not specified as the cause of death, code to the category provided for the combination, e.g., mixed sedatives (967.6). Otherwise if the components are classified to the same three-digit category, code to the appropriate subcategory for " Other "; if not, code to 977.8.

Combinations of medicinal agents with alcohol should be coded to the medicinal agent.

XI. *Expression indicating doubtful diagnosis*

Qualifying expressions indicating some doubt as to the accuracy of the diagnosis, such as " apparently ", " presumably ", " possibly ", etc., should be ignored, since entries without such qualification differ only in degree of certainty of the diagnosis.

PERINATAL MORTALITY

It is recommended that, where practicable, a separate certificate of cause of perinatal death should be adopted, in which the causes are set out in the following manner:

(a) Main disease or condition in fetus or infant
(b) Other diseases or conditions in fetus or infant
(c) Main maternal disease or condition affecting fetus or infant
(d) Other maternal diseases or conditions affecting fetus or infant
(e) Other relevant circumstances

The form of certificate should include identifying particulars with relevant dates and times, a statement as to whether the baby was born alive or dead, and information about autopsy.

For a thorough analysis of perinatal mortality, supplementary data on both mother and child is needed in addition to information about the causes of death. Consideration should be given to the collection of the following items as a minimum, not only for perinatal deaths but also for all live births, in order to provide denominators for the calculation of meaningful rates:

Mother

Date of birth
Number of previous pregnancies: live births/stillbirths/abortions
Outcome of last previous pregnancy: live birth/stillbirth/abortion and
    date
Present pregnancy:
    First day of last menstrual period (if unknown, then estimated
        duration of pregnancy in completed weeks)
    Antenatal care, two or more visits: yes/no/not known
    Delivery: normal spontaneous vertex/other (specify)

Child

Birthweight in grammes
Sex: boy/girl/indeterminate
Single birth/first twin/second twin/other multiple birth
If stillborn, when death occurred: before labour/during labour/not
    known

Other variables that might appear on the basic certificate include particulars of the birth attendant, as follows: physician/trained midwife/other trained person (specify)/other (specify).

The method by which the supplementary data is collected will vary according to the civil registration system obtaining in different countries. Where it can be collected at the registration of the stillbirth or early neonatal death, a form similar to the " Certificate of Cause of Perinatal Death " on page 732 could be used. Otherwise, special arrangements would need to be made (for example, by linking birth and death records) to bring together the supplementary data and the cause of death.

CERTIFICATE OF CAUSE OF PERINATAL DEATH

To be completed for stillbirths and live born infants dying within 168 hours (1 week) from birth

(Identifying Particulars)

☐ This child was live born on   at   hours
      and died on   at   hours

☐ This child was stillborn on   at   hours
and died Before labour ☐ During labour ☐ Not known ☐

Mother	Child

Mother

Date of birth ☐☐☐☐
or, if unknown, age (years) ☐

Number of previous pregnancies:
    Live births ☐
    Stillbirths ☐
    Abortions ☐

Outcome of last previous pregnancy:
    Live birth ☐
    Stillbirth ☐
    Abortion ☐
    Date ☐☐☐☐

1st day of last
menstrual period ☐☐☐☐
or, if unknown, estimated duration
of pregnancy
(completed weeks) ☐☐

Antenatal care, two or more visits
    Yes ☐
    No ☐
    Not known ☐

Delivery:
    Normal spontaneous vertex ☐
    Other (specify) . . . .

Child

Birthweight: . . . . . . grammes
Sex:
    Boy ☐ Girl ☐ Indeterminate ☐
Single birth ☐ First twin ☐
Second twin ☐ Other multiple ☐

Attendant at birth

Physician ☐ Trained midwife ☐
Other trained person (specify) . . . .
Other (specify) . . . .

CAUSES OF DEATH

a. Main disease or condition in fetus or infant

b. Other diseases or conditions in fetus or infant

c. Main maternal disease or condition affecting fetus or infant

d. Other maternal diseases or conditions affecting fetus or infant

e. Other relevant circumstances

The certified cause of death has been confirmed by autopsy ☐

Autopsy information may be available later ☐

Autopsy not being held ☐

I certify . . . .
. . . .
. . . .

Signature and qualification

Where civil registration requirements make it difficult to introduce a common death certificate for live born and stillborn infants, the problem could be met by *separate* certificates for stillbirths and early neonatal deaths, each incorporating the recommended format for the causes of death.

Statement of causes of death

The form of certificate provides five sections for the entry of causes of perinatal deaths, labelled (*a*) to (*e*). In sections (*a*) and (*b*) should be entered diseases or conditions of the infant or fetus, with the single most important one of these in section (*a*) and the remainder, if any, in section (*b*). By " the most important " is meant that pathological condition which in the opinion of the certifier made the greatest contribution to the death of the infant or fetus. The mode of death, e.g. heart failure, asphyxia, anoxia, should not be entered in section (*a*) unless it was the only fetal or infant condition known. This also holds true for prematurity.

In sections (*c*) and (*d*), the certifier should enter all diseases or conditions in the mother which in his opinion had some adverse effect on the infant or fetus. Again, the most important one of these should be entered in section (*c*) and the others, if any, in section (*d*). Section (*e*) is provided for the reporting of any other circumstance which the certifier considers to have a bearing on the death but which cannot be described as a disease or condition of the infant or the mother. An example of this might be delivery in the absence of an attendant.

The following examples illustrate the statement of the causes of death for the cases described:

Example 1. The mother, whose previous pregnancies had ended in spontaneous abortions at 12 and 18 weeks, was admitted when 24 weeks pregnant, in premature labour. There was spontaneous delivery of a 700 g infant which died during the first day of life. The main finding on autopsy was " pulmonary immaturity ".

Causes of perinatal death:

    (*a*) Pulmonary immaturity
    (*b*) —
    (*c*) Premature labour, cause unknown
    (*d*) Recurrent aborter
    (*e*) —

Example 2. A primigravida aged 26 years with a history of regular menstrual cycles. She received routine antenatal care starting at the 10th week of pregnancy. At 30-32 weeks, fetal growth retardation was noted clinically, and confirmed at 34 weeks. There was no evident cause apart from a symptomless bacteriuria. A caesarean section was performed and a liveborn boy weighing 1600 g was delivered. The placenta weighed 300 g and was described as infarcted. Respiratory distress syndrome developed which was responding to treatment. The baby died suddenly on the third day. Autopsy revealed extensive pulmonary hyaline membrane and massive intraventricular haemorrhage.

Causes of perinatal death:
   (a) Intraventricular haemorrhage
   (b) Respiratory distress syndrome
        Retarded fetal growth
   (c) Placental insufficiency
   (d) Bacteriuria in pregnancy
        Caesarean section
   (e) —

Example 3.   A known diabetic was controlled during her first pregnancy with difficulty. She developed megaloblastic anaemia at 32 weeks. Labour was induced at 38 weeks. There was spontaneous delivery of an infant weighing 3200 g. The baby developed hypoglycaemia. There was death on the second day. Autopsy showed truncus arteriosus.

Causes of perinatal death:
   (a) Truncus arteriosus
   (b) Hypoglycaemia
   (c) Diabetes
   (d) Megaloblastic anaemia
   (e) —

Example 4.   The patient was a 30 year old woman with a healthy four year old boy. There was a normal pregnancy apart from hydramnios. X-ray at 36 weeks suggested anencephaly. Labour was induced. A stillborn anencephalic fetus weighing 1500 g was delivered.

Causes of perinatal death:
   (a) Anencephaly
   (b) —
   (c) Hydramnios
   (d) —
   (e) —

Coding of causes of death

Each condition entered in sections (a), (b), (c) and (d) should be coded separately. Maternal conditions affecting the infant or fetus, entered in sections (c) and (d), should be coded to categories 760-763 and these codes should not be used for sections (a) and (b). Conditions in the fetus or infant, entered in sections (a) and (b), can be coded to any categories other than 760-763 but will most often be coded to categories 764-779 (Perinatal conditions) or 740-759 (Congenital anomalies). Only one code should be entered for sections (a) and (c), but for sections (b) and (d) as many codes should be entered as there are conditions reported.

Section (e) is provided not so much for statistical analysis as for review of individual perinatal deaths and will not therefore normally need to be coded. If, however, an attempt at statistical analysis of the circumstances entered in section (e) is desired, some suitable categories may exist in the E and V Codes; where this is not the case, users should devise their own coding system for this information.

The selection rules for general mortality do not apply to the perinatal death certificate. It may happen, however, that perinatal death certificates are received where the causes of death have not been entered in accordance with the guidelines on page 733. Such cases should, whenever possible, be referred to the certifier for correction, but where this is not possible, the following rules should be applied.

Rule P1.   Mode of death or prematurity entered in section (a). If heart cr cardiac failure, asphyxia or anoxia (any condition in 768.–) or prematurity (any condition in 765.–) is entered in section (*a*) and other conditions of the infant or fetus are entered either in sections (*a*) or (*b*), code the first-mentioned on these other conditions as if it had been entered alone in section (*a*) and code the condition actually entered in section (*a*) as if it had been entered in section (*b*).

Example 1: Liveborn; death at 4 days	Coding
(*a*) Prematurity	741.9
(*b*) Spina bifida	765.1
(*c*) Placental insufficiency	762.2
(*d*) —	

Prematurity is coded at (*b*) and spina bifida at (*a*).

Example 2: Liveborn; death at 50 minutes	Coding
(*a*) Severe birth asphyxia	742.3
Hydrocephalus	
(*b*) —	768.5
(*c*) Obstructed labour	763.1
(*d*) Severe pre-eclampsia	760.0

Severe birth asphyxia is coded at (*b*) and hydrocephalus at (*a*).

Rule P2.   Two or more conditions entered in sections (a) or (c). If two or more conditions are entered in section (*a*) or section (*c*), code the first-mentioned of these as if it had been entered alone in section (*a*) or (*c*) and code the others as if they had been entered in sections (*b*) or (*d*).

Example 3: Stillborn; death before onset of labour	Coding
(*a*) Severe fetal malnutrition	764.1
Light for dates	
Antepartum anoxia	
(*b*) —	768.0
(*c*) Toxaemia	760.0
Placenta praevia	
(*d*) —	762.0

Light for dates with fetal malnutrition is coded at (*a*) and antepartum anoxia at (*b*); toxaemia is coded at (*c*) and placenta praevia at (*d*).

Example 4: Liveborn; death at 2 days	Coding
(*a*) Subdural haemorrhage	767.0
Massive inhalation of meconium	
Intrauterine anoxia	

(b)	Hypoglycaemia	770.1
	Prolonged pregnancy	768.4
		775.6
		766.2
(c)	Toxaemia	760.0
(d)	Forceps delivery	763.2

Subdural haemorrhage is coded at (a) and the other conditions entered in (a) are coded at (b).

Rule P3. No entry in sections (a) or (c). If there is no entry in section (a) but there are conditions of the infant or fetus entered in section (b), code the first-mentioned of these as if it had been entered in section (a); if there are no entries in either section (a) or section (b), use code 779.9 (Unspecified perinatal cause) for section (a).

Similarly, if there is no entry in section (c) but there are maternal conditions entered in section (d), code the first-mentioned of these as if it had been entered in section (c); if there are no entries in either section (c) or section (d), use some artificial code (e.g. xxxx) for section (c) to indicate that no maternal condition was reported.

Example 5: Liveborn; death at 15 minutes   *Coding*

(a)	—	767.0
(b)	Tentorial tear	769
	Respiratory distress syndrome	
(c)	—	xxx.x
(d)	—	

Tentorial tear is coded at (a); xxx.x is coded at (c).

Example 6: Liveborn; death at 2 days   *Coding*

(a)	—	779.9
(b)	—	
(c)	—	760.0
(d)	Eclampsia (longstanding essential hypertension)	

Unspecified perinatal cause is coded at (a); eclampsia is coded at (c).

Rule P4. Conditions entered in wrong section. If a maternal condition (i.e. conditions in 760-763) is entered in sections (a) or (b) or if a condition of the infant or fetus is entered in sections (c) or (d), code the conditions as if they had been entered in the respective correct section.

If a condition classifiable as a condition of the infant or fetus or as a maternal condition is mistakenly entered in section (e), code it as an additional fetal or maternal condition in sections (b) or (d) respectively.

Example 7: Stillborn; death after onset of labour   *Coding*

(a)	Severe birth asphyxia	768.5
(b)	Persistent occipitoposterior	
(c)	—	763.1
(d)	—	763.2
(e)	Difficult forceps delivery	

Persistent occipitoposterior is coded at (c); difficult forceps delivery is coded at (d).

Rule P5.   Obstetrical complications recorded as causes of death before labour. If the certificate shows that the fetus died before the onset of labour and obstetrical complications that could not have affected the outcome are recorded as causes of death, ignore such causes.

Example 8:   Stillborn; death before onset of labour   *Coding*

   (*a*)   Anoxia   ·   768.0
   (*b*)   —
   (*c*)   Severe pre-eclampsia   760.0
   (*d*)   Accidental concealed antepartum haemorrhage   762.1
       Obesity   760.8
       Breech delivery

Breech delivery is not coded since the fetus died before labour started.

MORBIDITY

Earlier editions of the ICD, whilst making recommendations concerning the certification, and rules for the classification, of causes of mortality, have been silent on the subject of morbidity, leaving such methods and rules to be developed by individual users, or groups of users, of the classification.   This was partly in recognition of the diversity of types of medical record from which statistics and indexes based on the ICD are derived, and the fact that flexibility in recording and analysing the data is often essential.   Nevertheless, in many countries records of episodes of health care are now collected on a wide scale for routine analysis and the Ninth International Revision Conference considered that some recommendations for these kinds of statistics were now appropriate.

Mortality statistics are derived from medical certificates of causes of death which summarize the diseases, injuries and circumstances leading to death and, where there is more than one, categorize them so that one " underlying " cause can be selected for routine, single-cause analysis. Similarly, morbidity statistics relating to episodes of health-care are normally derived from a statistical abstract from each case-record.   In addition to personal details about the patient and administrative information, the statistical abstract sets out the diseases, injuries and other problems dealt with during the relevant episode of health care, and sometimes records the treatment given, especially surgery.   Until now, there has been no standard procedure, where more than one disease, injury or problem was present, of selecting one of them to be processed for routine, single-condition statistics.

The Conference accordingly made the following recommendations:

(i)   the condition to be selected for single-cause analysis from records of episodes of hospital or other health-care is the main condition treated or investigated during the relevant episode; if no diagnosis was made, the main symptom or problem should be selected;

(ii) the record should also show, separately, other conditions or problems dealt with during the relevant episode of care;

(iii) whenever possible, the choice of the main diagnosis, symptom or problem for tabulation should be exercised by the responsible medical practitioner or other health-care professional.

The Conference also considered it desirable that in addition to the selection of a single cause for tabulation purposes, multiple condition coding and analysis should be attempted wherever possible, particularly for data relating to episodes of health-care by hospitals (inpatient or outpatient), health clinics and family practitioners. For certain other types of data, such as from health examination surveys, multiple-condition analysis may be the only satisfactory method.

Recording of diagnoses for entry on case-record statistical abstract

In the majority of cases, by the end of an episode of hospital or other health care, some kind of diagnostic " labels " will have been formulated in relation to the various diseases, injuries, symptoms and problems which were dealt with. These have to be " captured " from the clinical information within the medical record itself for entry on the statistical abstract, where the " main " diagnosis treated or investigated during the relevant episode is to be distinguished from other diagnoses. The process is greatly facilitated if the information within the medical record is organized systematically and if standard recording methods are used which allow the responsible medical practitioner to indicate his choice of the " main " and " other " diagnoses, in conformity with the Revision Conference's recommendation. It is the concept of " main condition treated or investigated " which is important. The actual title may vary locally.

Each diagnostic label entered on the abstract should be as informative as possible and should include whatever detail is available about the site, variety, aetiology, etc. of a condition, e.g. transitional cell carcinoma of bladder; acute appendicitis, perforated; diabetic retinitis; cerebral degeneration associated with advanced carcinoma of uterus.

If the patient is treated or investigated on account of some symptom, sign or other abnormal finding which remains unexplained at the end of the episode of care, the symptom, sign or finding itself should be recorded as a " diagnosis ".

If an episode of care (including occupation of a hospital bed, consultation with a medical practitioner or other health-care professional) relates to some problem or circumstance which is not in itself a medical condition (e.g. prophylactic vaccination, plastic surgery for purely cosmetic reasons) or if some nonmedical circumstance or past history is thought to affect a patient's condition, these problems or circumstances may appear as " diagnoses ".

If a patient commences a spell of care for one condition, and the spell of care is prolonged by the necessity for treatment of an independent condition arising or discovered during treatment for the original condition, the condition " consuming " the greater amount of medical resources will usually be regarded as the " main " condition. Local development of standard recording methods, incorporating the above criteria and accompanied by relevant definitions, is to be encouraged.

Coding of the main condition treated or investigated, for single-cause analysis

The main condition treated or investigated, which is the one to be selected and coded, will already have been identified in the case-record statistical abstract and coding is in most cases straightforward.

Some abstracts may be received for coding in which the condition identified as the main condition treated or investigated appears to be grossly inconsistent with other information contained in the abstract, such as the specialty or other service responsible, the investigations or operations performed or the length of time under care, or is otherwise incorrectly completed. Examples of obviously incorrect selection are as follows:

(i) a minor condition is recorded as the main condition and a more significant condition, relevant to the specialty which cared for the patient and the treatment given, is recorded as an " other " condition;

(ii) several conditions are listed in the part of the record intended for the main condition;

(iii) the condition recorded as the main condition is obviously the presenting symptom of a diagnosed disease for which treatment was given;

(iv) a symptom or ill-defined condition (usually a condition codeable to Chapter XVI of ICD), is the only condition recorded, but other information in the abstract makes it seem likely that the cause of the symptom was found and treated.

Such cases should, whenever possible, be returned for correction to the person who abstracted the information from the original case-record. Where this is not possible, the following rules should be applied:

Rule MB1. Minor condition recorded as main condition ; treated, more significant condition recorded as " other " condition.

Where a minor or longstanding condition, or an incidental problem is recorded as the main condition, and a more significant condition, relevant to the specialty which cared for the patient and/or the treatment given, is recorded as an " other " condition, select the latter as the main condition.

Example 1:   Main condition: Acute sinusitis
             Other conditions: Carcinoma of endocervix
                                  Hypertension
             Patient in hospital for three weeks:
             Operation performed — total hysterectomy
             Specialty — gynaecology

Select carcinoma of endocervix (180.0)

Example 2:   Main condition: Rheumatoid arthritis
             Other conditions: Diabetes mellitus
                                  Strangulated femoral hernia
                                  Generalized arteriosclerosis
             Patient in hospital for three weeks
             Operation performed — herniorrhaphy
             Specialty — gastroenterological surgery

Select strangulated femoral hernia (552.0)

Example 3:   Main condition: Kidney graft in situ
             Other conditions: Impacted wisdom tooth
             Specialty — dentistry
             Procedure — removal of wisdom tooth

Select impacted wisdom tooth (520.6)

Example 4:   Main condition: Dental caries
             Other conditions: Rheumatic mitral stenosis
             Specialty — dentistry
             Procedure — dental extractions

Select dental caries (521.0). The rule does not apply. Although dental caries can be regarded as a minor condition and rheumatic mitral stenosis as a more significant condition, the latter was not the condition treated during this episode of care, and the abstract should not be questioned.

Rule MB2.   Several conditions listed under " main condition ".

If several conditions are listed in the part of the abstract intended for the main condition and other details on the record point to one of them as being obviously the main condition for which the patient received care, select that condition. Otherwise select the first mentioned.

Example 1:   Main condition: Dental caries
                                  Syphilitic meningitis
                                  Ischaemic heart disease
             Other conditions: —
             Patient in hospital for five weeks
             Specialty — neurology

Select syphilitic meningitis (094.2)

Example 2:   Main condition: Chronic obstructive bronchitis
                                  Hypertrophy of prostate
                                  Psoriasis
             Patient in the care of a dermatologist
             Twelve visits in a six-months' spell of care

Select psoriasis (696.1)

Example 3:   Main condition: Mitral stenosis
                                   Acute bronchitis
                                   Rheumatoid arthritis
             Other conditions: —
             Specialty — general medicine
             No information about therapy

Select mitral stenosis (394.0)

Rule MB3.   Condition recorded as the main condition obviously the presenting symptom of a diagnosed, treated condition

If a symptom or sign (usually a condition classifiable to Chapter XVI of ICD), or a problem classifiable to the Supplementary Classification (V code), is entered as the main condition and this is obviously the presenting sign, symptom or problem of a diagnosed condition listed on the record as an " other " condition, and care was given for the latter, select the diagnosed condition.

Example 1:   Main condition: Haematuria
             Other conditions: Papillomata of posterior wall of bladder
                                  Varicose veins of legs
             Specialty — genitourinary medicine
             Treatment — diathermy excision of papillomata

Select papillomata of posterior wall of bladder (188.4)

Example 2:   Main condition: Abnormal glucose tolerance test
             Other conditions: Ischaemic heart disease
                                  Otosclerosis
                                  Diabetes mellitus
             Specialty — endocrinology
             Care — establishment of correct dose of insulin

Select diabetes mellitus (250.0)

Rule MB4.   Specificity

Where the " main " diagnosis describes a condition in general terms and a term which provides more precise information about the site or nature of this condition is reported amongst the " other " diagnoses, select the latter condition.

Example 1:   Main condition: Cerebrovascular accident
             Other conditions: Diabetes mellitus
                                  Hypertension
                                  Cerebral haemorrhage

Select cerebral haemorrhage (431).

Example 2:   Main condition: Congenital heart disease
             Other conditions: Interventricular septal defect

Select interventricular septal defect (745.4).

Example 3:   Main condition: Enteritis
             Other conditions: Crohn's disease of ileum

Select Crohn's disease of ileum (555.0).

SPECIAL TABULATION LISTS

Basic Tabulation List

Mortality List of 50 Causes

Morbidity List of 50 Causes

The special tabulation lists which follow have been adopted by the World Health Assembly under Article 23 of the Constitution of the World Health Organization (*Off. Rec. Wld Hlth Org.*, 1976, **233**, 18).

SPECIAL TABULATION LISTS

The Lists A, B, C, D and P of the Eighth Revision have been replaced by a more flexible system allowing users to construct their own tabulation lists from the rubrics of a basic list. The Basic Tabulation List consists of 57 two-digit rubrics which add up to the " all causes " total. Within each two-digit rubric, up to 9 three-digit rubrics are identified, but these do *not* add up to the total of the two-digit rubric; if the frequency for the residue of the two-digit rubric is required it must be calculated as the difference between the two-digit total and the sum of its three-digit rubrics. The 10th three-digit rubric is always vacant so that any user can display some other item or items contained in the two-digit rubric; these should be given the numbers —9.0, —9.1, etc. The basic list contains 307 two- and three-digit rubrics and is intended to replace the previous lists A and D.

For the national display of mortality and morbidity data, countries are free to use any lists constructed from the items of the basic list, but to ensure a minimum of international comparability, any tabulation lists used for these purposes should contain the 50 rubrics of the attached Mortality and Morbidity Lists, which replace the previous lists B and C.

Where a diagnostic statement includes information about both aetiology and clinical manifestation, the Ninth Revision of the ICD provides two assignments, one according to aetiology and one according to manifestation, identified by the symbols † and * respectively (e.g. tuberculous meningitis 013.0† and 320.4*). Any list used for mortality data must be based on coding according to aetiology (†). Morbidity lists may be based on either coding method, but it is essential that the method used (aetiology or manifestation) be clearly stated when publishing the data, as frequency distributions from the same data would obviously vary considerably according to the method used (see Introduction, page XXVI).

BASIC TABULATION LIST

01	Intestinal infectious diseases	001-009
	010 Cholera	001
	011 Typhoid fever	002.0
	012 Shigellosis	004
	013 Food poisoning	003, 005
	014 Amoebiasis	006
	015 Intestinal infections due to other specified organism	007, 008
	016 Ill-defined intestinal infections	009

02	Tuberculosis	010-018
	020 Pulmonary tuberculosis	011
	021 Other respiratory tuberculosis	010, 012
	022 Tuberculosis of meninges and central nervous system	013
	023 Tuberculosis of intestines, peritoneum and mesenteric glands	014
	024 Tuberculosis of bones and joints	015
	025 Tuberculosis of genitourinary system	016

03	Other bacterial diseases	020-041
	030 Plague	020
	031 Brucellosis	023
	032 Leprosy	030
	033 Diphtheria	032
	034 Whooping cough	033
	035 Streptococcal sore throat, scarlatina and erysipelas	034, 035
	036 Meningococcal infection	036
	037 Tetanus	037
	038 Septicaemia	038

04	Viral diseases	045-079
	040 Acute poliomyelitis	045
	041 Smallpox	050
	042 Measles	055
	043 Rubella	056
	044 Yellow fever	060
	045 Arthropod-borne encephalitis	062-064
	046 Viral hepatitis	070
	047 Rabies	071
	048 Trachoma	076

05	Rickettsiosis and other arthropod-borne diseases		080-088
	050	Louse-borne typhus	080
	051	Other rickettsiosis	081-083
	052	Malaria	084
	053	Leishmaniasis	085
	054	Trypanosomiasis	086

06	Venereal diseases		090-099
	060	Syphilis	090-097
	061	Gonococcal infections	098

07 Other infectious and parasitic diseases and late effects of
infectious and parasitic diseases   100-139

	070	Non-syphilitic spirochaetal diseases	100-104
	071	Mycosis	110-118
	072	Schistosomiasis	120
	073	Echinococcosis	122
	074	Filarial infection and dracontiasis	125
	075	Ancylostomiasis and necatoriasis	126
	076	Other helminthiasis	121, 123, 124 127-129
	077	Late effects of tuberculosis	137
	078	Late effects of acute poliomyelitis	138

08	Malignant neoplasm of lip, oral cavity and pharynx		140-149

09	Malignant neoplasm of digestive organs and peritoneum		150-159
	090	Malignant neoplasm of oesophagus	150
	091	Malignant neoplasm of stomach	151
	092	Malignant neoplasm of small intestine, including duodenum	152
	093	Malignant neoplasm of colon	153
	094	Malignant neoplasm of rectum, rectosigmoid junction and anus	154
	095	Malignant neoplasm of liver, specified as primary	155.0
	096	Malignant neoplasm of pancreas	157

10	Malignant neoplasm of respiratory and intrathoracic organs		160-165
	100	Malignant neoplasm of larynx	161
	101	Malignant neoplasm of trachea, bronchus and lung	162

11		Malignant neoplasm of bone, connective tissue, skin and breast	170-175
	110	Malignant neoplasm of bone and articular cartilage	170
	111	Malignant melanoma of skin	172
	112	Other malignant neoplasm of skin	173
	113	Malignant neoplasm of female breast	174
12		Malignant neoplasm of genitourinary organs	179-189
	120	Malignant neoplasm of cervix uteri	180
	121	Malignant neoplasm of placenta	181
	122	Malignant neoplasm of uterus, other and unspecified	179, 182
	123	Malignant neoplasm of ovary and other uterine adnexa	183
	124	Malignant neoplasm of prostate	185
	125	Malignant neoplasm of testis	186
	126	Malignant neoplasm of bladder	188
13		Malignant neoplasm of other and unspecified sites	190-199
	130	Malignant neoplasm of brain	191
14		Malignant neoplasm of lymphatic and haemopoietic tissue	200-208
	140	Hodgkin's disease	201
	141	Leukaemia	204-208
15		Benign neoplasm	210-229
	150	Benign neoplasm of skin	216
	151	Benign neoplasm of breast	217
	152	Benign neoplasm of uterus	218, 219
	153	Benign neoplasm of ovary	220
	154	Benign neoplasm of kidney and other urinary organs	223
	155	Benign neoplasm of nervous system	225
	156	Benign neoplasm of thyroid	226
16		Carcinoma in situ	230-234
17		Other and unspecified neoplasm	235-239
18		Endocrine and metabolic diseases, immunity disorders	{ 240-259 270-279
	180	Disorders of thyroid gland	240-246
	181	Diabetes mellitus	250
	182	Hyperlipoproteinaemia	272.0, 272.1
	183	Obesity of non-endocrine origin	278.0

19	Nutritional deficiencies	260-269
190	Kwashiorkor	260
191	Nutritional marasmus	261
192	Other protein-calorie malnutrition	262, 263
193	Avitaminosis	264-269

20	Diseases of blood and blood-forming organs	280-289
200	Anaemias	280-285

21	Mental disorders	290-319
210	Senile and presenile organic psychotic conditions	290
211	Schizophrenic psychoses	295
212	Affective psychoses	296
213	Other psychoses	291-294 297-299
214	Neurotic and personality disorders	300, 301
215	Alcohol dependence syndrome	303
216	Drug dependence	304
217	Physiological malnutrition arising from mental factors	306
218	Mental retardation	317-319

22	Diseases of the nervous system	320-359
220	Meningitis	320-322
221	Parkinson's disease	332
222	Other degenerative and hereditary disorders of the central nervous system	330, 331, 333-336
223	Multiple sclerosis	340
224	Infantile cerebral palsy and other paralytic syndromes	343, 344
225	Epilepsy	345

23	Disorders of the eye and adnexa	360-379
230	Glaucoma	365
231	Cataract	366
232	Blindness and low vision	369
233	Conjunctivitis	372.0-372.3
234	Disorders of lacrimal system	375
235	Strabismus and other disorders of binocular eye movements	378

24	Diseases of the ear and mastoid process	380-389
240	Otitis media and mastoiditis	381-383
241	Deafness	389

25   Rheumatic fever and rheumatic heart disease   390-398

    250   Acute rheumatic fever   390-392
    251   Chronic rheumatic heart disease   393-398

26   Hypertensive disease   401-405

    260   Hypertensive heart disease   402, 404

27   Ischaemic heart disease   410-414

    270   Acute myocardial infarction   410

28   Diseases of pulmonary circulation and other forms of heart
      disease   415-429

    280   Pulmonary embolism   415.1
    281   Cardiac dysrhythmias   427

29   Cerebrovascular disease   430-438

    290   Subarachnoid haemorrhage   430
    291   Intracerebral and other intracranial haemorrhage   431, 432
    292   Cerebral infarction   433, 434
    293   Acute but ill-defined cerebrovascular disease   436
    294   Cerebral atherosclerosis   437.0

30   Other diseases of the circulatory system   440-459

    300   Atherosclerosis   440
    301   Arterial embolism and thrombosis   444
    302   Other diseases of arteries, arterioles and capillaries   { 441-443, 446-448
    303   Phlebitis, thrombophlebitis, venous embolism and
          thrombosis   451-453
    304   Varicose veins of lower extremities   454
    305   Haemorrhoids   455

31   Diseases of the upper respiratory tract   { 460-465, 470-478

    310   Acute tonsillitis   463
    311   Acute laryngitis and tracheitis   464
    312   Other acute upper respiratory infections   { 460-462, 465
    313   Deflected nasal septum and nasal polyps   470, 471
    314   Chronic pharyngitis, nasopharyngitis and sinusitis   472, 473
    315   Chronic diseases of tonsils and adenoids   474

32	Other diseases of the respiratory system	{ 466, 480-519
	320 Acute bronchitis and bronchiolitis	466
	321 Pneumonia	480-486
	322 Influenza	487
	323 Bronchitis, chronic and unspecified, emphysema and asthma	490-493
	324 Bronchiectasis	494
	325 Other chronic obstructive pulmonary disease	495, 496
	326 Pneumoconiosis and other lung disease due to external agents	500-508
	327 Pleurisy	511
33	Diseases of oral cavity, salivary glands and jaws	520-529
	330 Diseases of teeth and supporting structures	520-525
	331 Diseases of the jaws	526
34	Diseases of other parts of the digestive system	530-579
	340 Diseases of oesophagus	530
	341 Ulcer of stomach and duodenum	531-533
	342 Appendicitis	540-543
	343 Hernia of abdominal cavity	550-553
	344 Intestinal obstruction without mention of hernia	560
	345 Diverticula of intestine	562
	346 Other functional digestive disorders	564
	347 Chronic liver disease and cirrhosis	571
	348 Cholelithiasis and cholecystitis	574-575.1
35	Diseases of urinary system	580-599
	350 Nephritis, nephrotic syndrome and nephrosis	580-589
	351 Infections of kidney	590
	352 Urinary calculus	592, 594
	353 Cystitis	595
36	Diseases of male genital organs	600-608
	360 Hyperplasia of prostate	600
	361 Hydrocele	603
	362 Redundant prepuce and phimosis	605
	363 Infertility, male	606
37	Diseases of female genital organs	610-629
	370 Diseases of breast	610, 611
	371 Salpingitis and oophoritis	614.0-614.2

	372	Inflammatory diseases of pelvic cellular tissue and peritoneum	614.3-614.9
	373	Inflammatory diseases of uterus, vagina and vulva	615, 616
	374	Uterovaginal prolapse	618
	375	Menstrual disorders	626.0-626.5
	376	Infertility, female	628
38	Abortion		630-639
	380	Spontaneous abortion	634
	381	Legally induced abortion	635
	382	Illegally induced abortion	636
39	Direct obstetric causes		640-646, 651-676
	390	Haemorrhage of pregnancy and childbirth	640, 641 666
	391	Toxaemia of pregnancy	642.4-642.9 643
	392	Infections of genitourinary tract in pregnancy	646.6
	393	Obstructed labour	660
	394	Complications of the puerperium	670-676
40	Indirect obstetric causes		647, 648
41	Normal delivery		650
42	Diseases of skin and subcutaneous tissue		680-709
	420	Infections of skin and subcutaneous tissue	680-686
43	Diseases of the musculoskeletal system and connective tissue		710-739
	430	Rheumatoid arthritis, except spine	714
	431	Other arthropathies	710-713 715, 716
	432	Other disorders of joints	717-719
	433	Ankylosing spondylitis	720.0
	434	Other dorsopathies	720.1-724
	435	Rheumatism, excluding the back	725-729
	436	Osteomyelitis, periostitis and other infections involving bone	730
	437	Acquired deformities of limbs	734-736
44	Congenital anomalies		740-759
	440	Spina bifida and hydrocephalus	741, 742.3
	441	Other deformities of central nervous system	740 742.0-742.2 742.4-742.9

	442	Congenital anomalies of heart and circulatory system	745-747
	443	Cleft palate and cleft lip	749
	444	Other deformities of digestive system	750, 751
	445	Undescended testicle	752.5
	446	Congenital dislocation of hip	754.3
	447	Other congenital anomalies of musculoskeletal system	{ 754.0-754.2 754.4-756
45		Certain conditions originating in the perinatal period	760-779
	450	Maternal conditions affecting fetus or newborn	760
	451	Obstetric complications affecting fetus or newborn	761-763
	452	Slow fetal growth, fetal malnutrition and immaturity	764, 765
	453	Birth trauma	767
	454	Hypoxia, birth asphyxia and other respiratory conditions	768-770
	455	Haemolytic disease of fetus or newborn	773
46		Signs, symptoms and ill-defined conditions	780-799
	460	Pyrexia of unknown origin	780.6
	461	Symptoms involving heart	785.0-785.3
	462	Renal colic	788.0
	463	Retention of urine	788.2
	464	Abdominal pain	789.0
	465	Senility without mention of psychosis	797
	466	Sudden infant death syndrome	798.0
	467	Respiratory failure	799.1
47		Fractures	800-829
	470	Fracture of skull and face	800-804
	471	Fracture of neck and trunk	805-809
	472	Fracture of humerus, radius and ulna	812, 813
	473	Fracture of neck of femur	820
	474	Fracture of other parts of femur	821
	475	Fracture of tibia, fibula and ankle	823, 824
	476	Other fractures of limbs	{ 810-811 814-819 822, 825 829
48		Dislocations, sprains and strains	830-848
49		Intracranial and internal injuries, including nerves	{ 850-869, 950-957
	490	Concussion	850
	491	Other intracranial injuries	{ 851-854 950-951

50	Open wounds and injury to blood vessels	870-904
	500 Open wound of eye, ear and head	870-873
	501 Open wound of upper limb	880-887
	502 Open wound of lower limb	890-897
51	Effects of foreign body entering through orifice	930-939
52	Burns	940-949
	520 Burn confined to eye and adnexa	940
	521 Burn of wrist and hand	944
53	Poisonings and toxic effects	960-989
	530 Medicinal agents	960-979
54	Complications of medical and surgical care	996-999
55	Other injuries, early complications of trauma	910-929 958-959 990-995
56	Late effects of injuries, of poisonings, of toxic effects and of other external causes	905-909
E47	Transport accidents	E800-E848
	E470 Railway accidents	E800-E807
	E471 Motor vehicle traffic accidents	E810-E819
	E472 Other road vehicle accidents	E826-E829
	E473 Water transport accidents	E830-E838
	E474 Air and space transport accidents	E840-E845
E48	Accidental poisoning	E850-E869
	E480 Accidental poisoning by drugs, medicaments and biologicals	E850-E858
	E481 Accidental poisoning by other solid and liquid substances	E860-E866
	E482 Accidental poisoning by gases and vapours	E867-E869
E49	Misadventures during medical care, abnormal reactions, late complications	E870-E879
E50	Accidental falls	E880-E888
E51	Accidents caused by fire and flames	E890-E899
E52	Other accidents, including late effects	E900-E929
	E520 Accidents due to natural and environmental factors	E900-E909
	E521 Accidental drowning and submersion	E910
	E522 Foreign body accidentally entering orifice	E914, E915
	E523 Accidents caused by machinery, and by cutting and piercing instruments	E919, E920
	E524 Accidents caused by firearm missile	E922

E53   Drugs, medicaments causing adverse effects in therapeutic use   E930-E949

E54   Suicide and self-inflicted injury   E950-E959

E55   Homicide and injury purposely inflicted by other persons   E960-E969

E56   Other violence   E970-E999

    E560   Injury undetermined whether accidentally or purposely inflicted   E980-E989

    E561   Injury resulting from operation of war   E990-E999

V0   Other reasons for contact with health services   V00-V82

    V01   Supervision of pregnancy and puerperium   V22-V24

    V02   Healthy liveborn infants   V30-V39

    V03   Persons encountering health services for specific procedures and aftercare   V50-V59

    V04   Persons encountering health services for psychosocial reasons   V60-V62

    V05   Examinations and investigations of individuals and populations   V70-V82

MORTALITY LIST

01-56	All causes of death	001-999
01-07	Infectious and parasitic diseases	001-139
01	Intestinal infectious diseases	001-009
02	Tuberculosis	010-018
034	Whooping cough	033
036	Meningococcal infection	036
037	Tetanus	037
038	Septicaemia	038
041	Smallpox	050
042	Measles	055
052	Malaria	084
08-14	Malignant neoplasms	140-208
091	Malignant neoplasm of stomach	151
093	Malignant neoplasm of colon	153
094	Malignant neoplasm of rectum, rectosigmoid junction and anus	154
101	Malignant neoplasm of trachea, bronchus and lung	162
113	Malignant neoplasm of female breast	174
120	Malignant neoplasm of cervix uteri	180
141	Leukaemia	204-208
181	Diabetes mellitus	250
191	Nutritional marasmus	261
192	Other protein-calorie malnutrition	262, 263
200	Anaemias	280-285
220	Meningitis	320-322
25-30	Diseases of the circulatory system	390-459
250	Acute rheumatic fever	390-392
251	Chronic rheumatic heart disease	393-398
26	Hypertensive disease	401-405
27	Ischaemic heart disease	410-414
270	Acute myocardial infarction	410
29	Cerebrovascular disease	430-438
300	Atherosclerosis	440
321	Pneumonia	480-486
322	Influenza	487
323	Bronchitis, emphysema and asthma	490-493
341	Ulcer of stomach and duodenum	531-533
342	Appendicitis	540-543
347	Chronic liver disease and cirrhosis	571

350	Nephritis, nephrotic syndrome and nephrosis	500-589
360	Hyperplasia of prostate	600
38	Abortion	630-639
39	Direct obstetric deaths	{ 640-646 651-676
44	Congenital anomalies	740-759
45	Certain conditions originating in the perinatal period	760-779
453	Birth trauma	767
46	Signs, symptoms and ill-defined conditions	780-799
47-56	Injury and poisoning	800-999
47	Fractures	800-829
49	Intracranial and internal injuries, including nerves	{ 850-869 950-957
52	Burns	940-949
53	Poisonings and toxic effects	960-989
E47-E53	Accidents and adverse effects	E800-E949
E471	Motor vehicle traffic accidents	E810-E819
E50	Accidental falls	E880-E888
E54	Suicide	E950-E959
E55	Homicide	E960-E969

MORBIDITY LIST

01-56	All causes of morbidity	001-999
01 ·	Intestinal infectious diseases	001-009
02	Tuberculosis	010-018
036	Meningococcal infection	036
042	Measles	055
052	Malaria	084
06	Venereal diseases	090-099
08-14	Malignant neoplasms	140-208
091	Malignant neoplasm of stomach	151
093	Malignant neoplasm of colon	153
094	Malignant neoplasm of rectum, rectosigmoid junction and anus	154
101	Malignant neoplasm of trachea, bronchus and lung	162
113	Malignant neoplasm of female breast	174
120	Malignant neoplasm of cervix uteri	180
141	Leukaemia	204-208
152	Benign neoplasm of uterus	218, 219
180	Diseases of thyroid gland	240-246
181	Diabetes mellitus	250
19	Nutritional deficiencies	260-269
21	Mental disorders	290-319
223	Multiple sclerosis	340
23	Diseases of eye and adnexa	360-379
24	Diseases of ear and mastoid process	380-389
25-30	Diseases of the circulatory system	390-459
251	Chronic rheumatic heart disease	393-398
26	Hypertensive disease	401-405
270	Acute myocardial infarction	410
29	Cerebrovascular disease	430-438
304	Varicose veins of lower extremities	454
315	Chronic diseases of tonsils and adenoids	474
321	Pneumonia	480-486
322	Influenza	487
323	Bronchitis, emphysema and asthma	490-493
330	Diseases of teeth and supporting structures	520-525
341	Ulcer of stomach and duodenum	531-533
342	Appendicitis	540-543
343	Hernia of abdominal cavity	550-553
35	Diseases of urinary system	580-599

360	Hyperplasia of prostate	600
371	Salpingitis and oophoritis	614.0-614.2
374	Uterovaginal prolapse	618
38	Abortion	630-639
39	Direct obstetric conditions	{ 640-646 651-676
41	Normal delivery	650
43	Diseases of the musculoskeletal system and connective tissue	710-739
44	Congenital anomalies	740-759
47-56	Injury and poisoning	800-999
47	Fractures	800-829
49	Intracranial and internal injuries, including nerves	{ 850-869 950-957
52	Burns	940-949
53	Poisonings and toxic effects	960-989
E47-E53	Accidents and adverse effects	E800-E949
E471	Motor vehicle traffic accidents	E810-E819
E50	Accidental falls	E880-E888
E54	Suicide and self-inflicted injury	E950-E959
E55	Homicide and injury purposely inflicted by other persons	E960-E969

DEFINITIONS
AND RECOMMENDATIONS

The following definitions and recommendations have been adopted by the World Health Assembly under Article 23 of the Constitution of the World Health Organization (*Off. Rec. Wld Hlth Org.,* 1950, **28**, 17, 1967, **160**, 11 and Annex 18, and 1976, **233**, 18).

DEFINITIONS AND RECOMMENDATIONS

Definitions

1. *Live birth*

Live birth is the complete expulsion or extraction from its mother of a product of conception, irrespective of the duration of the pregnancy, which, after such separation, breathes or shows any other evidence of life, such as beating of the heart, pulsation of the umbilical cord, or definite movement of voluntary muscles, whether or not the umbilical cord has been cut or the placenta is attached; each product of such a birth is considered live born.

2. *Fetal death*

Fetal death is death prior to the complete expulsion or extraction from its mother of a product of conception, irrespective of the duration of pregnancy; the death is indicated by the fact that after such separation the fetus does not breathe or show any other evidence of life, such as beating of the heart, pulsation of the umbilical cord, or definite movement of voluntary muscles.

3. *Causes of death*

The causes of death to be entered on the medical certificate of cause of death are all those diseases, morbid conditions or injuries which either resulted in or contributed to death and the circumstances of the accident or violence which produced any such injuries.

4. *Underlying cause of death*

The underlying cause of death is (a) the disease or injury which initiated the train of events leading directly to death, or (b) the circumstances of the accident or violence which produced the fatal injury.

5. *Birthweight*

The first weight of the fetus or newborn obtained after birth. This weight should be measured preferably within the first hour of life before significant postnatal weight loss has occurred.

6. *Low birthweight*

Less than 2500 g (up to, and including 2499 g).

7. *Gestational age*

The duration of gestation is measured from the first day of the last normal menstrual period. Gestational age is expressed in completed days or completed weeks (e.g. events occurring 280 to 286 days after the onset of the last normal menstrual period are considered to have occurred at 40 weeks of gestation).

Measurements of fetal growth, as they represent continuous variables, are expressed in relation to a specific week of gestational age (e.g. the mean birthweight for 40 weeks is that obtained at 280-286 days of gestation on a weight-for-gestational age curve).

8. *Pre-term*

Less than 37 completed weeks (less than 259 days).

9. *Term*
From 37 to less than 42 completed weeks (259 to 293 days).

10. *Post-term*

Forty-two completed weeks or more (294 days or more).

11. *Maternal mortality*

A maternal death is defined as the death of a woman while pregnant or within 42 days of termination of pregnancy, irrespective of the duration and the site of the pregnancy, from any cause related to or aggravated by the pregnancy or its management but not from accidental or incidental causes.

Maternal deaths should be subdivided into two groups:

(1) Direct obstetric deaths: those resulting from obstetric complications of the pregnant state (pregnancy, labour and puerperium), from interventions, omissions, incorrect treatment, or from a chain of events resulting from any of the above.

(2) Indirect obstetric deaths: those resulting from previous existing disease or disease that developed during pregnancy and which was not due to direct obstetric causes, but which was aggravated by physiologic effects of pregnancy.

Recommendations

1. *Responsibility for medical certification of cause of death*

Medical certification of cause of death should normally be the responsibility of the attending physician. In the case of deaths certified by coroners or other legal authorities, the medical evidence supplied to the certifier should be stated on the certificate in addition to any legal findings.

2. Form of medical certificate of cause of death

The forms of medical certificate of cause of death should conform to the models appended [1] to these recommendations.

3. Confidentiality of medical information

In the statistical use of the medical certificate of cause of death and other medical records, administrative procedures should provide such safeguards as are necessary to preserve the confidential nature of the information given by the physician.

4. Selection of the cause for mortality tabulation

For the purpose of single-cause mortality coding, the cause for tabulation should be selected from the particulars entered on the medical certificate of cause of death in accordance with such rules as may be from time to time approved by the Assembly.

5. Use of the International Classification of Diseases

Mortality and morbidity statistics should be coded according to the Detailed List of three-digit categories of the International Classification of Diseases, with or without the fourth-digit sub-categories, using for the purpose the tabular list of inclusions and the alphabetical index. Save in exceptional circumstances, fourth-digit sub-categories, when published, should be those of the International Classification of Diseases; any additions or variations should be indicated in published statistical tables.

6. Perinatal mortality statistics

It is recommended that *national* perinatal statistics should include all fetuses and infants delivered weighing at least 500 g (or, when birth-weight is unavailable, the corresponding gestational age (22 weeks) or body length (25 cm crown-heel)), whether alive or dead. It is recognized that legal requirements in many countries may set different criteria for registration purposes, but it is hoped that countries will arrange the registration or reporting procedures in such a way that the events required for inclusion in the statistics can be identified easily. It is further recommended that less mature fetuses and infants should be excluded from perinatal statistics unless there are legal or other valid reasons to the contrary.

It is recommended above that national statistics should include fetuses and infants weighing between 500 g and 1000 g, both for their inherent value and because their inclusion improves the completeness of

---

[1] See pages 701 and 732.

reporting at 1000 g and over. Inclusion of this group of very immature births, however, disrupts international comparisons because of differences in national practices concerning their registration. Another factor affecting international comparisons is that all live-born infants, irrespective of birthweight, are included in the calculation of rates, whereas some lower limit of maturity is applied to infants born dead.

In order to eliminate these factors, it is recommended that countries should present, solely for *international* comparisons, " standard perinatal statistics " in which both the numerator and denominator of all rates are restricted to fetuses and infants weighing 1000 g or more (or, where birthweight is unavailable, the corresponding gestational age (28 weeks) or body length (35 cm crown-heel)).

7. *Maternal mortality statistics*

The maternal mortality rate, the direct obstetric death rate and the indirect obstetric death rate should be expressed as rates per 1000 live-births.

8. *Statistical tables*

The degree of detail in cross-classification by cause, sex, age, and area of territory will depend partly on the purpose and range of the statistics and partly on the practical limits as regards the size of particular tables. The following patterns, designed to promote international comparability, consist of standard ways of expressing various characteristics. Where a different classification is used (e.g., in age-grouping) in published tables, it should be so arranged as to be reducible to one of the recommended groupings.

(*a*) *Analysis by the International Classification of Diseases* should, as appropriate, be in accordance with:

    (i) the Detailed List of three-digit categories, with or without fourth-digit sub-categories;

    (ii) the Basic Tabulation List of 307 Causes;

    (iii) the Mortality List of 50 Causes;

    (iv) the Morbidity List of 50 Causes.

(*b*) *Age classification for general purposes*

    (i) Under 1 year, single years to 4 years, 5 year groups from 5 to 84 years, 85 years and over;

    (ii) Under 1 year, 1-4 years, 5-14 years, 15-24 years, 25-34 years, 35-44 years, 45-54 years, 55-64 years, 65-74 years, 75 years and over;

    (iii) Under 1 year, 1-14 years, 15-44 years, 45-64 years, 65 years and over.

(c) *Age classification for special statistics of infant mortaliy*

   (i) By single days for the first week of life (under 24 hours, 1, 2, 3, 4, 5, 6 days), 7-13 days, 14-20 days, 21-27 days, 28 days up to, but not including, 2 months, by single months of life from 2 months to 1 year (2, 3, 4 . . . 11 months);

   (ii) Under 24 hours, 1-6 days, 7-26 days, 28 days up to, but not including, 3 months, 3-5 months, 6 months but under 1 year;

   (iii) Under 7 days, 7-27 days, 28 days but under 1 year.

(d) *Age classification for early neonatal deaths*

   (i) Under 1 hour, 1-11 hours, 12-23 hours, 24-47 hours, 48-71 hours, 72-167 hours;

   (ii) Under 1 hour, 1-23 hours, 24-167 hours.

(e) *Birthweight classification for perinatal mortality statistics*

By weight intervals of 500 g, i.e. 1000-1499 g, 1500-1999 g, etc.

(f) *Gestational age classification for perinatal mortality statistics*

Under 28 weeks (under 196 days), 28-31 weeks (196-223 days), 32-36 weeks (224-258 days), 37-41 weeks (259-293 days), 42 weeks and over (294 days and over).

(g) *Classification by area* should, as appropriate, be in accordance with:

   (i) each major civil division;

   (ii) each town or conurbation of 1 000 000 population and over, otherwise the largest town with a population of at least 100 000;

   (iii) national aggregate of urban areas of 100 000 population and over;

   (iv) national aggregate of urban areas of less than 100 000 population;

   (v) national aggregate of rural areas.

Note 1. Statistics relating to (iii), (iv) and (v) should be accompanied by the definitions of urban and rural used in them.

Note 2. In countries where coverage of medical certification of cause of death is incomplete or limited to certain areas, separate figures should be published for medically certified and other deaths.

9. *Tabulation of causes of death*

Statistics of causes of death in respect of the territory as a whole should be in accordance with recommendation 8 (a) (i), or, if this is not possible, with recommendation 8 (a) (ii). They should preferably be classified by sex and the age-groups in recommendation 8 (b) (i).

Statistics of causes of death in respect of the areas in recommendation 8 (g) should be in accordance with recommendation 8 (a) (ii) or, if this is not possible, with recommendation 8 (a) (iii). They should preferably be classified by sex and the age-groups in recommendation 8 (b) (ii).

For statistics of perinatal mortality derived from the form of certificate recommended for this purpose (see page 732), full-scale multiple-cause analysis of all conditions reported will yield the maximum of benefit. Where this is impracticable, analysis of the main disease or condition in the fetus or infant (part (a)) and of the main maternal condition affecting the fetus or infant (part (c)) with cross-tabulation of groups of these two conditions should be regarded as the minimum. Where it is necessary to select only one condition (for example, when it is necessary to incorporate early neonatal deaths in single-cause tables of deaths at all ages), the main disease or condition in the fetus or infant (part (a)) should be selected.

REGULATIONS

The Nomenclature Regulations 1967 have been adopted by the World Health Assembly under Article 21(b) of the Constitution of the World Health Organization (*Off. Rec. Wld Hlth Org.*, 1967, **160**, 9).

WORLD HEALTH ORGANIZATION

REGULATIONS REGARDING NOMENCLATURE (INCLUDING THE COMPILATION AND PUBLICATION OF STATISTICS) WITH RESPECT TO DISEASES AND CAUSES OF DEATH

The Twentieth World Health Assembly,

Considering the importance of compiling and publishing statistics of mortality and morbidity in comparable form;

Having regard to Articles 2(s), 21(b), 22 and 64 of the Constitution of the World Health Organization,

ADOPTS, this twenty-second day of May 1967, the Nomenclature Regulations 1967; these Regulations may be cited as the WHO Nomenclature Regulations.

Article 1

Members of the World Health Organization for whom these Regulations shall come into force under Article 7 below shall be referred to hereinafter as Members.

Article 2

Members compiling mortality and morbidity statistics shall do so in accordance with the current revision of the International Statistical Classification of Diseases, Injuries and Causes of Death as adopted from time to time by the World Health Assembly. This Classification may be cited as the International Classification of Diseases.

Article 3

In compiling and publishing mortality and morbidity statistics, Members shall comply as far as possible with recommendations made by the World Health Assembly as to classification, coding procedure, age-grouping, territorial areas to be identified, and other relevant definitions and standards.

Article 4

Members shall compile and publish annually for each calendar year statistics of causes of death for the metropolitan (home) territory as a whole or for such part thereof as information is available, and shall indicate the area covered by the statistics.

Article 5

Members shall adopt a form of medical certificate of cause of death that provides for the statement of the morbid conditions or injuries resulting in or contributing to death, with a clear indication of the underlying cause.

Article 6

Each member shall, under Article 64 of the Constitution, provide the Organization on request with statistics prepared in accordance with these Regulations and not communicated under Article 63 of the Constitution.

Article 7

1. These Regulations shall come into force on the first day of January 1968.

2. Upon their entry into force these Regulations shall, subject to the exceptions hereinafter provided, replace as between the Members bound by these Regulations and as between these Members and the Organization, the provisions of the Nomenclature Regulations 1948 and subsequent revisions thereof.

3. Any revisions of the International Classification of Diseases adopted by the World Health Assembly pursuant to Article 2 of these Regulations shall enter into force on such date as is prescribed by the World Health Assembly and shall, subject to the exceptions hereinafter provided, replace any earlier classifications.

Article 8

1. The period provided in execution of Article 22 of the Constitution of the Organization for rejection or reservation shall be six months from the date of the notification by the Director-General of the adoption of these Regulations by the World Health Assembly. Any rejection or reservation received by the Director-General after the expiry of this period shall have no effect.

2. The provisions of paragraph 1 of this Article shall likewise apply in respect of any subsequent revision of the International Classification of Diseases adopted by the World Health Assembly pursuant to Article 2 of these Regulations.

Article 9

A rejection, or the whole or part of any reservation, whether to these Regulations or to the International Classification of Diseases or any revision thereof, may at any time be withdrawn by notifying the Director-General.

Article 10

The Director-General shall notify all Members of the adoption of these Regulations, of the adoption of any revision of the International Classification of Diseases as well as of any notification received by him under Articles 8 and 9.

Article 11

The original texts of these Regulations shall be deposited in the Archives of the Organization. Certified true copies shall be sent by the Director-General to all Members. Upon the entry into force of these Regulations, certified true copies shall be delivered by the Director-General to the Secretary-General of the United Nations for registration in accordance with Article 102 of the Charter of the United Nations.

IN FAITH WHEREOF, we have set our hands at Geneva this twenty-second day of May 1967.

(signed) V. T. H. GUNARATNE,
President of the World Health Assembly

(signed) M. G. CANDAU
Director-General of the World Health Organization

WHO publications may be obtained, direct or through booksellers, from:

ALGERIA: Entreprise nationale du Livre (ENAL), 3 bd Zirout Youcef, ALGIERS

ARGENTINA: Carlos Hirsch SRL, Florida 165, Galerías Güemes, Escritorio 453/465, BUENOS AIRES

AUSTRALIA: Hunter Publications, 58A Gipps Street, COLLINGWOOD, VIC 3066 — Australian Government Publishing Service (Mail order sales), P.O. Box 84, CANBERRA A.C.T. 2601; or over the counter from Australian Government Publishing Service Bookshops at: 70 Alinga Street, CANBERRA CITY A.C.T. 2600; 294 Adelaide Street, BRISBANE, Queensland 4000; 347 Swanston Street, MELBOURNE, VIC 3000; 309 Pitt Street, SYDNEY, N.S.W. 2000; Mt Newman House, 200 St. George's Terrace, PERTH, WA 6000; Industry House, 12 Pirie Street, ADELAIDE, SA 5000; 156–162 Macquarie Street, HOBART, TAS 7000 — R. Hill & Son Ltd, 608 St. Kilda Road, MELBOURNE, VIC 3004; Lawson House, 10–12 Clark Street, CROW'S NEST, NSW 2065

AUSTRIA: Gerold & Co., Graben 31, 1011 VIENNA I

BANGLADESH: The WHO Programme Coordinator, G.P.O. Box 250, DHAKA 5

BELGIUM: For books: Office International de Librairie s.a., avenue Marnix 30, 1050 BRUSSELS. For periodicals and subscriptions: Office International des Périodiques, avenue Louise 485, 1050 BRUSSELS — Subscriptions to World Health only: Jean de Lannoy, 202 avenue du Roi, 1060 BRUSSELS

BHUTAN: see India, WHO Regional Office

BOTSWANA: Botsalo Books (Pty) Ltd., P.O. Box 1532, GABORONE

BRAZIL: Biblioteca Regional de Medicina OMS/OPS, Sector de Publicações, Caixa Postal 20.381, Vila Clementino, 04023 SÃO PAULO, S.P.

BURMA: see India, WHO Regional Office

CANADA: Canadian Public Health Association, 1335 Carling Avenue, Suite 210, OTTAWA, Ont. K1Z 8N8. (Tel: (613) 725–3769. Télex: 21–053–3841)

CHINA: China National Publications Import & Export Corporation, P.O. Box 88, BEIJING (PEKING)

DEMOCRATIC PEOPLE'S REPUBLIC OF KOREA: see India, WHO Regional Office

DENMARK: Munksgaard Export and Subscription Service, Nørre Søgade 35, 1370 COPENHAGEN K (Tel: +45 1 12 85 70)

FIJI: The WHO Programme Coordinator, P.O. Box 113, SUVA

FINLAND: Akateeminen Kirjakauppa, Keskuskatu 2, 00101 HELSINKI 10

FRANCE: Librairie Arnette, 2 rue Casimir-Delavigne, 75006 PARIS

GERMAN DEMOCRATIC REPUBLIC: Buchhaus Leipzig, Postfach 140, 701 LEIPZIG

GERMANY, FEDERAL REPUBLIC OF: Govi-Verlag GmbH, Ginnheimerstrasse 20, Postfach 5360, 6236 ESCHBORN — Buchhandlung Alexander Horn, Friedrichstrasse 39, Postfach 3340, 6200 WIESBADEN

GHANA: Fides Entreprises, P.O. Box 1628, ACCRA

GREECE: G. C. Eleftheroudakis S.A., Librairie internationale, rue Nikis 4, ATHENS (T. 126)

HONG KONG: Hong Kong Government Information Services, Beaconsfield House, 6th Floor, Queen's Road, Central, VICTORIA

HUNGARY: Kultura, P.O.B. 149, BUDAPEST 62

INDIA: WHO Regional Office for South-East Asia, World Health House, Indraprastha Estate, Mahatma Gandhi Road, NEW DELHI 110002

INDONESIA: P.T. Kalman Media Pusaka, Pusat Perdagangan Senen, Block 1, 4th Floor, P.O. Box 3433/Jkt, JAKARTA

IRAN (ISLAMIC REPUBLIC OF): Iran University Press, 85 Park Avenue, P.O. Box 54/551, TEHERAN

IRELAND: TDC Publishers, 12 North Frederick Street, DUBLIN 1 (Tel: 744835–749677)

ISRAEL: Heiliger & Co., 3 Nathan Strauss Street, JERUSALEM 94227

ITALY: Edizioni Minerva Medica, Corso Bramante 83–85, 10126 TURIN; Via Lamarmora 3, 20100 MILAN; Via Spallanzani 9, 00161 ROME

JAPAN: Maruzen Co. Ltd, P.O. Box 5050, TOKYO International, 100–31

JORDAN: Jordan Book Centre Co. Ltd., University Street, P.O. Box 301 (Al-Jubeiha), AMMAN

KUWAIT: The Kuwait Bookshops Co. Ltd, Thunayan Al-Ghanem Bldg, P.O. Box 2942, KUWAIT

LAO PEOPLE'S DEMOCRATIC REPUBLIC: The WHO Programme Coordinator, P.O. Box 343, VIENTIANE

LUXEMBOURG: Librairie du Centre, 49 bd Royal, LUXEMBOURG

MALAWI: Malawi Book Service, P.O. Box 30044, Chichiti, BLANTYRE 3

MALAYSIA: The WHO Programme Coordinator, Room 1004, 10th Floor, Wisma Lim Foo Yong (formerly Fitzpatrick's Building), Jalan Raja Chulan, KUALA LUMPUR 05–10; P.O. Box 2550, KUALA LUMPUR 01 –02 — Parry's Book Center, 124–1 Jalan Tun Sambanthan, P.O. Box 10960, KUALA LUMPUR

MALDIVES: see India, WHO Regional Office

MEXICO: Librería Internacional, S.A. de C.V., av. Sonora 206, 06100-MÉXICO, D.F.

MONGOLIA: see India, WHO Regional Office

MOROCCO: Editions La Porte, 281 avenue Mohammed V, RABAT

NEPAL: see India, WHO Regional Office

NETHERLANDS: Medical Books Europe BV, Noorderwal 38, 7241 BL LOCHEM

NEW ZEALAND: New Zealand Government Printing Office, Publishing Administration, Private Bag, WELLINGTON; Walter Street, WELLINGTON; World Trade Building, Cubacade, Cuba Street, WELLINGTON. Government Bookshops at: Hannaford Burton Building, Rutland Street, Private Bag, AUCKLAND; 159 Hereford Street, Private Bag, CHRISTCHURCH; Alexandra Street, P.O. Box 857, HAMILTON; T & G Building, Princes Street, P.O. Box 1104, DUNEDIN — R. Hill & Son, Ltd, Ideal House, Cnr Gillies Avenue & Eden St., Newmarket, AUCKLAND 1

NORWAY: Tanum — Karl Johan A.S., P.O. Box 1177, Sentrum, N-0107 OSLO 1

PAKISTAN: Mirza Book Agency, 65 Shahrah–E–Quaid–E–Azam, P.O. Box 729, LAHORE 3

PAPUA NEW GUINEA: The WHO Programme Coordinator, P.O. Box 646, KONEDOBU

PHILIPPINES: World Health Organization, Regional Office for the Western Pacific, P.O. Box 2932, MANILA

PORTUGAL: Livraria Rodrigues, 186 Rua do Ouro, LISBON 2

REPUBLIC OF KOREA: The WHO Programme Coordinator, Central P.O. Box 540, SEOUL

SINGAPORE: The WHO Programme Coordinator, 144 Moulmein Road, SINGAPORE 1130; Newton P.O. Box 31, SINGAPORE 9122

SOUTH AFRICA: Contact major book stores

SPAIN: Ministerio de Sanidad y Consumo, Centro de Publicaciones, Documentación y Biblioteca, Paseo del Prado 18, 28014 MADRID — Comercial Atheneum S.A., Consejo de Ciento 130–136, 08015 BARCELONA; General Moscardó 29, MADRID 20 — Librería Díaz de Santos, P.O. Box 6050, 28006 MADRID; Balmes 417 y 419, 08022 BARCELONA

SRI LANKA: see India, WHO Regional Office

SWEDEN: For books: Aktiebolaget C.E. Fritzes Kungl. Hovbokhandel, Regeringsgatan 12, 103 27 STOCKHOLM. For periodicals: Wennergren-Williams AB, Box 30004, 104 25 STOCKHOLM

SWITZERLAND: Medizinischer Verlag Hans Huber, Länggassstrasse 76, 3012 BERN 9

THAILAND: see India, WHO Regional Office

UNITED KINGDOM: H.M. Stationery Office: 49 High Holborn, LONDON WCIV 6HB; 13 a Castle Street, EDINBURGH EH2 3AR; 80 Chichester Street, BELFAST BT1 4JY; Brazennose Street, MANCHESTER M6O 8AS; 258 Broad Street, BIRMINGHAM B1 2HE; Southey House, Wine Street, BRISTOL BS1 2BQ. All mail orders should be sent to: HMSO Publications Centre, 51 Nine Elms Lane, LONDON SW8 5DR

UNITED STATES OF AMERICA: Copies of individual publications (not subscriptions): WHO Publications Center USA, 49 Sheridan Avenue, ALBANY, NY 12210. Subscription orders and correspondence concerning subscriptions should be addressed to the World Health Organization, Distribution and Sales, 1211 GENEVA 27, Switzerland. Publications are also available from the United Nations Bookshop, NEW YORK, NY 10017 (retail only)

USSR: For readers in the USSR requiring Russian editions: Komsomolskij prospekt 18, Medicinskaja Kniga, MOSCOW — For readers outside the USSR requiring Russian editions: Kuzneckij most 18, Meždunarodnaja Kniga, MOSCOW G-200

VENEZUELA: Librería Médica Paris, Apartado 60.681, CARACAS 106

YUGOSLAVIA: Jugoslovenska Knjiga, Terazije 27/II, 11000 BELGRADE

Special terms for developing countries are obtainable on application to the WHO Programme Coordinators or WHO Regional Offices listed above or to the World Health Organization, Distribution and Sales Service, 1211 Geneva 27, Switzerland. Orders from countries where sales agents have not yet been appointed may also be sent to the Geneva address, but must be paid for in pounds sterling, US dollars, or Swiss francs. Unesco book coupons may also be used.

Price: Sw. fr. 40.— Prices are subject to change without notice. C/1/86